Cytokines

Cytokines
in Health and Disease

edited by
Steven L. Kunkel
Daniel G. Remick
The University of Michigan Medical School
Ann Arbor, Michigan

Marcel Dekker, Inc. **New York • Basel • Hong Kong**

Library of Congress Cataloging-in-Publication Data

Cytokines in health and disease / edited by Steven L. Kunkel, Daniel
G. Remick.
p. cm.
Includes bibliographical references and index.
ISBN 0-8247-8648-3 (alk. paper)
1. Cytokines. I. Kunkel, S. L. (Steven L.) II. Remick, Daniel
G.
[DNLM: 1. Cytokines. 2. Immunity, Cellular. QW 568 C9961]
QR185.8.C95C96 1992
616.07'9--dc20
DNLM/DLC
for Library of Congress 92-9990
CIP

This book is printed on acid-free paper.

MARCEL DEKKER, INC.
270 Madison Avenue, New York, New York 10016

Current printing (last digit):
10 9 8 7 6 5 4 3 2 1

PRINTED IN THE UNITED STATES OF AMERICA

PREFACE

Cytokines as a group may be defined as soluble mediators secreted by one cell that acts on another cell or organ. Within this broad definition, nearly any secreted cellular product may be considered a cytokine; however, the term is generally reserved for protein mediators. While there has always been great interest in the field, recent advances in molecular biology have provided researchers with sufficient amounts of purified recombinant material for engaging in exacting studies of the unique roles of cytokines. The availability of these purified products has also allowed for their use as biological response modifiers in the treatment of human diseases.

The field of cytokine research covers a wide spectrum of disciplines. Experts from pathology, physiology, surgery, microbiology, molecular biology, and cancer research have all made important and exciting contributions to our understanding of these mediators of inflammation. Cytokines themselves have also been documented to exert diverse effects both in vitro and in vivo, and their broad spectrum of activities further expands the field. Therefore, it represents a challenging task to compile a current, comprehensive text that does justice to this rich and varied field of research.

This book endeavors to provide, in a single, readable source, much of the currently available knowledge in the field of cytokines. There are four areas covered in this volume, including general overviews of each of the major cytokines, listings of the important interactions these cytokines have with inflammatory cells, discussions of current and future areas of important research, and descriptions of cytokine interactions with several of the major organ/systems.

Despite rapid advances in the field of cytokines, readers of this text will gain a firm grasp of the basic concepts and a foundation on which to build future ideas. The book should prove useful to clinicians looking for a reference work, and basic scientists seeking information on the role of cytokines in their field of interest.

Steven L. Kunkel
Daniel G. Remick

CONTENTS

CONTRIBUTORS

Timothy D. Anderson, Ph.D. Hoffmann-La Roche, Inc., Nutley, New Jersey

Monique A. Berman, Ph.D. California College of Medicine, University of California, Irvine, California

Darrell A. Campbell, Jr., M.D. The University of Michigan Medical School, Ann Arbor, Michigan

Michael S. Caplan, M.D. Evanston Hospital, Northwestern University Medical School, Chicago, Illinois

Stephen W. Chensue, M.D., Ph.D. The University of Michigan Medical School, Ann Arbor, Michigan

Lisa Colletti, M.D. The University of Michigan Medical School, Ann Arbor, Michigan

Gerard Cox McMaster University, Hamilton, Ontario, Canada

Elisabetta Dejana, Ph.D. Istituto di Richerche Farmacologiche Mario Negri, Milan, Italy

Deborah DeMarco, M.D. Temple University Hospital, Philadelphia, Pennsylvania

Steven N. Emancipator, Ph.D. Institute of Pathology, Case Western Reserve University, Cleveland, Ohio

Mark K. Eskandari, Ph.D. The University of Michigan Medical School, Ann Arbor, Michigan

Terje Espevik, M.D. Institute of Cancer Research, University of Trondheim, Trondheim, Norway

Jon S. Friedland, M.R.C.P. St. George's Hospital Medical School, London, England

Jack Gauldie, Ph.D. McMaster University, Hamilton, Ontario, Canada

Frank Gonzalez-Crussi, M.D. Children's Memorial Hospital, Northwestern University Medical School, Chicago, Illinois

Georges E. Grau, M.D. Centre Médical Universitaire, University of Geneva, Geneva, Switzerland

George E. Griffin, Ph.D., F.R.C.P. St. George's Hospital Medical School, London, England

John M. Ham, M.D. The University of Michigan Medical School, Ann Arbor, Michigan

Evan M. Hersh, M.D. Arizona Cancer Center, University of Arizona, Tucson, Arizona

Wei Hsueh, M.D., Ph.D. Children's Memorial Hospital, Northwestern University Medical School, Chicago, Illinois

Stanley C. Jordan, M.D. UCLA School of Medicine and Cedars-Sinai Medical Center, Los Angeles, California

Soverin Karmiol, Ph.D. The University of Michigan Medical School, Ann Arbor, Michigan

Steven L. Kunkel, Ph.D. The University of Michigan Medical School, Ann Arbor, Michigan

James W. Larrick, M.D., Ph.D. Palo Alto Institute for Molecular Medicine, Stanford, California

Joseph P. Lynch III, M.D. The University of Michigan Medical School, Ann Arbor, Michigan

Alberto Mantovani, M.D. Istituto di Ricerche Farmacologiche Mario Negri, Milan, Italy

Dominique Mazier, M.D. INSERM Unité, Paris, France

Kenneth McCurry, M.D. The University of Michigan Medical School, Ann Arbor, Michigan

Ian K. McNiece, Ph.D. Amgen Inc., Thousand Oaks, Calfornia

Andrew P. Metinko The University of Michigan Medical School, Ann Arbor, Michigan

Lyle L. Moldawer, Ph.D. The New York Hospital, Cornell University Medical Center, New York, New York

Brian J. Nickoloff, M.D., Ph.D. The University of Michigan Medical School, Ann Arbor, Michigan

Sem H. Phan, M.D., Ph.D. The University of Michigan Medical School, Ann Arbor, Michigan

Pierre-François Piguet, M.D. Centre Médical Universitaire, University of Geneva, Geneva, Switzerland

Pascal Pointaire, M.D. Centre Médical Universitaire, University of Geneva, Geneva, Switzerland

Daniel G. Remick, M.D. The University of Michigan Medical School, Ann Arbor, Michigan

Mark W. Rolfe, M.D. The University of Michigan Medical School, Ann Arbor, Michigan

Christy I. Sandborg, M.D. California College of Medicine, University of California, Irvine, California

Wendy E. Scales, M.D. The University of Michigan Medical School, Ann Arbor, Michigan

John R. Sedor, M.D. MetroHealth Medical Center, University Hospital, Case Western Reserve University, Cleveland, Ohio

Refaat Shalaby, Ph.D.* Institute of Cancer Research, University of Trondheim, Trondheim, Norway

Virginia L. Shepherd, Ph.D. Vanderbilt University and Veterans Administration Medical Center, Nashville, Tennessee

Theodore J. Standiford, M.D. The University of Michigan Medical School, Ann Arbor, Michigan

* *Current affiliation:* Genentech, Inc., South San Francisco, California

Robert M. Strieter, M.D. The University of Michigan Medical School, Ann Arbor, Michigan

Xiaoming Sun, M.D. Children's Memorial Hospital, Northwestern University Medical School, Chicago, Illinois

Charles W. Taylor, M.D. Arizona Cancer Center, University of Arizona, Tucson, Arizona

Frank M. Torti, M.D. Stanford University Medical Center and Palo Alto Veterans Administration Medical Center, Palo Alto, California

Yoshiaki Tsuji, Ph.D. Stanford University Medical Center and Palo Alto Veterans Administration Medical Center, Palo Alto, California

Thomas R. Ulich, M.D. School of Medicine, University of California, Irvine, California

Donata Vercelli, M.D. Children's Hospital, Harvard Medical School, Boston, Massachusetts

Anders Waage, M.D. Institute of Cancer Research, University of Trondheim, Trondheim, Norway

Jeffrey S. Warren, M.D., Ph.D. The University of Michigan Medical School, Ann Arbor, Michigan

John Westick, M.D. Hunterian Institute, Royal College of Surgeons of England, London, England

Mark D. Wewers, M.D. The Ohio State University, Columbus, Ohio

Susan C. Wright, M.D. Palo Alto Institute for Molecular Medicine, Stanford, California

Robert B. Zurier, M.D. University of Massachusetts Medical Center, Worcester, Massachusetts

CHAPTER 1

QUANTITATION OF THE BIOLOGICAL ACTIVITIES OF CYTOKINES

Mark K. Eskandari and Daniel G. Remick

The University of Michigan Medical School
Ann Arbor, Michigan

INTRODUCTION

This chapter briefly discusses the quantitation of the biological activity of cytokines. It is not intended to represent a complete description of the methodologies involved but to review the nature of the assays and potential pitfalls in interpreting the data. We describe the quantitation of biological activity of interleukins 1 through 6 and 8, as well as tumor necrosis factor.

Cytokines may also be assessed in immunological assays, either radioimmunoassays (RIA) or enzyme-linked immunoabsorbent assays (ELISA). Both these techniques are predicated on the ability of a specific antibody to recognize the cytokine in question. With RIAs, the radioactivity (usually ^{125}I) is detected in a gamma counter, and the radioactivity is then related to a standard curve used to calculate the amount of cytokine. The RIAs are rapid and easily quantifiable and may have exquisite sensitivity. They have the disadvantage of working with radioactivity, especially the gamma emitter ^{125}I. ELISAs are routinely performed in plates with 96 wells, and at the end of the reaction a color is developed in each well. The intensity of the color may be quantitated spectrophotometrically in each well with an ELISA reader and the degree of activity directly related to a standard curve. ELISAs are often easy to perform, and several of the steps may be automated. The assays generally take longer to run than RIAs and may not offer the same degree of sensitivity.

Since both RIAs and ELISAs depend on an antibody recognizing a specific antigen, they both have the same inherent shortcomings. Clearly, the antibody must be specific for the cytokine in question, and it should be a high-titer antibody. Monoclonal antibodies usually provide unmatched specificity, but their sensitivity may be lacking. Polyclonal antibodies may react with other factors present in the biological samples, to yield a false positive. This may be especially true in situations in which there is some structural homology between two cytokines, such as lymphotoxin and tumor necrosis factor (1). Last, the immunoassays may be detecting degraded peptide fragments that are immunoreactive but not biologically active. Thus, in certain disease settings, it is possible to have a positive immunoassay but a negative biological assay.

One method to differentiate between cytokines with structural similarity (and thus possible cross-reactivity of antibodies) is to perform a western blot analysis. For this procedure, the samples are first subjected to polyacrylamide gel electrophoresis, which separates the proteins based primarily on their molecular weight. The proteins are then transferred to a support matrix, usually nitrocellulose. The individual bands are detected with an antibody, the same antibody that would be used in the ELISA or RIA. With this method, the molecular size of the cytokine is known, which may give important information about which cytokine is being recognized by the antibody. Also, if multiple smaller bands are detected, it may indicate that there has been some breakdown.

With this brief description of the advantages and disadvantages of immunoassays, we now describe the biological assays. Limitations in interpretation of the data are discussed, although this is by no means a complete presentation of the potential pitfalls one may encounter when performing these complex assays.

GENERAL CONSIDERATIONS FOR BIOASSAYS

Bioassays require knowledge of tissue culture techniques. These are not difficult to learn, but they do require a considerable investment in equipment. It is absolutely critical to maintain sterility in the equipment, solutions, and cells. Bacterial overgrowth may make it impossible to interpret the data.

To set up a tissue culture facility requires purchase of or access to a sterile, laminar flow hood. All cell work should be performed in this hood to minimize the potential of contamination, and all solutions should be prepared and aliquoted in the laminar flow hood. A CO_2 incubator is used to grow the cells and is also used for conducting the bioassays. All material that comes into contact with the cells (i.e., tissue culture flasks, pipettes, and pipette tips) must be sterile. These items may be purchased as sterile or may be sterilized if an autoclave is available. Tissue culture media also may be prepared and then filter sterilized, or they may be purchased in an already sterile condition. Some cells require multiple, special additives for optimal growth. There may be great variation in quality, and the best supplier for each reagent must be determined. Some investigators assay for the best reagents and then buy a large quantity of the particular lot.

Bioassays are often performed using cell lines, that is, cells that may grown indefinitely in vitro. Cell lines are advantageous since they provide a uniform population that should respond to the cytokine in a similar manner. Many cell lines have an absolute requirement for a particular cytokine (i.e., they do not continue to grow in culture unless the cytokine is present). This forms the basis for the assay, since the cells die out if the sample does not contain the cytokine. Tumor necrosis factor (TNF) is measured by the opposite property: TNF kills the target cells, and cell death indicates the presence of the cytokine.

Cell lines may sometimes be obtained from other investigators. Another excellent source is the American Type Culture Collection (ATCC), a nonprofit organization in Rockville, Maryland. The ATCC serves as a central repository for cell lines, and frozen cells may be purchased for a minimal price. With this brief introduction to the dangers of cell culture we now discuss several different cytokine assays.

INTERLEUKIN-1 (IL-1)

The original assay for IL-1 was based on its ability to coinduce the proliferation of murine thymocytes (2,3). In this system, IL-1 was able to augment proliferation in conjunction with a suboptimal concentration of a lectin, either phytohemagglutinin (PHA) or concanavalin A. Since two mitogens were involved, this assay has also been called the comitogen, or coproliferation assay. The assay is done by performing dilutions of the samples to be tested and adding the samples to 96-well microtiter plates. Murine thymocytes are then prepared as a single-cell suspension, mixed with the appropriate, suboptimal concentration of lectin, and then added to the wells. Incubation of the thymocytes, IL-1, and lectin causes the production of IL-2, and IL-2 then induces proliferation of IL-2-responsive thymocytes. After 2 days of incubation at 37°C, the proliferation of the thymocytes is detected by pulsing the cells with [^{3}H-methyl]thymidine. As the cells proliferate, the radioactive thymidine is incorporated into the DNA of the cell. The amount of incorporated thymidine is determined by harvesting the cells on glass fiber filters. The DNA adheres to the filters, and the radioactivity may be counted in a scintillation counter. The activity in the sample is then ascertained by determining the dilution that induces a half-maximal response. (For a more complete discussion of half-maximal units, see the following section on IL-2.) The thymocyte coproliferation assay has several factors that may cause a false positive reaction. IL-6 also induces proliferation of thymocytes (4–6), and murine TNF, but not human TNF, also causes proliferation (7). Since the assay actually measures the response to IL-2, this cytokine also results in a false positive reaction (8). To determine if the thymocyte proliferation is truly due to IL-1, it is necessary either to use specific assays for IL-2, IL-6, and TNF to rule out their presence or to inhibit the proliferative activity with specific antibodies. Since either IL-1α or IL-1β will drive the assay, the use of antibodies has the advantage of being able to distinguish between the α and β forms.

Another assay for IL-1 activity that is similar in principle to the thymocyte assay utilizes cell lines instead of the heterogeneous thymocyte populations (9–11). For this assay, the lymphoma cell line LBRM is stimulated with IL-1 and PHA; this stimulation results in the production of IL-2. The supernatants are transferred to another plate, leaving the LBRM cells behind, and the IL-2 detected in a standard IL-2 assay using an IL-2-dependent cell line. Obviously, samples that contain IL-2 cause false positive results; however, IL-6 does not cause a positive reaction in this assay (12).

An additional cell line has been described that responds to IL-1 directly, the D10.G4.1 assay (13). In the presence of IL-1, these cells proliferate. A subclone of the D10 cell line has recently been described that is extremely sensitive to the effects of IL-1 and is not significantly affected by other cytokines, such as TNF,

IL-2, or IL-6 (14). The proliferation may be monitored by either incorporation of [^{3}H]thymidine (as in the thymocyte assay), or the degree of proliferation may be assessed by their ability to metabolize a tetrazolium dye, MTT-tetrazolium, described in greater detail in the section on IL-2.

IL-1 in biological samples may also be quantitated by determining its ability to inhibit the binding of radiolabeled IL-1 to the IL-1 receptor present on fibroblasts. This is a very sensitive assay that measures both IL-1α and β. It is similar in principle to a radioimmunoassay, but instead of evaluating binding to antibody one measures binding to receptors.

No discussion of IL-1 measurement would be complete without mentioning the presence of IL-1 inhibitors in biological samples (Ref. 15, comments). This is particularly a problem in blood products and has caused great difficulties in data interpretation. Various methods have been tried to remove the inhibitors, including performing serial dilutions, extraction with chloroform (16), and treatment with polyethylene glycol (17). The biological relevance of IL-1 values obtained from samples subjected to the treatments is not known with certainty.

INTERLEUKIN-2

IL-2 was originally described as a factor that would support the long-term growth of T cell clones. The most widely used biological assay today to test for the presence of IL-2 measures the ability of a sample to stimulate the proliferation of a cloned line of T cells. Two commonly employed lines are the HT-2 and the CTLL-2 (18). The CTLL-2 cell line is available from the ATCC (#TIB-214). The CTLL-2 line may be easily maintained in culture or frozen for long-term storage.

The proliferation of the cells may be measured either by the amount of [^{3}H]thymidine incorporated or by the ability of the cells to metabolize MTT-tetrazolium (3-[4,5-dimethylthiazol-2-yl-]2,5-diphenyltetrazolium bromide) (19, 20). The assay is based on the knowledge that the cell lines have a requirement for IL-2 to proliferate or remain viable for longer than 20 h. Furthermore, it has been demonstrated that many of the prostaglandins (PGE_2 and $PGF_2α$), and leukotrienes (LTB_4, LTC_4, LTD_4, and LTE_4) do not block the ability of IL-2 to induce CTLL proliferation (21). However, high-dose dexamethasone or cyclosporine A inhibits the ability of the assay to detect IL-2 (Fig. 1) (21). For either assay, samples are serially diluted in 96-well flat-bottomed microtiter plates in 0.1 ml volumes of tissue culture media. Since both cell lines are lymphocytes, it is critical to include 2β-mercaptoethanol in the media for optimal cell proliferation. Both cell lines are sufficiently sensitive to the effects of IL-2 that only 4000–10,000 cells per well are required. The samples are allowed to incubate at 37°C overnight, and the next morning they are pulsed for 4 h with either MTT-tetrazolium or [^{3}H]thymidine.

The amount of activity in the fluid that was assayed is usually expressed in terms of half-maximal units. These units are defined as the dilution that produces a half-maximal response (22). When using the [^{3}H]thymidine method, the counts per minute (cpm) are plotted against the dilutions, with both axes a logarithmic scale. Figure 2 shows a typical plot of a standard and unknown samples. In this example, the standard's maximum response was 16,000 cpm, the half-maximal

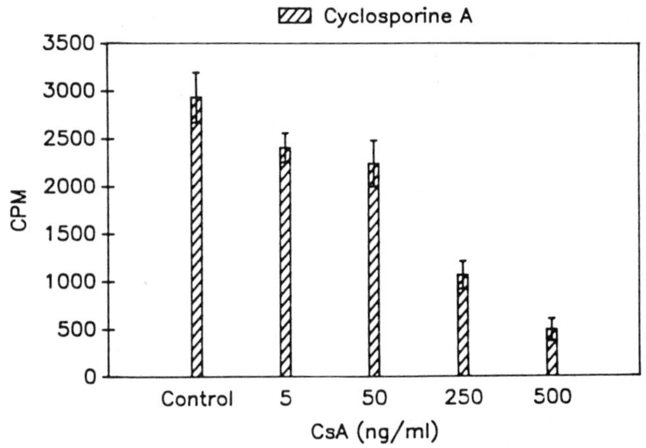

FIGURE 1 Cyclosporine A (CsA) inhibition of the CTLL assay. CsA was added to CTLL cells in the presence of interleukin-2, and the proliferation was determined after 20 h. CsA at doses above 250 ng/ml significantly inhibited the ability of the cells to respond to the IL-2.

was 8000 cpm, so the log of the half-maximal was 3.9. As can be seen on the graph, the standard (middle curve) plateaus at the maximum and then falls off in a linear fashion. Regression analysis of the curve discloses an R^2 value of 0.9999. The number of units is calculated by determining the equation of the line and then solving for the x value that corresponds to the y value, giving the half-maximal response. In this example, the standard has 40 units/ml. The sample

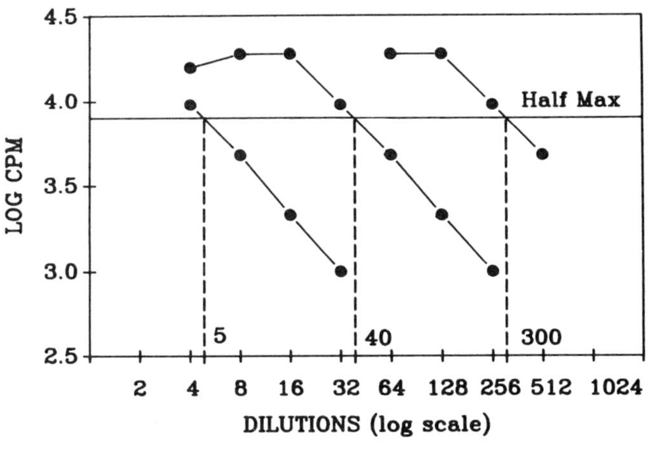

FIGURE 2 Determination of half-maximal units: calculation using the CTLL assay as an example; similar data analysis is performed for other interleukin assays. Half-maximal units are defined as the reciprocal of the dilution that results in half-maximal stimulation of the assay.

on the left is subjected to a similar analysis and has 5 units/ml; the sample on the right has 300 units/ml. This figure also shows the importance of calculating half-maximal units, since both the standard and the sample on the right produce the same maximal response, but they have markedly different activities.

Instead of using the radioactive [^{3}H]thymidine, the cells may be pulsed with MTT-tetrazolium. This is an extremely valuable method for quantitating cell proliferation, or cytotoxicity (19,20). With this method, MTT-tetrazolium is added to the wells and the cells are incubated an additional 4–6 h. As the cells undergo oxidative respiration, the dye is metabolized to form insoluble dark purple crystals. The crystals are dissolved by removing some of the supernatant and then adding an appropriate solvent, such as a detergent or acidified isopropanol (20). The 96-well plates are then conveniently read in a micro-ELISA reader. If the plate reader is interfaced with a computer, the data may then be easily analyzed. Figure 3 shows an example of a plate with samples of varying activity. As dilutions are continued across the plate, there is less biological activity and less color. Samples A, B, and D have less activity than samples E and F, since the color is less intense as one moves from left to right on the plate.

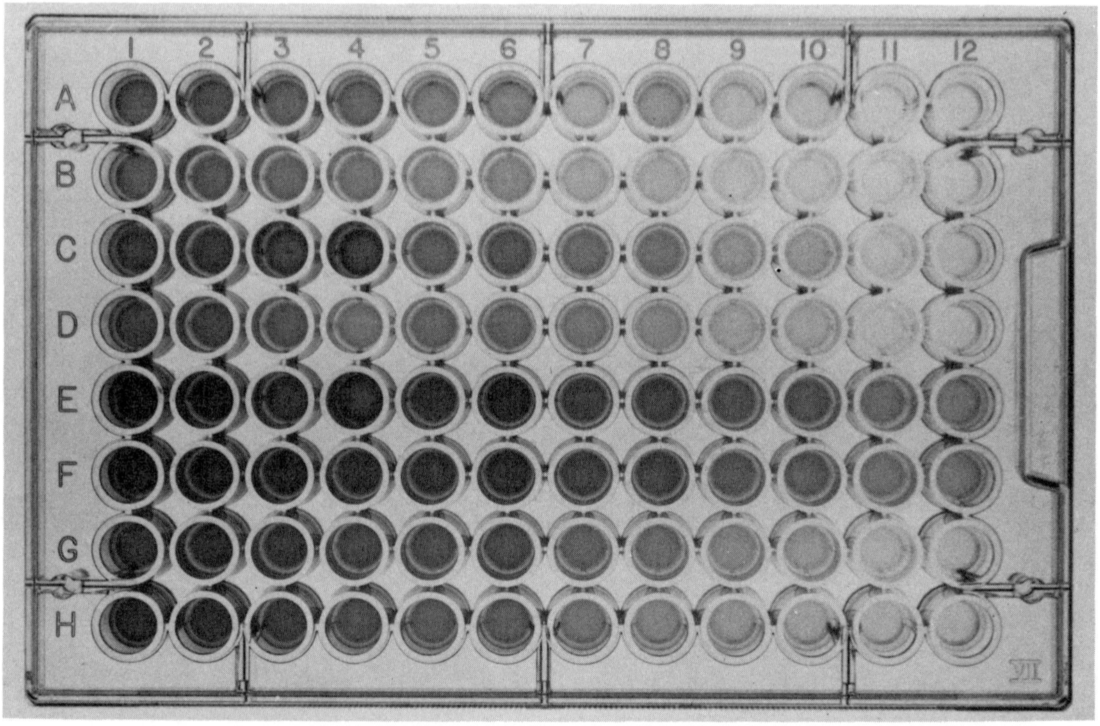

FIGURE 3 MTT-tetrazolium dye reduction. Serial dilutions of cytokines were placed in each well of this 96-well plate, in duplicate. Each row (A, B, C, and so on) is used for one sample, so there are six dilutions for each sample. If the assay is a cell proliferation assay, then the activity decreases as one moves from right to left (i.e., the sample becomes diluted). In this plate, samples E and F have the most activity, since the dye is still intense even in wells 7 and 8. Sample B has the least activity, since the dye is almost completely gone by wells 7 and 8.

Some lines of CTLL-2 cells also respond to IL-4 (23,24), and a positive assay may thus indicate the presence of either IL-2 or IL-4. To differentiate between these two possibilities, three approaches may be used. The first is to test the cell line with recombinant IL-4 and ascertain whether the cell line being used is sensitive to IL-4. The second approach is to inhibit any potential IL-4 using the 11B11 antibody, which blocks murine IL-4 (ATCC# HB188) (25). Last, anti-IL-2 receptor antibodies may be included to specifically inhibit the ability of IL-2 to induce proliferation. Additional information regarding measurement of IL-4 may be found in the section on interleukin-4.

INTERLEUKIN-3

Interleukin 3 has also been named multi-CSF to indicate that it has colony-stimulating activity for a several different cell lineages. A number of assays exist for the quantitation of IL-3 (26). These assays have included the induction of the enzyme 20α-hydroxysteroid dehydrogenase (SDH) in splenic lymphocytes from nude mice, induction of proliferation of IL-3-dependent T cell lines from long-term bone marrow cultures, induction of proliferation of mastlike cells, and colony formation in soft agar cultures. The least complex assay involves the use of IL-3-dependent T cell lines and measurement of proliferation induced by IL-3. The other assays may lack specificity; that is, induction of colonies in soft agar cultures may be due to other colony-stimulating factors or involve the expense of nude mice and the complexity of measuring the induction of 20α-SDH (27). Different cell lines have maintained their dependence on IL-3 for proliferation, such as prebasophil and prelymphoid cell lines; for this reason they have been used to assay this cytokine (28). However, some cell lines respond only to murine IL-3, not to human IL-3. An alternative is to enrich a population of bone marrow cells for MY-10-positive cells, which proliferate in response to IL-3. This may be done by adhering the antibody to plastic dishes, adding the bone marrow cells in suspension, and gently removing the nonadherent T cells (29). The MY-10 cells remain adherent to the dishes and may be removed by more vigorous pipetting and scraping. These cells are used in colony-forming assays as an indicator for the presence of IL-3. When long-term cell lines are used to assay IL-3, the degree of proliferation is assessed by [^{3}H]thymidine incorporation in the same fashion as described for the IL-1 assay, except that an IL-3-dependent cell line is used, such as the FDC-P cell line (30–32). The assay is then performed similarly to that described for IL-2.

It has recently been shown that interferon-γ (IFN-γ) inhibits the ability of the FDC-P cell line to respond to IL-3 (33). Since the same T cells that produce IL-3 also make IFN-γ, it is easy to mask the IL-3 activity unless specific antibodies are used to inhibit the IFN-γ material.

IL-3-dependent cell lines must be maintained in long-term cultures by adding an exogenous source of IL-3. This may be obtained by culturing an IL-3-producing cell line, such as the WEHI-3 (ATCC #TIB 68) for 48 h and collecting the supernatant. This supernatant is then used as the source of IL-3 for growth of the IL-3-dependent cell line. The optimal concentration of supernatant must be determined for each batch of conditioned media.

All the hematopoietic stimulating factors, or colony-stimulating factors, may be detected by determining their ability to stimulate colony formation in soft agar cultures. This is a complex assay procedure that requires not only expertise in tissue culture work but also the ability to differentiate the morphology of the cells growing in colonies. The basic protocol consists of collecting bone marrow cells from the femora of mice. The cells are resuspended in tissue culture media containing 0.4% agar. Serial dilutions of the samples to be tested are added to the cells in agar, and the samples are incubated for 3–7 days at 37°C. At the end of the assay, the number of colonies are counted and the types of cells in the colonies are determined.

INTERLEUKIN-4

One assay for the quantitation of IL-4 utilizes a costimulation assay, since IL-4 stimulates B cell proliferation in the presence of the polyclonal activator IgM (34). Briefly, B cells are purified from T cell-depleted mouse spleens, their purity confirmed, and the cells resuspended in tissue culture media and placed into 96-well plates. The cells are then stimulated with anti-μ chain, which serves as one stimulus. The samples containing IL-4 are serially diluted and also added to the well; this serves as the second stimulus. After 54 h of incubation, the wells are pulsed with [^{3}H]thymidine for 18 h and the degree of proliferation determined. A unit of IL-4 is expressed in terms of half-maximal units, as described for the IL-2 assay. IL-4 is species specific, and a different assay is used for quantitating human material. The assay is similar to that described for murine IL-4, but the B cells are isolated from blood, tonsils, or spleen and then preactivated with either anti-μ antibodies, or *Staphylococcus aureus* Cowan strain (35).

As mentioned in the section on IL-2, some CTLL-2 cell lines respond to IL-4 (23,24). Using an IL-4-responsive cell line allows detection of IL-4 if appropriate controls are included to ensure that one is not detecting IL-2. A cell line has been cloned that responds only to IL-4, the CT.4S (36). This variant of the CTLL-2 cells is very sensitive to IL-4 and does not respond to other cytokines (36); unfortunately, this cell line responds only to murine IL-4, not human IL-4. Since CT.4S cells do not respond to murine IL-2, these cells may be used to quantitate the presence of murine IL-4 directly. The other alternative is to use a cell line responsive to both IL-2 and IL-4 and use an antibody to inhibit the activity of either IL-2 or IL-4. If anti-IL-2 is used (a monoclonal rat antimurine IL-2 is available from ATCC, S4B6, #HB 8794), then the remaining CTLL-2 activity is due to IL-4.

The CT.4S cell line must be maintained by culturing in the presence of 100 units/ml of murine IL-4. This can be an expensive procedure since it requires the continued purchase of recombinant material. A much more economical approach is to obtain IL-4-rich supernatants and use these as a source of exogenous IL-4. Such supernatants may be obtained by stimulating D10.G4.1 cells (ATCC, #TIB 224) with concanavalin A (2.5 μg/ml) and collecting the overnight supernatant. The optimal concentration of the supernatant to maintain long-term growth of the CT.4S cells needs to be determined empirically.

INTERLEUKIN-5

Two assays may be used to detect the presence of IL-5 (37). In the first, purified B cells are distributed into 96-well plates, and the cells are stimulated with dextran sulfate along with serial dilutions of test supernatant. After 66 h of incubation, the wells are pulsed with [^{3}H]thymidine and harvested after 6 h. In the second assay, mouse lymphoma cells (BCL-1) are purified from the spleens of mice previously injected with the cell line. The cells are cultured with serial dilutions of supernatant with no other stimulus and then incubated and pulsed as with the normal B cells.

The second assay for IL-5 uses mouse B cell lymphoma cells (BCL_1) as the indicator cell line. These cells are prepared by injecting the cells intravenously into Balb/c mice. The mice are sacrificed 4–8 weeks later and the spleens dispersed in a sterile manner. T cells are removed from the suspension by incubation with anti-Thy-1.2 (ATCC #TIB 90) and anti-Lyt-2 (ATCC #TIB 105) antibodies and complement. Macrophages are removed by passage over Sephadex G-10 columns, and the dead cells and debris are removed by density centrifugation on Ficoll-Hypaque gradients. These purified BCL_1 cells are then aliquoted and frozen for future use. The actual assay is performed in a similar fashion to most of the other cytokine assays; serial dilutions are prepared, the BCL_1 cells are added, and the plates are incubated overnight. Routinely, the samples are then pulsed with [^{3}H]thymidine for 6 h, cells harvested, and the radioactivity counted.

The BCL_1 assay is not affected by IL-2 or granulocyte-macrophage colony-stimulating factor (38). However, it is augmented by IL-4 and inhibited by interferon-γ (39). Human IL-5 has considerably less activity in the BCL_1 assay compared to murine IL-5. IL-5 quickly loses activity if stored at 4°C.

Other assays for IL-5 are based on its ability to induce antibody secretion. These are generally indirect assays, with the IL-5 inducing antibody secretion and the actual assay detecting the presence of antibody. Antibody production is usually measured by plaque formation (40).

INTERLEUKIN-6

IL-6 has previously been called B cell stimulatory factor 2 (41), hybridoma growth factor (42,43), hepatocyte stimulating factor (44), and interferon-β_2 (45). IL-6 is responsible for a number of biological activities, and thus several different assays exist to quantitate its presence. These assays have recently been investigated, and the authors determined that the most sensitive and specific test for IL-6 is its hybridoma growth factor activity (46). Standard bioassays for the detection of IL-6 hybridoma growth-promoting activity involve the use of IL-6-dependent cell lines in a fashion similar to that already described for the other interleukins. Two such cell lines are the T1165 (47) and B9 (43), both of which are murine plasmacytomas. These cells have a requirement for IL-6 for growth, and in the absence of IL-6 they die over a 3 day period. Several interleukins have been tested in B9 cell line, and to date, IL-6 is the only interleukin that allows B9 cells to proliferate. However, high concentrations of lipopolysaccharide (10 μg/ml) result in a small degree of augmentation (48). The B9 cell line responds to IL-6 from multiple sources, including rat, mouse, and human.

To run the assay, samples are serially diluted in tissue culture media (either RPMI-1640 or Iscoves, although we have had considerably better success with B9 cells in Iscoves) containing fetal calf serum. Inclusion of fetal calf serum in the diluting media enhances the sensitivity of the assay since it provides a source of protein to prevent nonspecific adherence of the IL-6 to the plasticware. The diluted samples are placed in a 96-well plate and the cells are added on top. As with the CTLL-2 cells, it is important to include 2β-mercaptoethanol in the assay media since the cell lines are lymphocyte derived. After about 60–70 h of incubation at 37°C, the cells are pulsed with either [^{3}H]thymidine or MTT-tetrazolium and incubated an additional 6 h. The [^{3}H]thymidine is then counted or the color developed, and the units are calculated from the standard curve, which is always run on the same assay.

The B9 cells have an absolute requirement for the presence of IL-6 for continued growth. Several sources of IL-6 exist; the most expensive involves purchase of recombinant material. We have taken conditioned media from fibroblasts as a source of IL-6. Fibroblasts are grown to near confluence in tissue culture flasks. The medium is removed and fresh medium containing 10% fetal calf serum is added and the cells carried in culture without stimulus for an additional 1 or 2 days. This medium is then removed and used as a rich source of IL-6. The B9 cells proliferate quickly, and they may easily exhaust the medium of nutrients and IL-6 if not subcultured. We routinely split our cells three times a week.

INTERLEUKIN-8

IL-8 functions primarily as an activator of neutrophils and has additionally been described as neutrophil activating peptide or monocyte-derived neutrophil chemotactic factor (49,50). Since it functions as a neutrophil activator, most assays quantitate its presence by its ability to alter specific neutrophil functions. IL-8 has been shown to induce in neutrophils the following functions: chemotaxis, calcium fluxes, respiratory burst, chemokinesis, and release of several enzymes (51). Unlike most of the other cytokines, which use cloned cell lines, normal neutrophils are used for these assays and several factors exist that may also stimulate the neutrophils. To ascertain that the activity is due to IL-8, it is necessary either to perform careful fractionation of the activity into the appropriate molecular weight or to inhibit its activity with specific antibodies.

One of the more sensitive assays for quantitating IL-8 activity is the chemotaxis assay. There are several variations in the performance of the chemotaxis assay, but all essentially measure the ability of neutrophils to migrate toward a positive gradient of the chemotactic factor. The chemotaxis may be measured by the cell's ability to migrate in soft agar or, more commonly, to migrate through the pores of a membrane.

Recently a very sensitive and specific ELISA was described for IL-8 (52). This ELISA has the capability to detect as little as 50 pg IL-8 per ml, even in protein-rich fluids like plasma. The rabbit antibody has been shown to not cross-react with other cytokines reported to be chemotactic and also does not cross-react with other members of the IL-8 supergene family (53). This ELISA uses a single rabbit polyclonal antibody. Since there is only one antibody, the capture and developing antibody are the same, but the developing antibody is coupled to biotin. Avidin linked to horseradish peroxidase is then used for color development. Bioassays generally provide more information than immunoassays, but the IL-8 bioassays are very time consuming and may be difficult to interpret.

TUMOR NECROSIS FACTOR

There exist several assays for the detection of tumor necrosis factor, and they vary in sensitivity and specificity. The original assay involved the fibrosarcoma cell line L929 or LM (54). Samples are serially diluted and added to plates that already contain the adherent cells. A standard of recombinant TNF is also prepared and added to wells in the same assay. To enhance the sensitivity and increase the speed of the assay, an inhibitor of either RNA synthesis (actinomycin D) or protein synthesis (cycloheximide) is added. The cells are incubated overnight at 37°C, the supernatants and dead, nonadherent cells discarded, and the remaining viable cells are stained with crystal violet. The plates are washed with tap water, and the absorbance is measured at 620 nm. Units are calculated based on the recombinant standard. There exist conflicting reports regarding the ability of IL-1 to lyse TNF-sensitive target cells (55). The L929 cell line is also lysed by TNF-β (lymphotoxin), and to discriminate between these two structurally related cytokines it is necessary to use specific, neutralizing antibodies (56). Investigators should check the cell line they are using to determine if their targets are susceptible to lysis by IL-1, and if they are, appropriate controls should be used.

Samples that contain low levels of TNF activity, such as serum or plasma, may be measured with the highly sensitive cell line WEHI 164 subclone 13 (57). These cells are exquisitely sensitive to the lytic effects of TNF and can detect as little as 1 pg/ml (57,58). This assay is also run in the presence of actinomycin D to enhance its sensitivity. To perform this assay, the samples are serially diluted in the plates and the cells are added on top. After overnight incubation, MTT-tetrazolium is added, the plates placed back in the incubator for an additional 4 h, and the color developed with isopropanol. Units are calculated based on a recombinant standard run in the same assay. The WEHI 164 cells have been shown to respond both TNF-α and lymphotoxin and are not lysed by several other cytokines. Furthermore, there is no synergism with IFN-γ (58), which has been shown to potentiate the effects of TNF in some systems.

SUMMARY

There are obviously many ways to quantitate the bioactivity of IL-1, IL-2, IL-3, IL-4, IL-5, IL-6, IL-8, and TNF. ELISA assays are specific, but they require antibodies for each cytokine and there may be species specificity to the antibodies. Additionally, the reagents, or kits, may be extremely expensive. The cell line assays are less costly and generally easier to perform but require maintenance of the cell cultures between assays. One must be constantly vigilant with the cell lines, since they may be responding to yet-to-be-discovered cytokines. This chapter lists some of the more useful biological cytokine assays, and newer methodologies and cell lines are constantly being discovered.

ACKNOWLEDGMENTS

Supported in part by National Institutes of Health Grants HL-39339 and GM 44918 and a Grant-in-Aid from the American Heart Association of Michigan.

REFERENCES

1. Pennica D, Nedwin GE, Hayflick JS, et al. Human tumour necrosis factor: precursor structure, expression and homology to lymphotoxin. Nature 1984; 312:724–9.
2. Koopman WJ, Farrar JJ, Fuller-Bonar J. Evidence for the identification of lymphocyte activating factor as the adherent cell-derived mediator responsible for enhanced antibody synthesis by nude mouse spleen cells. Cell Immunol 1978; 35:92–8.
3. Mizel SB, Oppenheim JJ, Rosenstreich DL. Characterization of lymphocyte-activating factor (LAF) produced by the macrophage cell line, P388D1. I. Enhancement of LAF production by activated T lymphocytes. J Immunol 1978; 120:1497–503.
4. Helle M, Brakenhoff JP, De Groot ER, Aarden LA. Interleukin 6 is involved in interleukin 1-induced activities. Eur J Immunol 1988; 18:957–9.
5. Van Damme J, Van Beeumen J, Decock B, Van Snick J, De Ley M, Billiau A. Separation and comparison of two monokines with lymphocyte-activating factor activity: IL-1 beta and hybridoma growth factor (HGF). Identification of leukocyte-derived HGF as IL-6. J Immunol 1988; 140:1534–41.
6. Lotz M, Jirik F, Kabouridis P, et al. B-cell stimulating factor 2/interleukin 6 is a costimulant for human thymocytes and T-lymphocytes. J Exp Med 1988; 167: 1253–8.
7. Ranges GE, Zlotnik A, Espevik T, Dinarello CA, Cerami A, Palladino MA Jr. Tumor necrosis factor alpha/cachectin is a growth factor for thymocytes. Synergistic interactions with other cytokines. J Exp Med 1988; 167:1472–8.
8. Lowenthal JW, Cerottini JC, MacDonald HR. Interleukin 1-dependent induction of both interleukin 2 secretion and interleukin 2 receptor expression by thymoma cells. J Immunol 1986; 137:1226–31.
9. Gillis S, Mizel SB. T-cell lymphoma model for the analysis of interleukin 1-mediated T-cell activation. Proc Natl Acad Sci U S A 1981; 78:1133–7.
10. Larrick JW, Brindley L, Doyle MV. An improved assay for the detection of interleukin 1. J Immunol Methods 1985; 79:39–45.
11. Conlon PJ. A rapid biologic assay for the detection of interleukin 1. J Immunol 1983; 131:1280–2.
12. Suda T, Hodgkin P, Lee F, Zlotnik A. Biological activity of recombinant murine interleukin-6 in interleukin-1 T cell assays. J Immunol Methods 1989; 120:173–8.
13. Kaye J, Gillis S, Mizel SB, et al. Growth of a cloned helper T-cell line induced by a monoclonal antibody specific for the antigen receptor: interleukin 1 is required for the expression of receptors for interleukin 2. J Immunol 1984; 133:1339–45.
14. Orencole SF, Dinarello CA. Characterization of a subclone (D10S) of the D10.G4.1 helper T-cell line which proliferates to attomolar concentrations of interleukin-1 in the absence of mitogens. Cytokine 1989; 1:14–22.
15. Larrick JW. Native interleukin 1 inhibitors. Immunol Today 1989; 10:61–6.
16. Cannon JG, van der Meer JW, Kwiatkowski D, et al. Interleukin-1 beta in human plasma: optimization of blood collection, plasma extraction, and radioimmunoassay methods. Lymphokine Res 1988; 7:457–67.
17. Hopkins SJ, Holt I, Humphreys M. Removal of inhibitory activity and determination of biologically active interleukin-1 in biological fluids. In: Dinarello CA, Kluger MJ, Powanda MC, Opennheim JJ, eds. The physiological and pathological effects of cytokines. New York: Wiley-Liss, 1990:7–12.

18. Gillis S, Ferm MM, Ou W, Smith KA. T-cell growth factor: parameters of production and a quantitative microassay for activity. J Immunol 1978; 120:2027–32.
19. Mosmann T. Rapid colorimetric assay for cellular growth and survival: application to proliferation and cytotoxicity assays. J Immunol Methods 1983; 65:55–63.
20. Tada H, Shiho O, Kuroshima K, Koyama M, Tsukamoto K. An improved colorimetric assay for interleukin 2. J Immunol Methods 1986; 93:157–65.
21. Eskandari MK, Kunkel SL, Remick DG. Effects of arachidonic acid metabolites and other compounds on the CTLL assay for interleukin-2. J Immunol Methods 1989; 118:85–9.
22. Remick DG, Scales WE, Chensue SW, Kunkel SL. The pathophysiology of interleukins and tumor necrosis factors. In: Sayeed M, ed. Focus on cellular pathophysiology. Boca Raton, FL: CRC Press, 1989:41–83.
23. Powers GD, Abbas AK, Miller RA. Frequencies of IL-2- and IL-4-secreting T-cells in naive and antigen-stimulated lymphocyte populations. J Immunol 1988; 140: 3352–7.
24. Grabstein K, Eisenman J, Mochizuki D, et al. Purification to homogeneity of B-cell stimulating factor. A molecule that stimulates proliferation of multiple lymphokine-dependent cell lines. J Exp Med 1986; 163:1405–14.
25. Ohara J, Paul WE. Production of a monoclonal antibody to and molecular characterization of B-cell stimulatory factor-1. Nature 1985; 315:333–6.
26. Ihle JN. Biochemical and biological properties of interleukin-3: a lymphokine mediating the differentiation of a lineage of cells that includes prothymocytes and mast-like cells. Contemp Top Mol Immunol 1985; 10:93–119.
27. Gearing AJ, Johnstone AP, Thorpe R. Production and assay of the interleukins. J Immunol Methods 1985; 83:1–27.
28. Rennick DM, Lee FD, Yokota T, Arai KI, Cantor H, Nabel GJ. A cloned MCGF cDNA encodes a multilineage hematopoietic growth factor: multiple activities of interleukin 3. J Immunol 1985; 134:910–4.
29. Otsuka T, Miyajima A, Brown N, et al. Isolation and characterization of an expressible cDNA encoding human IL-3. Induction of IL-3 mRNA in human T-cell clones. J Immunol 1988; 140:2288–95.
30. Dexter TM, Garland J, Scott D, Scolnick E, Metcalf D. Growth of factor-dependent hemopoietic precursor cell lines. J Exp Med 1980; 152:1036–47.
31. Ihle JN, Keller J, Greenberger JS, Henderson L, Yetter RA, Morse III HC. Phenotypic characteristics of cell lines requiring interleukin 3 for growth. J Immunol 1982; 129:1377–83.
32. Le Gros GS, Gillis S, Watson JD. Induction of IL 2 responsiveness in a murine IL 3-dependent cell line. Immunology 1985; 135:4009–14.
33. Gajewski TF, Fitch FW. Anti-proliferative effect of IFN-gamma in immune regulation. IV. Murine CTL clones produce IL-3 and GM-CSF, the activity of which is masked by the inhibitory actin of secreted IFN-gamma. J Immunol 1990; 144:548–56.
34. Howard M, Farrar J, Hilfiker M, et al. Identification of a T-cell-derived B-cell growth factor distinct from interleukin 2. J Exp Med 1982; 155:914–23.
35. Muraguchi A, Fauci AS. Proliferative responses of normal human B-lymphocytes. Development of an assay system for human B-cell growth factor (BCGF). J Immunol 1982; 129:1104–8.
36. Hu-Li J, Ohara J, Watson C, Tsang W, Paul WE. Derivation of a T-cell line that is highly responsive to IL-4 and IL-2 (CT.4R) and of an IL-2 hyporesponsive mutant of that line (CT.4S). J Immunol 1989; 142:800–7.
37. Dutton RW, Wetzel GD, Swain SL. Partial purification and characterization of a BCGFII from EL4 culture supernatants. J Immunol 1984; 132:2451–6.

38. McKenzie DT, Filutowicz HI, Swain SL, Dutton RW. Purification and partial sequence analysis of murine B-cell growth factor II (interleukin 5). J Immunol 1987; 139:2661–8.
39. Lohoff M, Sommer F, Rollinghoff M. Suppressive effect of interferon-gamma on the BCL1 cell-dependent interleukin 5 bioassay. Eur J Immunol 1989; 19:1327–9.
40. Takatsu K, Harada N, Hara Y, et al. Purification and physicochemical characterization of murine T-cell replacing factor (TRF). J Immunol 1985; 134:382–9.
41. Hirano T, Yasukawa K, Harada H, et al. Complementary DNA for a novel human interleukin (BSF-2) that induces B-lymphocytes to produce immunoglobulin. Nature 1986; 324:73–6.
42. Van Snick J, Cayphas S, Vink A, et al. Purification and NH2-terminal amino acid sequence of a T-cell-derived lymphokine with growth factor activity for B-cell hybridomas. Proc Natl Acad Sci USA 1986; 83:9679–83.
43. Aarden LA, De Groot ER, Schaap OL, Lansdorp PM. Production of hybridoma growth factor by human monocytes. Eur J Immunol 1987; 17:1411–6.
44. Gauldie J, Richards C, Harnish D, Lansdorp P, Baumann H. Interferon-beta 2/B-cell stimulatory factor type 2 shares identity with monocyte-derived hepatocyte-stimulating factor and regulates the major acute phase protein response in liver cells. Proc Natl Acad Sci USA 1987; 84:7251–5.
45. Zilberstein A, Ruggieri R, Korn JH, Revel M. Structure and expression of cDNA and genes for human interferon-beta-2, a distinct species inducible by growth-stimulatory cytokines. EMBO J 1986; 5:2529–37.
46. Van Damme J, Van Snick J. Induction of hybridoma growth factor (HGF), identical to IL-6, in human fibroblasts by IL-1: use of HGF activity in specific and sensitive biological assays for IL-1 and IL-6. Dev Biol Stand 1988; 69:31–8.
47. Nordan RP, Pumphrey JG, Rudikoff S. Purification and NH2-terminal sequence of a plasmacytoma growth factor derived from the murine macrophage cell line P388D1. J Immunol 1987; 139:813–7.
48. Ulich TR, Guo K, Remick D, del Castillo J, Yin S. Endotoxin-induced cytokine gene expression *in vivo*. J Immunol 1991; 146:2316–1212.
49. Matsushima K, Oppenheim JJ. Interleukin 8 and MCAF: novel inflammatory cytokines inducible by IL-1 and TNF. Cytokine 1989; 1:2–13.
50. Baggiolini M, Walz A, Kunkel SL. Neutrophil-activating peptide-1/interleukin 8, a novel cytokine that activates neutrophils. J Clin Invest 1989; 84:1045–9.
51. Peveri P, Walz A, Dewald B, Baggiolini M. A novel neutrophil-activating factor produced by human mononuclear phagocytes. J Exp Med 1988; 167:1547–59.
52. DeForge LE, Remick DG. Sandwich ELISA for detection of picogram quantities of interleukin-8. Immun Invest 1991; 20:89–97.
53. DeForge LE, Remick DG. Kinetics of TNF, IL-6, and IL-8 gene expression in LPS-stimulated human whole blood. Biochem Biophys Res Commun 1991; 174:18–24.
54. Ruff MR, Gifford GE. Tumor necrosis factor. Lymphokines 1981; 2:235–40.
55. Onozaki K, Matsushima K, Aggarwal BB, Oppenheim JJ. Human interleukin1 is a cytocidal factor for several tumor cell lines. J Immunol 1985; 135:3962–8.
56. Bringman TS, Aggarwal BB. Monoclonal antibodies to human tumor necrosis factors alpha and beta: application for affinity purification, immunoassays, and as structural probes. Hybridoma 1987; 6:489–507.
57. Espevik T, Nissen Meyer J. A highly sensitive cell line, WEHI 164 clone 13, for measuring cytotoxic factor/tumor necrosis factor from human monocytes. J Immunol Methods 1986; 95:99–105.
58. Eskandari MK, Nguyen DT, Kunkel SL, Remick DG. WEHI 164 subclone 13 assay for TNF: sensitivity, specificity and reliability. Immun Invest 1990; 190:69–79.

CHAPTER 2

STRUCTURE AND FUNCTION OF INTERLEUKIN-1

Wendy E. Scales

The University of Michigan Medical School
Ann Arbor, Michigan

INTRODUCTION

Interleukin-1 (IL-1) is a fascinating, multifunctional, and complex molecule. The protein IL-1 (both α and β forms) is now known to be the same as a group of previously identified substances, each independently discovered and characterized and named according to the discrete biological activity associated with the given protein. These include endogenous pyrogen (EP), leukocyte endogenous mediator (LEM), lymphocyte activating factor (LAF), B cell activating factor (BAF), thymocyte proliferation factor (TPF), helper peak 1 (HP-1), mononuclear cell factor (MCF), osteoclast activating factor (OAF), and epidermal cell-derived thymocyte activating factor (ETAF). Based upon a number of technological advances and collaborative efforts, it became clear that in fact these were all properties of one protein or group of proteins, and thus in 1979, it was recommended at the Second International Lymphokine Workshop that interleukin-1 be used to refer to the protein or group of proteins previously identified as outlined here (1). Clearly this molecule possesses numerous biological activities, is capable of acting upon a multitude of target cell types, and, further, is synthesized by a variety of different cell populations within the body.

BIOCHEMISTRY

Considerable advances in our understanding of the IL-1 molecule were achieved with improvements in protein purification methodologies and cloning of the interleukin-1 genes. For the purposes of this discussion, attention is primarily focused on the human and murine interleukin-1. IL-1 is a heat-labile protein, inactivated by heat treatment at 70°C for 30 minutes. Interestingly, this property facilitated early investigations of endogenous pyrogen activity since heat lability provided a means of distinguishing the pyrogenic properties of IL-1 from those of heat-resistant endotoxins. The predominant form of IL-1 detected in stimulated cell supernatants is 17,000 daltons, derived from a precursor protein of approximately 31,000–33,000 daltons. Both larger and smaller species of IL-1 have been reported; the 50,000–75,000 dalton species are likely to reflect aggregates of smaller molecular weight sizes, and the 4000 and 2000 dalton fragments in urine and plasma may represent proteolytic cleavage products (2–4). Another potentially important form of IL-1, with a molecular weight of 23,000 daltons, has been demonstrated on the membranes of a variety of cells, including macrophages, monocytes, dendritic cells, and fibroblasts (5–9). This membrane-associated IL-1 may be critical for the action of IL-1 in antigen presentation to T cells and other local effects in an inflammatory lesion involving cell-cell interactions. Isoelectric focusing of IL-1 derived from both murine and human sources has revealed charge heterogeneity in the protein, with two forms, pI 5.0 and 7.0, designated IL-1α and IL-1β, respectively (10,11).

Cloning studies have provided additional insight into the two forms of the IL-1 protein. In 1984, Auron et al. (12) isolated a cDNA from lipopolysaccharide (LPS)-stimulated human peripheral blood monocytes coding for a 269 amino acid protein with a predicted molecular weight of 31,000 daltons. This gene product was deduced to be the pI 7.0 form of human IL-1, with cleavage of the larger precursor resulting in a 17,000 dalton protein (carboxy-terminal 152 amino acids), consistent with the predominant secreted biologically active form of IL-1. These investigators noted the absence of a strand of hydrophobic amino acids near the amino terminus common to the signal sequence of a traditional secreted protein. Further, March et al. (13) reported the isolation of two distinct human cDNAs from stimulated macrophages, IL-1α and IL-1β. These investigators demonstrated that the C-terminal 159 and 153 amino acids were sufficient for biological activity of IL-1α and IL-1β, respectively. This demonstration supports the concept of precursor cleavage to smaller, biologically active forms of the protein. Consistent with the report of Auron et al. (12) for IL-1β, March and coworkers also noted the absence of a typical signal sequence in either the human IL-1α or IL-1β molecules.

Another advance in the understanding of IL-1 was the cloning of murine IL-1α by Lomedico et al. (14) utilizing the murine macrophage cell line P388D1. Not unlike the human IL-1 molecule, these investigators demonstrated a polypeptide precursor of approximately 270 amino acids, with an associated molecular weight of about 33,000 daltons. Lomedico et al. further demonstrated that the carboxyl 156 amino acids of this murine IL-1α, pI 5.0, possessed biological activity. In 1986, Gray et al. (15) reported the cloning of murine IL-1β and demonstrated that this gene product, derived from the murine macrophage PU5-1.8 cell line, was a 269 amino acid protein (calculated molecular weight of 31,000 daltons). As seems to be the case for human IL-1α and IL-1β and for murine IL-1α, this precursor form of murine IL-1β is likely to be cleaved to a smaller 17,000 dalton moiety. Interesting observations derived from the cloning studies relate to the degree of homology between the forms and species of IL-1 described. At the amino acid level, there appears to be a closer relationship between the human and murine IL-1s of similar isoelectric points than between the two forms within a given species; human and murine IL-1β, 67% homology; human and murine IL-1α, 62% homology; human IL-1α and IL-1β, 26% homology; and murine IL-1α and IL-1β, 22% homology. The conservation of amino acid sequences between the murine and human species for the two forms of IL-1 may relate to the critical role (or roles) each form of the molecule plays with regard to immune cell interactions. The human interleukin-1 genes have been shown to be located on chromosome 2, with both IL-1α and IL-1β consisting of seven exons, and 12 and 9.7 kb in length, respectively (16,17).

Processing of the IL-1 proteins is an intriguing issue, since as mentioned the molecules lack the normal signal sequence of secreted proteins. Studies conducted by Murphy et al. (18) and Mizel (19) indicated that glycosylation of IL-1 is not a requisite step in the processing of the IL-1 molecule for biological activity. An interesting study by Matsushima et al. (7) examined the intracellular localization of IL-1 activity in LPS-stimulated monocytes. These investigators found that IL-1 activity was present in the greatest proportions in the cytosolic compartment, as opposed to the Golgi or particulate fractions. High-performance liquid chromotography of this IL-1 activity suggested a molecular weight of approximately 23,000 daltons, with lesser amounts at 31,000 daltons. IL-1 activity detected in the cell supernatants in these studies was found to be the 17,000 dalton form of IL-1. The IL-1 molecule appears to be posttranslationally processed either before or during release from macrophages. An additional finding from this study was that treatment of IL-1 producing cells with trypsin or plasmin resulted in the release of biologically active IL-1 (23,000 daltons), which supports the concept of biologically active IL-1 present on the outer surface of stimulated cell membranes. These authors postulate that some processing of IL-1 precursor (31,000) may occur intracellularly to yield the 23,000 dalton form observed in the cytosolic and cell membrane fractions. The cell surface-bound IL-1 is likely to perform important functions in cell-cell immune interactions. Further enzymatic action by tissue plasminogen activator and serum enzymes, such as plasmin, may be involved in the actual release of IL-1 from stimulated IL-1-producing cells. A related but alternative hypothesis was advanced by Giri et al. (20). These investigators examined the 33,000 dalton precursor and conversion to a lower molecular weight form of murine IL-1 in P388D1 cells and peritoneal murine macrophages. They proposed the idea that a 33,000 dalton IL-1 precursor is actually secreted in precursor form and then rapidly converted to a lower molecular weight by proteases of macrophage origin.

CELLULAR SOURCES AND STIMULI FOR IL-1 PRODUCTION

Reflective of the multifaceted nature of the IL-1 molecule, numerous cell types are capable of synthesizing the IL-1 protein; further, numerous stimuli directly and indirectly participate in the induction of IL-1 from these cell types. The initial studies of lymphocyte activating factor by Gery et al. (21,22) identified the macrophage as the cell source of this soluble factor. Cells typically thought of as participating in immune responses are capable of making IL-1, the most prominant being circulating blood monocytes and tissue macrophages, including alveolar macrophages, Kupffer cells of the liver, synovial cells, and peritoneal macrophages. Lymphocytes, including B cells, natural killer (NK) cells, and helper T cells, are additional sources of IL-1. A variety of other cell types have been shown to produce IL, some perhaps unexpectedly. In the central nervous system, astrocytes, microglia, and glioma cells make IL-1; vascular smooth muscle cells and endothelial cells also synthesize IL-1. Neutrophils, fibroblasts, chondrocytes, epithelial cells, keratinocytes, Langerhans cells, and renal mesangial cells are among the other cell types that have been demonstrated to produce IL-1 (see reviews, Refs. 23–25). It is possible that most nucleated cells possess the capacity to upregulate the expression and synthesis of IL-1 in response to the appropriate stimulation.

Both exogenous and endogenous agents provide adequate stimuli for the induction of IL-1. Cytokines may serve as inducing signals for IL-1, including IL-2, granulocyte-macrophage colony-stimulating factor (GM-CSF), transforming growth factor β (TGF-β), TNFα, interferons (IFNα, β, and γ, and IL-1 itself may actually stimulate further IL-1 production in certain cell types (see reviews, Refs. 26 and 27). Cell-to-cell contact involving antigen presentation by macrophages to T cells requires participation and thus synthesis of macrophage IL-1. Microbial products, such as endotoxins, peptidoglycans, muramyl dipeptide, virus, yeast, and zymosan, serve as IL-1 stimulating agents. Among other stimuli for IL-1 production are endogenous agents, such as antigen-antibody complexes, the Fc region of IgG, and C5A; other nonspecific exogenous agents include silica, urate crystals, and ultraviolet (UV) radiation. It is important to appreciate the complexity of the cytokine network and the interactions contributing to the inflammatory cascade. For example, a given stimulus for IL-1 production from peripheral blood monocytes and tissue macrophages may both directly and indirectly result in the expression and synthesis of other cytokines, such as TNF and interleukin-6. These cytokines have effects on other cell populations as well as monocytes-macrophages. Further, endogenous regulators of cytokine production, such as products of arachidonate metabolism, may also be generated under the described conditions. LPS and IL-1-treated macrophages have been demonstrated to release prostaglandin E_2 (PGE_2) in a time-dependent manner. A number of investigators have demonstrated a dose-dependent suppression of macrophage IL-1 and TNF production by PGE_2 (28–33). Many cytokines in addition to IL-1 are multifaceted, with multiple biological activities, and hence it is far too simplistic to view a single stimulus and target cell resulting in the generation of one cytokine product.

IL-1 RECEPTOR

With a multitude of biological activities ascribed to the IL-1 molecule, an understanding of the IL-1 receptor on target tissues may provide insight into this diversity. Technological advances providing pure and recombinant preparations of IL-1 have greatly facilitated this endeavor. In 1985, Dower et al. (34) described IL-1-specific receptors on the T lymphoma LBRM 33 1A5 cell line. These investigators presented evidence for specific high-affinity binding of ^{125}I-IL-1 to these cells (0.2–2 × 10^{10} per M), with 500 receptors per cell. The plasma membrane IL-1 receptor they characterized was found to exhibit a molecular weight of approximately 80,000 daltons, as analyzed by sodium dodecyl sulfate–polyacrylamide gel electrophoresis (SDS-PAGE). In the cell types tested, the most significant binding of IL-1 to receptor was found to be on cells of lymphoid origin or fibroblast or epithelial types. Binding of recombinant murine IL-1α to EL4 thymoma cells was investigated by Kilian et al. (35). IL-1 was shown to stimulate IL-2 production by EL4 cells. Specific and saturable binding of ^{125}I-IL-1 was demonstrated with a $K_d = 2.6 \times 10^{-10}$ M and the estimated number of binding sites as 1200 binding sites per cell. Further, recombinant human IL-1α and IL-1β (17,500 dalton forms) competed equally with recombinant IL-1α for binding to these receptors. This point is of interest considering the relatively low extent of homology between these forms and species of IL-1; perhaps part of the conserved sequence involves the receptor binding site important for signal transduction and biological response in target cells. Lowenthal et al. (36) in 1986 investigated the binding of IL-1 to EL4–6.1 thymoma cells, a cell line that simultaneously secretes IL-2 and expresses IL-2 receptor in the presence of IL-1. This cell type was shown to possess high numbers of IL-1 receptors on the cells (approximately 20,000 per cell), and further, these could be resolved into two classes based upon affinity for ligand. These investigators found that 98–99% of the receptors had affinities with a K_d of approximately 200–500 pM, whereas 1–2% of the receptors characterized displayed a K_d of approximately 3–8 pM, with the associated ability to internalize the IL-1–receptor complex. It was proposed that the biological action of IL-1 could only be attributed to the interaction of IL-1 with the high-affinity receptor population, since the IL-1 concentration giving half-maximal biological activity in EL4–6.1 cells corresponds exactly to the K_d of this class of receptor. Mosley et al. (37) investigated the binding of both the precursor and processed forms of human IL-1α and IL-1β to murine T cell lines EL4 and LBRM 33 1A5. Both processed human IL-1α and IL-1β (17,500 dalton) forms were biologically active and bound specifically to receptors on these cells. Only IL-1α precursor bound to receptor with associated biological activity. Clearly, the initial IL-1β translation product must be processed further before receptor interaction and biological response. A major achievement in the study of the IL-1 receptor was the cloning of this entity from EL46.1 C10 cells by Sims et al. (38). In this study, the cloned IL-1 receptor was shown to comigrate on SDS polyacrylamide gels with receptor from EL46.10 C10 cells at a molecular weight of 80,000 daltons. Further, binding to the cloned receptor could be inhibited by an excess of unlabeled IL-1β or IL-1α. The receptor was demonstrated to consist of 576 amino acids, comprised of a 319 amino acid extracellular portion with seven potential glycosylation sites, a 21-residue transmembrane region, and a C-terminal 217 amino acid cytoplasmic portion of the molecule. The predicted molecular weight of the receptor was 64,598 daltons. Previous studies have demonstrated that removal of carbohydrate from the 80,000 dalton receptor using *N*-glycanase decreases the receptor size to approximately 62,000 daltons (39). Sims et al. (38) indicated that the extracellular portion of the IL-1 receptor was organized into three domains, similarly to the immunoglobulin gene superfamily. No mechanisms for IL-1 signal transduction were proposed by these investigators. A follow-up study with the cloned murine IL-1 receptor by Dower et al. (40) involved construction of a cDNA clone encoding the 319 amino acid carbohydrate containing extracellular region (that region suggested to contain the IL-1 binding site). Expression of this clone in HeLa cells led to soluble IL-1α binding protein in the cell supernatants. This study gives further support to the concept of the 21-residue hydrophobic transmembrane anchor portion of the receptor.

IN VIVO ACTIVITIES

One of the biologic actions of IL-1 in vivo is the induction of fever upon injection into experimental animals. Some of the earliest investigations of interleukin-1 centered around the endogenous pyrogenic activity of the molecule (41). To date there is no evidence that the IL-1 molecule crosses the blood-brain barrier to act directly upon thermosensitive hypothalamic neurons to bring about an elevation in temperature. This protein is likely to exert its pyrogenic action by interaction with the endothelial cells of the vascularized hypothalamus, resulting in the generation of prostaglandins of the E series. Prostaglandins then act at the level of the hypothalamus to alter the firing rates of thermosensitive neurons, resulting in an elevation in body temperature (42,43). Antipyretic drugs, such as indomethacin and aspirin, owe their effectiveness to the inhibition of the cyclooxygenase enzyme involved in the metabolism of arachidonic acid to prostaglandins. The development of fever is considered an evolutionarily conserved nonspecific host defense response to infection, and further, many immune reactions and activities are potentiated at elevated (febrile) temperatures. Other cytokines in addition to IL-1 have been demonstrated to possess endogenous pyrogen activity. Thus it is possible that the "true" endogenous pyrogen is not merely one protein, but is rather a cocktail of proteins released from cells in the development of an inflammatory response, all of which may act to bring about a febrile state in the infected organism.

Another component of the nonspecific host defense response to infection involves changes in several plasma trace metal concentrations. Specific alterations include an elevation in plasma copper and depression in both plasma zinc and iron concentrations. Many of these alterations in the storage and binding of trace metals have been attributed to the activity of IL-1 (44–47). This response of the host may too be adaptive, particularly in combination with an elevation in body temperature, as was elegantly demonstrated by Kluger and Rothenburg (48). Redistribution of iron may provide the host with a mechanism to reduce the quantities of iron available for microbial proliferation, establishing a kind of competition between the host and the microbe for iron. Redistribution of zinc resulting in reduced plasma concentrations may accomplish similar goals.

The increased synthesis of hepatic acute-phase proteins and the associated decrease in albumin synthesis is another hallmark of inflammation. Early investigations of the leukocyte endogenous mediator properties of IL-1 implicated a role for this cytokine in the induction of the acute-phase response. Clearly, the injection of pure preparations of IL-1 into experimental animals results in an elevation of many hepatic acute-phase proteins. An interesting development associated with the availability of recombinant and pure proteins is the discovery that the cytokine IL-6 may in fact be the predominant mediator of the acute-phase response during inflammation. Both IL-1 and TNF have been demonstrated to stimulate the synthesis of IL-6 from fibroblasts and other target cells. In vitro studies utilizing recombinant preparations of IL-1, TNF, and IL-6 and hepatic cell lines suggest differential induction of acute-phase proteins by these cytokines. Specifically, Castell et al. (49) examined the effect of recombinant human IL-1β, TNF-α, and IL-6 on human primary hepatocyte acute-phase protein synthesis. Only IL-6 was found by these investigators to induce a full spectrum of acute-phase protein synthesis and secretion from these cells, including C-reactive protein, serum amyloid A, fibrinogen, α_1-antitrypsin, α_1-antichymotrypsin, and haptoglobin, with an associated reduction in albumin, transferrin, and fibronectin. IL-1β and TNF were found to similarly inhibit the synthesis and secretion of fibronectin, albumin, and transferrin but failed to induce serum amyloid A and C-reactive protein in this system. Andus et al. (50) investigated the differential induction of acute-phase proteins by recombinant human IL-6, IL-1β, and TNF-α in the rat hepatoma cell line Fao. In the presence of 10^{-6} M dexamethasone, all three cytokines were shown to cause a reduction in albumin synthesis from this cell line; however, only rIL-6 induced significant levels of β-fibrinogen mRNA. Further, IL-6 was shown to be only a weak stimulus for α_1-acid glycoprotein mRNA induction, but both TNF and IL-1 caused profound elevations in this acute-phase protein from the Fao cell line. Many other studies provide additional examples of differential induction of acute-phase proteins by various cytokines. Undoubtedly, IL-1 participates in the acute-phase response, directly stimulating the synthesis of some acute-phase proteins itself but also indirectly via the stimulation of IL-6 synthesis and secretion.

Somnolence and reduction in food appetite are common manifestations of acute infectious illness. Krueger et al. (51,52) demonstrated that central administration of IL-1 will induce slow-wave sleep in experimental animals. McCarthy et al. (53) demonstrated an anorexigenic effect of injection of IL-1 in experimental animals, and in vitro studies have demonstrated that IL-1 suppresses lipoprotein lipase activity (54). A property of IL-1 characterized by Kampschmidt and Pullian (47) during investigation of leukocyte endogenous mediator properties of the molecule is the ability of IL-1 to cause a mobilization of neutrophils from the bone marrow upon injection into experimental animals, resulting in a neutrophilia.

Considerable evidence has accumulated in recent years implicating interactions between the immune system and the neuroendocrine axis. An example of this interplay is the demonstration by Besedovsky et al. (55) that injection of rats and mice with pure or recombinant IL-1 preparations results in increased blood levels of adrenocorticotropic hormone (ACTH) and corticosterone. TNF, IL-2, and IFN-γ were shown to be without these effects. Hence, these authors postulate an immunoregulatory feedback circuit involving IL-1 as an afferent signal and the glucocorticoid response as the efferent hormone limb of the circuit.

The ability of IL-1 to induce colony-stimulating activity in vivo was demonstrated by Vogel et al. (56). In these studies, intraperitoneal injection of rIL-1α induced dose- and time-dependent CSF activity (a mixture of granulocyte and macrophage colonies) within 3 h of administration. This effect of IL-1 may be critical in the hematopoietic alterations associated with inflammation. Further, this property of IL-1 may relate to the radioprotective effects of the cytokine. Neta et al. in 1986 (57) demonstrated the dose-dependent protection of mice from the effects of ionizing radiation with intraperitoneal IL-1 pretreatment 20 h before irradiation. This protection could correlate with a shift in the cell cycle of granulocyte and monocyte progenitors, rendering them less susceptible to the effects of the irradiation, or alternatively, the IL-1 may accelerate the hematopoietic recovery in irradiated mice.

IL-1 may participate in a number of pathologic disorders, as discussed later in this volume. Pettipher et al. (58) examined the inflammatory changes in the knee joints of New Zealand white rabbits injected intraarticularly with IL-1. Such treatment caused a marked cellular infiltrate into the synovium and significant loss of proteoglycan from the articular cartilage. This response was not associated with swelling of the joint or skin, and further the investigators were unable to demonstrate a stimulation of eicosanoid synthesis (the response was not blunted by the administration of inhibitors of PGE_2 synthesis). IL-1 may directly activate degradative enzymes that result in the destruction of the joint tissues. Based upon this kind of evidence, IL-1 may be a key mediator in the development of chronic destructive arthritis.

IN VITRO EFFECTS

Numerous in vitro activities have been documented for IL-1. Perhaps one of the most noteworthy is the lymphocyte activating factor property of IL-1 described by Gery et al. (21,22) in 1972. These investigators examined the macrophage participation in the immunologic response of lymphocytes to antigen and found that IL-1 augmented the response of T lymphocytes to suboptimal concentrations of mitogens, such as phytohemagglutinin and concanavalin A. IL-1 interaction with T lymphocytes is also associated with IL-2 production and IL-2 receptor expression (59), and these combined effects of IL-1 suggest that this cytokine is likely to be a key participant in the clonal expansion of lymphocytes as part of the cell-mediated immune response. IL-1 may act with such factors as IL-2 and interferon to enhance natural killer cell activity (60). B cells are also responsive to the effects of IL-1. These actions include maturation, proliferation, and differentiation of B cells (including enhancement of antibody secretion), with the particular action dependent upon the maturational state of the target B cell (61).

The interaction of IL-1 with the vascular endothelium should no doubt be considered a proinflammatory interaction. It must be pointed out, however, that many of the described effects of IL-1 on endothelial cells are not unique to IL-1; TNF and LPS, as well as other cytokines, may also produce such responses. The endothelial cell stands in a unique position between the formed and soluble elements of the blood and tissue sites of inflammation. Perhaps one of the most pivotal roles played by IL-1 (or other cytokines) and endothelial cells is to promote adhesiveness for polymorphonuclear neutrophils, monocytes, lymphocytes, eosinophils, and basophils to the endothelial cell (62–64). This has been shown to involve interaction between the leukocyte adhesion molecules (CD11/CD18 complex) on leukocytes and leukocyte adhesion receptor complexes on endothelial cells (ICAM-1 and ELAM-1) (62,65). By inducing expression of ICAM-1 and ELAM-1 on endothelial cells, IL-1 provides a key step in the extravasation of leukocytes to sites of local inflammation and injury. Other manifestations of IL-1–endothelial cell interactions include PGE_2, prostacyclin, and platelet-activating factor production, as well as secretion of a variety of colony-stimulating factors. These responses are likely to facilitate mobilization and activation of appropriate leukocyte cell populations for participation in specific localized immune interactions. Further cytokine (including IL-1) action on endothelial cells involves a shift toward thrombosis and a procoagulant state by the downregulation of the fibrinolytic system and enhancement of plasminogen activator inhibitor and tissue factor-like procoagulant activity (66,67).

IL-1 has been shown to have effects on both bone and cartilage. IL-1 stimulates the resorption of bone (this activity was originally called osteoclast activating factor) (68), and a stimulation of PGE_2 synthesis is also associated with the interaction of this cytokine with bone. The effects of IL-1 on cartilage were mentioned with regard to the degradative effects on cartilage proteoglycan, perhaps implicating IL-1 in some of the destruction and inflammation of joints associated with rheumatoid arthritis. Schmidt et al. (11) demonstrated IL-1 stimulation of fibroblast proliferation and suggested the involvement of this monokine in the establishment of fibrosis associated with chronic granulomatous lesions.

SUMMARY AND CONCLUSION

Interleukin-1 is certainly a multifaceted molecule, with numerous cell sources and activities on target cell populations. This review by no means exhaustively documents all cell sources, stimuli, and activities of this molecule. Topics not included here of particular interest with regard to the IL-1 molecule include the signal transduction pathways involved subsequent to the IL-1-receptor interaction at target cells. Achievements with the study of the IL-1 receptor on target cells will no doubt advance this area of investigation. A number of inhibitors of IL-1 action have been documented, including corticosteroids, α-melanocyte stimulating hormone, PGE_2, urine-derived inhibitors, and products of virally infected macrophages (see review, Ref. 69). The roles of these various inhibitors and regulators of IL-1 in the dynamics of cytokine interactions continue to be an intriguing area of investigation. Interleukin-1 shares a number of functions with other cytokines. Elucidation of the dominant roles played by the various cytokines and how these mediators impact on the expression and production of other proteins pivotal to a successful inflammatory response are important areas for contemplation and experimentation. Continued investigation of the IL-1 protein at the level of the gene, messenger RNA and processed protein, and both in vivo and in vitro activities will enhance our understanding of the role of this particular cytokine in health and disease.

REFERENCES

1. Aarden LA, Brunner TK, Cerottini JC, et al. Revised nomenclature for antigen nonspecific T-cell proliferation and helper factors. J Immunol 1979; 123:2928–9.
2. Dinarello CA, Clowes GHA, Gordon HA, Saravis CA, Wolff SM. Cleavage of human interleukin 1: isolation of a peptide fragment from plasma of febrile humans and activated monocytes. J Immunol 1984; 133:1332–8.
3. Cannon JG, Dinrello CA. Increased plasma interleukin 1 activity in women after ovulation. Science 1985; 227:1247–9.
4. Kimball ES, Pickeral SF, Oppenheim JJ, Rossio JL. Interleukin 1 activity in normal human urine. J immunol 1984; 133:256–60.
5. Kurt-Jones EA, Beller DI, Mizel SB, Unanue ER. Identification of membrane-associated interleukin 1 in macrophages. Proc Natl Acad Sci U S A 1985; 82:1204–8.
6. Kurt-Jones EA, Virgin HW, Unanue ER. In vivo and in vitro expression of mac-

rophage membrane interleukin 1 in response to soluble and particulate stimuli. J Immunol 1986; 137:10–4.
7. Matsushima K, Taguchi M, Kovacs EJ, Young HA, Oppenheim JJ. Intracellular localization of human monocyte associated IL1 activity and release of biologically active IL1 from monocytes by trypsin and plasmin. J Immunol 1986; 136:2883–90.
8. Nagelkerker LM, Peter JC, van Breda V. Membrane-associated IL1 like activity on rat dendritic cells. J Immunol 1986; 136:2164–70.
9. Le J, Weinstein D, Gubler V, Vilcek J. Induction of membrane associated interleukin 1 by tumor necrosis factor in human fibroblasts. J Immunol 1987; 138:2137–42.
10. Wood DD, Bayne EK, Goldring MB, et al. The 4 biochemically distinct species of human interleukin 1 all exhibit similar biological activities. J Immunol 1985; 134:895–903.
11. Schmidt JA, Mizel SB, Cohen D, Green I. Interleukin 1: a potential regulator of fibroblast proliferation. J Immunol 1982; 128:2177–82.
12. Auron PE, Webb AC, Rosenwasser LJ, et al. Nucleotide sequences of human monocyte interleukin 1 precursor cDNA. Proc Natl Acad Sci U S A 1984; 81:7907–11.
13. March CJ, Mosley B, Larsen A, et al. Cloning, sequence and expression of two distinct human interleukin 1 complentary DNAs. Nature 1985; 315:641–7.
14. Lomedico PT, Gubler U, Hellmann CP, et al. Cloning and expression of murine interleukin 1 cDNA in *Escherichia coli*. Nature 1984; 312:458–62.
15. Gray PW, Glaister D, Chen E, Goeddel DV, Pennica D. Two interleukin 1 genes in the mouse: cloning expression of the cDNA for murine interleukin 1. J Immunol 1986; 137:3644–8.
16. Furutani Y. Notake M, Fukui T, et al. Complete nucleotide sequence of the gene for human interleukin1 alpha. Nucleic Acids Res 1986; 14:3167–79.
17. Clark BD, Collins KL, Gandy MS, Webb AC, Auron PE. Genomic sequence for human prointerleukin 1 beta: possible evolution from a reverse transcribed prointerleukin 1 alpha gene. Nucleic Acids Res 1986; 14:7897–914.
18. Murphy PA, Cebula TA, Windle BE. Heterogeneity of rabbit endogenous pyrogen is not attributable toglycosylated variants of a single polypeptide chain. Infect Immun 1981; 34:184–91.
19. Mizel SB. Physicochemical characterization of lymphocyte activating factor (LAF). J Immunol 1979; 122:2167–72.
20. Giri JG, Lomedico PT, Mizel SB. Studies on the synthesis and secretion of interleukin 1. I. A 33,000 molecular weight precursor for interleukin 1. J Immunol 1985; 134(1):343–8.
21. Gery I, Gershon RK, Waksman BH. Potentiation of the T-lymphocyte response to mitogens. I. The responding cell. J Exp Med 1972; 136:128–42.
22. Gery I, Waksman BH. Potentiation of the T-lymphocyte response to mitogens. II. The cellular source of potentiating mediator(s). J Exp Med 1972; 136:143–55.
23. Dinarello CA. Interleukin 1. Rev Infect Dis 1984; 6:51–95.
24. Oppenheim JJ. Interleukins and interferons in inflammation. Current concepts. Kalamazoo, MI: Upjohn Company, 1986.
25. Oppenheim JJ, Kovacs EJ, Mastsushima K, Durum SK. There is more than one interleukin 1. Immunol Today 1986; 7:45–55.
26. di Giovine FS, Duff GW. Interleukin 1: the first interleukin. Immunol Today 1990; 11(1):13–20.
27. Muegge K, Kurum SK. The role of interleukin 1 in the immune response. In: Bomford R, Henderson B, eds. Interleukin 1, inflammation and disease. Amsterdam: Elsevier, 1989:107–22.
28. Dinarello CA, Marnoy SO, Rosenwasser LJ. Role of arachidinate metabolism in the immunoregulatory function of human leukocytic pyrogen/lymphocyte-activating factor/interleukin 1. J Immunol 1983; 130(2):890–5.

29. Kunkel SL, Wiggins RC, Larrick J. Regulation of macrophage tumor necrosis factor production by prostaglandin E_2. Biochem Biophys Res Commun 1986; 137:404–10.
30. Kunkel SL, Chensue SW, Phan SH. Prostaglandins as endogenous mediators of interleukin-1 production. J Immunol 1986; 136(1):186–92.
31. Kunkel SL, Spengler M, Kwon G, May MS, Remick DG. Production and regulation of tumor necrosis factor alpha. A cellular and molecular analysis. Mech Achiev Exp Pathol 1988; 13:240–59.
32. Kunkel SL, Spengler M, May MA, Spengler R, Larrick J, Remick D. Prostaglandin E_2 regulates macrophage-derived tumor necrosis factor gene expression. J Biol Chem 1988; 263(11):5380–4.
33. Scales WE, Chensue SW, Otterness I, Kunkel SL. Regulation of monokine gene expression: prostaglandin E_2 suppresses tumor necrosis factor but not interleukin 1α or β mRNA and cell associated bioactivity. J Leukoc Biol 1989; 45:416–21.
34. Dower SK, Kronheim SR, March CJ, et al. Detection and characterization of high affinity plasma membrane receptors for human interleukin 1. J Exp Med 1985; 162:501–15.
35. Kilian PL, Kaffka KJ, Stern AS, et al. Interleukin 1α and interleukin 1β bind to the same receptor on T cells. J Immunol 1986; 136(12):4509–14.
36. Lowenthal JW, MacDonald HR. Binding and internalization of interleukin 1 by T cells. Direct evidence for high and low affinity classes of interleukin 1 receptor. J Exp Med 1986; 164:1060–74.
37. Mosley B, Urdal DL, Prickett KS, et al. The interleukin 1 receptor binds the human interleukin 1α precursor but not the interleukin 1β precursor. J Biol Chem 1987; 262(7):2941–4.
38. Sims JE, March CJ, Cosman D, et al. cDNA expression cloning of the IL1 receptor: a member of the immunoglobulin superfamily. Science 1988; 241:585–9.
39. Bron C, MacDonald HR. Identification of the plasma membrane receptor for interleukin 1 on mouse thymoma cells. FEBS Lett 1987; 219(2):365–8.
40. Dower SK, Wignall JM, Schooley K, et al. Retention of ligand binding activity by the extracellular domain of the IL1 receptor. J Immunol 1989; 142(12):4314–20.
41. Atkins E. Pathogenesis of fever. Physiol Rev 1960; 40:580–646.
42. Stitt JT. Prostaglandin E as the neural mediator of the febrile response. Yale J Biol Med 1986; 59:137–49.
43. Bernheim HA. Is prostaglandin E_2 involved in the pathogenesis of fever? Effects of interleukin 1 on the release of prostaglandins. Yale J Biol Med 1986; 59:151–8.
44. Kampschmidt RF, Upchurch HF. Lowering of plasma iron concentration in the rat with leukocytic extracts. Am J Physiol 1969; 216:1287–91.
45. Pekarek RS, Beisel WR. Characterization of endogenous mediator(s) of serum zinc and iron depression during infection and other stresses. Proc Soc Exp Biol Med 1971; 138:728–32.
46. Merriman CR, Pulliam LA, Kampschmidt RF. Comparison of leukocytic pyrogen and leukocyte endogenous mediator. Proc Soc Exp Biol Med 1977; 154:224–7.
47. Kampschmidt RF, Pulliam LA. The effect of human monocyte pyrogen on plasma iron, plasma zinc and blood neutrophils in rabbits and rats. Proc Soc Exp Biol Med 1978; 158:32–5.
48. Kluger MJ, Rothenburg BA. Fever and reduced iron: their interaction as a host defense response to bacterial infection. Science 1979; 203:374–6.
49. Castell JV, Gofmez-Lechon MJ, David M, et al. Interleukin 6 is the major regulator of acute phase protein synthesis in adult human hepatocytes. FEBS Lett 1989; 242(2):237–9.
50. Andus T, Geiger T, Hirano T, Kishimoto T, Heinrich PC. Action of recombinant human interleukin 6, interleukin 1 beta and tumor necrosis factor alpha on the mRNA induction of acute phase proteins. Eur J Immunol 1988; 18(5):739–46.

51. Krueger JM, Walter J, Dinarello CA, Wolff SM, Chedid L. Sleep promoting effects of endogenous pyrogen (interleukin 1). Am J Physiol 1984; 246:R994–9.
52. Walter J, Davenne D, Shoham S, Dinarello CA, Krueger JM. Brain temperature changes coupled to sleep states persist during interleukin 1 enhanced sleep. Am J Physiol 1986; 250:R96–103.
53. McCarthy DO, Kluger MJ, Vander AJ. Suppression of food intake during infection: is interleukin 1 involved? Am J Clin Nutr 1985; 42:1179–82.
54. Beutler BA, Cerami A. Recombinant interleukin 1 suppresses lipoprotein lipase acitivity in 3T3L1 cells. J Immunol 135:3969–71.
55. Besedovsky H, delRey A, Sorkin E, Dinarello CA. Immunoregulatory feedback between interleukin 1 and glucocorticoid hormones. Science 1986; 233:652–4.
56. Vogel SN, Douches SD, Kaufman EN, Neta R. Induction of colony stimulting factor in vivo by recombinant interleukin 1 alpha and recombinant tumor necrosis factor alpha. J Immunol 1987; 138:2143–8.
57. Neta R, Douches S, Oppenheim JJ. Interleukin 1 is radioprotector. J Immunol 1986; 136:2483–5.
58. Pettipher ER, Higgs GA, Henderson B. Interleukin-1 induces leukocyte infiltration and cartilage protoglycan degradation in the synovial joint. Proc Natl Acad Sci U S A 1986; 83:8749–53.
59. Mannel DN, Mizel SB, Diamantstein T, Falk W. Induction of interleukin 2 responsiveness in thymocytes by synergistic action of interleukin 1 and interleukin 2. J Immunol 1985; 134:3108–10.
60. Dempsey RA, Dinarello CA, Mier JW, et al. The differential effects of human leukocytic pyrogen/lymphocyte-activting factor, T cell growth factor, and interferon on human natural killer activity. J Immunol 1982; 129:2504–10.
61. Jelinek DF, Lipsky PE. Regulation of human B lymphocyte activation, proliferation and differentiation. Adv Immunol 1987; 40:1–59.
62. Haskard DO. Interleukin 1 and the vascular endothelial cell in inflammation. In: Bomford R, Henderson B, eds. Interleukin 1, inflammation and disease. Amsterdam: Elsevier, 1989:123–42.
63. Cavender DE, Haskard DO, Joseph B, Ziff M. Interleukin 1 increases the binding of human B and T lymphocytes to endothelial cell monolayers. J Immunol 1986; 136:203–7.
64. Schleimer RP, Rutledge BK. Cultured human vascular endothelial cells acquire adhesiveness for neutrophils after stimulation with interleukin-1, endotoxin and tumor promoting pharbol diesters. J Immunol 1986; 136:649–54.
65. Pohlman TH, Stanness KA, Beatty PG, Ochs HD, Harlan JM. An endothelial cell surface factor(s) induced in vitro by lipopolysaccharide, interleukin 1 and tumor necrosis factor alpha increases neutrophil adherence by a CDW18 dependent mechanism. J Immunol 1986; 136:4548–53.
66. Bevilacqua MP, Pober JS, Majeau GR, Fiers W, Cotran RS, Gimbrone MA. Recombinant tumor necrosis factor induces procoagulant activity in cultured human vascular endothelium: characterization and comparison with the actions of interleukin 1. Proc Natl Acad Sci U S A 1986; 83:4533–7.
67. Nachman RL, Hajjar KA, Silverstein RL, Dinarello CA. Interleukin 1 induces endothelial cell synthesis of plasminogen activator inhibitor. J Exp Med 1986; 163:1595–600.
68. Gowen M, Wood DD, Ihrie EJ, McGuire MKB, Russell GG. An interleukin-1 like factor stimulates bone resorption in vitro. Nature 1983; 306:378–80.
69. Larrick JW. Native interleukin 1 inhibitors. Immunol Today 1989; 10(2):61–6.

CHAPTER 3

STRUCTURE AND FUNCTION OF INTERLEUKIN-2

Timothy D. Anderson

Hoffmann-La Roche, Inc.
Nutley, New Jersey

INTRODUCTION

Interleukin-2 (IL-2) is a naturally occurring lymphocytotrophic cytokine of 133 amino acids produced by antigen- or mitogen-activated T lymphocytes (T cells). IL-2 was one of the first immunologic hormones to be discovered and characterized and was originally described as a factor capable of maintaining the long-term growth of T cells in culture (T cell growth factor, TCGF). Probably more information is available on IL-2 regarding its in vitro effects, its effects in preclinical animal studies, and its effects in human clinical studies than exists for any other cytokine.

IL-2 exerts regulatory effects on virtually all cell types participating in immune responses and has a pivotal role in the antigen-specific clonal proliferation of T cells. Like polypeptide hormones, IL-2 acts by binding to specific cell surface receptors. IL-2 has been shown to stimulate the proliferation and differentiation of both B and T lymphocytes, the activation and proliferation of nonspecific cytolytic effector cells, including natural killer (NK) and lymphokine-activated killer (LAK) cells, and the activation of monocytes-macrophages. Additionally, the functional, activational, or proliferative state of nonimmune cells, including such diverse cell types as brain glial cells, osteoclasts, and pituitary cells, can be altered by IL-2. IL-2 can stimulate the production and secretion of other cytokines, such as interferon-γ and tumor necrosis factors, from lymphocytes, NK cells, and macrophages.

Research on IL-2 has progressed to the point that the in vivo effects of IL-2 in multiple animal species have been characterized, the respective IL-2 molecules of the feline, bovine, rat, mouse, and sheep have been purified and characterized or expressed in recombinant form, and mice transgenic for and expressing IL-2 or the IL-2 receptor (IL-2R) have been constructed and characterized.

The IL-2 receptor binding proteins have been molecularly and functionally characterized, and alterations in the functional state, cellular expression, or serum levels of IL-2 and/or IL-2R have shown great clinical relevance in many disease states. Finally, the therapeutic values of IL-2 are being evaluated in human tumor immunotherapy, as immunotherapy in immunodeficiency diseases, and as a vaccine adjuvant. A number of reviews regarding nearly every aspect of IL-2 and its biology have been published (1–3).

HISTORICAL BACKGROUND

A virtual explosion of research has occurred in the last decade that is related to characterization of the in vitro or in vivo effects of IL-2 or reports research possible only because of the T cell growth activity of IL-2. A reliable measure of the importance of IL-2 in immunological research can be gained by examining the numbers of scientific articles published. In 1977, only two articles regarding a T cell growth factor were published, whereas in 1989 nearly 200 scientific articles per month were published characterizing either the effects of IL-2 or reporting research dependent upon IL-2-dependent T cells (Fig. 1). Complete historical reviews of the discovery and development of IL-2 have been recently published (4,5). This section presents a brief overview of the highlights in the IL-2 story and provides a timeline of IL-2 development (Table 1).

Observations that culture media "conditioned" by proliferating lymphocytes contained an unidentified substance that enhanced lymphocyte growth when antigen was present were first reported in 1965 (6). Many reports regarding

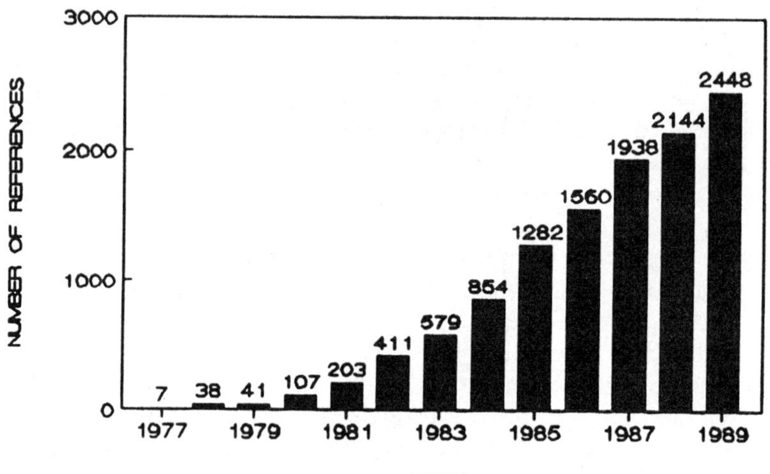

FIGURE 1 Published scientific articles that contain IL-2 or TCGF in their title, abstract, or key words from 1977 to 1989. Data were obtained from MEDLINE services (via DIALOG) on May 10, 1990 using the search terms IL-2, interleukin-2, TCGF, and T cell growth factor.

TABLE 1 Historical Background of Interleukin-2[a]

Date	Event	References
1965	Mitogenic factors for T cells present in LCM	6, 230
1976	Long-term culture of antigen-nonspecific T cells	7
1977	Long-term culture of antigen-specific CTL cells	8
1978	Description of TCGF biological characteristics and bioassay for TCGF	231
1978	T cells established as source of IL-2	231
1979	Normal CTL clones established with LCM	9
1979	Proposal to rename TCGF as IL-2	10
1981	Biochemical and molecular characterization of IL-2	27
1981	Description of IL-2Rp55 on T cells	11
1981	Isolation of antibody to IL-2Rp55 (anti-Tac)	12, 13
1983	IL-2 purified to homogeneity, N-terminal sequence determined, monoclonal antibodies to IL-2 developed	232
1983–4	Isolation of cDNA and genomic DNA IL-2 genes, cloning, and sequence analysis	22, 24, 233
1983	Clinical studies of natural, purified IL-2 begin	234
1983	Clinical studies of recombinant IL-2 begin	235–237
1984	Cloning, sequence, and expression of gene encoding IL-2Rp55	14, 15, 151
1986–7	Three-dimensional structure of IL-2 determined	25, 238
1984–7	Two separate IL-2 binding peptides described	16
1987	High-, intermediate-, and low-affinity IL-2R defined	18–20
1988–9	Isolation of gene encoding IL-2Rp75	21, 152

[a] LCM, lymphocyte-conditioned media; CTL, cytolytic T cells; TCGF, T cell growth factor; IL-2R, IL-2 receptor.

lymphocyte growth-enhancing substances occurred over the next decade. However, these reports were largely ignored by immunologists because it was believed that antigens were the sole agents responsible for lymphocyte proliferation and it was not understood how a cellularly released factor could stimulate the growth of antigen-stimulated lymphocytes without also expanding the entire lymphocyte population.

In 1976 Doris Morgan reported that normal human T cells could be cultured without antigen for up to 9 months, provided that a lymphocyte-conditioned medium was added to the cultures at regular intervals (7). This was followed, in 1977, by a report from Kendall Smith's group on the long-term culture of functional, immunologically relevant, tumor antigen-specific, cytotoxic T cells despite antigen removal from the culture (8). Subsequent utilization of lymphocyte-conditioned-medium led to the establishment of the first normal cytotoxic T cell clones in 1979 (9). The establishment of IL-2-responsive and homogeneous T cell clones led to the development of quantitative assays and the subsequent biological and biochemical characterization of the T cell growth factor named IL-2 in 1979 (10).

IL-2 was shown to bind specifically to activated T cells in 1981 (11). These studies showed that an IL-2 and IL-2 receptor interaction was necessary for the mediation of IL-2's biological effects and were the first studies to demonstrate that lymphokines exert their biological effects by mechanisms similar to the classic hormone-receptor interactions described for endocrinology, enzymology, and pharmacology. Also in 1981, a monoclonal antibody (anti-Tac) was isolated that reacted specifically with activated T cells, inhibited their proliferation, and was reported to react with IL-2R (12,13).

The isolation of a gene encoding an IL-2 low-affinity receptor protein (IL-2Rp55) was reported by Warren J. Leonard and others in Thomas A. Waldmann's laboratory and by Tasuku Honjo and Junji Yodoi in 1984 (14,15). During 1984–1987 there were several reports suggesting that a second IL-2 binding peptide existed (16,17). In 1986, Keisuke Teshigawara and Mitsuru Tsudo independently discovered this second, larger IL-2 receptor chain. In 1987 a distinction between high-, intermediate-, and low-affinity binding sites was established (18–20), and by 1988 Tsudo had identified and isolated the gene encoding this 75 kilodalton IL-2 receptor chain (IL-2Rp75) (21).

The first cDNA clone encoding IL-2 was isolated from the Jurkat cell line and sequenced by Tadatsugu Taniguchi and his colleagues in 1983 (22). Also in 1983, a cDNA clone coding for IL-2 was isolated from lymphocytes, expressed in *Escherichia coli*, and a 15,000 dalton peptide with IL-2 activity was demonstrated in bacterial lysates (23). Subsequent investigators cloned cDNA encoding IL-2, also from the Jurkat cell line, inserted it into *E. coli*, obtained recombinant IL-2, and showed that the recombinant IL-2 was biologically active in vitro and in vivo (24). The subsequent cloning of the IL-2 gene and the availability of large quantities of recombinant IL-2 enabled David B. McKay and his group to grow crystals of IL-2 and to derive the three-dimensional structure of the IL-2 molecule by x-ray crystallography in 1987 (25).

Recombinant IL-2 was shown to be useful for tumor immunotherapy in several animal tumor models in 1983. The first clinical trials with natural and recombinant IL-2 occurred in 1983. Clinical assessment of IL-2, principally in tumor immunotherapy, has continued and expanded to the current day.

MOLECULAR PROPERTIES OF INTERLEUKIN-2

Natural IL-2

Before the availability of recombinant IL-2 (rIL-2), definitive studies of the biological role of IL-2 required the use of natural IL-2 (nIL-2) (26). Six molecular species of nIL-2 have been purified to homogeneity from stimulated peripheral blood mononuclear cells. Human nIL-2, with a molecular weight of 15,000, was purified from Jurkat, a leukemic cell line, by affinity chromatography using a monoclonal antibody and high-performance liquid chromatography (HPLC). Early studies were hampered by the extremely small quantities of nIL-2 produced by activated cells, that is, early recovery of nIL-2 was about 40 μg nIL-2 starting from 100 liters culture fluid (26). Even in the high-producing cell lines, such as Jurkat, it was difficult to obtain adequate quantities of the purified material.

Natural IL-2 (nIL-2) comprises a group of proteins with molecular weights of

13,000–17,500, resulting in multiple isoelectric forms with pI values ranging from 6.6 to 8.2 (26). The heterogenity of the nIL-2 molecule was suggested to be due to the variable degree of glycosylation (27).

Recombinant IL-2

The ability to produce recombinant human IL-2 (rIL-2) was first reported in 1983 and 1984 when the gene encoding human IL-2 was cloned from the Jurkat cell line and expressed in eukaryotic cells and *E. coli* (22,24). The physicochemical and biological properties of purified rIL-2 are quite similar to those of nIL-2 except that rIL-2, which is not glycosylated in *E. coli* expression systems, lacks carbohydrate. Both nIL-2 and rIL-2 have similar in vitro and in vivo activities as judged by their ability to (a) support long-term proliferation of IL-2-dependent human peripheral blood lymphocytes (PBL), mouse killer T cell lines (NRB), and mouse natural killer cell lines; (b) generate lymphokine-activated killer cells from resting murine and human PBL; (c) to induce antibody-forming cells in nude mouse spleen cells; and (d) to provide helper activity in the generation of murine cytolytic cells (24,26).

Purification of rIL-2 preparations from *E. coli* results in two molecular species. In addition to a molecular species with the amino-terminal alanine (rIL-2), the purified preparations contained another molecular species (rMet-IL-2) having an additional methionine residue at the amino terminus. The relative amount of rMet-IL-2 varies depending on host-vector combinations, expression levels, and culture conditions. The presence of methionine at the amino terminus of recombinant human IL-2 produced in *E. coli* is consistent with the evidence that formylmethionine initiates protein synthesis in *E. coli* and that the formyl group is enzymatically cleaved from the newly synthesized polypeptide chain. The chromatographic behavior on gel-filtration, ion-exchange chromatography, and reversed-phase-HPLC for both rIL-2 and rMET-IL-2 were identical; however, the two proteins differed in gel isoelectric focusing and isoelectric points. The in vitro biological activity of rIL-2 and rMet-IL-2, as assessed by the ability to stimulate the growth of NKC3 cells, was the same (26,28).

The α-carbon backbone of IL-2 has been resolved to 3Å resolution by x-ray crystallography. IL-2 has an approximately 60% α-helical structure but contains no β-strands or β-sheets (25). Crystallographic studies of rIL-2 have revealed six helices, of which three, the A, B, and B′ helices, are thought to be involved in the binding of IL-2 to its receptor. Site-directed mutagenesis, substituting Asp-20 or deleting Phe-124, resulted in analogs that bind only to the IL-2Rp55 subunit of IL-2R; modification of Arg-38 to an Ala resulted in the loss of binding to the IL-2Rp55 subunit. Substitutions for Leu-17, Trp-21, or Phe-44 resulted in loss of all bioactivity and was attributed to loss of conformation of the IL-2 molecule as assessed by circular dichroism (29,30).

IN VITRO ACTIVITY OF IL-2

IL-2 has effects on many cell types, predominantly those of the immune system (Table 2). The cells most affected by IL-2 are T cells of all types but B cells, NK cells, monocytes, macrophages, and cells of nonimmune lineage are also affected by interactions with IL-2.

Table 2 Reported In Vitro Activity of IL-2

T cells
Induction of cytotoxic T cells (33,225)
Cause proliferation of T cells (32–37,39,40)
Intrathymic maturation of T cell precursors (38,138)
Regulation of lymphocyte TNF receptors (240)
Induce secretion of other cytokines (79,241)
Induction of suppressor T cells (242)
B cells
Induced to assemble and secrete IgM (55,56)
Stimulate proliferation and differentiation (57,243)
Regulate immunoglobulin response (54)
NK cells
Stimulate proliferation (76)
Enhance cytolytic activity (244,245)
Stimulate serine protease (granzyme) production (246)
Macrophages
Augment cytotoxic and lytic activity (67,247,248)
Induction of TNF secretion and macrophage activation (65,68)
Enhance LPS-stimulated prostaglandin synthesis (73)
Induce Kupffer's cells to suppress hepatocyte protein synthesis (70)
Other cells
Initiate expression of LAK phenomenon (24,88,89)
Induce proliferation and differentiation of glial cells (95,96)
Osteoclasts; stimulate osteoclastic activity (97)
Stimulate growth of *Leishmania* (protozoan) (101)
Inhibition of erythropoiesis (249)
Pituitary cells; release of corticotropin (99)
Basophils and mast cells; expression of IL-2Rp55 (100)

T Lymphocytes

The biological activity originally associated with IL-2 was its ability to cause the proliferation of activated T cells. The importance of IL-2 to normal T cell growth and development is apparent when one considers that only three parameters are important for regulating T cell proliferation after antigen activation: the concentration of IL-2, the density of IL-2 receptors on the cell surface, and the duration of the IL-2–receptor interaction (16).

The T cell growth-promoting activity of IL-2 has been utilized to support the long-term growth of activated T cell lines in vitro. Indeed, the most widely used assays for quantitating IL-2 bioactivity measure its ability to cause the dose-dependent proliferation of T cell lines (31). IL-2 has been shown to cause the proliferation of mitogen-activated primary T lymphoblasts (32), cytolytic T cells (33), helper T cells (33,34), and suppressor T cells (35). In addition to causing the proliferation of "activated" T lymphocytes, rIL-2 has been reported to cause dose-dependent proliferation of thymocytes (36,37), maturation of intrathymic T cell precursors (38), and proliferation of "resting" peripheral T lymphocytes (39,40) in the apparent absence of other activation stimuli.

IL-2 enhances cytolytic T cell responses, indirectly through its effects on helper T cells and directly via effects on cytolytic T cells (CTL). IL-2 facilitates the generation of both murine (41) and human (41) specific CTL responses. At high concentrations IL-2 is sufficient by itself to stimulate cytolytic responses of CTL precursors to allogeneic cells (42). At lower concentrations IL-2 acts synergistically with other cytokines to facilitate CTL responses (41,43–46).

In addition to causing the proliferation of T cells, IL-2 has been shown to stimulate cytokine production by activated T cells. IL-2 has been reported to stimulate the production of interferon-γ (47–49), B cell growth factor (50), tumor necrosis factor (51), and even additional IL-2 (52).

B Lymphocytes

Resting B cells express few, if any, receptors for IL-2, whereas activated B cells can express receptors for and respond to IL-2. Either IL-4 or IL-5 can induce IL-2R expression by B cells, with a resultant proliferative response by the B cells to IL-2 (53). A role probably exists for IL-2 in the activation, maturation, and differentiation of antigen-specific naive B cells in their response to T cell antigens as IL-2 can increase numbers and IgG-producing ability of antigen-specific B cells in vitro (54).

IL-2 can stimulate antigen-activated B lymphocytes to progress through the cell cycle and to differentiate into antibody-secreting cells (55–57). An IL-2-inducible B lymphoma line has been described and used to characterize the signaling mechanisms operation in growth and differentiation (58). IL-2 may be part of the complex T cell controls that regulate IgE-committed B cells as IgE-committed B cells are principally able to express receptors for and respond to IL-2 (59).

A small number of circulating or resting B cells express the IL-2Rp55 IL-2 receptor (60). IL-2Rp55 is expressed by many B cell lines derived from patients with Burkitt's lymphoma and on all B cell lines containing the human T cell leukemia virus type I (HTLV-I) genome. Certain malignant as well as activated normal B lymphocytes can be induced to express IL-2Rp55, IL2-Rp75, and high-affinity IL-2R (61–64).

Monocytes-Macrophages

The exact role of IL-2 in the modulation of macrophage activity is unknown, although it appears that a pathway for macrophage activation by IL-2 exists in vitro and in vivo (65). IL-2 directly augments the cytotoxicity of and induces IL-1 mRNA expression in human monocytes (66,67). Purified human and murine monocytes can be activated in vitro by IL-2 to secrete TNF (68) both in vitro and in vivo (69). Rat Kupffer's cells can be primed and triggered by IL-2 to suppress hepatocyte protein synthesis. This response was similar to that induced by lipopolysaccharide, suggesting an important role for IL-2 in regulating macrophage responses to septic stimuli (70).

Human monocytes activated by lipopolysaccharide or interferon express surface IL-2 receptors (71,72) and can release soluble IL-2R (73). IL-2Rp55 has been detected on cells of the monocyte-macrophage series, including cultured monocytes, Langerhan's cells of the skin, Kupffer's cells of the liver, cultured lung macrophages, and Reed-Sternberg cells in Hodgkin's disease (71) and on intestinal lamina proprial macrophages in inflammatory bowel disease (74). IL-2Rp75 has been detected in circulating $CD14^+$ monocytes (60), and human peripheral blood monocytes can express IL-2R (65,75).

Natural Killer and Lymphokine-Activated Killer Cells

As early as 1981 it was reported that cells with natural killer activity were stimulated by IL-2 (76). IL-2 enhances the cytolytic and proliferative activity of murine (77) and human NK cells (78). Like activated T cells, NK and LAK cells can be stimulated by IL-2 to secrete cytokines, including interleukin-1, interferon-γ, and tumor necrosis factor (78,79).

Unlike T cells, NK cells have no antigen receptors but express the IL-2Rp75 receptor and are activated by IL-2 (80–82). Initial activation of NK or of LAK precursors by IL-2 appears to result from the interaction of IL-2 with the IL-2Rp75 component of the IL-2 receptor, which is expressed on these cells in the absence of IL-2Rp55 (83). IL-2Rp75 has been proposed as the sole receptor responsible for the IL-2-mediated activation of NK cells (84,85). IL-2 induces the expression of serine protease enzymes and genes in NK and in nonspecific T killer cells that correlated with increased lytic activity (86).

IL-2 directly activates a heterogenous population of cytotoxic lymphocytes that mediate the destruction of fresh tumor cells and a variety of natural killer cell-resistant cultured tumor cell lines. This has been designated the lymphokine-activated killer phenomenon and is a cellular effector system separate from the NK and CTL systems. Although the exact origin and nature of LAK cells is currently being defined, it appears that the LAK cell may represent NK cells in a unique stage of activation (87).

The LAK system is unique in its simplicity of activation, since culture of non-adherant peripheral blood lymphocytes for a minimum of 3 days in lectin-free lymphokine preparations is the only requirement. LAK cells generated in vitro from human, mouse, or rat lymphocytes have a broad range of cytotoxic activity, unrestricted by major histocompatibility complex determinants and against multiple tumor targets and with low-level but significant activity against normal, nonmalignant cells (88–91). In animal models, adoptively transferred LAK cells have been shown to mediate the regression of established hepatic and pulmonary metastasis when concomitant IL-2 is given (92,93). Although IL-2 is sufficient for induction of LAK cytotoxic activity, the magnitude of the response can be positively or negatively regulated by other cytokines, including TNF and IL-4 (94).

Other Cell Types

The range of other cells on which IL-2 has been reported to have some effect include such diverse cell types as oligodendrocytes, osteoclasts, neurons, pituitary cells, and even protozoan parasites. IL-2 stimulates the in vitro proliferation and differentiation of neonatal rat oligodendrocytes and brain glial cells (95,96). Based on these data it was proposed that IL-2 may have a role in the inflammatory neural lesions of multiple sclerosis patients and in the growth of brain glial cells during injury or disease.

Osteoclasts are activated in vitro by IL-2 to increase acid production and osteoclastic activity (97). In the rat brain, there are IL-2 binding sites and IL-2-like immunoreactive material associated with the neuronal cholinergic system, suggesting a role for IL-2 as a mediator of brain–immune system interactions (98). Pituitary cells express a protein related to IL-2Rp55 and are stimulated by IL-2 to release corticotropin (ACTH) (99). Human mast cells and basophils are reported to express surface IL-2Rp55 in normal and pathological tissue and under in vitro conditions (100).

Nonmammalian cells are also affected by IL-2. IL-2 has been reported to enhance the in vitro growth of *Leishmania mexicana* and to exacerbate the in vivo lesion formation in murine cutaneous leishmaniasis (101).

IN VIVO ACTIVITY OF IL-2

The cloning and expression of the IL-2 gene have permitted the production of large quantities of rIL-2. The systemic or local administration of IL-2 has been assessed in animals and humans, particularly to assess its role in tumor immunotherapy. In animals and in humans several in vivo responses were predictable, that is, enhancement of the immune system. However, more types of in vivo responses were unpredicted based on knowledge of the in vitro activity of IL-2. In both animals and humans, there are reports of the systemic administration of IL-2 affecting nearly every organ system.

Interleukin-2 in Animals

There does not appear to be a significant species specificity to the biological activity of human IL-2. The biological activity of human rIL-2, or cloning of the respective species IL-2, has been reported in mice, rats, cats, dogs, and sheep (Table 3).

In general, the effects of rIL-2 administration in rodents resembles those effects seen with rIL-2 therapy in humans, that is, antitumor effects and high-dose toxicities. Administration of rIL-2 to mice causes proliferation of both adoptively transferred T cell lines (102,103) and endogenous T lymphocytes (104,105) and enhances the activity of endogenous NK/LAK cells (104,106,107). The endogenous proliferation of endogenous, IL-2-activated lymphocytes in mice treated with rIL-2 is associated with splenomegaly (lymphoid hyperplasia) and lymphoid infiltration of multiple tissues but primarily in perivascular areas of the lung and liver (106,108).

In mice, the intravenous injection of LAK cells in conjunction with rIL-2 can mediate the regression of established pulmonary metastasis from a variety of sarcomas as well as from the B16 melanoma (93,109). Additionally, the systemic administration of high doses of rIL-2 in mice leads to the generation of LAK cells in the spleens of treated mice and mediates the regression of established pulmonary metastases and subcutaneous implants from a variety of established

Table 3 Bioactivity of Human and Animal IL-2 in Animals[a]

Bioactivity	References
Mice	
Stimulate endogenous lymphoid proliferation	104
Enhance natural killer cell function	250–252
Augment alloantigen responsiveness	251
Mediate antitumor effects	92, 105
Improve host defense in bacterial infections	253, 254
In vivo proliferation of adoptively transferred LAK cells	255
Induction of LAK activity	251, 256, 257
Augment adoptively transferred CTL activity	258
Inhibition of pregnancy viability	259
Vascular leak syndrome (pulmonary edema, ascites)	108, 116, 260
Adjuvant activity with viral vaccines	207
Induction of NK activity	261
Myelostimulatory	262
Rats	
Induction of LAK activity	263
Systemic toxicity of multiple organ systems	108, 117, 264
Mediate tumor regression	265
Altered cholinergic neuron discharge in hypothalmus	266
Alteration in blood-brain barrier	267
Induction of NK activity	261
Altered neuron discharge hypothalamic nuclei	115
Feline	
Altered blood-brain barrier integrity	268
Induction of cytolytic large granular lymphocytes	122
Feline IL-2 maintains long-term culture of feline PBL	121
Canine	
Induction of antitumor activity by canine PBL	132
Sheep	
Cardiopulmonary dysfunction	123–127, 269
Induction of LAK activity in sheep PBL	270
Bovine	
Expression of IL-2R on bovine lymphocytes infected by *Theileria* sp.	271
Augment immunity and resistance to bovine herpesvirus	130
Guinea pigs	
Lung injury	272

[a] CTL, cytolytic T cells; NK, natural killer cells; PBL, peripheral blood lymphocytes.

tumors. Tumor regression appears to be mediated by endogenously activated lymphocytes, presumably LAK cells, present at the tumor site and in the organs of mice receiving high-dose rIL-2 (105,110). In murine tumor models, LAK effectors derived from asialo GM_1^+ precursors (NK-LAK cells) are responsible for the elimination of some tumor types regardless of tumor immunogenicity, whereas Lyt-2^+ cells (cytotoxic-suppressor T cells) mediate the elimination of weakly immunogenic sarcomas (111).

Treatment of rat bone marrow progenitors, or rat thymocytes, with human IL-2 results in the generation of LAK and NK activity (112–114). Injection of IL-2 into the third ventricle of rats is followed by a marked decrease in neuronal discharge frequency in the ventromedial nucleus of the hypothalamus and a marked increase in supraoptic and paraventricular nuclei. Because of the secretion by these nuclei of antidiuretic hormone, it was proposed that the action of IL-2 on these neuronal nuclei offer a partial explanation of the water retention observed in human patients receiving IL-2 immunotherapy (115).

Mice and rats given appropriate dosing regimens of rIL-2 exhibit many of the toxicities associated with high-dose rIL-2 therapy in humans, including "vascular leak syndrome," hepatotoxicity, hematological effects (anemia, lymphocytosis, and eosinophilia), and infiltration of multiple tissues with lymphocytes and eosinophils (108,116,117). In mice the toxicity of IL-2 appears at least in part to be mediated by IL-2-activated NK cells (118), by cells expressing the asialo GM_1 phenotype (108), or by endogenous secretion of tumor necrosis factor (119).

Up to 22% of feline peripheral blood lymphocytes express a surface receptor that reacts with antihuman IL-2Rp55 chain (Anti-tac) (120). The conditions for the production of feline IL-2 from feline PBL and partial characterization of feline IL-2 have been described (121). IL-2-dependent cytotoxic lymphocytes, with the morphology of large granular lymphocytes, can be derived by treating feline PBL with human or gibbon IL-2 (122).

Sheep have been utilized in the study of the cardiopulmonary responses to systemic IL-2 administration. Sheep treated with human IL-2 develop multiple effects in the cardiovascular and respiratory systems, including a decrease in systemic vascular resistance, increased pulmonary microvascular leakage, alterations in peripheral blood leukocyte numbers, and hypotension (123–127). Ovine IL-2 has been purified from concanavalin A (ConA)-stimulated PBL, and levels of ovine IL-2 were reported to be decreased in lymph node supernatants from sheep with clinical and pathological evidence of retrovirus-induced ovine progressive pneumonia and lymphoproliferation (128).

Bovine IL-2, secreted by bovine PBL stimulated with concanavalin A, has been purified and characterized. Bovine IL-2 supported the growth of bovine, buffalo, and goat lymphocytes but not that of sheep lymphocytes (129). Bovine recombinant IL-2 augments the immunity and resistance of calves vaccinated and challenged with bovine herpesvirus type 1 (130).

Canine IL-2, with a molecular weight of 27,000, has been purified from peripheral blood leukocytes stimulated with phytohemagglutin (PHA) (131). Canine peripheral blood mononuclear cells can be activated by human recombinant IL-2 to express cytolytic activity against a variety of allogeneic and xenogeneic neoplastic cells (132).

Bioactivity in Humans

Administration of rIL-2 to humans for purposes of tumor immunotherapy has been associated with systemic immune activation, antitumor effects in selected cases, and other effects on the cardiovascular, respiratory, neurological, dermatological, hematological, renal, and other systems (Table 4).

TABLE 4 Effects Associated with Administration of rIL-2 to Humans

Effect	References
Cardiovascular: Hypotension, tachycardia, vasodilation, cardiac dysfunction	205, 273–278
Respiratory: Pulmonary edema	279
Dermatological: Macular erythema, burning, pruritus	280
Immune activation	
Increase mRNA in lymphocytes for other cytokines	281
Increased NK cytolytic activity	282, 283
LAK cell generation	88, 89, 284
Development of anti-IL-2 antibodies	285
Antitumor effects	201, 205, 286, 287
Elevated serum levels of soluble IL-2R and interferon	288
Hematological: Anemia, lymphocytosis, lymphopenia, eosinophilia	289
Neuroendocrine	
Increase in β-endorphin, ACTH, cortisol	290
Neuropsychiatric	291
Hypothyroidism	292
Increased neuropeptides in ascitic fluid	293
Increased brain water	294
Renal: Prerenal azotemia	295
Endothelial activation	296
Vascular leak syndrome	274
Intrahepatic cholestasis	297
Altered tryptophan and neopterin metabolism	298
Hypocholesterolemia: decreased HDL and LDL	299
Neutrophil chemotactic defect	300
Activation of complement system	301

NK, natural killer cells; ACTH, adrenocorticotropic hormone.

Mice Transgenic for IL-2 or IL-2R

Transgenic mice bearing cDNA for human IL-2 or the IL-2Rp55 chain have been constructed. The expression of these cDNAs was directed by the constitutive H-2Kd promoter. Unstimulated spleen cells of the IL-2Rp55 transgenic mice had approximately 120 high-affinity binding sites for IL-2 per cell and proliferated in vitro in the presence of exogenous human rIL-2, indicating the constitutive expression of the IL-2Rp75 chain in unstimulated normal spleen cells. No abnormalities were observed in this transgenic mouse constitutively expressing human IL-2Rp55 (133).

In contrast, transgenic mice expressing cDNA for human IL-2 developed alopecia and pneumonia, their sera contained 30–500 pM human IL-2, and they died within 1 year after birth (134).

Hybrid mice that carried both human IL-2 and IL-2Rp55 chain transgenes were produced by crossing these two strains of transgenic mice. The hybrid mice showed severe growth retardation and died by 4 weeks of age. The spleens of the mice contained an unusually large number of large granular lymphocytes that had elevated NK activity. In contrast to the marked increase in NK cell activity, there was no evidence of T cell expansion. Pathological changes in the hybrid mice included severe lymphoid interstitial pneumonia, lymphocyte depletion of the T cell-dependent areas of the spleen, and a selective loss of Purkinje's cells of the cerebellum (135). The severe interstitial lymphoid pneumonia was considered the cause of death in the hybrid mice. Interestingly, the cause of death in mice given high doses of human rIL-2 is also considered secondary to lymphoid interstitial pneumonia and pulmonary edema (108).

INTERLEUKIN-2 RECEPTOR

The activation of T lymphocytes by IL-2 is mediated by specific cell surface receptors to which IL-2 binds. Just as the interaction of appropriately presented antigen with its specific receptors on T cells confers specificity for an immune response, the interaction of IL-2 with high-affinity IL-2 receptors determines its magnitude and duration (136). Resting T cells do not produce IL-2 or express high-affinity IL-2 receptors; however, both IL-2 and its receptor are rapidly expressed on T cells after appropriately processed and presented antigen interacts with the complex T cell antigen receptor. Failure of IL-2 and IL-2R production results in failure of the immune response (136). Additionally, in the mouse, IL-2R and IL-2 interactions provide signals crucial to the intrathymic development of mature T cells (137,138). Several excellent reviews of the IL-2 receptor complex have been published (136,139).

Structure of the IL-2 Receptor Complex

The high-affinity, multisubunit human IL-2 receptor complex (IL-2R) consists of at least two IL-2 binding peptides, one a 55 kD transmembrane glycoprotein (IL-2Rp55, Tac, α, or L chain) and the second a 70–75kD chain (IL-2Rp75, β, or H1 chain). A multisubunit model for the high-affinity IL-2 receptor has been proposed in which independently existing IL-2Rp55 or IL-2Rp75 peptides create low- or intermediate-affinity receptors, respectively, whereas high-affinity receptors consist of IL-2Rp55 and IL-2Rp75 noncovalently associated in a multisubunit, high-affinity IL-2 receptor complex (140–143).

The receptor structure operating in the IL-2 system is unique in that two structurally distinct membrane molecules, the IL-2Rp55 and IL-2Rp75 chains, both bind IL-2 independently. The IL-2Rp55 and IL-2Rp75 differ in the site of the IL-2 molecule that they bind, in the kinetics of their association and disassociation with IL-2, and in their potential role in signal transduction (1,17).

IL-2Rp55 constitutes the low-affinity receptor form and is not functional in IL-2 internalization and signal transduction unless it is associated with the IL-2Rp75 peptide (144–148). IL-2Rp55 is composed of a 33 kD (251 amino acid) peptide precursor that is posttranslationally glycosylated, sulfated, and phosphorylated in its mature 55 kD form (136,149,150). The IL-2Rp55 peptide has a 219 amino acid extracellular domain, a 19 amino acid membrane-spanning domain, and a short 13 amino acid intracytoplasmic domain. The intracytoplasmic domain of the IL-2Rp55 IL-2 receptor differs from other growth factor receptors in that the intracytoplasmic domain is much shorter and lacks the tyrosine kinase activity necessary for transmembrane signal transduction (14,15,151). It has been proposed that the principal and perhaps sole physiological role of IL-2Rp55 is to augment the binding of IL-2 to biologically active IL-2Rp75 (84).

The IL-2Rp75 IL-2 binding peptide constitutes the intermediate-affinity receptor (18,140), is responsible for internalization of bound IL-2 (152), has one or more domains responsible for driving the intracellular transduction pathways (148,153,154), and is responsible for the IL-2 stimulation of intracellular tyrosine kinase activities (155,156). The association of IL-2Rp75 with IL-2Rp55 results in the high-affinity IL-2 receptor. The isolation, structural analysis, and expression of the cDNAs encoding the human IL-2Rp75 chain have been reported (152). The overall primary structure of IL-2Rp75 shows no apparent homology to other known receptors. The mature form of IL-2Rp75 consists of 525 amino acids divided into a 214 amino acid extracellular domain, a 25 amino acid membrane-spanning domain, and a 286 amino acid cytoplasmic domain (152). Unlike the IL-2Rp55 chain, the IL-2Rp75 peptide has a large cytoplasmic region in which a functional domain (or domains) mediating an intracellular signal transduction pathway may be embodied (152).

Unlike many other cytokine receptors, the IL-2Rp55 and IL-2Rp75 peptides do not belong to the immunoglobulin superfamily (152). Significant structural similarity consisting of two conserved motifs separated by a unique sequence of amino acids is present in the external domain of IL-2Rp75 and in the external domains of the receptors for IL-3, IL-4, IL-6, and erythropoietin. It has been proposed that these cytokine receptors may belong to a new gene family and may have evolved from a common ancestor (157,158).

The IL-2Rp55 and IL-2Rp75 peptides each binds IL-2; however, each peptide reacts with IL-2 with distinct kinetic and equilibrium binding constants, each of which is also different from the binding affinity and dissociation rate of the high-affinity IL-2 receptor (IL-2Rp55–IL-2Rp75 complex). The on and off rates for IL-2 binding to the IL-2Rp55 protein are very rapid (i.e., 5–10 s); the on and off rates for IL-2 binding to the IL-2Rp75 protein are markedly slower (20–50 minutes). The kinetic data obtained when high-affinity IL-2Rp55-IL-2Rp75 receptor complex are analyzed show that the association rate of this receptor is dependent upon the fast-reacting IL-2Rp55 Tac chain, whereas the dissociation rate is derived from the slow-releasing IL-2Rp75 chain. Since the affinity of binding at equilibrium is determined by the ratio of the dissociation and the association rate constants, the kinetic cooperation between the low-affinity (IL-2Rp55) and intermediate-affinity (IL-2Rp75) IL-2 binding sites results in a receptor with a very high affinity for IL-2 (17,136).

The probable sites of human IL-2 involved in receptor binding have been determined by utilizing monoclonal antibodies directed toward defined regions of IL-2, by deletional analysis, and by site-specific mutagenesis of IL-2 in neutralization and binding assays. The IL-2Rp55 and IL-2Rp75 peptides have been shown to interact with different regions of the IL-2 molecule, with amino acids 11–20 of IL-2 required for biological activity and for binding to IL-2Rp75 and amino acids 33–56 being most likely required for binding to IL-2Rp55 (30,159). Additionally, the carboxy-terminal residues 131–133 and two of the three cysteine residues (58 and 105) are required for full biological activity and binding (30).

There is evidence for a third 95 kD IL-2 binding peptide (p95) involved in the multisubunit high-affinity IL-2 receptor with IL-2Rp55 and IL-2Rp75 (142,160,161). Fluorescence photobleaching and flow cytometry energy transfer studies on human T cells have indicated that p95 and IL-2Rp55 are associated and physically interact on the surface of at least some activated T cells and are in proximity to the HLA class I antigen (160,161). A 90–100 kD IL-2 binding peptide associated with the IL-2Rp55-IL-2Rp75 complex, which is unreactive with anti-IL-2Rp55 (anti-Tac) antibodies, has been demonstrated in mouse T cell blasts, the CTLL-16 cell line, and the mouse EL-4 cell line transfected with IL-2Rp55 cDNA (142).

Expression of IL-2R

Two-color flow cytometric analysis has demonstrated that IL-2Rp55 and IL-2Rp75 subunits are differentially expressed on various cell populations of resting PBL (60). Most resting or circulating T cells, B cells, and monocytes do not display IL-2 receptors (IL-2Rp55 chain). Depending on the sensitivity of the assay system, it has been shown that from 5 to 45% of freshly isolated, unstimulated human peripheral blood lymphocytes (T and B cells) express the IL-2Rp55 chain (162). Additionally, most T lymphocytes can be induced to express IL-2Rp55 by interaction with lectins, monoclonal antibodies to the T cell antigen-receptor, complex, or alloantigen stimulation (61).

Messenger RNA for IL-2Rp75 is detectable in unstimulated peripheral blood lymphocytes. This expression pattern is quite different from that of the IL-2Rp55 chain whose mRNA expression requires the mitogenic stimulation of PBLs, suggesting the presence of distinct mechanisms of gene expression between the IL-2Rp55 and IL-2Rp75 genes (152,163).

The IL-2Rp75 peptide, but not IL-2Rp55, is expressed on and is the receptor for IL-2 on both circulating T cells (84) and large granular lymphocytes (LGL) (84,85,140) in quantities approximately proportional to their responsiveness to IL-2. Interaction of IL-2 with IL-2Rp75 on resting or circulating T cells and LGLs induces transcription of the IL-2Rp55 gene, expression of IL-2Rp55 on the LGL surface, expression of the high-affinity IL-2Rp55–IL-2Rp75 IL-2 receptor complex, cell proliferation, and triggering of LGLs to become efficient natural killer and lymphokine-activated killer cells (84,85,163). IL-2Rp75 has been identified on the surface of a B cell that secretes immunoglobulin in response to IL-2 (20).

IL-2R expression is strongly associated with several forms of human lymphoproliferative disease in which it may play a pathogenetic role, including adult T cell leukemia-lymphoma, hairy cell leukemia, Hodgkin's disease, B cells in non-Hodgkin's lymphoma, histiocytic proliferations, and peripheral T cell lymphoma (164). Fresh leukemic cells and cells from established leukemic lines of T cells, B cells, and myeloid origin constitutively express the IL-2Rp75 binding protein (165).

Circulating and Free IL-2R

IL-2p55 is released in soluble form from the cell surface of lymphocytes activated either in vitro or in vivo. The release of soluble IL-2Rp55 appears to be a characteristic marker of T cell activation and may serve an immunoregulatory function during both normal and abnormal cell growth and differentiation. Soluble IL-2Rp55 chains are released into culture medium following in vitro lectin and antigen stimulation of normal lymphocytes as well as from certain tumor cell lines (166).

Soluble IL-2Rp55 IL-2 receptor is still capable of binding IL-2 and can be released by virtually all cells expressing the IL-2Rp55 chain (166,167). The released form of IL-2Rp55 has been characterized as a 45,000 molecular weight molecule lacking the transmembrane and the cytoplasmic portion of the cell surface-expressed IL-2Rp55 chain (168). Proteolytic cleavage of surface IL-2Rp55, differential splicing of the IL-2Rp55 chain encoding mRNA, or an additional unknown mechanism has been suggested as possible mechanisms underlying the receptor release (166,168,169). The released IL-2R has a peptide backbone approximately 10 kD smaller than the membrane associated IL-2R but does efficiently bind IL-2 without the need for accessory molecules (170). Circulating soluble IL-2R can be detected in the serum of healthy individuals at low levels and at greatly elevated levels in the serum of patients with certain malignant diseases, particularly those with the HTLV-I-positive adult T cell leukemia (ATL) (167). Released IL-2R is constitutively produced at high levels by cell lines infected with human T lymphocytotrophic virus type I (61,170).

Clinical Relevance of IL-2R and IL-2R Antagonists

In general, high systemic levels of IL-2Rp55 reflect widespread in vivo immunological (lymphoid) activation associated either with immunoenhancement therapy or with stage of disease progression in autoimmune disorders, with T cell neoplasia, or with T cell-mediated pathology in viral diseases. Elevated serum levels of IL-2Rp55 occur in many conditions, including in humans whose lymphocytes are activated by high-dose IL-2 therapy (171,172), those with high tumor burden in various lymphoid malignancies (173), in acute renal, liver, or heart and lung allograft rejection (174–176), in actopic eczema (177), in renal dysfunction (178), and with viral or protozoan infections (179,180).

Because IL-2 receptors are present on both normally and abnormally activated T cells but not on normal resting cells, the IL-2 receptor is a potential target for pharmacological manipulation of IL-2 antagonism in many disease states. Clinical trials are currently utilizing unmodified monoclonal anti-Tac antibodies (anti-IL-2Rp55), anti-Tac antibodies conjugated to toxins, toxin–IL-2 conjugates, isotopic chelates of anti-Tac, or recombinant "humanized" antibodies to the IL-2 receptor. These monoclonal antibodies and IL-2 toxin conjugates are directed toward the IL-2 receptors expressed on leukemia and lymphoma cells, autoreactive T cells of certain patients with autoimmune disorders, and host T cells responding to foreign histocompatibility antigens of organ allografts (136,181).

Use of antibodies directed against the rat IL-2Rp55 protein have been effective in preventing acute rejection of cardiac, renal, pancreatic islet, small bowel, and peripheral nerve transplants in rats (181,182) and have decreased the severity of autoimmune diabetes in BB rats (182). Anti-IL-2Rp55 antibodies, in a rat model of cardiac allograft transplant, prevented graft rejection by elimination, rather than functional inhibition, of the immune cells bearing surface IL-2R (169).

Human T cell lymphotrophic virus type I-associated adult T cell leukemia cells constitutively express very large numbers of IL-2 receptors. Recent studies have linked this disordered expression of IL-2 receptors in this retrovirus-induced T cell leukemia with the action of a trans-activator gene product (*tax*-1) encoded by the virus. The Tax protein may play a role in HTLV-I-induced malignancy both by augmenting viral transcription and by deregulating the expression of the cellular genes encoding IL-2 and the IL-2Rp55 IL-2 receptor peptide, which control T cell proliferation (183).

Viral diseases associated with elevations in serum IL-2R include human immunodeficiency virus (HIV), human T cell lymphotrophic virus (HTLV-I), hepatitis, and cytomegalovirus. Soluble IL-2R levels increase with disease progression in patients infected with HIV, are most pronounced in patients with HIV-induced acquired immunodeficiency syndrome (AIDS), and may be involved in the down-regulation of IL-2-dependent immune functions in AIDS (184). Additionally, elevated serum levels of soluble IL-2R are present in patients with HTLV-I-associated myelopathy and are correlated with disease progression and level of tumor burden (185). Elevated levels of serum IL-2R in patients with chronic hepatitis closely parallel disease activity (186).

IL-2R in Animals

IL-2 binding proteins have been reported in the mouse and rat (187–189). In the mouse, two molecules have been described that, together with the IL-2Rp55 or L chain, comprise a high-affinity IL-2R (142,187). As in humans, the release of IL-2 binding proteins derived from IL-2Rp55 has been reported for virtually all cells bearing IL-2Rp55 in both mice and rats. Two distinct forms of the rat IL-2Rp55 IL-2R chain, one an intact molecule of 50,000–55,000 molecular weight and a second molecule of 40,000 molecular weight are released by rat lymphocytes (190). Small levels of soluble IL-2R are detectable in the sera of normal mice (191). Equivalent amounts of IL-2 activity, IL-2 mRNA levels, and IL-2R expression are present in young and aged rats (192). Antibodies to human IL-2R do not cross-react with murine IL-2R; however, antibodies to both mouse and rat IL-2R are available and have been shown effective in promoting allograft survival (193,194) and in preventing disease progression (182,195,196).

CLINICAL UTILITY OF IL-2

The primary focus of current clinical activity with rIL-2 has been in the area of tumor immunotherapy. IL-2 has no direct cytotoxic or cytostatic effect on most neoplastic cells. Its antitumor effect is derived from its ability to activate or stimulate the production of lytic cells (NK or LAK cells) that are cytotoxic to a broad range of neoplastic and transformed tissues as well as of some normal tissues. Clinical studies utilizing very high doses of IL-2 combined with in vitro activated LAK cells, or combined with "tumor-infiltrating lymphocytes" (TIL) (197), have demonstrated tumor regression in selected patients, particularly with melanoma and renal cell carcinoma. IL-2 immunotherapy may provide a base for the development of practical, effective biological treatments for some cancer patients. Many reviews regarding the preclinical and clinical evaluation of IL-2 in tumor immunotherapy have been published (197–205).

Additional therapeutic uses of IL-2's immunomodulatory activities are as an adjuvant or immunoenhancement factor in live virus vaccines (206,207) and as immunoenhancement therapy in the treatment of T cell dysfunction (208) or severe combined immunodeficiency disease (209), and in such infectious diseases as leprosy (210).

ROLE OF IL-2 IN SPONTANEOUS DISEASE

The essential nature of IL-2 and IL-2 receptors for the generation of a normal immune response is demonstrated by the existence of spontaneous disease in animals and in humans, characterized in part by a deficiency in the IL-2 production or response system (199). There is evidence to suggest that a endogenously hyperactivated or hyperreactive IL-2–IL-2R system is likely to be involved in autoimmunity in chickens, animals, and humans (211).

Defective IL-2 production has been reported in patients with severe combined immunodeficiency (SCID) or Nezelof's syndrome (212), acquired immunodeficiency syndrome (213,214), type I diabetes mellitus (215), systemic lupus erythematosus (216), and following bone marrow transplantation (217). Disorders of IL-2 receptor expression have been described in patients with AIDS (218), hypogammaglobulinemia (219), multiple sclerosis (220), protozoan infection (221), and adult T cell leukemia (222). There is diminished IL-2 production and IL-2 unresponsiveness in humans with pulmonary tuberculosis (223) and in *Mycobacterium*-infected mice (224).

Immunodeficient athymic mice were found to lack the ability to produce IL-2 but could respond to IL-2 when it was given exogenously (225). IL-2 can enhance the development and severity of some disease models, including spontaneous insulin-dependent diabetes in BB rats (226).

There are reports of serum inhibitors of IL-2 production and/or activity that are secreted under normal and pathological conditions by macrophages and endothelial cells (227). Serum inhibitory activity has been reported during ontogeny, in systemic lupus erythematosus, in rheumatoid arthritis (228), and with some systemic infections. Some tumor cells may generate IL-2 inhibitory activity, which diminishes NK activity against the tumor. The clinical and pathological relevance of IL-2 inhibitors remains to be determined (229); however, it appears that they regulate IL-2-related functions by a suppressive action on the T cell (227).

CONCLUSION

The disciplines of molecular biology, immunology, pharmacology, medicine, and protein biochemistry have contributed to a vast expansion of knowledge regarding the in vitro and in vivo effects of IL-2 and have affirmed its profound relevance in all higher mammalian life forms. IL-2 has proven to be a molecule essential for the normal immune response but is also active, either directly or indirectly, on several types of nonimmune cells and on nearly every organ system of the body. Undoubtedly, future research will disclose as yet unexpected properties, effects, and potential therapeutic applications of IL-2.

ACKNOWLEDGMENT

Grateful appreciation is expressed to Dr. M. Gately and Dr. T. J. Hayes for helpful suggestions and manuscript review, to Ms. J. Becker for help with manuscript preparation, and to my wife Heidi for her patience and the final manuscript review.

REFERENCES

1. Smith K. Interleukin 2: inception, impact, and implications. Science 1988; 240:1169–76.
2. Mertelsmann R, Welte K. Human interleukin-2: molecular biology, physiology, and clinical possibilities. Immunobiology 1986; 172:400–19.
3. Fletcher M, Goldstein AL. Recent advances in the understanding of the biochemistry and clinical pharmacology of interleukin-2. Lymphokine Res 1987; 6:45–56.
4. Smith KA. Interleukin 2: A 10-year perspective. In: Smith KA, ed. Interleukin 2. San Diego: Academic Press, 1988; 1–35.
5. Smith KA. Interleukin-2. Sci Am 1990; 262(3):50–7.
6. Gordon J, McLean LD. A lymphocyte-stimulating factor produced in vitro. Nature 1965; 208:795–7.
7. Morgan DA, Ruscetti FW, Gallo R. Selective in vitro growth of T lymphocytes from normal human bone marrows. Science 1976; 193:1007–9.
8. Gillis S, Smith KA. Long term culture of tumour-specific cytotoxic T cells (letter). Nature 1977; 268:154–6.
9. Baker PE, Gillis S, Smith KA. Monoclonal cytolytic T-cell lines. J Exp Med 1979; 149:273–8.
10. Letter to the editor. Revised nomenclature for antigen-nonspecific T cell proliferation and helper factors. J Immunol 1979; 123:2928–9.
11. Robb RJ, Munck A, Smith KA. T cell growth factor receptors. Quantitation, specificity, and biological relevance. J Exp Med 1981; 154:1455–74.
12. Uchiyama T, Broder S, Waldmann TA. A monoclonal antibody (anti-Tac) reactive with activated and functionally mature human T cells. I. Production of anti-Tac monoclonal antibody and distribution of Tac(+) cells. J Immunol 1981; 126:1393–7.
13. Uchiyama T, Nelson DL, Fleisher TA, Waldmann TA. A monoclonal antibody (anti-Tac) reactive with activated and functionally mature human T cells. II. Expression of Tac antigen on activated cytotoxic killer T cells, suppressor cells, and on one of two types of helper T cells. J Immunol 1981; 126:1398–403.
14. Leonard WJ, Depper JM, Crabtree GR, et al. Molecular cloning and expression of cDNAs for the human interleukin-2 receptor. Nature 1984; 311:626–31.
15. Nikaido T, Shimizu A, Ishida N, et al. Molecular cloning of cDNA encoding human interleukin-2 receptor. Nature 1984; 311:631–5.
16. Smith KA, Cantrell DA. Interleukin 2 regulates its own receptors. Proc Natl Acad Sci U S A 1985; 82:864–8.
17. Wang H, Smith KA. The interleukin 2 receptor. Functional consequences of its bimolecular structure. J Exp Med 1987; 166:1055–69.
18. Teshigawara K, Wang HM, Kato K, Smith KA. Interleukin 2 high-affinity receptor expression requires two distinct binding proteins. J Exp Med 1987; 165:223.
19. Robb RJ, Rusk CM, Yodoi J, Greene WC. Interleukin 2 binding molecule distinct from the Tac protein: analysis of its role in formation of high-affinity receptors. Proc Natl Acad Sci U S A 1987; 84:2002–6.
20. Dukovich M, Wano Y, Thuy LTB, et al. A second human interleukin-2 binding

protein that may be a component of high-affinity interleukin-2 receptors. Nature 1987; 327:518–21.

21. Hatakeyama M, Tsudo M, Minamoto S, et al. Interleukin-2 receptor beta chain gene: generation of three receptor forms by cloned human alpha and beta chain cDNA's. Science 1989; 244:551–6.
22. Taniguchi T, Matsui H, Fujita T, et al. Structure and expression of a cloned cDNA for human interleukin-2. Nature 1983; 302:305–10.
23. Devos R, Plaetinck G, Cheroutre H, et al. Molecular cloning of human interleukin 2 cDNA and its expression in *E. coli*. Nucleic Acids Res 1983; 11:4307.
24. Rosenberg SA, Grimm EA, McGrogan M et al. Biological activity of recombinant human interleukin-2 produced in *Escherichia coli*. Science 1984; 22:1412–5.
25. Brandhuber BJ, Boone TJ, Kenney WC, McKay DB. Three dimensional structure of interleukin-2. Science 1987; 238:1707–9.
26. Kato K. Characteristics of natural and recombinant human interleukin 2. In: Smith Kendall A, ed. Interleukin 2. San Diego, CA: Academic Press, 1988:37–66.
27. Robb RJ, Smith KA. Heterogeneity of human T-cell growth factor(s) due to variable glycosylation. Mol Immunol 1981; 18:1087–94.
28. Kato K, Yamada T, Kwahara K, et al. Purification and characterization of recombinant human interleukin-2 produced in *Escherichia coli*. Biochem Biophys Res Commun 1985; 130:692–9.
29. Rees RC, Wiltrout RH. The biology and clinical applications of interleukin 2. Immunol Today 1990; 11:36–8.
30. Ju G, Collins L, Kaffka KL, et al. Structure-function analysis of human interleukin-2. J Biol Chem 1987; 262:5723–31.
31. Gearing AJH, Johnstone A, Thorpe R. Production and assay of the interleukins. J Immunol Methods 1985; 83:1–27.
32. Katzen D, Chu E, Terhost C, et al. Mechanisms of human T cell response to mitogens: IL 2 induces IL 2 receptor expression and proliferation but not IL 2 synthesis in PHA-stimulated T cells. J Immunol 1985; 135:1840–5.
33. Palacios R, Leu T. Both cloned interleukin 2 and purified interleukin 1 are required for optimal growth of purified $L3T4^+$ and lyt 2^+ lymphocytes initiated by concanavalin A. Cell Immunol 1985; 94:369–82.
34. Fernandez-Botran R, Sanders VM, Mosmann TR, Vitetta ES. Lymphokine-mediated regulation of the proliferative response of clones of T helper 1 and T helper 2 cells. J Exp Med 1988; 168:543–58.
35. Fox EJ, Lewis DE, Deemer KP, El Masry MN, Rich RR. T suppressor cell growth factor and anti-CD-3 antibodies stimulate reciprocal subsets of T Lymphocytes. J Exp Med 1987; 166:404–18.
36. Raulet DH. Expression and function of interleukin-2 receptors on immature thymocytes. Nature 1985; 314:102–3.
37. de la Hera A, Toribio ML, Marquez C, Martinez-A C. Interleukin 2 promotes growth and cytolytic activity in human $T3^+4^-8^-$ thymocytes. Proc Natl Acad Sci U S A 1985; 82:6268–71.
38. Toribio ML, de la Hera A, Borst J, et al. Involvement of the interleukin 2 pathway in the rearrangement and expression of both alpha/beta and gamma/delta T cell receptor genes in human T cell precursors. J Exp Med 1988; 168:2231–49.
39. Lakhanpal S, Gonchoroff NJ, Handwerger BS. Interleukin 2 induces proliferation of normal "resting" human T cells in the absence of other known external stimulation. Cell Immunol 1987; 106:62–75.
40. Bich-Thuy LT, Dukovich M, Peffer NJ, Fauci AS, Kehrl JH, Greene WC. Direct activation of human resting T cells by IL 2: the role of an IL 2 receptor distinct from the Tac protein. J Immunol 1987; 139:1550–6.

41. Gately MK, Wilson DE, Wong HL. Synergy between recombinant interleukin 2 (rIL-2) and IL-2-depleted lymphokine-containing supernatants in facilitating allogeneic human cytolytic T lymphocyte responses in vitro. J Immunol 1986; 136:1274–82.
42. Erard F, Nabholz M, MacDonald HR. Antigen stimultion of cytolytic T lymphocyte precursors: minimal requirements for growth and acquisition of cytolytic activity. Eur J Immunol 1985; 15:798–803.
43. Takai Y, Herrmann S, Greenstein JL, Spitalny GL, Burakoff SJ. Requirement for three distinct lymphokies for the induction of cytotoxic T lymphocytes from thymocytes. J Immunol 1986; 137:3494–500.
44. Biasi G, Rivarollo R, Colmagro R, Ronchese F, Collavo D. Lymphokine-induced cytotoxic cell generation in thymus and spleen cel cultures. J Biol Regul Homeost Agents 1987; 1:119–25.
45. Gately MK, Jenson JC, Benjamin WR. Role of cytokines in T and B cell mediated immunity. Concepts Immunopathol 1987; 3:74–108.
46. Wong HL, Wilson DE, Jenson JC, Familletti PC, Stremlo DL, Gately MK. Characterization of a factor(s) which synergizes with recombinant interleukin 2 in promoting allogeneic human cytolytic T lymphocyte responses in vitro. Cell Immunol 1988; 111:39–54.
47. Farrar WL, Ruscetti FW, Young HA. 5-Azacytidine treatment of a murine cytotoxic T cell line alters interferon-gamma gene induction by interleukin 2. J Immunol 1985; 135:1551–4.
48. Grabstein K, Dower S, Gillis S, Urdal D, Larsen A. Expression of interleukin 2, interferon-gamma, and the Il-2 receptor by human peripheral blood lymphocytes. J Immunol 1986; 136:4503–8.
49. Kelly CD, Welte K, Murray HW. Antigen-induced human interferon-gamma production. Differential dependence on interleukin 2 and its receptor. J Immunol 1987; 139:2325–8.
50. Howard M, Matis L, Malek TR, et al. Interleukin-2 induces antigen-reactive T cell lines to secrete BOGF-I. J Exp Med 1983; 158:2024–31.
51. Turner M, Londei M, Feldmann M. Human T cells from autoimmune and normal individuals can produce tumor necrosis factor. Eur J Immunol 1987; 17:1807–14.
52. Hu J, Vaquero C, Huet S, Bernard M, Sterkers G. Interleukin 2 up-regulates its own production. J Immunol 1987; 139:4109–15.
53. Loughnan MS, Nossal GJ. Interleukins 4 and 5 control expression of IL-2 receptor on murine B cells through independent induction of its two chains. Nature 1989; 340:76–9.
54. Isakov N, Morrow PR. Interleukin 2 regulates antigen-specific immunoglobulin response of naive murine B cells. Cell Immunol 1989; 120:366–74.
55. Blackman MA, Tigges MA, Minie ME, Koshland ME. A model system for peptide hormone action in differentiation: interleukin 2 induces a B lymphoma to transcribe the J chain gene. Cell 1986; 47:609.
56. Brooks K, Yuan D, Uhr JW, Krammer PH, Vitetta ES. Lymphokine-induced IgM secretion by clones of neoplastic B cells. Nature 1983; 302:825.
57. Zubler RH, Loventhal JW, Erard F, Hashimoto N, Devos R, McDonald HR. Activted B cells express receptors for and proliferate in response to pure interleukin 2. J Exp Med 1984; 160:1170.
58. Tigges MA, Casey LS, Elliott M, Koshland E. Mechanisms of interleukin-2 signaling: mediation of different outcomes by a single receptor and transduction pathway. Science 1989; 243:781–6.
59. Chan MA, Dosch HM. Human IgE response: virus-activated IgE secretors are interleukin-2-dependent cells. Int Arch Allergy Appl Immunol 1989; 89:90–7.

60. Ohashi Y, Takeshita T, Nagata N, Mori S, Sugamura K. Differential expression of the IL-2 receptor subunits, p55 and p75 on various populations of primary peripheral blood mononuclear cells. J Immunol 1989; 143:3548.
61. Waldmann TA. The structure, function, and expression of interleukin-2 receptors on normal and malignant lymphocytes. Science 1986; 232:727–32.
62. Waldmann TA, Goldman CK, Robb RJ, et al. Expression of interleukin 2 receptors on activated human B cells. J Exp Med 1984; 160:1450.
63. Tsudo M, Uchiyama T, Uchino H. Expression of Tac antigen on activated normal human B cells. J Exp Med 1984; 160:612.
64. Tanaka T,Saiki O, Doi S, et al. Functional interleukin 2 receptors on B cells lacking Tac antigens. Eur J Immunol 1987; 17:1379.
65. Economou JS, McBride WH, Essner R, et al. Tumour necrosis factor production by IL-2-activated macrophages in vitro and in vivo. Immunology 1989; 67:514–9.
66. Kovacs EJ, Young HA, Ruscetti FW. Interleukin-2 induction of interleukin-1 mRNA expression in human monocytes. J Leukocyte Biol 1987; 42:368.
67. Malkovsky MB, Loveland B, North M, et al. Recombinant interleukin-2 directly augments the cytotoxicity of human monocytes. Nature 1987; 325:262.
68. McBride WH, Economou JS, Nayersina R, Comora S, Essner R. Influences of interleukins 2 and 4 on tumor necrosis factor production by murine mononuclear phagocytes. Cancer Res 1990; 50:2949–52.
69. Economous JS, McBride WH, Essner R, et al. Tumor necrosis factor production by interleukin-2 activated macrophages in vitro and in vivo. Immunology 1989; 67:514–9.
70. Curran RD, Billiar TR, West MA, Bentz BG, Simmons RL. Effect of interleukin 2 on Kupffer cell activation. Interleukin 2 primes and activates Kupffer cells to suppress hepatocyte protein synthesis in vitro. Arch Surg 1988; 123:1373–8.
71. Herrmann F, Cannistra SA, Levine H, Griffin JD. Expression of interleukin 2 receptors and binding of interleukin 2 by gamma interferon-induced human leukemic and normal monocytic cells. J Exp Med 1985; 162:1111–6.
72. Holter W, Goldman CK, Casabo L, Nelson DL, Greene WC, Waldmann TA. Expression of functional interleukin-2 receptors by lipopolysaccharide and interferon-stimulated human monocytes. J Immunol 1987; 138:2917.
73. Valitutti S, Carbone A, Castellino F, et al. The expression of functional IL-2 receptor on activated macrophages depends on the stimulus applied. Immunology 1989; 67:44–50.
74. Mahida YR, Patel S, Wu K, Jewell DP. Interleukin 2 receptor expression by macrophages in inflammatory bowel disease. Clin Exp Immunol 1988; 74:382–6.
75. Holter W, Grunow R, Stockinger H, Knapp W. Recombinant interferon-gamma induces interleukin 2 receptors on human peripheral blood monocytes. J Immunol 1987; 136:2171–5.
76. Henney CS, Kuribayashi K, Kern DE, Gillis S. Interleukin-2 augments natural killer cell activity. Nature 1981; 291:335–8.
77. Brunda M, Tarnowski D, Davatelis V. Interaction of recombinant interferons with recombinant interleukin-2: differential effects on natural killer cell activity and interleukin-2-activated killer cells. Int J Cancer 1986; 37:787–93.
78. Ortaldo JR, Mason AT, Gerard JP, et al. Effects of natural and recombinant IL 2 on regulation of IFN gamma production and natural killer cell activity: lack of involvement of the Tac antigen for these immunoregulatory effects. J Immunol 1984; 133:779–83.
79. Kovacs EJ, Beckner SK, Longo DL, Varesio L, Young HA. Cytokine gene expression during the generation of human lymphokine-activated killer cells: early induction of interleukin-1B by interleukin 2. Cancer Res 1989; 49:940–4.

80. Mohamed-Habib BA, Moire N, Metivier D, et al. IL-2 receptors on circulating natural killer cells and T lymphocytes: similarity in number and affinity but difference in transmission of the proliferation signal. J Immunol 1989; 142:490.
81. Kehrl JH, Dukovich M, Whalen G, Katz P, Fauci AS, Greene WC. Novel interleukin 2 (IL-2) receptor appears to mediate IL-2-induced activation of natural killer cells. J Clin Invest 1988; 81:200.
82. Phillips JH, Takeshita T, Sugamura K, Lanier LL. Activation of natural killer cells via the p75 interleukin 2 receptor. J Exp Med 1989; 170:291.
83. Phillips JH, Takeshita T, Sugamura , Lanier LL. Activation of natural killer cells via the p75 interleukin 2 receptor. J Exp Med 1989; 170:291–6.
84. Siegel JP, Sharon M, Smith PL, Leonard WJ. The IL-2 receptor b chain (p70): role in mediating signals for LAK, NK, and proliferative activities. Science 1987; 238:75–8.
85. Tsudo T, Goldman CK, Bongiovanni KF, et al. The p75 peptide is the receptor for interleukin 2 expressed on large granular lymphocytes and is responsible for the interleukin 2 activation of these cells. Proc Natl Acad Sci U S A 1987; 84: 5394–8.
86. Manyak CL, Norton GP, Lobe OG, et al. IL-2 induces expression of serine protease enzymes and genes in natural killer and nonspecific T killer cells. J Immunol 1989; 142:3707–13.
87. Kanamori H, Suzuki N, Ishida N, Honjo T. Transcriptional regulation alone does not explain the constitutive expression of the interleukin 2 receptor (Tac/L-chain) in HTLV-1 infected cells. Immunol Lett 1989; 20:293–8.
88. Grimm EA, Mazumder A, Zhang HZ, Rosenberg SA. Lymphokine-activated killer cell phenomenon. Lysis of natural killer-resistant fresh solid tumor cells by interleukin 2-activated autologous human peripheral blood lymphocytes. J Exp Med 1982; 155:1823–41.
89. Grimm EA, Ramsey KM, Mazumder A, Wilson DJ, Djeu JY, Rosenberg SA. Lymphokine-activated killer cell phenomenon. II. Precursor phenotype is serologically distinct from peripheral T lymphocytes, memory cytotoxic thymus-derived lymphocytes, and natural killer cells. J Exp Med 1983; 157:884–97.
90. Sondel PM, Hank JA, Kohler PC, Chen BP, Minkoff DZ, Molenda JA. Destruction of autologous human lymphocytes by interleukin 2-activated cytotoxic cells. J Immunol 1986; 137:502–11.
91. Grimm EA, Wilson DJ. The human lymphokine activated killer cell system. V. Purified recombinant interleukin-2 activated cytotoxic lymphocytes which lyse both natural killer resistant autologous and allogeneic tumors and trinitrophenyl modified autologous periperal blood lymphocytes. Cell Immunol 1985; 94:568.
92. Lafreniere R, Rosenberg SA. Successful immunotherapy of murine experimental hepatic metastases with lymphokine-activated killer cells and recombinant interleukin 2. Cancer Res 1985; 45:3735–41.
93. Mule JJ, Shu S, Schwarz SL, Rosenberg SA. Adoptive immunotherapy of established pulmonary metastases with LAK cells and recombinant interleukin-2. Science 1984; 225:1487–9.
94. Blay JY, Bertoglio J, Fradelizi D, Chouaib S. Functional interactions of IL2 and TNF in the differentiation of LGL into LAK effectors. Int J Cancer 1989; 44:598–604.
95. Benveniste EN, Merrill JE. Stimulation of oligodendroglial proliferation and maturation by interleukin-2. Nature 1986; 321:610.
96. Merrill JE, Kutsunai S, Mohlstrom C, Hofman F, Groopman J, Golde DW. Proliferation of astroglia and oligodendroglia in response to human T cell-derived factors. Science 1984; 224:1428.

97. Ries WL, Seeds MC, Key LL. Interleukin-2 stimulates osteoclastic activity: increased acid production and radioactive calcium release. J Periodont Res 1989; 24:242–6.
98. Araujo DM, Lapchak PA, Collier B, Quirion R. Localization of interleukin-2 immunoreactivity and interleukin-2 receptors in the rat brain: interaction with the cholinergic system. Brain Res 1989; 498:257–66.
99. Smith LR, Brown SL, Blalock JE. Interleukin-2 induction of ACTH secretion: presence of an interleukin-2 receptor alpha-chain-like molecule on pituitary cells. J Neuroimmunol 1989; 21:249–54.
100. Maggiano N, Colotta F, Castellino F, et al. Interleukin-2 receptor expression in human mast cells and basophils. Int Arch Allergy Appl Immunol 1990; 91:8–14.
101. Mazingue C, Cottrez-Detoeuf F, Louis J, Kweider M, Auriault C, Capron A. In vitro and in vivo effects of interleukin 2 on the protozoan parasite leishmania. Eur J Immunol 1989; 19:487–91.
102. Cheever MA, Thompson JA, Kern DE, Greenberg PD. Interleukin 2 (IL 2) administered in vivo: influence of IL 2 route and timing on T cell growth. J Immunol 1985; 134:3895–900.
103. Klarnet JP, Matis LA, Kern DE, et al. Antigen-driven T cell clones can proliferate in vivo, eradicate disseminated leukemia, and provide specific immunologic memory. J Immunol 1987; 138:4012–7.
104. Ettinghausen SE, Lipford EH, Mule JJ, Rosenberg SA. Systemic administration of recombinant interleukin 2 stimulates in vivo lymphoid cell proliferation in tissues. J Immunol 1985; 135:1488–97.
105. Rosenberg SA, Mule JJ, Spiess PJ, Reichert CM, Schwarz SL. Regression of established pulmonary metastases and subcutaneous tumor mediated by the systemic administration of high-dose recombinant interleukin 2. J Exp Med 1985; 161:1169–88.
106. Gately MK, Anderson TD, Hayes TJ. Role of asialo-GM_1-positive lymphoid cells in mediating the toxic effects of recombinant IL-2 in mice. J Immunol 1988; 141:189–200.
107. Wiltrout RH, Pilaro AM, Gruys ME, et al. Augmentation of mouse liver-associated natural killer activity by biologic response modifiers occurs largely via rapid recruitment of large granular lymphocytes from the bone marrow. J Immunol 1989; 143:372–8.
108. Anderson TD, Hayes TJ, Gately MK, Bontempo JM, Stern LL, Truitt GA. Toxicity of human recombinant interleukin-2 in the mouse is mediated by interleukin-activated lymphocytes. Lab Invest 1988; 59:598–612.
109. Mazumder A, Rosenberg SA. Successful immunotherapy of natural killer cell-resistant established pulmonary melanoma metastasis by the intravenous adoptive transfer of syngeneic lymphocytes activated in vitro by interleukin 2. J Exp Med 1984; 159:495.
110. Hinuma S, Naruo K, Ootsu K, Houkan T, Shiho O, Tsukamoto K. Suppression of pulmonary tumour metastasis in mice by recombinant human interleukin-2:role of asialo GM1-positive cells. Immunology 1987; 60:173–9.
111. Mule JJ, Yang JC, Afreniere RL, Shu S, Rosenberg SA. Identification of cellular mechanisms operational invivo during the regression of established pulmonary metastases by the systemic administration of high-dose recombinant interleukin 2. J Immunol 1987; 139:285–94.
112. Vujanovic NL, Herberman RB, Olszowy MW, et al. Lymphokine-activated killer cells in rats: analysis of progenitor and effector cell phenotype and relationship to natural killer cells. Cancer Res 1988; 48:884–90.
113. Sarneva M, Vujanovic NL, Van den Brink MR, Herberman RB, Hiserodt JC. Lymphokine-activated killer cells in rats: generation of natural killer cells and

lymphokine-activted killer cells from bone marrow progenitor cells. Cell Immunol 1989; 118:448–57.
114. Imaya H, Matsuura H, Kudo M, Nakazawa S. Induction of lymphokine-activated killer cells from rat thymocytes using recombinant human interleukin-2. Cancer Immunol Immunother 1988; 27:13–6.
115. Bindoni M, Perciavalle V, Berretta S, Belluardo N, Diamantstein T. Interleukin 2 modifies the bioelectric activity of some neurosecretory nuclei in the rat hypothalamus. Brain Res 1988; 462:10–4.
116. Rosenstein M, Ettinghausen SE, Rosenberg SA. Extravasation of intravascular fluid mediated by the systemic administration of recombinant interleukin 2. J Immunol 1986; 137:1735–42.
117. Anderson TD, Hayes TJ. Toxicity of human recombinant interleukin-2 in rats. Pathologic changes are characterized by marked lymphocytic and eosinophilic proliferation and multisystem involvement. Lab Invest 1989; 60:331–46.
118. Peace DJ, Cheever MA. Toxicity and therapeutic efficacy of high-dose interleukin 2. J Exp Med 1989; 169:161–73.
119. Fraker DL, Langstein HN, Norton JA. Passive immunization against tumor necrosis factor partially abrogates interleukin 2 toxicity. J Exp Med 1989; 170:1015–20.
120. Iwamoto K, Takeishi M, Takagi K, et al. Expression of interleukin-2 receptor (IL-2R) in feline peripheral blood lymphocytes. Cell Mol Biol 1989; 35:279–84.
121. Bauer RM, Olsen RG. Parameters of production and partial characterization of feline interleukin 2. Vet Immunol Immunopathol 1988; 19:173–83.
122. Tompkins MB, Pang VF, Michaely PA, et al. Feline cytotoxic large granular lymphocytes induced by recombinant human IL-2. J Immunol 1989; 143:749–54.
123. Klausner JM, Paterson IS, Morel NML, et al. Role of thromboxane in interleukin 2-induced lung injury in sheep. Cancer Res 1989; 49:3542–9.
124. Glauser FL, DeBlois GG, Bechard DE, et al. Cardiopulmonary effects of recombinant interleukin-2 infusion in sheep. J Appl Physiol 1988; 64(3):1030–7.
125. Glauser FL, De Blois GG, Bechard DE, et al. A comparison of the cardiopulmonary effects of continuous versus bolus infusion of recombinant interleukin-2 in sheep. Cancer Res 1988; 48:2221–5.
126. Zeilender S, Davis D, Fairman RP, Glauser FL. Inotropic and vasoactive drug treatment of interleukin 2 induced hypotension in sheep. Cancer Res 1989; 49:4423–6.
127. Jesmok GJ, Gunther RA. In vivo biology of recombinant interleukin-2 infusion in sheep: cardiopulmonary manifestations of an intravascular immune-inflammatory response. Inflammation 1989; 13:267–84.
128. Ellis JA, DeMartini JC. Ovine interleukin-2: partial purification and assay in normal sheep and sheep with ovine progressive pneumonia. Vet Immunol Immunopathol 1985; 8:5–25.
129. Arunachalam B, Subba Rao MV, Ram GC. Bovine interleukin 2: biochemical and biological characterization. Vet Immunol Immunopathol 1989; 23:377–83.
130. Reddy PG, Blecha F, Minocha HC, et al. Bovine recombinant interleukin-2 augments immunity and resistance to bovine herpesvirus infection. Vet Immunol Immunopathol 1989; 23:61–74.
131. Daemen AJ, Buurman WA, Linden CJ, Groenewegen G, Kootstra G. Canine Il–2: characterization and optimal conditions for production. Vet Immunol Immunopathol 1984; 5:247–58.
132. Jardine JH, Jackson HJ, Lotzova E, Savary CA, Small SM. Tumoricidal effect of interleukin-2-activated killer cells in canines. Vet Immunol Immunopathol 1989; 21:153–60.

133. Nishi M, Yasamasa Y, Honjo T. Expression of functional interleukin-2 receptors in human light chain/Tac transgenic mice. Nature 1988; 331:267–9.
134. Ishida Y, Nishi O, Taguchi O, et al. Effects of the deregulated expression of human interleukin-2 in transgenic mice. Int Immunol 1989; 1:113.
135. Ishida Y, Nishi M, Taguchi O, et al. Expansion of natural killer cells but not T cells in human interleukin 2/interleukin 2 receptor (Tac) transgenic mice. J Exp Med 1989; 170:1103–15.
136. Waldmann TA. The multi-subunit interleukin-2 receptor. Annu Rev Biochem 1989; 58:875–911.
137. Jenkinson EJ, Kingston R, Owen JJT. Importance of Il-2 receptors in intra-thymic generation of cells expressing T-cell receptors. Nature 1987; 329:160–2.
138. Tentori L, Longo D, Zuniga-Pflucker JC, Wing C, Kruisbeek AM. Essential role of the interleukin 2-interleukin 2 receptor pathway in thymocyte maturation in vivo. J Exp Med 1988; 168:1741–7.
139. Wano Y, Dukovich M, Kehrl JH, Greene WC. New perspectives on the structure of the human high-affinity interleukin-2 receptor. In: Smith KA, ed. Interleukin-2. San Diego: Academic Press, 1988:99–112.
140. Tsudo M, Kozak RW, Goldman CK, Waldmann TA. Contribution of a p75 interleukin 2 binding peptide to a high-affinity interleukin 2 receptor complex. Proc Natl Acad Sci U S A 1987; 84:4215–8.
141. Sharon M, Klausner RD, Cullen BR, Chizzonite R, Leonard WJ. Novel interleukin-2 receptor subunit detected by cross-linking under high-affinity conditions. Science 1986; 234:859–63.
142. Saragovi H, Malek TR. The murine interleukin 2 receptor. Irreversible cross-linking of radiolabeled interleukin 2 to high affinity interleukin 2 receptors reveals a non-covalently associated subunit. J Immunol 1987; 139:1919–26.
143. Hermann T, Diamantstein T. The human intermediate-affinity interleukin 2 receptor consists of two distinct, partially homologous glycoproteins. Eur J Immunol 1988; 18:1051.
144. Hatakeyama M, Minamoto S, Uchiyama T, Hardy RR, Yamada G, Taniguchi T. Reconstitution of functional receptor for human interleukin-2 in mouse cells. Nature 1985; 318:467–70.
145. Greene WC, Robb RJ, Svetlik PB, Rusk CM, Depper JM, Leonard WJ. Stable expression of cDNA encoding the human interleukin 2 receptor in eukaryotic cells. J Exp Med 1985; 162:363–8.
146. Kondo S, Shimizu A, Maeda M, Tagaya Y, Yodoi J, Honjo T. Expression of functional human interleukin-2 receptor in mouse T cells by cDNA transfection. Nature 1986; 320:75.
147. Robb RJ. Conversion of low-affinity interleukin 2 receptors to a high-affinity state following fusion of cell membranes. Proc Natl Acad Sci U S A 1986; 83:3992.
148. Robb RJ, Greene WC. Internalization of interleukin 2 is mediated by the B chain of the high-affinity interleukin 2 receptor. J Exp Med 1987; 165:1201.
149. Leonard WJ, Depper JM, Uchiyama T, Smith KA, Waldmann TA, Greene WC. A monoclonal antibody that appears to recognize the receptor for human T-cell growth factor; partial characterization of the receptor. Nature 1982; 300:267–9.
150. Leonard WJ, Depper JM, Robb RJ, Waldmann TA, Greene WC. Characterization of the human receptor for T-cell growth factor. Proc Natl Acad Sci U S A 1983; 80:6957–61.
151. Cosman D, Ceretti DP, Larsen A, et al. Cloning, sequence and expression of human interleukin-2 receptor. Nature 1984; 312:768–71.
152. Hatakeyama M, Tsudo M, Minamoto S, et al. Interleukin-2 receptor B chain gene:

generation of three receptor forms by cloned human alpha and beta chain cDNA's. Science 1989; 244:551–6.
153. Hatakeyama H, Doi T, Kono T, et al. Transmembrane signaling of interleukin 2 receptor conformation and function of human interleukin 2 receptor (p55)/insulin receptor chimeric molecules. J Exp Med 1987; 166:362.
154. Kondo S, Kinoshita M, Shimizu A, et al. Expression and functional characterization of artificial mutants of interleukin-2 receptor. Nature 1987; 327:64.
155. Ferris DK, Willette-Brown J, OrtaldoJR, FarrarWL. IL-2 regulation of tyrosine kinase activity is mediated through the p70–75 beta-subunit of the IL-2 receptor. J Immunol 1989; 143:870–6.
156. Farrar WL, Ferris DK. Two-dimensional analysis of interleukin 2-regulated tyrosine kinase activation mediated by the p70–75 beta subunit of the interleukin 2 receptor. J Biol Chem 1989; 264:12562–7.
157. D'Andrea AD, Fasman GD, Lodish HF. Erythropoietin receptor and interleukin-2 receptor beta chain: a new receptor family. Cell 1989; 58:1023–4.
158. Itoh N, Yonehara Y, Schreurs J, et al. Cloning of an interleukin-3 receptor gene: a member of a distinct receptor gene family. Science 1989; 247:324–7.
159. Collins L, Tsien WH, Seals C, et al. Identification of specific residues of human interleukin 2 that affect binding to the 70-kDa subunit of the interleukin 2 receptor. Proc Natl Acad Sci U S A 1988; 85:7709.
160. Szollosi J, Damjanovich S, Goldman CK, et al. Flow cytometric resonance energy transfer measurements support the association of a 95-kDa peptide termed T27 with the 55-kDa Tac peptide. Proc Natl Acad Sci U S A 1987; 84:7246–51.
161. Edidin M, Aszalos A, Damjanovich S, Waldmann TA. Lateral diffusion measurements give evidence for association of the Tac peptide of the IL-2 receptor with the T27 peptide in the plasma membrane of HUT-102-B2 T cells. J Immunol 1988; 141:1206–10.
162. Zola H, Mantzioris BX, Webster J, Kette FE. Circulating human T and B lymphocytes express the p55 interleukin-2 receptor molecule (TAC, CD25). Immunol Cell Biol 1989; 67:233–7.
163. Yagita H, Nakata M, Azuma A, et al. Activation of peripheral blood T cells via the p75 interleukin 2 receptor. J Exp Med 1989; 170:1445–50.
164. Strauchen JA. Interleukin receptors in lymphoid lesions. Relevance to diagnosis, biology, and therapy. Pathol Annu 1989; 24(Part 2):149–65.
165. Allouche M, Sahraoui Y, Augery-Bourget Y, et al. Presence of a p70 IL-2-binding peptide on leukemic cells from varius hemopoietic lineages. J Immunol 1989; 143:2223–9.
166. Rubin LA, Kurman CC, Fritz ME, et al. Soluble interleukin 2 receptors are released by activated human lymphoid cells in vitro. J Immunol 1985; 135:3172.
167. Rubin LA, Kurman CC, Fritz ME, Yarchoan R, Nelson DL. Identification and characterization of a released form of the interleukin 2 receptor. In: Oppenhein JJ, ed. The role of leukocytes in host defense. New York: Alan R. Liss, 1985:95.
168. Robb RJ, Kutny RM. Structure-function relationship for the IL-2 receptor system. IV. Analysis of the sequence and ligand binding properties of soluble Tac protein. J Immunol 1987; 139:855.
169. Tanaka K, Hancock WW, Osawa H, et al. Mechanism of action of anti-IL-2 monoclonal antibodies. ART-18 prolongs cardiac allograft survival in rats by elimination of IL-2+ mononuclear cells. J Immunol 1989; 143:2873–9.
170. Rubin LA, Jay G, Nelson DL. The released interleukin 2 receptor binds interleukin 2 efficiently. J Immunol 1986; 137:3841–4.
171. Voss SD, Hank JA, Nobis CA, Fisch P, Sosman JA, Sondel PM. Serum levels of the

low-affinity interleukin-2 receptor molecule (TAC) during IL-2 therapy reflect systemic lymphoid mass activation. Cancer Immunol Immunother 1989; 29:261–9.

172. Lotze MT, Custer MC, Sharrow SO, Rubin LA, Nelson DL, Rosenberg SA. In vivo administration of purified interleukin-2 to patients with cancer: development of interleukin-2 receptor positive cells and circulating soluble interleukin-2 receptors following interleukin-2 administration. Cancer Res 1987; 47:2188.
173. Pui CH. Serum interleukin-2 receptor: clinical and biological implications. Leukemia 1989; 3:323–7.
174. Perkins JD, Nelson DL, Rakela J, Grambsch PM, Krom RAF. Soluble interleukin-2 receptor level as an indicator of liver allograft rejection. Transplantation 1989; 47:77–81.
175. Colvin RB, Preffer FI, Fuller T, et al. A critical analysis of serum and urine interleukin 2 receptor assays in renal allograft recipients. Transplant Proc 1989; 21:1863.
176. Lawrence EC, Holland VA, Young JB, et al. Dynamic changes in soluble interleukin-2 receptor levels after lung or heart-lung transplantation. Am Rev Respir Dis 1989; 140:789–96.
177. Colver GB, Symons JA, Duff GW. Soluble interleukin 2 receptor in atopic eczema. Br Med J 1989; 298:1426–8.
178. Takamatsu T, Yasuda N, Ohno T, Kanoh T, Uchino H, Fujisawa A. Soluble interleukin-2 receptors in the serum of patients with chronic renal failure. Tohoku J ExpMed 1988; 155:343–7.
179. Voss SD, Hank JA, Nobis CA, Fisch P, Sosman JA, Sondel PM. Serum levels of the low-affinity interleukin-2 receptor molecule (TAC) during IL-2 therapy reflect systemic lymphoid mass activation. Cancer Immunol Immunother 1989; 29:261–9.
180. Deloron P, Lepers JP, Coulanges P. Evolution of the levels of soluble interleukin-2 receptors during *Plasmodium falciparum* and *P. vivax* malaria. J Clin Microbiol 1989; 27:1887–9.
181. Diamantstein T, Kupiec-Weglinski JW, Storm TB, Tileny NL. Current stage of interleukin 2 receptor targeted therapy. Exp Clin Endocrinol 1989; 93:114–24.
182. Hahn HJ, Gerdes J, Lucke S, et al. Phenotypical characterization of the cells invading pancreatic islets of diabetic BB/OK rats: effect of interleukin 2 receptor-targeted immunotherapy. Eur J Immunol 1988; 18:2037–42.
183. Doi T, Hatakeyama M, Itoh S, Taniguchi T. Transient induction of IL-2 receptor in cultured T cell lines by HTLV-1 LTR-linked *tax*-1 gene. EMBO J 1989; 8:1953–8.
184. Honda M, Kitamura K, Matsuda K, et al. Soluble IL-2 receptor in AIDS. Correlation of its serum level with the classification of HIV-induced diseases and its characterization. J Immunol 1989; 142:4248–55.
185. Yamaguchi K, Nishimura Y, Kiyokawa T, Takatsuki K. Elevated serum levels of soluble interleukin-2 receptors in HTLV-I-associated myelopathy. J Lab Clin Med 1989; 114:407–10.
186. Alberti A, Chemello L, Fattovich G, et al. Serum levels of soluble interleukin-2 receptors inacute and chronic viral heptitis. Dig Dis Sci 1989; 34:1559–63.
187. Herrmann T, Diamantstein T. The mouse high affinity IL-2 receptor complex. Evidence for a third molecule, the putative gamma-chain, associated with alpha and or beta chain of the receptor. Immunobiology 1987; 175:145.
188. Mouzaki A, Osawa H, Diamantstein T. An ELISA that detects cell-associated and released rat interleukin 2 receptors in a soluble form. J Immunol Methods 1987; 100:243.
189. Osawa H, Josimovic-Akasevic O, Diamantstein T. Interleukin 2 receptors are released by cells in vitro and in vivo. I. Detection of soluble IL-2 receptors in cell

culture supernatents and in the serum of mice by an immunoradiometric assay. Eur J Immunol 1986; 16:467.
190. Herrmann T, Josimovic-Alasevic O, Mouzaki A, Diamantstein T. Demonstration of two distinct forms of released low affinity-type rat IL-2 receptors. Immunology 1989; 66:384–7.
191. Diamantstein T, Osawa H, Mouzaki A, Josimovic-Alasevic O. Regulation of interleukin-2 receptor expression and receptor release. Mol Immunol 1986; 23:1165–72.
192. Holbrook NJ, Chopra RK, McCoy MT, et al. Expression of interleukin 2 and the interleukin 2 receptor in aging rats. Cell Immunol 1989; 120:1–9.
193. Kupiec-Weglinski JW, Diamanstein T, Tilney NL, Strom TB. Therapy with monoclonal antibody to interleukin 2 receptor spares suppressor T cells and prevents or reverses acute allograft rejection in rats. Proc Natl Acad Sci U S A 1986; 83: 2624–7.
194. Kirkman RL, Barrett LV, Gaulton GN, Kelley VE, Ythier A, Strom TB. Administration of an anti-interleukin 2 receptor monoclonal antibody prolongs cardiac alograft survival in mice. J Exp Med 1985; 162:358–62.
195. Kelly VE, Gaulton GN, Hattori M, Ikegami H, Eisenbarth G, Strom TB. Anti-interleukin 2 receptors antibody suppresses murine diabetic insulitis and lupus nephritis. J Immunol 1988; 140:59–61.
196. Banerjee S, Wei BY, Hillman K, Luthra HS, David CS. Immunosuppression of collagen-induced arthritis in mice with an anti-IL-2 receptor antibody. J Immunol 1988; 141:1150–4.
197. Rosenberg SA, Spiess P, Lafreniere R. A new approach to the adoptive immunotherapy of cancer with tumor-infiltrating lymphocytes. Science 1986; 233:1318–21.
198. Rosenberg SA. The development of new immunotherapies for the treatment of cancer using Interleukin-2. Ann Surg 1988; 208:121–35.
199. Malkovsky M, Sondel PM, Strober W, Dagleish AG. The interleukins in acquired disease. Clin Exp Immunol 1988; 74:151–61.
200. Rosenberg SA. Immunotherapy of cancer using interleukin 2: current status and future prospects. Immunol Today 1988; 9:58–62.
201. Rosenberg SA, Lotze MT, Muul IM, et al. A progress report on the treatment of 157 patients with advanced cancer using lymphokine-activated killer cells and interleukin-2 or high-dose interleukin-2 alone. N Engl J Med 1987; 316:889–97.
202. Herberman RB. Interleukin-2 therapy of human cancer: potential benefits versus toxicity. J Clin Oncol 1989; 7:1–4.
203. van Haelst-Pisani CM, Pisani RJ, Kovach JS. Cancer immunotherapy: current status of treatment with interleukin 2 and lymphokine-activated killer cells. Mayo Clin Proc 1989; 64:451–65.
204. Richards JM. Therapeutic uses of interleukin-2 and lymphokine-activated killer (LAK) cells. Blood Rev 1989; 3:110–9.
205. Rosenberg SA, Lotze MT, Yang JC, et al. Experience with the use of high-dose interleukin-2 in the treatment of 652 cancer patients. Ann Surg 1989; 210:474–5.
206. Ramshaw IA, Andrew ME, Phillips SM, Boyle DB, Coupor BEH. Recovery of immunodeficient mice from a vaccinia virus/IL-2 recombinant infection. Nature 1987; 329:545.
207. Nunberg JH, Doyle MV, York SM, York CJ. Interleukin 2 acts as an adjuvant to increase the potency of inactivated rabies virus vaccine. Proc Ntl Acad Sci U S A 1989; 86:4240–3.
208. Herrod HG. Interleukins in immunologic and allergic diseases. Ann Allergy 1989; 63:269–72.

209. Pahwa R, Chatila T, Pahwa S, et al. Recombinant interleukin 2 therapy in severe combined immunodeficiency disease. Proc Natl Acad Sci U S A 1989; 86:5069–73.
210. Kaplan G, Kiesling R, Teklemariam S, et al. The reconstitution of cell-mediated immunity in the cutaneous lesions of lepromatous leprosy by rcombinant interleukin 2. J Exp Med 1989; 169:893–907.
211. Kroemer G, Wick G. The role of interleukin 2 in autoimmunity. Immunol Today 1989; 10:246–51.
212. Flomenberg N, Welte K, Mertelsmann R, et al. Immunologic effects of interleukin 2 in primary immunodeficiency diseases. J Immunol 1983; 130:2644.
213. Murray HW, Welte K, Jacobs JL, Rubin BY. Production of and in vitro response to interleukin 2 in the acquired immunodeficiency syndrome. J Clin Invest 1985; 76:1959.
214. Borzy MS. Interleukin 2 production and responsiveness in individuals with acquired immunodeficiency syndrome and the generalized lymphadenopathy syndrome. Cell Immunol 1987; 104:142.
215. Kaye WA, Adri MNS, Soeldner JS, et al. Acquired defect in interleukin-2 production in patients with type I diabetes mellitus. N Engl J Med 1986; 315:920.
216. Linker-Israeli M, Bakke AC, Kitridou RC, Gendler S, Gillus S, Horwitz DA. Defective production of interleukin 1 and interleukin 2 in patients with systemic lupus erythematosus (SLE). J Immunol 1983; 130:2651.
217. Welte K, Ciobanu N, Moore MAS, Gulati S, O'Reilly RJ, Mertelsmann R. Defective interleukin 2 production in patients after bone marrow transplantation and in vitro restoration of defective T lymphocyte proliferation by highly purified interleukin 2. Blood 1984; 64:380.
218. Tsang KY, Fudenberg HH, Galbraith GMP, Donnelly RP, Bishop LR, Koopman WR. Partial restoration of impaired interleukin-2 production and Tac antigen (putative interleukin-2 receptor) expression in patients with acquired immune deficiency syndrome by isoprinosine treatment in vitro. J Clin Invest 1985; 75:1538.
219. Malkovsky M, Jira M, Gao L, et al. Reduced expression of interleukin-2 receptors in hypogammaglobulinaemia: a possible cause of higher cancer incidence. Lancet 1986; 1:1442.
220. DeFreitas FC, Sandberg-Wollheim M, Schonely K, Boufal M, Koprowski H. Regulation of interleukin 2 receptors on T cells from multiple sclerosis patients. Proc Natl Acad Sci U S A 1986; 83:2637.
221. Kierszenbaum F, Sztein MB, Beltz LA. Decreased human IL-2 receptor expression due to a protozoan pathogen. Immunol Today 1989; 10:129–31.
222. Depper JM, Leonard WJ, Kronke M, Waldmann TA, Greene WC. Augmented T-cell growth factor receptor expression in HTLV-I-infected human leukemic T cells. J Immunol 1984; 133:1691.
223. Toosi Z, Kleinhenz ME, Ellner JJ. Defective interleukin-2 production and responsiveness in human pulmonary tuberculosis. J Exp Med 1986; 1986:1162.
224. Turcotte R, Lemieux S. Unresponsiveness to ConA in spleen cell cultures of *M. lepraemurium*-infected mice is dependent on a defective expression of high-affinity IL-2 receptors rather than on a lack of IL-2 production. Clin Exp Immunol 1989; 76:126–31.
225. Gillis S, Union NA, Baker PE, Smith KA. The in vitro generation and sustained culture of nude mouse cytolytic T-lymphocytes. J Exp Med 1979; 149:1460–76.
226. Kolb H, Zielasek J, Treichel U, Freytag G, Wrann M, Kiesel U. Recombinant interleukin 2 enhances spontaneous insulin-dependent diabetes in BB rats. Eur J Immunol 1986; 16:209–12.
227. Kashiwado T, Oppenheimer-Marks N, Ziff M. T cell inhibitor secreted by macrophages and endothelial cells. Clin Immunol Immunopathol 1989; 53:137–50.

228. Emery P, Gentry KC, Kelso A, Mackay IR. Interleukin 2 inhibitor in synovial fluid. Clin Exp Immunol 1988; 72:60–6.
229. Kucharz EJ, Goodwin JS. Minireview. Serum inhibitors of Interleukin-2. Life Sci 1988; 42:1485–91.
230. Kasakura S, Lowenstein L. Nature 1965; 208:894–6.
231. Gillis S, Ferm MM, Ou W, Smith KA. T cell growth factor: parameters of production and a quantitative microassay for activity. J Immunol 1978; 120:2027–32.
232. Smith KA, Favata MF, Oroszlan S. Production and characterization of monoclonal antibodies to human interleukin 2: strategy and tactics. J Immunol 1983; 131:1808–15.
233. Fujita T, Takaoka C, Matsui H, Taniguchi T. Proc Natl Acad Sci U S A 1983; 80:7437–41.
234. Lotze MT, Frana LW, Sharrow SO, Robb RJ, Rosenberg SA. In vivo administration of purified human interleukin 2. I. Half life and immunologic effects of the Jurkat cell line derived IL-2. J Immunol 1985;134:157.
235. Lotze MT, Matory YL, Ettinghausen SE, et al. In vivo administration of purified human interleukin 2 II. Half life, immunologic effects, and expansion of peripheral lymphoid cells in vivo with recombinant IL 2. J Immunol 1985; 135:2865–75.
236. Rosenberg SA. Immunotherapy of cancer by systemic administration of lymphoid cells plus interleukin-2. J Biol Response Mod 1984; 3:501–11.
237. Lotze MT, Rosenberg SA. Results of clinical trials with the administration of interleukin-2 and adoptive immunotherapy with activated cells in patients with cancer. Immunobiology 1986; 172:420–37.
238. Cohen FE, Kosen PA, Kuntz ID, Epstein LB, Ciardelli TC, Smith KA. Structure-activity studies of interleukin-2. Science 1986; 234:349–52.
239. Mookerjee BK, Pauly JL. Mitogenic effect of interleukin-2 on unstimulated human T cells: an editorial review. J Clin Lab Anal 1990; 4:138–49.
240. Owen-Schaub LB, Crump WL, Morin GI, Grimm EA. Regulation of lymphocyte tumor necrosis factor receptors by IL-2. J Immunol 1989; 143:2236–41.
241. Numorof RP, Aronsen FR, Mier JW. IL-2 stimulates the production of IL-1α and IL-1β by human peripheral blood mononuclear cells. J Immunol 1988; 141: 4250–7.
242. Hirohata S, Davis LS, Lipsky PE. Role of IL-2 in the generation of $CD4^+$ suppressors of human B cell responsiveness. J Immunol 1989; 142:3104–12.
243. Punnonen J, Viljanen MK. Interleukin 2 and interferon-gamma affect human B cells at different stages of activation. APMIS 1989; 97:200–6.
244. Chun M, Krim M, Granelli-Piperno A, et al. Enhancement of cytotoxic activity of natural killer cells by interleukin 2, and antagonism between interleukin 2 and adenosine cyclic monophosphate. Scand J Immunol 1985; 22:375–81.
245. Savary CA, Lotzova E, Klostergaard J. Interleukin 2-activated large granular lymphocytes: cytotoxic efficiency and mechanism of killing of tumor cell lines. Immunol Lett 1989; 21:145–51.
246. Velotti F, Palmieri G, Morrone S, Piccoli M, Frati L, Santoni A. Granzyme A expression by normal rat natural killer (NK) cells in vivo and by interleukin 2-activted NK cells in vitro. Eur J Immunol 1989; 19:575–8.
247. Kakita T, Sasada M. Moriguchi T, Nishimura T, Yamamoto K, Uchino H. Lysis of human leukemic cells by monocyte-derived macrophages activated with interferon-gamma and interleukin-2. Jpn J Cancer Res 1989; 80:59–64.
248. Malkovsky M, Loveland B, North M, et al. Recombinnt interleukin-2 directly augments the cytotoxicity of human monocytes. Nature 1987; 325:262.
249. Burdach S, Levitt L. T cell regulated hematopoiesis—molecular interactions in hematopoietic control by CD2 and interleukin 2. Behring Inst Mitt 1988; 56–67.

250. Talmadge JE, Phillips H, Schindler J, Tribble H, Pennington R. Systematic preclinical study on the therapeutic properties of recombinant human interleukin-2 for the treatment of metastatic disease. Cancer Res 1987; 47:5725–32.
251. Chang AE, Hyatt CL, Rosenberg SA. Systemic administration of recombinant human interleukin-2 in mice. J Biol Response Mod 1984; 3:561–72.
252. Piguet PF, Grau G, Irle C, Vassalli P. Administration of recombinant interleukin 2 to mice enhances production of hemopoietic and natural killer cells. Eur J Immunol 1986; 16:1257–61.
253. Eduardo L, Bermudez M, Stevens P, Kolonoski P, Wu M, Young LS. Treatment of experimental disseminated *Mycobacterium avium* complex infection in mice with recombinant IL-2 and tumor necrosis factor. J Immunol 1989; 143:2996–3000.
254. Haak-Frendscho M, Young KM, Czuprynski CJ. Treatment of mice with human recombinant interleukin-2 augments resistance to the facultative intracelular pathogen *Listeria monocytogenes*. Infect Immun 1989; 57:3014–21.
255. Ettinghausen SE, Lipford EH, Mule JJ, Rosenberg SA. Recombinant interleukin 2 stimulates in vivo proliferation of adoptively transferred lymphokine-activated killer (LAK) cells. J Immunol 1985; 135:3623–35.
256. Hinuma S, Naruo K, Shiho O, Tsukamoto K. Characteristics of murine non-specific killer cells induced in vivo by recombinant human interleukin-2. Immunology 1986; 59:251–9.
257. Kelland T, Belfrage H, Bhiladvala P, Hedlund G. Analysis of the murine lymphokine-activated killer (LAK) cell phenomenon: dissection of effectors and progenitors into NK and T-like cells. J Immunol 1987; 138:3640–5.
258. Cheever MA, Greenberg PD, Fefer A, Gillis S. Augmentation of the anti-tumor therapeutic efficacy of long-term cultured T lymphocytes by in vivo administration of purified interleukin 2. J Exp Med 1982; 155:968–80.
259. Tezabwala BU, Johnson PM, Rees RC. Inhibition of pregnancy viability in mice following IL-2 administration. Immunology 1989; 67:115–9.
260. Ettinghausen SE, Puri RK, Rosenberg SA. Increased vascular permeability in organs mediated by the systemic administration of lymphokine-activated killer cells and recombinant interleukin-2 in mice. J Natl Cancer Inst 1988; 80:177–88.
261. Sarin A, Saxena RK. Interleukin-2 induced activation of natural killer cells in rats and mice: a comparative study. Asian Pac J Allergy Immunol 1988; 6:88–94.
262. Talmadge JE, Schneider M, Keller J, et al. Myelostimulatory activity of recombinant human interleukin-2 in mice. Blood 1989; 73:1458–67.
263. Vujanovic NL, Herberman RB, Olszowy MW, et al. Lymphokine-activated killer cells in rats: analysis of progenitor and effector cell phenotype and relationship to natural killer cells. Cancer Res 1988; 48:884–90.
264. Matory YL, Chang AE, Lipford EH, et al. Toxicity of recombinant human interleukin-2 in rats folowing intravenous infusion. J Biol Response Mod 1985; 4:377–90.
265. Fairman RP, Glauser FL, Merchant RE, Bechard D, Fowler AA. Increase of rat pulmonary microvascular permeability to albumin by recombinant interleukin-2. Cancer Res 1987; 47:3528–32.
266. Bindoni M, Perciavalle V, Berretta S, Belluardo N, Diamantstein T. Interleukin 2 modifies the bioelectric activity of some neurosecretory nuclei in the rat hypothalamus. Brain Res 1988; 462:10–4.
267. Watts RG, Wright JL, Atkinson LL, Merchant RE. Histopathological and blood-brain barrier changes in rats induced by an intracerebral injection of human recombinant interleukin 2. Neurosurgery 1989; 25:202–8.
268. Ellison MD, Povlishock JT, Merchant RE. Blood-brain barrier dysfunction in cats following recombinant interleukin-2 infusion. Cancer Res 1987; 47:5765–70.

269. Klausner JM, Paterson IS, Morel NM, et al. Role of thromboxane in interleukin 2-induced lung injury in sheep. Cancer Res 1989; 49:3542–9.
270. Duke SS, King LS, Jones MR, Newman JH, Brigham KL, Forbes JT. Human recombinant interleukin 2-activated sheep lymphocytes lyse sheep pulmonary microvascular endothelial cells. Cell Immunol 1989; 122:188–99.
271. Coquerelle TM, Eichhorn M, Magnuson NS, Reeves R, Williams RO, Dobbelaere DA. Expression and characterization of the interleukin 2 receptor in *Theileria parva*-infected bovine lymphocytes. Eur J Immunol 1989; 19:655–9.
272. Ishizaka A, Hatherill JR, Harada H, et al. Prevention of interleukin 2-induced acute lung injury in guinea pigs by pentoxifylline. J Appl Physiol 1989; 67:2432–7.
273. Lee RE, Lotze MT, Skibber JM, et al. Cardiorespiratory effects of immunotherapy with interleukin-2. J Clin Oncol 1989; 7:7–20.
274. Glauser FL, DeBlois G, Bechard D, Fowler AA, Merchant R, Fairman RP. Cardiopulmonary toxicity of adoptive immunotherapy (review). Am J Med Sci 1988; 296:406–12.
275. Ognibene FP, Rosenberg SA, Lotze M, et al. Interleukin-2 administration causes reversible hemodynamic changes and left ventricular dysfunction similar to those seen in septic shock. Chest 1988; 94:750–4.
276. Gaynor ER, Vitek L, Sticklin L, et al. The hemodynamic effects of treatment with interleukin-2 and lymphokine-activated killer cells. Ann Intern Med 1988; 109:953–8.
277. Silverman HJ, Arbrams J, Rubin LJ. Effects of interleukin-2 on oxygen delivery and consumption in patients with advanced malignancy. Chest 1988; 94:816–21.
278. Samlowski WE, Ward JH, Craven CM, Freedman RA. Severe myocarditis following high-dose interleukin-2 administration. Arch Pathol Lab Med 1989; 113:838–41.
279. Conant EF, Fox KR, Miller WT. Pulmonary edema as a compliction of interleukin-2 therapy. Am J Radiol 1989; 152:749–52.
280. Gaspari AA, Lotze MT, Rosenberg SA, Stern JB, Katz SI. Dermatologic changes associated with interleukin 2 administration. JAMA 1987; 258:1624–9.
281. Kasid A, Director EP, Rosenberg SA. Induction of endogenous cytokine-mRNA in circulating peripheral blood mononuclear cells by IL-2 administration to cancer patients. J Immunol 1989; 143:736–9.
282. Hank JA, Kohler PC, Weil-Hillman G, et al. In vivo induction of the lymphokine-activated killer phenomenon: interleukin 2-dependent human non-major histocompatibility complex-restricted cytotoxicity generated in vivo during administration of human recombinant interleukin 2. Cancer Res 1988; 48:1965–71.
283. Walewski J, Paietta E, Dutcher J, Wiernik PH. Evaluation of natural killer and lymphokine-activated killer (LAK) cell activity in vivo in patients treated with high-dose interleukin-2 and adoptive transfer of autologous LAK cells. J Cancer Res Clin Oncol 1989; 115:170–4.
284. Sano T, Saijo N, Sasaki Y, et al. Three schedules of recombinant human interleukin-2 in the treatment of malignancy: side effects and immunologic effects in relation to serum level. J J Cancer Res 1988; 79:131–43.
285. Allegretta M, Atkins MB, Dempsey RA, et al. The development of anti-interleukin-2 antibodies in patients treated with recombinant human interleukin-2 (IL-2). Clin Immunol 1986; 6:481–90.
286. Lotze MT, Chang AE, Seipp CA, Simpson C, Vetto JT, Rosenberg SA. High-dose recombinant interleukin 2 in the treatment of patients with disseminated cancer. JAMA 1986; 256:3117–24.
287. Rosenberg SA, Lotze MT, Muul IM, et al. Observations on the systemic administration of autologous lymphokine-activated killer cells and recombinant interleukin-2 to patients with metastatic cancer. N Engl J Med 1985; 313:1485–92.

288. Giannella G, Pelosi-Testa E, Carlini P, et al. Fluctuations of plasma beta 2-microglobulin, soluble interleukin 2 receptor and interferon-gamma concentrations after adoptive immunotherapy with high-dose interleukin 2 and lymphokine-activated killer cells. Immunobiology 1989; 178:305–15.
289. Ettinghausen SE, Moore JG, White DE, Platanias L, Young NS, Rosenberg SA. Hematologic effects of immunotherapy with lymphokine-activated killer cells and recombinant interleukin-2 in cancer patients. Blood 1987; 69:1654–60.
290. Denicoff KD, Kurkin TM, Lotze MT, et al. The neuroendocrine effects of interleukin-2 treatment. J Clin Endocrinol Metab 1989; 69:402–10.
291. Denicoff KD, Rubinow DR, Papa MZ, et al. The neuropsychiatric effects of treatment with interleukin-2 and lymphokine-activated killer cells. Ann Intern Med 1987; 107:293–300.
292. Atkins MB, Mier JW, Parkinson DR, Gould JA, Berkman EM, Kaplan MM. Hypothyroidism after treatment with interleukin-2 and lymphokine-activated killer cells. N Engl J Med 1988; 318:1557–63.
293. Schiogolev SA, Goetzel EJ, Urba WJ, Longo DL. Appearance of neuropeptides in ascitic fluid after peritoneal therapy with interleukin-2 and lymphokine-activated killer cells for intraabdominal malignancy. J Clin Immunol 1989; 9:169–73.
294. Saris SC, Patronas NJ, Rosenberg SA, et al. The effect of intravenous interleukin-2 on brain water content. J Neurosurg 1989; 71:169–74.
295. Belldegrun A, Webb DE, Austin HA, et al. Effects of interleukin-2 on renal function in patients receiving immunotherapy for advanced cancer. Ann Intern Med 1987; 106:817–22.
296. Cotran RS, Pober JS, Gimbrone MA, et al. Endothelial activation during interleukin 2 immunotherapy. A possible mechanism for the vascular leak syndrome. J Immunol 1987; 12:1883–8.
297. Hoffman M, Mittelman A, Dworkin B, et al. Severe intrahepatic cholestasis in patients treated with recombinant interleukin-2 and lymphokine-activated killer cells. J Cancer Res Clin Oncol 1989; 115:175–8.
298. Brown RR, Lee CM, Kohler PC, Hank JA, Storer BE, Sondel PM. Altered tryptophan and neopterin metabolism in cancer patients treated with recombinant interleukin 2. Cancer Res 1989; 49:4941–44.
299. Wilson DE, Birchfield GR, Hejazi JS, Ward JH, Samlowski WE. Hypocholesterolemia in patients treated with recombinant interleukin-2: appearance of remnant-like lipoproteins. J Clin Oncol 1989; 7:1573–7.
300. Klempner MS, Noring R, Mier JW, Atkins MB. An acquired chemotactic defect in neutrophils from patients receiving interleukin-2 immunotherapy. N Engl J Med 1990; 322:959–65.
301. Thijs LG, Hack CE, Strack van Schijndel RJ, et al. Activation of the complement system during immunotherapy with recombinant IL-2. Relation to the development of side effects. J Immunol 1990; 144:2419–24.

CHAPTER 4

STRUCTURE AND FUNCTION OF INTERLEUKIN-3, ERYTHROPOIETIN, AND THE COLONY-STIMULATING FACTORS

Ian K. McNiece

Amgen Inc.
Thousand Oaks, California

INTRODUCTION

In 1966, two groups independently developed techniques for the cloning of mouse bone marrow cells in a semisolid agar system (1,2). To grow the bone marrow cells, feeder layers of thymus, spleen, kidney, liver, or embryo cells were required (1). Media conditioned by embryo fibroblasts were capable of replacing the feeder layers, and it was concluded that the cells used in the feeder layers or in conditioning the media produced an essential growth factor (2). As this factor stimulated the bone marrow cells to form colonies in the agar cultures, it was termed colony-stimulating factor (CSF).

Subsequent studies using the mouse bone marrow colony forming assay described four distinct CSFs based upon the colony morphology that resulted: (a) macrophage CSF (M-CSF or CSF-1) stimulates the formation of macrophage colonies (3); (b) granulocyte CSF (G-CSF) stimulates the formation of neutrophilic granulocyte colonies (4); (c) granulocyte-macrophage CSF (GM-CSF) stimulates the formation of mixed neutrophilic granulocyte and macrophage colonies (5); and (d) multi-CSF or interleukin-3 (IL-3) stimulates the formation of mixed colonies of neutrophilic granulocytes, macrophages, megakaryocytes, and erythrocytes (6,7). The human analogs of each of the mouse CSFs have been identified and recombinantly cloned (8–12). A summary of the cell types stimulated by these molecules is presented in Fig. 1 and Tables 1 and 2.

With the purification of the CSFs to homogeneity, sufficient material became available to begin preliminary characterization of the CSFs in vitro; however, the lack of in vivo characterization led many scientists to doubt the validity of the

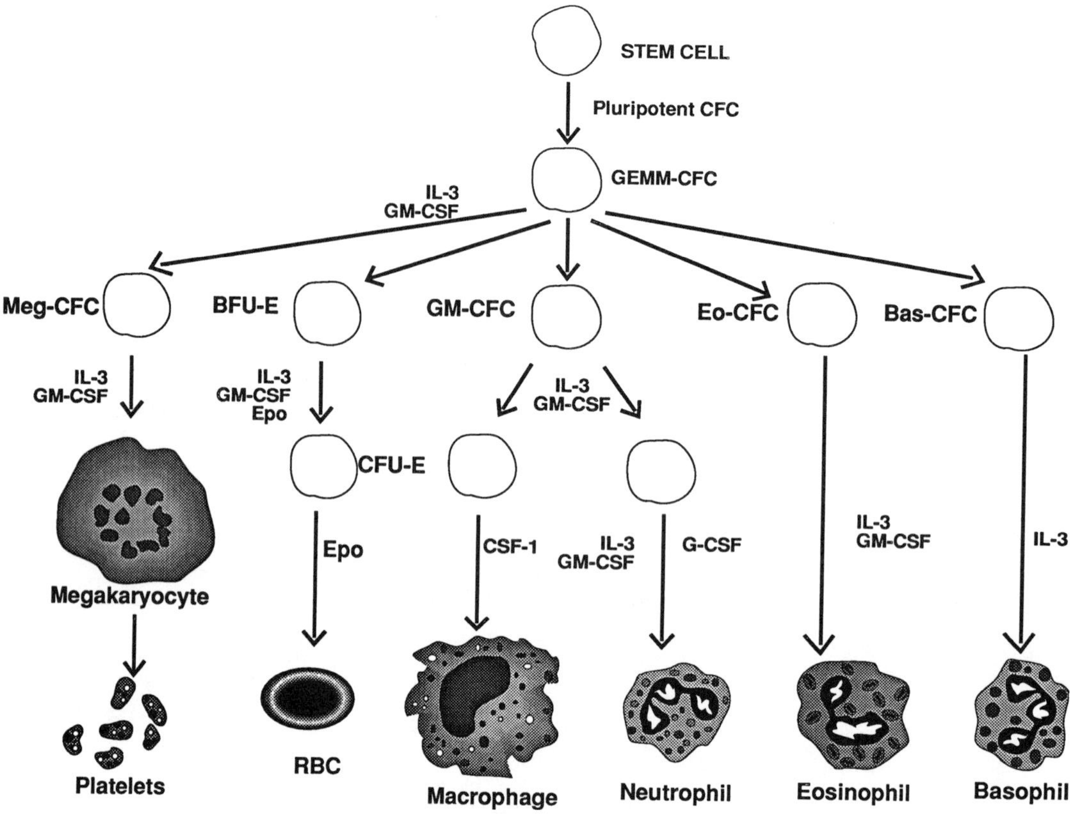

FIGURE 1 Model of differentiation of hematopoietic cells and the stages at which the CSFs and Epo stimulate various progenitor cells.

TABLE 1 Lineage Potential of CSFs and Epo[a]

Growth factor	Progenitor cell	Lineage[a]
CSF-1	GM-CFC, M-CFC, Mk-CFC, HPP-CFC[b]	Mac, Meg
G-CSF	GM-CFC, G-CFC, HPP-CFC,[b] Mk-CFC,[b] CFU-blast[b]	Gran, Meg
GM-CSF	GM-CFC, M-CFC, G-CFC, Mk-CFC, HPP-CFC,[b] CFU-GEMM,[b] BFU-Mk, BFU-E,[b] Eo-CFC	Gran, Mac, Meg Eryth, Eos
IL-3	GM-CFC, M-CFC, G-CFC, Mk-CFC, HPP-CFC,[b] CFU-GEMM,[b] BFU-Mk, BFU-E,[b] CFU-blast, CFU-S, Mast-CFC	Gran, Mac, Meg Eryth, Mast
Epo	CFU-E, BFU-E, Mk-CFC	Eryth, Meg

[a] Gran, granulocytes; Mac, macrophages; Meg, megakaryocytes; Eryth, erythrocytes; Eo, eosinophils; Mast, mast cells.

[b] The CSFs alone do not stimulate these progenitor cells; however, they do act in combination with one or more growth factors to stimulate the progenitor cells.

Table 2 Tissue and Cell Sources of CSFs and Epo

Growth factor	Molecular weight	Sources
CSF-1	45,000 (human) 70,000 (mouse)	Urine, MIA PaCa cells, fibroblasts, monocytes, endothelial cells, L cells, uterine glandular epithelial cells
G-CSF	25,000–30,000 (human 25,000 (mouse)	5637 cells, monocytes, fibroblasts, endothelial cells, mouse lung cells
GM-CSF	22,000 (human) 23,000 (mouse)	Mo cells, monocytes, T cells, endothelial cells, mouse lung cells
IL-3	14,000–28,000 (human) 23,000–28,000 (mouse)	WEHI-3B cells, T cells, keratinocytes
Epo	30,400 (human)	Human urine, proximal tubular cells of the kidney

CSFs. It was not until the advent of biotechnology that sufficient quantities of purified recombinant protein became available to enable in vivo studies to be undertaken. These studies have certainly validated the importance of the CSFs to the stage that a number have entered into clinical trials and are expected to be approved for the treatment of a variety of diseases in the near future. Other authors discuss the in vivo studies in this book. The present chapter concentrates on the in vitro properties of the CSFs and attempts to summarize the biological actions and biochemical properties of the CSFs.

Initially the CSFs, with the exception of IL-3, were thought to be specific for a single lineage; for example, G-CSF was thought to act exclusively in the neutrophil lineage. However, a number of recent studies have shown that combinations of CSFs can act synergistically to stimulate primitive cell types and act on multiple lineages rather than being exclusive to a single lineage. A further complication is that a range of cell types can be induced by one CSF to produce a secondary CSF. This highlights the need to confirm in vitro studies using cell populations that are devoid of accessory cell types, such as macrophages and fibroblasts, which produce multiple growth factors in response to various inducers. Research in this area is entering an extremely interesting time, with several laboratories approaching the isolation of purified stem cells (13–15). These techniques will enable detailed studies of the effects of purified recombinant CSFs at a single-cell level.

MACROPHAGE COLONY-STIMULATING FACTOR

The stimulatory actions of CSF-1 were originally described for the mononuclear phagocyte series (16). CSF-1 was shown to stimulate the proliferation of monocytes, macrophages, and their committed bone marrow progenitors (M-CFC, macrophage colony-forming cells) (3,16). More recent studies have demonstrated synergistic effects of CSF-1 on primitive hematopoietic progenitor cells in combination with other hematopoietic growth factors, such as IL-3, GM-CSF, G-CSF, IL-1α, and IL-6 (17–22). CSF-1 has also been shown to stimulate mRNA expression of platelet factor 4 in megakaryocytes, suggesting a possible role in platelet production (23). CSF-1 affects the function of mature monocytes and macrophages, it enhances the production of IL-1, tumor necrosis factor (TNF), G-CSF, and interferon and potentiates the release of prostaglandins and biocidal oxygen metabolites (8,24,25).

CSF-1 is produced by mesenchymal cells, including stromal cells of the bone marrow, fibroblasts, and endothelial cells (3,26,27). Peripheral blood monocytes and macrophages can be induced to express CSF-1 by phorbol esters, GM-CSF, interferon-γ, or tumor necrosis factor α (28–31). In addition to its role in hematopoiesis, CSF-1 synthesized by normal uterine glandular epithelial cells in response to ovarian hormones during pregnancy, appears to stimulate receptor-bearing trophoblasts of the adjacent placenta (32–34), suggesting a role of CSF-1 in placental development.

In semisolid agar culture of mouse bone marrow cells, both mouse- and human-derived CSF-1 stimulate the formation of colonies of mature macrophages. Mouse-derived CSF-1 has no activity on human bone marrow progenitors or human monocytes or macrophages. Surprisingly, human CSF-1 also has very little effect on human bone marrow progenitors, stimulating only cluster formation (colonies containing less than 50 cells) in semisolid agar cultures of human bone marrow cells (8). This finding complicates our understanding of the role of CSF-1 in humans.

Native human and mouse CSF-1 are heavily glycosylated dimer proteins of 45,000–70,000 daltons. The unglycosylated subunits of murine and human urinary CSF-1 are reported to have a size of 14,500 daltons (26), whereas the human cDNA predicts a polypeptide of 26,000 daltons. Removal of the carbohydrate moieties from CSF-1 does not affect its biological activity; however, reduction in the disulfide bonds abrogates all activity (26,35). At least two differentially spliced mRNAs for human CSF-1 are expressed from a common gene, and each encodes a different CSF-1 precursor. Additional processing and glycosylation result in at least two forms: a 70,000–90,000 glycoprotein consisting of a 35,000–45,000 dalton subunit, and a 40,000–50,000 dalton glycoprotein consisting of a dimer of a 20,000–25,000 dalton subunit. The two resulting proteins are 554 and 256 amino acids in length, respectively. In mouse cells only a 552 amino acid form has been found thus far (36,37).

CSF-1 has been shown to bind to a single class of high-affinity cell surface receptors expressed primarily on mature mononuclear phagocytes and their immature bone marrow precursors (38–41). Sherr and colleagues (42) demonstrated that the CSF-1 receptor is the product of the c-*fms* protooncogene. Binding of CSF-1 to its receptor activates the receptor kinase and leads to autophosphorylation of the receptor on tyrosine (42–44), internalization and degradation of the receptor-ligand complexes (39,45,46), and phosphorylation of a series of cellular proteins (46). CSF-1 receptors can be trans-downmodulated by IL-3, GM-CSF, and CSF-1 at 37°C but not by G-CSF (47).

GRANULOCYTE-MACROPHAGE COLONY-STIMULATING FACTOR

GM-CSF was originally described by its ability to stimulate the proliferation and differentiation of progenitor cells for neutrophilic granulocyte and macrophage lineages (48). Subsequent studies demonstrated the ability of GM-CSF to also stimulate progenitor cells, giving rise to eosinophils and megakaryocytes (49,50). GM-CSF also shows additive and synergistic effects with many other growth factors. In combination with erythropoietin (Epo), human or mouse GM-CSF stimulates early erythroid progenitor cells (BFU-E) and with CSF-1, IL-3, or G-CSF stimulates early myeloid progenitors (high proliferative potential CFC, HPP-CFC) (21,51–53). GM-CSF has additive effects with IL-3 in stimulating maximal numbers of eosinophil, erythroid, and megakaryocyte colonies to develop (50,54,55). In human cultures, GM-CSF synergizes with CSF-1 or G-CSF to stimulate increased colony numbers of macrophages or granulocytes, respectively (56,57).

Mouse GM-CSF stimulates only mouse bone marrow cells, not human bone marrow cells; human GM-CSF stimulates only human bone marrow, not mouse bone marrow cells. In addition to the stimulatory effects of GM-CSF on a wide range of progenitor cells, it also stimulates the functional activity of mature cells. GM-CSF inhibits the migration of neutrophils, it is directly chemotactic for neutrophils and monocytes, and it enhances the ability of neutrophils to kill antibody-coated tumor cells and to phagocytose bacteria, parasites and yeast (58–64). GM-CSF has similar effects on monocytes and macrophages, stimulating the antibody-dependent cytotoxicity of macrophages and the killing of parasites (65,66).

GM-CSF is produced by a range of cell types, including T cells, endothelial cells, and fibroblasts (67–69). Keratinocytes and the Hodgkin's tumor cell line L428KSA have also been found to produce GM-CSF (70,71). IL-1, tumor necrosis factor α, and lipopolysaccharide (LPS) have all been shown to induce the expression of GM-CSF in endothelial and macrophage cells (72–76).

Mouse GM-CSF was originally detected and isolated from medium conditioned by lung tissue from mice previously injected with endotoxin (5,77,78). The mouse GM-CSF was purified from lung tissue and the cDNA for GM-CSF isolated from lung mRNA (79,80). In 1985, two groups isolated cDNA clones encoding human GM-CSF using functional expression in mammalian cells. Wong and colleagues isolated a cDNA library from the human T lymphoblast cell line Mo (11); Lee and colleagues isolated a cDNA library from a concanavalin A (ConA)-stimulated human helper T cell clone T7 (12).

Although natural GM-CSF is glycosylated, *Escherichia coli*-derived GM-CSF, which is nonglycosylated, has high levels of biological activity (81). Mature mouse GM-CSF consists of 124 amino acids encoding a 14,000 dalton protein; the human GM-CSF contains an additional 3 amino acids between residues 21 and 22 (11,80). The mouse and human GM-CSF have only approximately 56% amino acid sequence homology (11), consistent with the lack of activity of human GM-CSF on mouse bone marrow.

Equilibrium binding studies have demonstrated low numbers of high-affinity binding sites on myeloid leukemic cells and on normal monocytes and neutrophils (82). GM-CSF receptors have also been demonstrated on nonhematopoietic tissues, including small lung carcinoma and malignant neural tissue (83). Cross-linking studies suggest that the GM-CSF receptor is an 84 kD polypeptide (83). GM-CSF induces a rapid internalization of its receptor followed by slow degradation of GM-CSF and receptor recycling. After binding to its receptor, GM-CSF stimulates the serine-specific phosphorylation of a 68 kD cytosolic protein and a 68 kD membrane protein as well as the tyrosine-specific phosphorylation of a 90 kD membrane protein (84).

GRANULOCYTE COLONY-STIMULATING FACTOR

Mouse G-CSF was first described as a factor in the serum of endotoxin-injected mice that induced terminal differentiation of the mouse myelomonocytic leukemic cell line WEHI-3 D^+ (85). G-CSF was soon purified from media conditioned by lungs from endotoxin-treated mice (86). Human G-CSF was subsequently purified from the bladder carcinoma cell line 5637 (87). The amino acid sequence was determined for both the human and mouse G-CSF by direct sequencing of the purified protein (88,89). The mouse G-CSF consists of 178 amino acids (molecular weight 19,000), and the human consists of 174 amino acids (molecular weight 18,600). Both mouse and human G-CSF are glycoproteins that have two disulfide bonds that stabilize the molecules (90,91).

Almost all murine tissues produce G-CSF when cultured in vitro (92). Endotoxin or the products of endotoxin-induced cells have been shown to stimulate macrophages, endothelial cells, and fibroblasts to increase G-CSF production (93–95). In semisolid agar culture of mouse bone marrow cells, both human and mouse G-CSF stimulate colony formation of predominantly (greater than 90%) neutrophilic granulocytes. Human bone marrow cells are similarly stimulated by human and mouse G-CSF to form neutrophil colonies (85,87). Recombinant human G-CSF has been shown to synergize with multiple factors, including CSF-1, IL-3, GM-CSF, and IL-1α, to form mature macrophage cells (21,96,97). G-CSF has not been reported to affect megakaryocyte formation alone but has been shown to augment the megakaryocyte-stimulating ability of IL-3 (98). Similarly, blast colony formation stimulated by IL-3 is augmented by G-CSF, but G-CSF alone has no stimulatory effect on blast cell formation (99). In preliminary data, G-CSF has been implicated in the generation of mouse pre-B cells; however, this effect may be mediated through accessory cells (100). G-CSF is a unique CSF: both mouse and human G-CSF stimulate mouse and human cells, suggesting strong conservation of the active regions of these molecules (101). Mouse and human G-CSF stimulate both bone marrow-derived and peritoneal exudate mouse neutrophils in their ability to demonstrate antibody-dependent cell-mediated cytotoxicity against coated mouse thymoma cells (60). G-CSF has also been shown to prime human neutrophils for enhanced responsiveness to other agents, such as ionophore or chemoattractants (102).

Binding studies reveal one class of high-affinity receptors on normal and leukemic myeloid cells, and cross-linking studies indicate that the G-CSF receptor is a single subunit protein of molecular weight 150 kD (103). The cDNA cloning of the G-CSF receptor was recently achieved by Fukunaga and colleagues (104) using expression cloning techniques. The G-CSF receptor is an 812 amino acid polypeptide with a molecular weight of 90,814 and contains a single transmembrane domain. The extracellular domain consists of 601 amino acids, with 220 amino acids closely resembling the rat prolactin receptor. The cytoplasmic domain shows a significant simularity with parts of the cytoplasmic domain of the murine IL-4 receptor (104).

INTERLEUKIN-3

Initially IL-3 was defined as a factor inducing the enzyme 20α-hydroxysteroid dehydrogenase, which was believed to be a unique marker for T cell maturation, and so IL-3 was thought to act in early T cell differentiation (105,106). IL-3 was subsequently purified to homogeneity in the early 1980s by Ihle and colleagues (107), and the purified protein was shown to be identical to a number of molecules reported to have vastly different biological actions (6). IL-3 was shown to be identical to burst promoting activity [BPA (108)], stem cell activating factor (109), P cell stimulating factor (110), mast cell growth factor (111), synergistic factor (19), and multi-CSF (7). In vitro IL-3 stimulates (a) granulocyte and/or macrophage colony formation, (b) erythroid burst-forming cells, (c) CFC that contain granulocyte, macrophages, erythroid cells, and megakaryocytes, (d) spleen colony forming cell (CFU-S) generation, (e) eosinophil colony formation, (f) mast cell colony formation, and (g) the proliferation of factor-dependent mast cell lines (6,112).

The cDNA encoding mouse IL-3 was isolated from WEHI-3-derived mRNA by Fung and colleagues in 1984, utilizing functional expression in oocytes and using the IL-3-dependent cell line 32Dcl-23 to detect biological activity (113). Recombinant IL-3 has been found to have biological and biochemical properties identical to those of the native IL-3 protein (112,114).

The mouse IL-3 cDNA predicts a mRNA of 851 bases that encodes a polypeptide of 166 amino acids (115). The mature mouse IL-3 has a molecular weight of approximately 16,000 dalton but native IL-3 has a molecular weight of 28,000, probably due to glycosylation (116).

In addition to the many activities of IL-3 on various mature cell types, it also synergizes with a number of other growth factors to stimulate primitive progenitor cells. In combination with erythropoietin, IL-3 stimulates early erythroid progenitors (6). The combination of IL-3 with G-CSF, CSF-1, GM-CSF, and IL-1 plus CSF-1 stimulates early myeloid progenitors termed high proliferative potential colony-forming cells (18,19,21,52). G-CSF augments the megakaryocyte-stimulating activity of IL-3, as does megakaryocyte potentiator (94,117). Ogawa and colleagues have demonstrated that IL-3 synergizes with G-CSF, IL-1, and IL-6 to stimulate primitive cells termed blast cells (95,118).

Identification of human IL-3 was complicated by the low level of homology between the mouse and human amino acid sequences [only 23% (10)]. Using mRNA from a gibbon T cell line the gibbon IL-3 cDNA was isolated, and using the cDNA as a probe the human IL-3 gene was isolated from a human genomic library (10). The homology between the mouse and human IL-3 is very low and is reflected in the lack of cross-reactivity between the two molecules, with human IL-3 stimulating only human cells and mouse IL-3 stimulating only mouse cells.

The predominant source of IL-3 appears to be activated T cells (119); however, other reports suggest that epidermal cells, yolk sac, and astrocytes may produce IL-3 (120–122). The best known source of IL-3 is the WEHI-3B cell line, which produces IL-3 constitutively. WEHI-3B is a myelomonocytic leukemic cell line that was induced in Balb/c mice and was the source used by Ihle and colleagues (107) to purify mouse IL-3. More recent studies utilizing polymerase chain reaction (PCR) technology have detected transcripts for IL-3 in cDNA prepared from total cytoplasmic RNA from normal human long-term bone marrow cultures in the absence of mature T cells (123).

The mouse IL-3 receptor was isolated by Krystal and colleagues (124) using the IL-3-dependent cell line B6SutA1. The IL-3 receptor is proposed to be 140 kD glycoprotein that is cleaved to a 70 kD surface protein by a receptor-associated protease.

CSFs AND NONHEMATOPOIETIC CELLS

Initially the CSFs were thought to act exclusively on cells of hematopoietic origin. However, recent reports from a number of laboratories suggest that the CSFs may be capable of stimulating cells from a variety of tissue origins. Berdel and colleagues (125) demonstrated that rhIL-3, rhGM-CSF, and rhG-CSF all stimulate the growth of the human colonic adenocarcinoma cell lines HTB-38 and CCL 187. GM-CSF receptors have been demonstrated on nonhematopoietic tissues, including small lung carcinoma and malignant neural tissue (83). Studies with in situ hybridization techniques demonstrated the expression of CSF-1 receptor genes in the maternal endometrium of pregnant mice (126). IL-3 has been shown to enhance neurite outgrowth and elevate choline acetyltransferase activity (127). Taken together with the production of CSFs by a number of nonhematopoietic cells, it seems reasonable to propose that the CSFs may have functions on cells of nonhematopoietic origin.

ERYTHROPOIETIN

Erythropoietin represents the first description of a hematopoietic growth factor, with the postulation in 1906 by Carnot (128) of an erythroid humoral factor produced in response to anemia. It was not until the 1950s that more formal proof was provided. The vascular systems of two rats were connected, and one rat was exposed to low oxygen levels, causing an increase in red cell production in both rats and suggesting a blood-borne factor had passed between the pair (129). Definitive studies were performed by Erslev and colleagues (130), who rendered rabbits anemic by bleeding and collected plasma from the anemic rabbits. This plasma was injected into normal rabbits, and increased red cell production was observed.

In 1957 it was demonstrated that plasma Epo levels of nephrectomized rats did not rise in response to hypoxia, and it was concluded that the kidneys are the site of Epo production (131). It was later demonstrated that anephric animals produce low levels of Epo in response to hypoxia and also that anephric fetal and neonatal animals produce normal levels of Epo predominantly in the liver (132–134). A number of chemical agents have been shown to trigger the production of Epo and include adenosine, eicosanoids, oxygen-derived free radicals, such as hydrogen peroxide, superoxide ion, and β_2-adrenergic agonists (135–138). These chemicals are probably released during hypoxia.

Epo was first purified to homogeneity from the urine of patients with aplastic anemia. The purified human urine Epo, which was shown to be homogeneous by sodium dodecyl sulfate (SDS) gel electrophoresis, consisted of two forms that varied in their carbohydrate content (139,140). Human urine Epo contains two internal disulfide bonds that are required for activity (141). Enzymic hydrolysis demonstrated that Epo contained three N-linked sugars and one O-linked sugar (142,143). The amino acid sequence of Epo was determined by direct sequencing of human urine Epo, and subsequent studies revealed a high degree of conservation between the human, monkey, and mouse predicted secondary sequences. The amino acid sequence of the human and monkey Epo are 92% identical, the human to mouse are 80% identical, and the monkey to mouse 82% identical (143,144). The peptide molecular weight of Epo is 18,398 based upon the amino acid sequence; the carbohydrate containing form has a molecular weight of 30,400 (145). Although human Epo was purified from urine in 1977, it was not until 1985 that the gene encoding Epo was cloned and expressed (146). Active recombinant human Epo has been expressed in CHO cells, and the purified Epo has properties identical to the native protein (145).

In the adult erythropoietin is mainly produced by the kidneys; it circulates in the plasma and is excreted in the urine. Epo induces red cell production by stimulating the proliferation and differentiation of erythroid progenitors (147). Red blood cells are produced from a mature progenitor population, termed erythroid colony-forming cells, which are directly stimulated by Epo (147,148). A more immature progenitor population, termed erythroid burst-forming cells, is stimulated by Epo in combination with IL-3 or GM-CSF (147–149). The combination of Epo with IL-3 or GM-CSF is thought to stimulate BFU-E, which differentiate to form CFU-E, which are responsive to Epo alone and give rise to mature red cells.

Epo affects target cells by binding to a specific receptor that has been identified on mouse erythroleukemic cells and normal human CFU-E (150,151). The Epo receptor was recently identified as a 507 amino acid polypeptide with a single transmembrane domain (152). No similarity to known proteins or nucleic acids has been identified from the sequence of the Epo receptor when compared to data bases. Both high-affinity (30 pM) and low-affinity (210 pM) receptors are expressed in COS cells containing the Epo receptor cDNA.

SUMMARY

The development of bone marrow colony-forming assays more than 20 years ago has enabled the study in vitro of the CSFs and other factors controlling blood cell production. These studies have led us to the present, when Epo is now being used clinically in the treatment of anemia associated with renal dialysis. Many of the in vivo effects of the other CSFs and interleukins are discussed in other chapters in this book and give great promise to further factors being used in clinical settings in the near future.

REFERENCES

1. Bradley TR, Metcalf D. The growth of mouse bone marrow cells in vitro. Aust J Exp Biol Med Sci 1966; 44:287.
2. Pluznik DH, Sachs L. The cloning of normal "mast" cells in tissue culture. J Cell Comp Physiol 1965; 66:319.
3. Stanley ER, Heard PM. Factors regulting macrophage production and growth. Pu-

rification and some properties of the colony stimulating factor from medium conditioned by mouse L cells. J Biol Chem 1977; 252:4305.

4. Nicola NA, Metcalf D. Analysis of purified fetal liver haemopoietic progenitor cells inliquid culture. J Cell Physiol 1982; 112:257.
5. Burgess AW, Camakaris J, Metcalf D. Purification and properties of colony-stimulating factor from mouse lung-conditioned medium. J Biol Chem 1977; 252:1998.
6. Ihle JN,Keller J, Oroszlan S, et al. Biological properties of homogeneous interleukin 3. J Immunol 1983; 131:282.
7. Cutler RL, Metcalf D, Nicola NA, Johnson GR. Purification of a multipotential colony-stimulating factor from pokeweed mitogen-stimulated mouse spleen cell conditioned medium. J Biol Chem 1985; 260:6579.
8. Ralph P, Warren MK, Ladner MD, Kawasaki ES, Boosman A, White TJ. Molecular and biological properties of human growth factor, CSF-1. Cold Spring Harbor Symp Quant Biol 1986; 51:679.
9. Souza LM, Boone TC, Gabrilove J, et al. Recombinant granulocyte colony-stimulating factor: effects on normal and leukemic myeloid cells. Science 1986; 232:61.
10. Yang YC, Ciarletta AB, Temple PA, et al. Human IL-3 (multi-CSF): identification by expression cloning of a novel hematopoietic growth factor related to murine IL-3. Cell 1986; 47:3.
11. Wong GG, Witek JS, Temple PA, et al. Human GM-CSF: molecular cloning of the complementary DNA and purification of the natural and recombinant proteins. Science 1985; 228:810.
12. Lee F, Yokota T, Otsuka L, et al. Isolation of a cDNA for a human granulocyte-macrophage colony stimulating factor by functional expression in mammalian cells. Proc Natl Acad Sci U S A 1985; 82:4360.
13. Spangrude GJ, Heimfeld S, Weissman IL. Purification and characterization of mouse hematopoietic stem cells. Science 1988; 241:58.
14. Bertoncello I, Hodgson GS, Bradley TR. Multiparameter analysis of transplantable hemopoietic stem cells. I. The separation and enrichment of stem cells homing to marrow. J Immunol 1987; 139:1096.
15. Visser JWM, deVries P. Isolation of spleen-colony forming cells (CFU-s) using wheat germ agglutinin and rhodamine 123 labelling. Blood Cells 1988; 14:369.
16. Stanley ER, Guilbert LJ, Tushinski RJ, Bartelmez SH. CSF-1—a mononuclear phagocyte lineage-specific hemopoietic growth factor. J Cell Biochem 1983; 21:151.
17. Bradley TR, Hodgson GS. Detection of primitive macrophage progenitor cells in mouse bone marrow. Blood 1979; 54:1446.
18. Bartelmez SH, Stanley ER. Synergism between hemopoietic growth factors (HGFs) detected by their effects on cells bearing receptors for a lineage specific HGF: assay of hemopoietin-1. J Cell Physiol 1984; 13:329.
19. McNiece IK, Kriegler AB, Hapel AJ, et al. Recombinant interleukin-3 exhibits synergistic factor activity. Cell Biol Int Rep 1984; 8:812.
20. McNiece IK, Kriegler AB, Bradley TR, Hodgson GS. Subpopultions of mouse bone marrow high-prolifertive-potential colony-forming cells (HPP-CFC). Exp Hematol 1986; 14:856.
21. McNiece IK, Stewart FM, Deacon DM, Quesenberry PJ. Synergistic interactins between hematopoietic growth factors as detected by in vitro mouse bone marrow colony formation. Exp Hematol 1988; 16:383.
22. Rennick D, Jackson J, Yang G, Wideman J, Lee F, Hudak S. Interleukin-6 interacts with interleukin-4 and other hematopoietic growth factors to selectively enhance the growth of megakaryocytic, erythroid, myeloid, and multipotential progenitor cells. Blood 1989; 73:1828.
23. Hunt P, personal communication 1990.

24. Metcalf D, Nicola NA. Synthesis by mouse peritoneal cells of G-CSF, the differentiation inducer for myeloid leukemia cells: stimulation by endotoxin, M-CSF, and multi-CSF. Leuk Res 1985;9:35.
25. Warren MK,Ralph P. Macrophage growth factor CSF-1 stimulates human monocyte production of interferon, tumor necrosis factor, and colony stimulating activity. J Immunol 1986; 137:2281.
26. Das SK, Stanley ER. Structure-function studies of a colony stimulating factor (CSF-1). J Biol Chem 1982; 257:13679.
27. Tushinski RJ, Oliver IT, Guilbert lJ, Tynan PW, Warner JR, Stanley ER. Survival of mononucler phgocytes depends on a lineage-specific growth factor that the differentiated cells selectively destroy. Cell 1982; 28:71.
28. Horiguchi J, Warren MK, Kufe D. Expression of the macrophage-specific colony-stimulating factor in human monocytes treated with granulocyte-macrophage colony-stimulating factor. Blood 1987; 69:1259.
29. Horiguchi J, Warren MK, Ralph P, Kufe D. Expression of the macrophage specific colony stimulating factor (CSF-1) during human monocytic differentiation. Biochem Biophys Res Commun 1986; 141:924.
30. Rambaldi A, Young DC, Griffin JD. Expression of the M-CSF (CSF-1) gene by human monocytes. Blood 1987; 69:1409.
31. Oster WA, Lindermann A, Horn S, Mertelsmann R, Herrmann F. Tumor necrosis factor (TNF)-alpha but not TNF-beta induces secretion of colony stimulating factor for macrophages (CSF-1) by human monocytes. Blood 1987; 70:1700.
32. Rettenmier CW, Roussel MF, Ashmun RA, Ralph P, Price K, Sherr CJ. Synthesis of membrane-bound colony-stimulating factor-1 (CSF-1) and downmodulation of CSF-1 receptors in NIH 3T3 cells transformed by cotransfection of the human CSF-1 and *c-fms* (CSF-1 receptor) genes.Mol Cell Biol 1987; 7:2378.
33. Bartocci A, Pollard JW, Stanley ER. Regulation of colony-stimulating factor 1 during pregnancy. J Exp Med 1986; 164:956.
34. Pollard JW, Bartocci R, Arceci R, Orlofsky A, Ladner MB, Stanley ER. Apparent role of the macrophage growth factor, CSF-1, in placental development. Nature 1987; 330:484.
35. Das SK, Stanley ER, Guilbert LJ, Forman LW. Human colony-stimulating factor (CSF-1) radioimmunoassay: resolution of three subclasses of human colony-stimulating fctors. Blood 1981; 58:630.
36. Wong GG, Temple PA, Leary AC, et al. Human CSF-1: molecular cloning and expression of 4kb cDNA encoding the human urinary protein. Science 1987; 235:1504.
37. Kawasaki ES, Ladner MB, Wang AM, et al. Molecular cloning of a complimentary DNA encoding human macrophage specific colony stimulating factor (CSF-1). Science 1985; 230:291.
38. Guilbert LJ, Stanley ER. Specific interaction of murine colony-stimulating factor with mononuclear phagocytic cells. J Cell Biol 1980; 85:153.
39. Guilbert LJ, Stanley ER. The interaction of ^{125}I-colony-stimulating factor-1 with bone marrow-derived macrophages. J Biol Chem 1986; 261:4024.
40. Byrne PV, Guilbert LJ, Stanley ER. Distribution of cells bearing receptors for a colony-stimulating factor (CSF-1) in murine tissues. J Cell Biol 1981; 91:848.
41. Morgan CJ, Stanley ER. Chemical crosslinking of the mononuclear phagocytic specific growth factor CSF-1 to its receptor at the cell surface. Biochem Biophys Res Commun 1984; 119:35.
42. Sherr CJ, Rettenmier CW, Sacca R, Roussel MF, Look AT, Stanley ER. The *c-fms* proto-oncogene product is related to the receptor for the mononuclear phagocyte growth factor, CSF-1. Cell 1985; 41:665.

43. Sacca R, Stanley ER, Sherr CJ, Rettenmeir CW. Specific binding of the mononuclear phagocyte colony-stimulating factor CSF-1 to the product of the v-*fms* oncogene. Proc Natl Acad Sci U S A 1986; 83:3331.
44. Yeung YG, Jubinsky PT, Sengupta A, Yeung DCY, Stanley ER. Purification of the colony-stimulating factor 1 receptor and demonstration of its tyrosine kinase activity. Proc Natl Acad Sci U S A 1987; 84:1268.
45. Wheeler EF, Rettenmier CW, Look AT, Sherr CJ. The v-*fms* oncogene induces factor independence and tumorigenicity in CSF-1 dependent macrophage cell line. Nature 1986; 324:377.
46. Downing JR, Rettenmeir CW, Sherr CJ. Ligand-induced tyrosine kinase activity of the colony stimulating factor-1 receptor in a murine macrophage cell line. Mol Cell Biol 1988; 8:1795.
47. Walker F, Nicola NA, Metcalf D. Hierachial downmodulation of hemopoietic growth factor receptors. Cell 1985; 43:269.
48. Metcalf D. Hemopoietic colonies. In: In vitro cloning of normal and leukemic cells. Berlin: Springer-Verlag, 1977:
49. Metcalf D, Burgess AW, Johnson GR, et al. In vitro actions on hemopoietic cells of recombinant murine GM-CSF purified after production in *E. coli*: comparison with purified native GM-CSF. J Cell Physiol 1986; 128:421.
50. Robinson BE, McGrath HE, Quesenberry PJ. Recombinant murine granulocyte macrophage colony-stimulating factor has megakaryocyte colony-stimulation activity and augments megakaryocyte colony stimulation by interleukin 3. J Clin Invest 1987; 79:1648.
51. Metcalf D, Johnson GR, Burgess AW. Direct stimulation by purified GM-CSF of the proliferation of multipotential and erythroid precursor cells. Blood 1980; 55:138.
52. Migliaccio AR, Bruno M, Migliaccio G. Evidence for direct action of human biosynthetic (recombinant) GM-CSF on erythroid progenitors in serum-free culture. Blood 1987; 70:1867.
53. McNiece IK, Stewart FM, Deacon DM, et al. Detection of a human CFC with a high proliferative potential. Blood 1989; 74:609.
54. Mazur EM, Cohne JL, Wong GG, Clark SC. Modest stimulating effect of recombinant human GM-CSF on colony growth from peripheral blood human megakaryocyte progenitor cells. Exp Hematol 1987; 15:1128.
55. Messner HA, Yamasaki K, Jamal N, et al. Growth of human hemopoietic colonies in response to recombinant gibbon interleukin 3: comparison with human recombinant granulocyte and granulocyte-macrophage colony-stimulating factor. Proc Natl Acad Sci U S A 1987; 84:6765.
56. Caracciolo D, Shirshat N, Wong GG,Lange B, Clark S, Rovera G. Recombinant human macrophage colony-stimulating factor (M-CSF) requires subliminal concentrations of granulocyte/macrophage (GM)-CSF for optimal stimulation of human macrophage colony formation in vitro. J Exp Med 1987; 166:1851.
57. McNiece I, Andrews R, Stewart M, Clark S, Boone T, Quesenberry P. Action of interleukin-3, G-CSF, and GM-CSF on highly enriched human hematopoietic progenitor cells: synergistic interaction of GM-CSF plus G-CSF. Blood 1989; 41:110.
58. Burgess AW, Begley CG, Johnson GR, et al. Purification and properties of bacterially synthesized human granulocyte-macrophage colony stimulating factor. Blood 1987; 69:43.
59. Fleischmann J, Golde DW, Weisbart RH, Gasson JC. Granulocyte-macrophage colony-stimulating factor enhances phagocytosis of bacteria by human neutrophils. Blood 1986; 68:708.
60. Lopez AF, Nicola NA, Burgess AW, et al. Activation of granulocyte cytotoxic function by purified mouse colony-stimulating factors. J Immunol 1983; 131:2983.

61. Vadas MA, Nicola NA, Metcalf D. Activation of antibody-dependent cell-mediated cytotoxicity of human neutrophils and eosinophils by separate colony stimulating factors. J Immunol 1983; 130:795.
62. Villalta F, Kierszenbaum. Effects of human colony-stimulating factor on the uptake and destruction of a pathogenic parasite (*Trypanosoma cruzi*) by human neutrophils. J Immunol 1986; 137:1703.
63. Weisbart RM, Golde DW, Clark SC, Wong GG, Gasson JC. Human granulocyte-macrophage colony-stimulating factor is a neutrophil activator. Nature 1985; 314:361.
64. Williamson DJ, Brown TC. Enhancement of neutrophil-mediated phagocytosis by human granulocyte-macrophage colony-stimulating factor demonstrated using a novel mathematical mode. Immunol. Cell Biol 1987; 65:329.
65. Grabstein KH, Urdal DL, Tushinski RJ, et al. Induction of macrophage tumoricidal activity by granulocyte-macrophage colony-stimulating factor. Science 1986; 232:506.
66. Handman E, Burgess AW. Stimulation by granulocyte-macrophage colony stimulating factor of *Leishmania tropica* killing by macrophages. J Immunol 1979; 122:1134.
67. Kelso A, Gough N. Expression of hemopoietic growth factor genes in murine T lymphocytes. In: Webb DR, Goeddel DV, eds. The lymphokines, Vol. 3. New York: Academic Press, 1987:209.
68. Koury MJ, Pragnell IB. Retroviruses induce granulocyte-macrophage colony-stimulating activity in fibroblasts. Nature 1982; 299:638.
69. Quesenberry PJ, Gimbrone MA. Vascular endothelium as a regulator of granulopoiesis. Production of colony-stimulting activity by cultured human endothelial cells. Blood 1980; 56:1060.
70. Chodakewitz JA, Kupper TS, Coleman DL. Keratinocyte-derived granulocyte/macrophage colony-stimulating factor induces DNA synthesis by peritoneal macrophages. J Immunol 1988; 140:832.
71. Byrne PV, Heit WF, March CJ. Human granulocyte-macrophage colony-stimulating factor purified from a Hodgkin's tumor cell line. Biochim Biophys Acta 1986; 874:266.
72. Broudy VC, Kaushansky K, Segal GM, Harlan JM, Adamson JW. Tumor necrosis factor type alpha stimulates human endothelial cells to produce granulocyte/macrophage colony stimulating factor. Proc Natl Acad Sci U S A 1986; 83:7467.
73. Munker R, Gasson J, Ogawa M, Koeffler HP. Recombinant human TNF induces production of granulocyte-monocyte colony-stimulating factor. Nature 1986; 323:79.
74. Seelentag WK, Mermod J-J, Montesano R, Vassali P. Additive effects of interleukin 1 and tumor necrosis factor-alpha on the accumulation of the three granulocyte and macrophage colony-stimulating factor mRNA's in human endothelial cells. EMBO J 1987; 6:2261.
75. Seiff CA, Tsai S, Faller DV. Interleukin-1 induces cultured human endothelial cell production of granulocyte-macrophage colony stimulating factor. J Clin Invest 1987; 79:48.
76. Zsebo KM, Yuscenkoff VN, Schiffer S, et al. Vascular endothelial cells and granulopoiesis: interleukin-1 stimulates release of G-CSF and GM-CSF. Blood 1988; 71:99.
77. Sheridan JW, Metcalf D. Purification of mouse lung-conditioned medium colony stimulating factor (CSF). Proc Soc Exp Biol Med 1974; 146:218.
78. Sheridan JW, Metcalf D, Stanley ER. Further studies on the factor in lung-conditioned medium stimulating granulocyte and monocyte colony formation in vitro. J Cell Physiol 1974; 84:147.

79. Sparrow LG, Metcalf D, Hunkapiller MW, Hood LE, Burgess AW. Purification and partial amino acid sequence of asialo murine granulocyte-macrophage colony stimulating factor. Proc Natl Acad Sci U S A 1985; 82:292.
80. Gough NM, Gough J, Metcalf D, et al. Molecular cloning of cDNA encoding a murine haemopoietic growth regulator, granulocyte-macrophage colony stimulating factor. Nature 1984; 309:763.
81. DeLarmarter JF, Mermod J-J, Liang C-M, Eliason JF, Thatcher DR. Recombinant murine GM-CSF from *E. coli* has biological activity and is neutralized by a specific antiserum. EMBO J 1985; 4:2575.
82. DiPersio J, Billing P, Kaufman S, Eghtesady P, Williams RE, Gasson JC. Characterization of the human granulocyte-macrophage colony-stimulating factor receptor. J Biol Chem 1988; 263:1834.
83. Baldwin GC, Gasson JC, Kaufman SE, et al. Nonhematopoietic tumor cells express functional GM-CSF receptors. Blood 1989; 73:1033.
84. Sorenson PH, Mui AL-F, Murphy SC, Krystal G. Interleukin-3, GM-CSF, and TPA induce distinct phosphorylation events in an interleukin 3-dependent multipotential cell line. Blood 1989; 73:406.
85. Burgess AW, Metcalf D. Characterization of a serum factor stimulating the differentiation of myelomonocytic leukemic cells. Int J Cancer 1980; 39:647.
86. Nicola NA, Metcalf D, Matsumoto M, Johnson GR. Purification of a factor inducing differentiation in murine myelomonocytic leukemia cells. Identification as granulocyte colony-stimulating factor. J Biol Chem 1983; 258:9017.
87. Welte K, Platzer E, Lu L, et al. Purification and biochemical characterization of human pluripotent hematopoietic colony-stimulating factor. Proc Natl Acad Sci U S A 1985; 82:1526.
88. Simpson RJ, Nice EC, Nicola NA. Structural studies on the murine granulocyte colony-stimulating factor. Biol Chem Hope Seyler 1987; 368:1327.
89. Nagata S, Tsuchiya M, Asano S, et al. Molecular cloning and expression of cDNA for human granulocyte colony-stimulating factor. Nature 1986; 319:415.
90. Nicola NA, Metcalf D. Differentiation induction in leukemic cells by normal growth regulators: molecular and binding properties of purified granulocyte colony-stimulting factor. In: Bishop JM, Rowley JD, Greaves M, eds. Genes and cancer. New York: Alan R. Liss, 1984:591.
91. Nicola NA. Granulocyte-colony-stimulting factor. Methods Enzymol 1987; 116:600.
92. Nicola NA, Metcalf D. Biochemical properties of differentiation factors for murine myelomonocytic leukemic cells in organ conditioned media. Separation from colony-stimulting factors. J Cell Physiol 1981; 112:257.
93. Vadas MA, Lopez AF. Regulation of granulocyte function by colony-stimulating factors and monoclonal antibodies. Lymphokines 1985; 12:179.
94. Koeffler HP, Gasson J, Raynard J, Souza L, Shepherd M, Munker R. Recombinant human TNF alpha stimulates production of granulocyte colony-stimulating factor. Blood 1987; 70:55.
95. Rennick D, Yang G, Gemmell L, Lee F. Control of hemopoiesis by a bone marrow stromal cell clone: lipopolysaccharide and interleukin-1-inducible production of colony-stimulating factors GM-CSF and G-CSF. Blood 1987; 69:682.
96. McNiece IK, Kriegler AB, Quesenberry PJ. Studies on the myeloid synergistic factor from 5637: comparison with interleukin-1 alpha. Blood 1989; 73:919.
97. Moore MAS, Warren DJ. Synergy of interleukin 1 and granulocyte colony-stimulating factor: in vivo stimulation of stem-cell recovery and hematopoietic regeneration following 5-fluorouracil treatment of mice. Proc Natl Acad Sci U S A 1987; 84:7134.
98. McNiece IK, McGrath HE, Quesenberry PJ. Granulocyte colony stimulating factor

augments in vitro megakaryocyte colony formation by interleukin-3. Exp Hematol 1988; 16:807.

99. Ikebuchi K, Clark S, Ihle JN, Souza LM, Ogawa M. Granulocyte colony-stimulating factor enhances interleukin-3 dependent proliferation of multipotential hemopoietic progenitors. Proc Natl Acad Sci U S A 1988; 85:3445.
100. Woodward TA, McNiece IK, Witte PL, et al. Further studies on growth factor production by the TC-1 stromal cell line: pre-B stimulating activity. Blood 1990; 75:2130.
101. Nicola NA, Begley CG, Metcalf D. Identification of the human analogue of a regulator that induces differentiation in murine leukaemic cells. Nature 1985; 314:625.
102. Avalos BR, Hedzat C, Baldwin GC, Golde DW, Gasson JC, DiPersio JF. Biological activities of human G-CSF and characterization of the human G-CSF receptor. Blood 1987; 70(Suppl. 1):165a.
103. Avalos BR, Gasson JC, Connors LG, Golde DW, Souza LM, Slamn DJ. Molecular characterization of the human G-CSF receptor. J Cell Biochem Suppl 1989; 13C:22.
104. Fukunaga R, Ishizaka-Ikeda E, Seto Y, Nagata S. Expression cloning of a receptor for murine granulocyte colony-stimulating factor. Cell 1990; 61:341.
105. Ihle JN, Pepersack L, Rebar L. Regulation of T-cell differentiation: in vitro induction of 20alpha-hydroxysteroid dehydrogenase in splenic lymphocytes from athymic mice by a unique lymphokine. J Immunol 1981; 126:2184.
106. Ihle JN, Rebar L, Kellar J, Lee JC, Hapel AJ. Interleukin 3: possible roles in the regulation of lymphocyte differentiation and growth. Immunol Rev 1982; 63:5.
107. Ihle JN, Keller J, Henderson L, Klein F, Palaszynski E. Procedures for the purification of interleukin 3 to homogeneity. J Immunol 1982b; 129:2431.
108. Iscove NN, Roitsch CA, Williams N, Guilbert LJ. Molecules stimulating early red cell, granulocyte, macrophage and megakaryocyte precursors in culture: similarity in size, hydrophobicity and charge. J Cell Physiol Suppl 1982; 1:65.
109. Wagemaker G, Merchav S, Burger H. Multiplication of pluripotent hemopoietic stem cells induced by purified stem cell activating factor (SAF) in serum free suspension cultures. Exp Hematol 1982; 10(Suppl. 11):162.
110. Clark-Lewis I, Kent SBH, Schrader JW. Purification to apparent homogeneity of a factor stimulating the growth of multiple lineages of hemopoietic cells. J Biol Chem 1984; 259:7488.
111. Yung YP, Eger R, Tertian G, Moore MAS. Long-term in vitro culture of murine mast cells. II. Purification of a mast cell growth factor and its dissociation from TCGF. J Immunol 1981; 127:794.
112. Hapel AJ, Fung MC, Johnson RM, Young IG, Johnson GR, Metcalf D. Biological properties of molecularly cloned and expressed murine interleukin 3. Blood 1985; 65:1453.
113. Fung MC, Hapel AJ, Ymer S, et al. Molecular cloning of cDNA for murine interleukin-3. Nature 1984; 307:233.
114. Rennick DM, Lee FD, Yokota T, Arai K-I, Cantor H, Nabel GJ. A cloned MCGF cDNA encodes a multilineage hematopoietic growth factor: multiple activities of interleukin 3. J Immunol 1985; 134:910.
115. Lee F, Abrams J, Arai K, et al. The expression and characterization of recombinant mouse IL-3. In: Schrader JW, ed. Lymphokines, Vol. 15, San Diego: Academic Press, 1988:163.
116. Ihle JN. Biochemical and biological properties of interleukin-3: a lymphokine mediating the differentiation of a lineage of cells that includes prothymocytes and mastlike cells. Contemp top Mol Immunol 1984; 10:93.
117. Oon SH, Williams N. Biochemical characterization of an in vitro murine megakaryocyte growth activity: megakaryocyte potentiator. Leuk Res 1986; 10:403.

118. Ikebuchi K, Wong GG, Clark SC, Ihle JN, Hirai Y, Ogawa M. Interleukin 6 enhancement of interleukin 3-dependent proliferation of multipotential hemopoietic progenitors. Proc Natl Acad Sci U S A 1987; 84:9035.
119. Kelso A, Metcalf D. Clonal heterogeneity in colony stimulating factor production by murine T-lymphocytes. J Cell Physiol 1985; 123:101.
120. Luger TA, Wirth U, Kock A. Epidermal cells synthesize a cytokine with interleukin-3-like properties. J Immunol 1985; 134:915.
121. Labastie MC, Thiery JP, Le Douarin NM. Mouse yolk sac and intra embryonic tissues produce factors able to elicit differentiation of erythroid burst-forming units and colony-forming units respectively. Proc Natl Acad Sci U S A 1984; 81:1453.
122. Frei K, Bodmer S, Scherdel C, Fontana A. Astrocyte-derived interleukin-3 as a growth factor for microglia cells and peritoneal macrophages. J Immunol 1986; 137:3521.
123. Barge AJ, Johnson GA, Simmons P, Torok-Storb B. Interleukin 3 transcript, bioactivity and protein is detectable in normal bone marrow stroma in the absence of mature T-lymphocytes. Blood 1989; 74(Suppl. 1):115a.
124. Murthy SC, Mui AL-F, Krystal G. Characterization of the interleukin 3 receptor. Exp Hematol 1990; 18:11.
125. Berdel WE, Danhauser-Riedl S, Steinhauser G, Winton EF. Various human hematopoietic growth factors (interleukin-3, GM-CSF, G-CSF) stimulate clonal growth of nonhematopoietic tumor cells. Blood 1989; 73(1):80.
126. Kamegai M, Niijima K, Kunishita T, et al. Interleukin 3 as a trophic factor for central cholinergic neurons in vitro and in vivo. Neuron 1990; 4:429.
127. Regenstreif LJ, Rossant J. Expression of the c-*fms* proto-oncogene and the cytokine, CSF-1, during mouse embryogenesis. Dev Biol 1989; 133:284.
128. Carnot P. Sur le mechanisme d'hyperglobulie provoquee par le serum d'animaux en renovation sanguine. CR Acad Sci (Paris) 1906; 111:344.
129. Reissmann KR. Studies on the mechanism of erythropoietic stimulation in parabiotic rats during hypoxia. Blood 1950; 5:372.
130. Erslev AJ, Lavietes PH, Van Wagenen G. Erythropoietic stimulation induced by "anemic" serum. Proc Soc Exp Biol Med 1953; 83:548.
131. Jacobson LO, Goldwasser E, Fried W, Plzak L. Role of the kidney in erythropoiesis. Nature 1957; 179:622.
132. Mirand AC, Prentice TC. Presence of plasma erythropoietin in hypoxic rats with or without kidneys and/or spleen. Proc Soc Exp Biol Med 1957; 96:49.
133. Carmena AO, Howard D, Stohlman F. Regulation of erythropoietin. XXII. Production in the newborn animal. Blood 1968; 32:376.
134. Zanjani ED, Foster I, Burlington H, Wasserman LR. Liver as the primary site of erythropoietin formation in the fetus. J Lab Clin Med 1977; 89:640.
135. Miller WL, Thomas RA, Berne RM, Rubio M. Adenosine production in the ischemic kidney. Circ Res 1978; 43:390.
136. Ueno J, Brookins J, Beckman B, Fisher JW. A1 and A2 adenosine receptor regulation of erythropoietin production. Life Sci 1988; 43:229.
137. McCord JM. Oxygen-derived free radicals in post-ischemic tissue injury. N Engl J Med 1985; 312:159.
138. Fink GD, Fisher JW. Stimulation of erythropoiesis by beta adrenergic agonists. I. Characterization of activity in polycythemic mice. J Pharmacol Exp Ther 1977; 202:192.
139. Miyake T, Kung CK-H, Goldwasser E. Purification of human erythropoietin. J Biol Chem 1977; 252:5558.
140. Dordal MS, Wang FF, Goldwasser E. The role of carbohydrate in erythropoietin action. Endocrinology 1985; 116:2293.

141. Wang FF, Kung CK-H, Goldwasser E. Some chemical properties of human erythropoietin. Endocrinology 1985; 116:2286.
142. Egrie J, Strickland TW, Lane J, et al. Characterization and biological effects of recombinant human erythropoietin. Immunobiology 1986; 172:213.
143. Lai PH, Everett R, Wang FF, Arakawa T, Goldwasser E. Structural characterization of human erythropoietin. J Biol Chem 1986; 261:3116.
144. McDonald J, Lin FK, Goldwasser E. Cloning, sequencing and evolutionary analysis of the mouse erythropoietin gene. Mol Cell Biol 1986; 6:842.
145. Davis JM, Arakawa T, Strickland TW, Yphantis DA. Characterization of recombinant human erythropoietin produced in Chinese hamster ovary cells. Biochemistry 1987; 26:2633.
146. Lin FK, Suggs S, Lin CH, et al. Cloning and expression of the human erythropoietin gene. Proc Natl Acad Sci U S A 1985; 82:7580.
147. Iscove NN. The role of erythropoietin in regulation of population size and cell cycling of early and late erythroid precursors in mouse bone marrow. Cell Tissue Kinet 1977; 10:323.
148. Axelrad AA, McLeod DL, Shreeve MM, Heath DS. Properties of cells that produce erythrocytic colonies in vitro. In: Robinson WA, ed. Proceedings of the second international workshop on hemopoiesis in culture. Washington, DC: Government Printing Office, 1974:226.
149. Gregory CJ. Erythropoietin sensitivity as a differentiation marker in the hemopoietic system: studies of three erythropoietic colony responses in culture. J Cell Physiol 1976; 89:289.
150. Krantz SB, Goldwasser E. Specific binding of erythropoietin to spleen cells infected with the anemia strain of Friend virus. Proc Natl Acad Sci U S A 1984; 81:7574.
151. Sawada K, Krantz SB, Kans JS. Purification of human erythroid colony-forming units and demonstration of specific binding of erythropoietin. J Clin Invest 1987; 80:357.
152. D'Andrea AD, Lodish HF, Wong GG. Expression cloning of the murine erythropoietin receptor. Cell 1989; 57:277.

CHAPTER 5

STRUCTURE AND FUNCTION OF INTERLEUKIN-4 AND INTERLEUKIN-5

Donata Vercelli

Harvard Medical School
Boston, Massachusetts

INTRODUCTION

Interleukins 4 and 5 (IL-4 and IL-5) are cytokines involved in the stimulation of inflammatory cells. As with several other cytokines, these mediators were originally described by multiple different names, each reflecting the biological activity attributed to the cytokine. IL-4 acts on B cells and has been described as B cell growth factor or B cell stimulating factor. More recent work has established a role for IL-4 in the regulation of IgE isotype switching and synthesis (described later). The principal function of IL-5 appears to be related to eosinophil differentiation and has been termed eosinophil differentiation factor or eosinophil colony-stimulating factor. Research on the roles of IL-4 and IL-5 moves at a rapid pace, and the availability of purified recombinant material allows better definition of the roles of these important cytokines.

CLONING, STRUCTURE, AND SYNTHESIS OF INTERLEUKIN-4

An expression cloning approach was used to isolate cDNA clones for murine IL-4 from a concanavalin A (ConA)-induced T cell line known to secrete factors with the biological characteristics of BSF-1/IL-4 (induction of major histocompatibility complex class II antigens on mouse B cells and stimulation of T cell growth) (1). Isolation of the mouse IL-4 cDNA clone led to the isolation of a human IL-4 cDNA clone from cDNA libraries obtained from activated human T cell clones (2). The human helper T cell clone 2F1 secretes B cell growth factor, T cell growth factor, GM-CSF (granulocyte-macrophage colony-stimulating factor) and interferon-γ (IFN-γ) activities after stimulation by either ConA or anti-

CD3 antibody and phorbol 12-myristate 13-acetate (PMA). Using cDNA libraries prepared with mRNA isolated from ConA-stimulated 2F1 cells or from PMA- and ConA-stimulated human peripheral blood lymphocytes, several cDNA clones were isolated using the mouse IL-4 cDNA as a probe. Analysis by restriction endonuclease cleavage showed that each of the hybridizing clones was identical in structure, and these clones were designated as human IL-4 cDNAs.

The cDNA insert of the human IL-4 clone is 615 bp long and contains a single open reading frame of 153 codons. Comparison of the IL-4 coding regions in humans and mice revealed that the human IL-4 coding sequences from amino acid 1 to 90 and from amino acid 129 to 149 share ~50% homology with the mouse sequences, whereas little homology is detectable between amino acid 91 and 128 (3). Despite the extensive amino acid sequence homology, IL-4 is highly species specific (4).

Cleavage of the precursor polypeptide for human IL-4 occurs following the glycine residue at position 24. Therefore, the mature polypeptide is 129 amino acids long, beginning with a histidine residue. There are two potential N-glycosylation sites in human IL-4 at positions 62–64 and 129–131. The human cDNA clone transfected in COS7 cells directs the synthesis of proteins of molecular weight 15,000, 18,000 and 19,000. This heterogeneity is thought to result from a difference in the degree of glycosylation, because endoglycosidase treatment abolished the heterogeneity (3).

The IL-4 gene is present in a single copy in the human haploid genome, and with its size of about 10 kb is the largest among known lymphokine genes. It consists of four exons and three introns. Intron 2, the longest, contains a unique feature, TG repeats interrupted by TA sequences, which may play a role in the modulation of gene expression. A conventional TATA-like sequence is located 27 bp upstream of the putative transcription initiation site. Several patches of sequences are found in the 5′-flanking region of the human IL-4 gene that are homologous to sequences upstream of the IL-2, IL-3, IL-5, and GM-CSF genes (3).

The human IL-4 gene has been mapped on chromosome 5 at bands q23–31. It should be noted that the GM-CSF, CSF-1 (macrophage colony-stimulating factor, M-CSF), and *c-fms* (the M-CSF receptor) genes are also assigned to bands q23–31, q33.1, and q33.2–33.3, respectively, on chromosome 5 (3). Deletion of the long arm of chromosome 5 has been observed in malignant cells of patients with acute nonlymphocytic leukemia arising either de novo or secondarily to chemotherapy for cancer. Furthermore, the IL-3 and IL-5 genes were assigned to human chromosome 5. It is tempting to speculate that a family of genes encoding hematopoietic growth factors and their receptors may be clustered within limited regions of a chromosome, thereby coordinately regulating hemopoiesis.

IL-4 was initially recognized as a T cell product. In mice, cloned T cells can be grouped into two subsets based on their ability to secrete different sets of lymphokines. Th1 cells produce IL-2, IFN-γ, and lymphotoxin but not IL-4 or IL-5. In contrast, Th2 cells produce IL-4 and IL-5 but not IL-2 or IFN-γ (5). Differential production of lymphokines has been correlated with in vivo activities of these clones. Th1 are thought to mediate delayed hypersensitivity reactions; Th2 clones are thought to provide help for humoral responses. In humans, however, the Th1/Th2 dichotomy does not seem to exist: most T cell clones in humans are able to secrete IL-4 as well as IL-2 and IFN-γ (6,7). The IL-4 and IL-5 genes are not always coexpressed in activated human T cells: host-reactive T cell clones isolated from a human chimera were unable to produce IL-4 but secreted IL-5, IL-2, IFN-γ, and GM-CSF (8). Interestingly, IL-4 production in T cells is developmentally regulated. In neonatal $CD4^+$ cells, the synthesis of IL-4 is lower compared to adult cells and IL-4 transcription is undetectable (9).

More recently, it has been shown that murine mast cells secrete IL-4 in response to cross-linkage of the high-affinity receptor for IgE or to calcium ionophores (10). Furthermore, Fcε receptor-mediated IL-4 synthesis has been detected in a population of murine spleen cells that lack B cell, T cell, and natural killer (NK) cell markers (11) and are highly enriched in basophils (12). A cell population with similar characteristics has been recently identified in humans (Romagnani S, personal communication). These non-T cells may represent a local source of IL-4 and may be important in such pathological conditions as hyper-IgE syndrome (13) and atopic dermatitis.

FUNCTIONAL PROPERTIES OF HUMAN IL-4

Like all lymphokines, IL-4 is characteristically able to modulate the function of different cell types at different maturation stages.

B Cells

The differentiation of resting B lymphocytes into immunoglobulin-secreting plasma cells occurs through sequential steps: activation (passage from G_0 into G_1 phase), proliferation, and differentiation. Human IL-4 was found to induce human B cell activation as expressed by a small but significant increase in the volume of resting B cells, accompanied by weak stimulation of RNA and protein synthesis (14). In the mouse, stimulation of B cells with IL-4 induces expression of c-*fos* and c-*myc*. Nuclear run-on assays show that c-*myc* expression is primarily regulated posttranscriptionally, whereas c-*fos* expression is regulated at the level of transcription (15). No such data are yet available for human B cells.

Incubation of resting B cells with IL-4 induced a strong expression of the CD23 antigen, the low-affinity receptor for IgE (FcεRII) (16), which is considered a B cell activation marker, and enhanced HLA-DR expression. Concomitant activation of the B cells with anti-IgM antibody, phorbol ester, or *Staphyloccocus aureus* Cowan strain I (SAC) increased the number of cells expressing CD23, as well as the surface density of CD23 (16). The induction of CD23 on normal B cells was specific for IL-4, since IL-1, IL-2, IL-3, IL-5, IFN-γ, and GM-CSF were not active. IL-4-induced CD23 expression was strongly inhibited by IFN-α, IFN-γ, or prostaglandin E_2 (PGE_2) and by pharmacological agents increasing intracellular levels of cAMP.

Human IL-4 was found to modulate B cell proliferation by acting as a costimulant with suboptimal concentrations of anti-IgM antibody and to induce the growth of B cells preactivated with either anti-IgM antibody or SAC (17). Moreover, combinations of IL-4 and anti-CD40 monoclonal antibody (MAb) induced a strong proliferation of B cells preactived with phorbol ester and ionomycin (18). These findings demonstrate that human IL-4 acts as a B cell growth factor.

IL-4 has complex effects on B cell differentiation. SAC-activated B cell blasts were found to secrete IgM and IgG when stimulated with IL-4. No Ig were produced in the absence of in vitro preactivation (19). In contrast, IL-4 selectively suppresses the IL-2-dependent differentiation (but not the proliferation) of antigen-activated human B cells, although IL-4 per se induces substantial proliferation of antigen-activated B cells (20). A blockage of the upregulation of IL-2 receptors (both high and low affinity) induced by IL-2 in normal human B cells activated with SAC may mediate inhibition of IL-2-dependent differentiation by IL-4 (21).

Isotype Switching and IgE Synthesis

The effects of IL-4 on IgE isotype switching deserve a separate discussion because induction of IgE synthesis by IL-4 represents the only well-characterized model of lymphokine-directed immunoglobulin switching in humans to date.

During an immune response, a B lymphocyte can express different heavy-chain isotypes sharing the same VDJ region. This phenomenon (heavy-chain class switching) allows a single B cell clone to produce antibodies that retain variable region specificity in association with a different C_H region gene, that is, with a different effector function. Class switching is thought to result from a recombination event that juxtaposes a downstream C_H gene to the expressed V(D)J gene. Intervening sequences, including the previously expressed C_H gene, are deleted. Recombination involves characteristic repetitive sequences (switch regions, S regions) located 5′ of the $C\mu$ gene and corresponding S regions located immediately 5′ of each C_H gene, except $C\delta$. S regions are 2–10 kb in length, and their sequence consists of short tandem repeats (e.g., GAGCT and GGGCT). S-region recombination sites are not flanked by obvious consensus elements, and joining has been observed at various locations within the S regions (reviewed in Refs. 22 and 23). Switch recombination has generally been thought to occur within one chromosome. However, recent studies in transgenic mice carrying an Ig μ heavy chain transgene show that switch recombination can occur between two different chromosomes (24).

Several studies have suggested that isotype switching is a nonrandom process, directed by mitogens and lymphokines. These agents are thought to control class switching by modulating the accessibility of specific S regions to a putative common switch recombinase (25–29).

Recent studies from various laboratories, including our own, have identified in the cytokine IL-4 a crucial factor for isotype switching to IgE. The role played by IL-4 in the induction of IgE synthesis first became evident in 1986, when it was shown that rIL-4 could induce IgE production by lipopolysaccharide (LPS)-stimulated murine B cells (30,31). More recently, it was shown that IL-4 is by itself sufficient to activate transcription through the ϵ locus. In murine B cells, stimulation with IL-4 induces the appearance of germline C_ϵ transcripts (29,32). The transcripts initiate ~2 kb upstream of the S region involved in switch recombination and are processed to an mRNA in which a 100–500 bp upstream exon (designated exon I) is spliced to the C_H coding exons. The resulting germline transcripts do not appear capable of initiating the synthesis of a mature protein because exon I contains stop codons in all three reading frames. Therefore, germline transcripts are also referred to as "sterile" transcripts. Because exon I is usually 200–300 bp shorter than the VDJ exon present in mature transcripts, germline transcripts are usually 0.2–0.3 kb smaller than mature transcripts.

The ϵ germline transcripts expressed by human B cells following stimulation with IL-4 consist of a ~140 bp I_ϵ exon spliced to $C_{\epsilon 1}$ by removal of the intervening sequences from the primary transcript (33). The germline transcript contains all four $C\epsilon$ exons, as well as the 3′-untranslated region. Interestingly, ϵ germline transcripts were also induced in resting B cells isolated by Percoll density gradients, indicating that no previous in vivo activation is required for expression of ϵ germline transcripts following IL-4 stimulation (34).

The precise role of germline transcripts in isotype switching remains to be defined. All germline transcripts initiate 5′ of the switch region, consistent with the possibility that transcription through a targeted region may be directly involved in promoting accessibility. However, other possibilities, not necessarily mutually exclusive, should be considered. Transcription may be a by-product of other events (e.g., binding of specific factors) involved in promoting recombinational accessibility. In addition, germline transcripts may themselves play a role in recombination events. The germline transcripts characterized thus far share a similar general structure: each consists of a 5′ exon derived from germline sequences upstream of the corresponding S region that is spliced to the C_{H1} gene immediately downstream. These structural similarities suggest an analogous function, although the different transcripts contain no significant sequence homologies. Germline RNA transcription may result in increased accessibility of the downstream S region for deletional switch recombination. Alternatively, germline transcripts could conceivably be used in interchromosomal RNA transsplicing, whereby transcripts from rearranged V(D)J exons are joined to C_H germline transcripts (35). This process, which would result in heavy-chain class switching in the absence of deletional DNA rearrangement in the heavy-chain locus, was recently identified as the mechanism underlying multiple Ig isotype expression in a transgenic mouse model (36). For an extensive review of the molecular mechanisms underlying IgE synthesis, see Ref. 37.

T Cells

Human IL-4 promoted the growth of T cell blasts (both $CD4^+$ and $CD8^+$) preactivated with phytohemagglutinin (PHA) (2). An analysis of the responsiveness of a series of $CD4^+$ and $CD8^+$ T cell clones with different functions and specificities revealed that almost all clones can respond to IL-4 (38). In addition, low but significant growth promotion by IL-4 was observed with $CD3^-$NK clones. The growth-promoting effect of IL-4 seems to require preactivation of T cells, since highly purified resting T cells that do not express HLA-DR or transferrin receptor do not respond to human IL-4 (38).

IL-4 increases IL-2 production in response to accessory cell-independent stimuli (plate-bound anti-CD3), although it is not essential for IL-2 production in response to accessory cell-dependent stimuli (soluble anti-CD3 and mitogens) (39). In contrast, IL-4 is a potent inhibitor of IL-2-induced proliferation of normal human T cells stimulated with a low concentration of anti-CD3 MAb. Inhibition is associated (and likely mediated) with a marked reduction of IL-2 receptor expression (40). Interestingly, activation and culturing of human $CD4^+$ T cell clones in IL-4 resulted in the acquisition of CD8 due to de novo synthesis. IL-4-induced expression of CD8 is reversible in that CD8 disappeared from double-positive T cell clones isolated in IL-4, when they were cultured in IL-2. CD8 was functional because an anti-CD8 MAb inhibited cytotoxicity mediated by a double-positive clone (41).

Human IL-4 is unable to induce lymphokine activated killing (LAK) activity against target cells that are not sensitive to fresh NK activity and strongly inhibits the IL-2-mediated induction of LAK cell activity (14). Moreover, IL-4 also inhibited the induction of LAK activity induced in $CD3^-$ NKH-1^+ cells, suggesting that the LAK precursor cell is the target of the inhibitory effect of IL-4. IL-4 did not inhibit the activity of LAK cells once they were activated by IL-2, since lymphocytes activated for 24–48 h with IL-2 and subsequently incubated with IL-2 plus IL-4 developed LAK activity similar to that in cells incubated only with IL-2. Moreover, incubation of T cell clones that have all the phenotypic characteristics of LAK cells ($CD3^-$NKH-1^+ or $CD3^+CD16^+$NKH-1^+) with IL-4 did not affect the cytotoxicity of these clones against the NK-insensitive target cell Daudi. Interestingly, IL-4 inhibited the induction of IL-4-mediated cytotoxic activities of thymocytes against NK-insensitive target cells and also against the NK-sensitive target cell K562 (14). This latter observation suggests that IL-4 plays a negative regulatory role in the differentiation of NK cells.

IL-4 did not inhibit the generation of antigen-specific cytotoxic T cells (CTL) in mixed leukocyte cultures (MLC) but rather enhanced this activity. In contrast, antigen-nonspecific cytotoxic activities that are generated in MLC are strongly blocked when IL-4 is present during the MLC. These results suggest that nonspecific cytotoxic activities in MLC are generated via IL-2 produced by the responder T cells. More importantly, these findings demonstrate that IL-4 is not an inhibitor of the generation of cytotoxic activities in general but that this activity of IL-4 is only restricted to those cytotoxic activities induced by IL-2 (14). The mechanism of this inhibition of IL-2-mediated induction of cytotoxic activity by IL-4 is still unclear.

Monocytes

IL-4 has an important role in the downregulation of monocyte-mediated inflammatory responses. IL-4 inhibits human mononuclear phagocyte superoxide anion production, and it promotes phagocyte differentiation (42). Furthermore, IL-4 inhibits the synthesis of the chemotactic peptide IL-8 by human monocytes stimulated with LPS, IL-1, and tumor necrosis factor (TNF) (43), but it decreases the membrane expression of Fcγ receptors I, II, and III; this effect correlated with a decrease in FcγR-mediated cytotoxic activity (44).

IL-4 downregulates the expression of CD14 (45), a glycosylphosphatidylinositol-linked protein expressed on mature monocytes. CD14 is the receptor for the LPS/LPS-binding protein complex and, furthermore, plays an important role in monocyte activation (46) and monocyte-T cell interactions (47).

IL-4 induces the expression of CD23 on normal human monocytes. CD23 induction was detectable both by flow cytometry and by immunoprecipitation.

CD23 was fully expressed after a 24 h incubation with rIL-4 and was still detectable after 72 h from the addition of IL-4. This effect was specific, because none of the other recombinant interleukins tested (IL-1, IL-2, IL-3, IL-5, IL-6, GM-CSF, and IFN-γ) could induce FcεR2/CD23, either alone or in various combinations. No synergism was observed between IL-4 and other interleukins. IFN-γ was not able to inhibit the IL-4-induced expression of CD23 on monocytes, neither when added to the culture together with IL-4 nor when added 36 h earlier (48). IL-4 selectively augments the expression of HLA-DR and HLA-DP antigens, but not HLA-DQ (49).

Other Cells

IL-4 suppresses IgG-mediated but not IgE-mediated human eosinophil degranulation, as well as eosinophil-mediated antibody-dependent killing of schistosomula of *Schistosoma mansoni*. Furthermore, IL-4 suppresses IgG receptor expression but not IgE receptor expression. Taken together, these results indicate a mechanism for T lymphocyte suppression of IgG-stimulated eosinophil functions via IL-4 (50).

IL-4 increases the adhesiveness of human endothelial cells for T cells, but not for neutrophils. Increased binding results from induction of an as yet unidentified receptor on the endothelial cell membrane (51). Furthermore, IL-4 synergizes with TNF and IFN-γ in causing a change in shape to a more fibroblastic morphology (52). IL-4 may thus play a role in the selective recruitment of T cells into sites of immune-mediated chronic inflammation, as well as in the development and maintenance of chronic inflammatory responses.

IL-4 also affects skin fibroblasts: IL-4 decreases the TNF-dependent synthesis of factor B, whereas the TNF-dependent synthesis of C3 is increased (53). IL-4 induces expression of intercellular adhesion molecule-1 (ICAM-1) antigen and ICAM-1 RNA in human mast cells. IL-4 also upregulates ICAM-1 expression in monocyte-macrophages but not in basophils, fibroblasts, or lymphocytes (54).

IL-4 acts on hematopoietic progenitors. It synergizes with erythropoietin and granulocyte colony-stimulating factor to enhance the formation of erythroid and granulocytic colonies, respectively (55), whereas it inhibits macrophage colony formation in response to GM-CSF or macrophage CSF (56). This last effect may be due to the blockage of proliferation of monocyte-committed progenitor cells and may be related to the ability of IL-4 to induce differentiation of mononuclear phagocytes (see earlier).

Interactions Between IL-4 and Other Lymphokines

Several lymphokines have been reported to functionally interact with IL-4. The most pervasive interaction is perhaps the one described for IFN-γ. Interferon-γ has been reported to inhibit IL-4-dependent IgE synthesis in both mice (30) and humans (57,58). IFN-γ also antagonizes the effects of IL-4 in other systems; for example, it blocks the IL-4-dependent induction of FcεR2/CD23 on B cells (16), although not on monocytes (48). The mechanisms by which IFN-γ antagonizes IL-4-dependent effects are not well understood. IFN-γ profoundly suppressed the expression of ε germline transcripts in murine B cells stimulated with IL-4 and LPS (59). In contrast, no inhibition was observed when IFN-γ was added to highly purified human B cells stimulated with IL-4 (33), suggesting that activation of germline transcription and switch recombination may not be necessarily coupled. Unlike IFN-γ, the lymphokine TGF-β has been recently reported to suppress both ε germline transcription and IgE synthesis in human B cells stimulated with IL-4 (de Vries, personal communication). For isotypes other than IgE, TGF-β is known to inhibit the switch from the membrane form to the secreted form of Ig mRNA (60). It is unclear whether this effect plays a role in TGF-β-dependent inhibition of IgE induction.

IL-4 induces IL-6 production by B cells (61) and endothelial cells and is thus likely to play a role in vascular inflammation (62). Furthermore, endigenous IL-6 is critical for IL-4-dependent induction of IgE synthesis both in T cell-dependent (63) and T cell-independent (64,65) systems. IL-6 is known to act at a late stage in B cell differentiation, with no isotype preference (66). IL-6 induces the secretion of IgG_1 by coordinated transcriptional activation, selective accumulation of mRNA for the secreted form of IgG, and possibly differential mRNA stabilization (67). IL-6 may amplify IgE secretion by similar mechanisms.

IL-4 inhibits IL-1β production by normal human monocytes both at the transcriptional level (by suppressing the formation of new transcripts), as well as posttranscriptionally (by decreasing IL-1 message stability). These effects require protein synthesis (68). IL-4 also suppresses TNF-α production by monocytes (69,70).

IL-4 and Disease

A clue to a potential role of IL-4 in disease has been provided by recent studies with T cell clones obtained from patients with atopic disease and parasitic infections. $CD4^+$ T cell clones established from atopic patients and specific for *Dermatophagoides pteronyssinus* and *Lolium perenne* produced very highly levels of IL-4 and IL-5 and very low levels of IFN-γ compared to $CD4^+$ T cell clones from the same patients not specific for allergens or $CD4^+$ clones from healthy individuals. These allergen-specific, IL-4-producing T cell clones strongly supported the induction of IgE synthesis (71–73). Furthermore, the vast majority of helper T cell clones isolated from patients with filariasis, toxocariasis, and ascaridiasis produced high levels of IL-4 (74). Because IL-4 production is known to require repeated antigen stimulation (75), these data seem to suggest that chronic stimulation by selected antigens (allergens) may select for allergen-specific T cells in individuals whose T cells are intrinsically prone to secrete large amounts of IL-4 upon activation. Furthermore, it has been reported that Th2-like T cell clones, which produce IL-4 but not IFN-γ and provide help for IgE synthesis, accumulate in the conjunctiva of patients with vernal conjunctivitis, and may play a role in the pathogenesis of the disease (76).

Another disease in which IL-4 may be implicated is the hyperimmunoglobulin E (HIE) syndrome, a complex disorder characterized by high levels of serum IgE, chronic dermatitis, and recurrent serious infections (77). The etiology of the HIE syndrome is unknown. HIE patients have very large numbers of circulating IgE-secreting B cells (~1:100,000 B lymphocytes, compared to 0.4:100,000 in normal subjects and ~10:100,000 in patients with lymphatic filariasis) (78). This suggests that clonal expansion of IgE-producing B cells may be a major mechanism underlying elevated IgE production in HIE syndrome. There is evidence to suggest that HIE patients have T cell defects, which include impaired in vivo and in vitro T cell-mediated responses to specific antigens and defective antibody responses, particularly to polysaccharides (reviewed in Refs. 79 and 80). The mechanisms responsible for increased IgE production in the HIE syndrome are unknown. We investigated the role played by cellular interactions and lymphokines in the regulation of spontaneous IgE synthesis by PBMC from patients with the HIE syndrome. Our data indicated that spontaneous in vitro IgE synthesis in the HIE syndrome is largely independent of endogenous lymphokines (IL-4 and IL-6) and T-B cell cognate interactions and is likely to be due to a terminally differentiated B cell population, no longer sensitive to regulatory signals known to modulate IgE induction in normals (13).

A definitive conclusion is difficult to draw at the present time, however, because IL-4 secretion in vitro could only be detected following activation with PMA and ionophore, a rather nonphysiological type of stimulation. Thus, although no simple causal relation is to be established between increased IgE production and lymphokine secretion in HIE patients, we cannot rule out the possibility that hyperproduction of IL-4 (absolute or relative to IFN-γ) may occur in vivo at a local and/or peripheral level, escaping our detection. In this respect, it has been observed that most circulating B cells from patients with hyper-IgE states bear CD23 on the membrane (T. Kishimoto, unpublished observation). This indirectly suggests that IL-4 may be abnormally secreted in HIE patients because the expression of FcϵR2b on B cells is IL-4 dependent (81). The frequent finding of eosinophilia in patients with the HIE syndrome (80) also supports this hypothesis because eosinophil differentiation is induced by IL-5 (82), which is produced by T cell clones concomitantly with IL-4 (83,84).

Finally, the intriguing possibility should be considered that IL-4 in HIE syndrome be derived, at least in part, from a local non-T cell source, such as mast cells and/or basophils (see earlier). The B cell activating signal required for IgE synthesis may be provided by polyclonal activators (such as Epstein-Barr virus EBV or other viruses or CD40 ligands yet to be identified) acting directly on B cells (64,85,86). It is tempting to speculate that hyperproduction of IgE in the HIE syndrome may derive, at least in part, from T cell-independent mechanisms.

CLONING, STRUCTURE, AND SYNTHESIS OF INTERLEUKIN-5

Cloning of human IL-5 was achieved following the same strategy that led to isolation of human IL-4. The human helper T cell clone HG120 produces a B cell growth factor activity distinct from that of IL-4 following stimulation by anti-CD3 antibody and PMA. By screening $\sim 10^4$ independent cDNA clones from stimulated HG120 cells, two clones were obtained that hybridized with the mouse IL-5 cDNA probe. As expected, the product of the human IL-4 cDNA has T cell and B cell stimulatory activities, whereas the human IL-5 cDNA enhances IgA production and acts as a colony-stimulating factor for eosinophils (87).

The nucleotide sequences of human IL-5 (clone 115) is 815 base pairs long and contains a single open reading frame of 134 codons (87). Cleavage of the human IL-5 precursor would occur following the alanine residue at positions 19. Therefore, the mature polypeptide of human IL-5 would be 125 amino acid residues long in the secreted molecule with a molecular weight of ~14,000 and would begin with an isoleucine residue. Biosynthetic labeling of proteins of COS-7 cells transfected with the human IL-5 clone produced a protein in the cultured supernatants with an apparent molecular weight of 20,000 under reducing conditions. The discrepancy between the predicted and observed sizes of IL-5 may be due to glycosylation of the molecules, which is predicted by the presence of two potential N-glycosylation sequences (Asn-Xaa-Thr or Asn-Xaa-Ser at positions 47–49 and 90–92). Under nonreducing conditions, human IL-5 migrates with an apparent molecular weight of 45,000, suggesting that it exists as a dimer. The activity of IL-5 is relatively nonspecies specific; that is, mouse IL-5 can stimulate human target cells and human IL-5 can react with mouse target cells (87). In contrast, activity of mouse and human IL-4 is species specific (88).

Functional Properties of Human IL-5

The ability to induce eosinophil differentiation is the most distinctive functional property of human IL-5. By using suspension cultures of mononuclear cells from human cord blood and bone marrow, it was shown that IL-5 induced the selective differentiation and proliferation of eosinophils. After 3 weeks in culture with IL-5, essentially all nonadherent cells in those cultures became eosinophilic myelocytes, whereas culture of the same cells with IL-4 resulted in the selective growth of $CD3^+$ lymphocytes (82). The primary role of IL-5 in the development of the eosinophilic lineage was further confirmed by the finding of markedly increased levels of IL-5 in patients with helminth-induced eosinophilia (but IL-3 and GM-CSF were normal) (89) and in patients with idiopathic hypereosinophilic syndrome (90). Furthermore, it was shown that purified T cells from asthmatic patients spontaneously secrete factors that prolong the life span of eosinophils in vitro and that are identical to IL-5 and GM-CSF (91).

We recently studied an alloreactive human T cell clone, A1, that was analogous to a murine Th2 clone in that it produced IL-4 and IL-5, but not IL-2 or IFN-γ (83). Supernatants from clone A1 induced the differentiation of eosinophil progenitors present in normal human cord blood into mature eosinophils. Electron microscopy studies demonstrated that mature eosinophils, displaying motile shapes and diminished numbers of large specific granules, developed in cultures of human umbilical cord blood mononuclear cells grown for 5 weeks in A1 supernatants (83).

The coordinate synthesis and secretion by a single alloreactive T cell clone of IL-4 and IL-5 has important implications for the amplification of the immune response. Indeed, IL-4 induces not only IgE synthesis but also the expression of low-affinity Fcε receptors (FcεR2/CD23) on B cells (16) and monocytes (48). The interaction between IgE and FcεR2/CD23 induces the release of such monocyte mediators as leukotrienes (92) and has been postulated to modulate signal transduction by B cell growth factors (93,94). Finally, IL-5 induces eosinophil maturation. Thus, the synthesis of both IL-4 and IL-5 by a single T cell clone may be important in the activation of multiple components of the immune response.

IgA is the predominant Ig class expressed in mucosal secretions. The regulation of B cell differentiation into IgA production has been extensively investigated, in particular at the level of Peyer's patches (PP) in the mouse model. Several studies have shown that, in PP, IgM B cells undergo differentiation, which results in an isotype switch to IgA. Switching is regulated by "switch" and "postswitch" T cells, of which PP represent a very rich source. Induction of polyclonal IgA secretion was found to be dependent on the interaction of B cells with a mixture of dendritic cells and T cells derived from PP, but not from the spleen (95). Furthermore, PP T cells, but not spleen T cells, induce LPS-stimulated slgM$^+$ B cells to switch to slgA$^+$ cells (96).

In 1987, it was reported that the lymphokine IL-5, produced by either PP T cells or T cell clones, selectively enhances IgA secretion by LPS-triggered murine B cells. The magnitude of the IL-5-dependent IgA response was increased by IL-4 (97–100). The stage of B cell differentiation at which IL-5 acts is at present under investigation, but conflicting evidence has come from different experimental systems. In LPS-stimulated cultures of PP B cells, IL-5 induces the secretion of large amounts of IgA by sIgA$^+$, but not by sIgA$^-$ cells, without affecting cell proliferation or the expression of sIgA by sIgM$^+$ B cell (101). This indicates that IL-5 is a "postswitch" IgA B cell differentiation factor, which acts on B cells that have already undergone isotype switch to IgA.

Furthermore, a comparison of the effects of IL-4 and IL-5 on isotype secretion by PP and splenic B cells, stimulated with LPS or autoreactive T cells, has indicated that PP and splenic B cells show a similar increase in IgA secretion upon LPS stimulation; T cell-stimulated cultures of PP cells show a higher IgA response than splenic B cells. The majority of secreted IgA comes from sIgA$^-$ cells in LPS-driven cultures and from sIgA$^+$ cells in cultures stimulated by T cells (102). On the other hand, another study indicates that, in the absence of any additional B cell trigger, PP B cell, but not splenic B cell cultures, synthesize IgA in response to rIL-5. Under such conditions, rIL-4 does not upregulate the IL-5-dependent IgA response. The PP B cell subset that responds to IL-5 by secreting IgA is in cell cycle and expresses IgA on the surface (103). Despite the discrepancies, all these results point at the crucial role of IL-5 in IgA differentiation. Further studies are necessary to define the targets and mechanisms of action of this lymphokine, and its precise role in IgA-specific isotype switching.

In conclusion, it should be added that IL-5 also seems to play a role in IgE synthesis. We have shown that IL-5 upregulates the IgE response induced by IL-4 in unfractionated mononuclear cells. IgE upregulation by rIL-5 was more evident when suboptimal concentrations of rIL-4 were used.

REFERENCES

1. Lee F, Yokota T, Otsuka T, et al. Isolation and characterization of a mouse interleukin cDNA clone that expresses B-cell stimulatory factor 1 activities and T-cell- and mast-cell-stimulating activities. Proc Natl Acad Sci U S A 1986; 83:2061.
2. Yokota T, Otsuka T, Mosmann T, et al. Isolation and characterization of a human interleukin cDNA clone, homologous to mouse B-cell stimulatory factor 1, that expresses B-cell- and T-cell-stimulating activities. Proc Natl Acad Sci U S A 1986; 83:5894.
3. Arai N, Nomura D, Villaret D, et al. Complete nucleotide sequence of the chromosomal gene for human IL-4 and its expression. J Immunol 1989; 142:274.
4. Mosmann TR, Yokota T, Kastelein R, Zurawski SM, Arai N, Takebe Y. Species-specificity of T cell stimulating activities of IL-2 and BSF-1 (IL-4): comparison of

normal and recombinant mouse and human IL-2 and BSF-1 (IL-4). J Immunol 1987; 138:1813.

5. Mosmann TR, Cherwinski H, Bond, MW, Giedlin M, Coffman RL. Two types of murine helper T cell clone. I. Definition according to profiles of lymphokine activities and secreted proteins. J Immunol 1986; 136:2348.
6. Umetsu DT, Jabara HH, DeKruyff R, Abbas AK, Abrams JS, Geha RS. Functional heterogeneity among human inducer T cell clones. J Immunol 1988; 140:4211.
7. Paliard X, de Waal Malefijt R, Yssel H, Blanchard D, Chretien I, Abrams J, de Vries JE, Spits H. Simultaneous production of IL-2, IL-4, and IFN-γ by activated human $CD4^+$ and $CD8^+$ T cell clones. J Immunol 1988; 141:849.
8. Bacchetta R, de Waal Malefijt R, Yssel H, et al. Host-reactive $CD4^+$ and $CD8^+$ T cell clones isolated from a human chimera produce IL-5, IL-2, IFN-γ and granulocyte/macrophage-colony-stimulating factor but not IL-4. J Immunol 1990; 144:902.
9. Lewis DB, Yu CC, Meyer J, English BK, Kahn SJ, Wilson CB. Cellular and molecular mechanisms for reduced interleukin 4 and interferon-γ production by neonatal cells. J Clin Invest 1991; 87:194.
10. Plaut M, Pierce JH, Watson CJ, Hanley-Hyde J, Nordan RP, Paul WE. Mast cell lines produce lymphokines in response to cross-linkage of FcεRI or to calcium ionophores. Nature 1989; 339:64.
11. Ben-Sasson SZ, Le Gros G, Conrad DH, Finkelman FD, Paul WE. Cross-linking Fc receptors stimulate splenic non-B, non-T cells to secrete interleukin 4 and other lymphokines. Proc Natl Acad Sci U S A 1990; 87:1421.
12. Seder RA, Paul WE, Dvorak AM, et al. Mouse splenic and bone marrow cell populations that express high-affinity Fcε receptors and produce interleukin 4 are highly enriched in basophils. Proc Natl Acad Sci U S A 1991; 88:2835.
13. Vercelli D, Jabara HH, Cunningham-Rundles C, et al. Regulation of Immunoglobulin (Ig)E synthesis in the Hyper-IgE syndrome. J Clin Invest 1990; 85:1666.
14. Yokota T, Arai N, de Vries J, et al. Molecular biology of interleukin 4 and interleukin 5 genes and biology of their products that stimulate B cells, T cells and hemopoietic cells. Immunol Rev 1988; 102:137.
15. Klemsz MJ, Justement LB, Palmer E, Cambier JC. Induction of *c-fos* and *c-myc* expression during B cell activation by IL-4 and immunoglobulin binding ligands. J Immunol 1989; 143:1032.
16. Defrance T, Aubry J, Rousset F, et al. Human recombinant interleukin 4 induces Fcε receptors (CD23) on normal B lymphocytes. J Exp Med 1987; 165:1459.
17. Defrance T, Vanbervliet B, Aubry JP, et al. B cell growth-promoting activity of recombinant human interleukin 4. J Immunol 1987; 139:1135.
18. Clark EA, Shu GL, Lüscher B, et al. Activation of human B cells—comparison of the signal transduced by IL-4 to four different competence signals. J Immunol 1989; 143:3873.
19. Defrance T, Vanbervliet B, Pene J, Banchereau J. Human recombinant IL-4 induces activated B lymphocytes to produce IgG and IgM. J Immunol 1988; 141:2000.
20. Llorente L, Mitjavi F, Crevon M-C, Galanaud P. Dual effects of interleukin 4 on antigen-activated human B cells: induction of proliferation and inhibition of interleukin-2-dependent differentiation. Eur J Immunol 1990; 20:1887.
21. Lee HK, Xia X, Choi YS. IL-4 blocks the up-regulation of IL-2 receptors induced by IL-2 in normal human B cells. J Immunol 1990; 144:3431.
22. Blackwell TK, Alt FW. In: Hames BD, Glover DM, eds. Molecular immunology. Oxford: IRL Press, 1988:1.
23. Esser C, Radbruch A. Immunoglobulin class switching: molecular and cellular analysis. Annu Rev Immunol 1990; 8:717.

24. Gerstein RM, Frankel WN, Hsieh C-L, et al. Isotype switching of an immunoglobulin heavy chain transgene occurs by DNA recombination between different chromosomes. Cell 1990; 63:537.
25. Yancopoulos GD, DePinho RA, Zimmerman KA, Lutzker SG, Rosenberg N, Alt FW. Secondary genomic rearrangement events in pre-B cells: V_HDJ_H replacement by a LINE-1 sequence and directed class switching. EMBO J 1986; 5:3259.
26. Stavnezer-Nordgren J, Sirlin S. Specificity of immunoglobulin heavy chain switch correlates with activity of germline heavy chain genes prior to switching. EMBO J 1986; 5:95.
27. Lutzker S, Rothman P, Pollock R, Coffman R, Alt FW. Mitogen- and IL-4-regulated expression of germ-line Ig γ2b transcripts: evidence for directed heavy chain class switching. Cell 1988; 53:177.
28. Lutzker S, Alt FW. Structure and expression of germ line immunoglobulin γ2b transcripts. Mol Cell Biol 1988; 8:1849.
29. Stavnezer J, Radcliffe G, Lin Y-C, et al. Immunoglobulin heavy-chain switching may be directed by prior induction of transcripts from constant-region genes. Proc Natl Acad Sci U S A 1988; 85:7704.
30. Coffman RL, Carty J. A T cell activity that enhances polyclonal IgE production and its inhibition by Interferon-γ. J Immunol 1986; 136:949.
31. Coffman RL, Ohara J, Bond MW, Carty J, Zlotnik A, Paul WE. B cell stimulatory factor-1 enhances the IgE response of lipopolysaccharide-activated B cells. J Immunol 1986; 136:4538.
32. Rothman P, Lutzker S, Cook W, Coffman R, Alt FW. Mitogen plus interleukin 4 induction of Cε transcripts in B lymphoid cells. J Exp Med 1988; 168:2385.
33. Gauchat J-F, Lebman DA, Coffman RL, Gascan H, de Vries JE. Structure and expression of germline ε transcripts in human B cells induced by interleukin 4 to switch to IgE production. J Exp Med 1990; 172:463.
34. Shapira SK, Vercelli D, Jabara HH, Fu SM, Geha RS. Molecular analysis of the induction of IgE synthesis in human B cells by IL-4 and engagement of CD40 antigen. J Exp Med (in press).
35. Durdik J, Gerstein RM, Rath S, Robbins PF, Nisonoff A, Selsing E. Isotype switching by a microinjected μ immunoglobulin heavy chain gene in transgenic mice. Proc Natl Acad Sci U S A 1989; 86:2346.
36. Shimizu A, Nussenzweig MC, Han H, Sanchez M, Honjo T. Trans-splicing as a possible molecular mechanism for the multiple isotype expression of the immunoglobulin gene. J Exp Med 1991; 173:1385.
37. Vercelli D, Geha RS. Regulation of IgE synthesis in humans: a tale of two signals. J Allergy Clin Immunol 1991;
38. Spits H, Yssel H, Takebe Y, et al. Recombinant interleukin 4 promotes the growth of human T cells. J Immunol 1987; 139:1142.
39. Tanaka T, Ben-Sasson SZ, Paul WE. IL-4 increases IL-2 production by T cells in response to accessory cell-independent stimuli. J Immunol 1991; 146:3831.
40. Martinez OM, Gibbons RS, Garovoy MR, Aronson FR. IL-4 inhibits IL-2 receptor expression and IL-2-dependent proliferation of human T cells J Immunol 1990; 144:2211.
41. Paliard X, de Waal Malefijt R, de Vries JE, Spits H. Interleukin-4 mediates CD8 induction on human $CD4^+$ T-cell clones. Nature 1988; 335:642.
42. Abramson SL, Gallin JI. IL-4 inhibits superoxide production by human mononuclear phagocytes. J Immunol 1990; 144:625.
43. Standiford TJ, Strieter RM, Chensue SW, Westwick J, Kasahara K, Kunkel SL. IL-4 inhibits the expression of IL-8 from stimulated human monocytes. J Immunol 1990; 145:1435.

44. Te Velde AA, Huijbens RJF, de Vries JE, Figdor CG. IL-4 decreases FcγR membrane expression and FcγR-mediated cytotoxic activity of human monocytes. J Immunol 1990; 144:3046.
45. Lauener RPL, Goyert SM, Geha RS, Vercelli D. Interleukin 4 down-regulates the expression of CD14 in normal human monocytes. Eur J Immunol 1990; 20:2375.
46. Lauener RP, Geha RS, Vercelli D. Engagement of the monocyte surface antigen CD14 induces lymphocyte function-associated antigen-1/intercellular adhesion molecule-1-dependent homotypic adhesion. J Immunol 1990; 145:1390.
47. Lue K-H, Lauener RP, Winchester RJ, Geha RS, Vercelli D. Engagement of CD14 on human monocytes terminates T cell proliferation by delivering a negative signal to T cells. J Immunol 1991;
48. Vercelli D, Jabara HH, Lee B, Woodland N, Geha RS, Leung DYM. Human recombinant interleukin 4 induces FcεR2/CD23 on normal human monocytes. J Exp Med 1988; 167:1406.
49. Gerrard TL, Dyer DR, Mostowski HS. IL-4 and granulocyte-macrophage colony-stimulating factor selectively increase HLA-DR and HLA-DP antigens but not HLA-DQ antigens on human monocytes. J Immunol 1990; 4670.
50. Baskar P, Silberstein DS, Pincus SH. Inhibition of IgG-triggered human eosinophil function by IL-4. J Immunol 1990; 144:2321.
51. Thornhill MH, Kyan-Aung U, Haskard DO. IL-4 increases human endothelial cell adhesiveness for T cells but not for neutrophils. J Immunol 1990; 144:3060.
52. Thornhill MH, Haskard DO. IL-4 regulates endothelial cell activation by IL-1, tumor necrosis factor, or IFN-γ. J Immunol 1990; 145:865.
53. Katz Y, Strunk RC. Enhanced synthesis of factor B induced by tumor necrosis factor in human skin fibroblasts is decreased by IL-4. J Immunol 1990; 144:4675.
54. Valent P, Bevec D, Maurer D, et al. Interleukin 4 promotes expression of mast cell ICAM-1 antigen. Proc Natl Acad Sci U S A 1991; 88:3339.
55. Bronxmeyer HE, Lu L, Cooper S, et al. Synergistic effects of purified recombinant human and murine B cell growth factor-1/IL-4 on colony formation in vitro by hematopoietic progenitor cells. J Immunol 1988; 141:3852.
56. Jansen JH, Wientjens G-JHM, Fibbe WE, Willemze R, Kluin-Nelemans HC. Inhibition of human macrophage colony formation by interleukin 4. J Exp Med 1989; 170:577.
57. Pene J, Rousset F, Briere F, et al. IgE production by normal human lymphocytes is induced by interleukin 4 and suppressed by interferons γ and α and prostaglandin E_2. Proc Natl Acad Sci U S A 1988; 85:6880.
58. Del Prete GF, Maggi E, Parronchi P, et al. IL-4 is an essential factor for the IgE synthesis induced in vitro by human T cell clones and their supernatants. J Immunol 1988; 140:4193.
59. Severinson E, Fernandez C, Stavnezer J. Induction of germ-line immunoglobulin heavy chain transcripts by mitogens and interleukins prior to switch recombination. Eur J Immunol 1990; 20:1079.
60. Kehrl JH, Thevenin C, Rieckmann P, Fauci AS. Transforming growth factor-β suppresses human B lymphocyte Ig production by inhibiting synthesis and the switch from the membrane form to the secreted form of Ig mRNA. J Immunol 1991; 146:4016.
61. Smeland EB, Blomhoff HK, Funderud S, Shalaby RR, Espevik T. Interleukin 4 induces selective production of interleukin 6 from normal human B lymphocytes. J Exp Med 1989; 170:1463.
62. Howells G, Pham P, Taylor D, Foxwell B, Feldmann M. Interleukin 4 induces interleukin 6 production by endothelial cells: synergy with interferon-γ. Eur J Immunol 1991; 21:97.

63. Vercelli D, Jabara HH, Arai K, Yokota T, Geha RS. Endogenous IL-6 plays an obligatory role in IL-4 induced human IgE synthesis. Eur J Immunol 1989; 14:1419.
64. Jabara HH, Fu SM, Geha RS, Vercelli D. CD40 and IgE: synergism between anti-CD40 mAb and IL-4 in the induction of IgE synthesis by highly purified human B cells. J Exp Med 1990; 172:1861.
65. Jabara HH, Ahern DJ, Vercelli D, Geha RS. in press. Hydrocortisone and IL-4 induce IgE isotype switching in human B cells. J Immunol
66. Muraguchi A, Hirano T, Tang B, et al. The essential role of B cell stimulatory factor 2 (BSF-2/IL-6) for the terminal differentiation of B cells. J Exp Med 1988; 167:332.
67. Raynal M-C, Liu Z, Hirano T, Mayer L, Kishimoto T, Chen-kiang S. Interleukin 6 induces secretion of IgG_1 by coordinated transcriptional activation and differential mRNA accumulation. Proc Natl Acad Sci U S A 1989; 86:8024.
68. Donnelly RP, Fenton MJ, Kaufman JD, Gerrard TL. IL-1 expression in human monocytes is transcriptionally and posttranscriptionally regulated by IL-4. J Immunol 1991; 146:3431.
69. Essner R, Rhoades K, McBride WH, Morton DL, Economou JS. IL-4 down-regulates IL-1 and TNF gene expression in human monocytes. J Immunol 1989; 142:3857.
70. Hart PH, Vitti GF, Burgess DR, Whitty GA, Piccoli DS, Hamilton JA. Potential antiinflammatory effects of interleukin 4: suppression of human monocyte tumor necrosis factor α, interleukin 1, and prostaglandin E_2. Proc Natl Acad Sci U S A 1989; 86:3803.
71. Wierenga EA, Snoek M, Bos JD, Jansen HM, Kapsenberg ML. Comparison of diversity and function of house dust mite-specific T lymphocyte clones from atopic and non-atopic donors. Eur J Immunol 1990; 20:1519.
72. Wierenga EA, Snoek M, de Groot C, et al. Evidence for compartimentalization of functinal subsets of $CD4^+$ T lymphocytes in atopic patients. J Immunol 1990; 144:4651.
73. Parronchi P, Macchia D, Piccinni M-P, et al. Allergen- and bacterial antigen-specific T-cell clones established from atopic donors show a different profile of cytokine production. Proc Natl Acd Sci U S A 1991; 88:4538.
74. Romagnani S. Regulation and deregulation of human IgE synthesis. Immunol Today 1990; 11:316.
75. Powers GD, Abbas AK, Miller RA. Frequencies of IL-2- and IL-4-secreting T cells in naive and antigen-stimulated lymphocyte populations. J Immunol 1988; 140:3352.
76. Maggi E, Biswas P, Del Prete GF, et al. Accumulation of Th-2-like helper T cells in the conjunctiva of patients with vernal conjunctivitis. J Immunol 1991; 146:1169.
77. Buckley RH, Becker WG. Abnormalities in the regulation of human IgE synthesis. Immunol Rev 1978; 41:288.
78. King CL, Pointdexter RW, Ragunathan J, Fleisher TA, Ottesen EA, Nutman TB. Frequency analysis of IgE-secreting B lymphocytes in persons with normal or elevated serum IgE levels. J Immunol 1991; 146:1478.
79. Leung DYM, Geha RS. Clinical and immunologic aspects of the hyperimmunoglobulin E syndrome. Hematol Oncol Clin North Am 1988; 2:81.
80. Geha RS, Leung DYM. Hyper immunoglobulin E syndrome. Immunodeficiency Rev 1989; 1:155.
81. Yokota A, Kikutani H, Tanaka T. Two species of human Fcε receptor II (FcεRII/CD23): tissue specific and interleukin 4-specific regulation of the gene expression. Cell 1988; 55:611.
82. Saito H, Hatake K, Dvorak A, et al. Selective differentiation and proliferation of hematopoietic cells induced by recombinant human interleukins. Proc Natl Acad Sci U S A 1988; 85:2288.

83. Jabara HH, Ackerman SJ, Vercelli D, et al. Induction of interleukin-4 dependent IgE synthesis and interleukin-5 dependent eosinophil differentiation by supernatants of a human helper T cell clone. J Clin Immunol 1988; 8:437.
84. Vercelli D, Geha RS. Regulation of IgE synthesis in man. J Clin Immunol 1989; 9:75.
85. Thyphronitis G, Tsokos GC, June CH, Levine AD, Finkelman FD. IgE secretion by Epstein-Barr virus-infected purified human B lymphocytes is stimulated by interleukin 4 and suppressed by interferon γ. Proc Natl Acad Sci U S A 1989; 86:5580.
86. Jabara HH, Schneider LC, Shapira SK, et al. Induction of germ-line and mature $C\epsilon$ transcripts in human B cells stimulated with rIL-4 and EBV. J Immunol 1990; 145:3468.
87. Yokota T, Coffman RL, Hagiwara H, et al. Isolation and characterization of lymphokine cDNA clones encoding mouse and human IgA-enhancing factor and eosinophil colony-stimulating factor activities: relationship to interleukin 5. Proc Natl Acad Sci U S A 1987; 84:7388.
88. Mosmann TR, Bond MW, Coffman RL, Ohara J, Paul WE. T-cell and mast cell lines respond to B-cell stimulatory factor 1. Proc Natl Acad Sci U S A 1986; 83:5654.
89. Limaye AP, Abrams JS, Silver JE, Ottesen EA, Nutman TB. Regulation of parasite-induced eosinophilia: selectively increased interleukin 5 production in helminth-infected patients. J Exp Med 1990; 172:399.
90. Owen WF, Rothenberg ME, Petersen J, et al. Interleukin 5 and phenotypically altered eosinophils in the blood of patients with the idiopathic hypereosinophilic syndrome. J Exp Med 1989; 170:343.
91. Walker C, Virchow J-C, Bruijnzeel PLB, Blaser K. T cell subsets and their soluble products regulate eosinophilia in allergic and nonallergic asthma. J Immunol 1991; 146:1829.
92. Rankin JA, Hitchcock M, Merrill W, Bach MK, Brashler JR, Askenase AW. IgE-dependent release of leukotriene C4 from alveolar macrophages. Nature 1982; 297:329.
93. Wang F, Gregory CD, Rowe M, et al. Epstein-Barr virus nuclear antigen 2 specifically induces expression of the B cell activation antigen CD23. Proc Natl Acad Sci U S A 1987; 84:3542.
94. Calender A, Billaud M, Aubry J-P, Banchereau J, Vuillaume M, Lenoir GM. Epstein-Barr virus (EBV) induces expression of B-cell activation markers on *in vitro* infection of EBV-negative B-lymphoma cells. Proc Natl Acad Sci U S A 1987; 84:8060.
95. Spalding DM, Griffin JA. Different pathways of differentiation of pre-B cell lines are induced by dendritic cells and T cells from different lymphoid tissues. Cell 1986; 44:507.
96. Kawanishi H, Saltzmann L, Strober W. Mechanisms regulating IgA class-specific immunoglobulin production in murine gut-associated lymphoid tissues. I. T cells derived from Peyer's patches that switch sIgM B cells to sIgA B cells in vitro. J Exp Med 1983; 157:437.
97. Murray PD, McKenzie DT, Swain SL, Kagnoff MF. Interleukin 5 and interleukin 4 produced by Peyer's patch T cells selectively enhance immunoglobulin A expression. J Immunol 1987; 139:2669.
98. Coffman RL, Shrader B, Carty J, Mosmann TR, Bond MW. A mouse T cell product that preferentially enhances IgA production. I. Biologic characterization. J Immunol 1987; 139:3685.
99. Bond MW, Shrader B, Mosmann TR, Coffman RL. A mouse T cell product that preferentially enhances IgA production. I. Physicochemical characterization. J Immunol 1987; 139:3691.

100. Harriman G, Strober W. Interleukin 5, a mucosal lymphokine? J Immunol 1987; 139:3553.
101. Harriman G, Kunimoto DY, Elliott JF, Paetkau V, Strober W. The role of IL-5 in B cell differentiation. J Immunol 1988; 140:3033.
102. Lebman DA, Coffman RL. The effects of IL-4 and IL-5 on the IgA response by murine Peyer's patch B cell subpopulations. J Immunol 1988; 141:2050.
103. Beagley KW, Eldridge JH, Kiyono H, et al. Recombinant murine IL-5 induces high rate IgA synthesis in cycling IgA-positive Peyer's patch B cells. J Immunol 1988; 141:2035.

CHAPTER 6

STRUCTURE AND FUNCTION OF INTERLEUKIN-6

Gerard Cox and Jack Gauldie

McMaster University
Hamilton, Ontario, Canada

INTRODUCTION

Interleukin-6 is the name given to a highly pleotropic cytokine (1) whose history and discovery typifies the complex nature of cell-derived factors and the limitations of the systems we have to study their characteristics. In retrospect (it is amazing we are comfortable in retrospection after only a few years!) this cytokine was discovered many times during the 1980s. It is an excellent example of factor discovery as summarized by Hotta and Baird (2) in their article on transforming growth factor β (TGF-β): "Physiological functions of many, if not all, growth promoting and growth inhibiting substances may have no correlation with activities for which they were first described." That so many groups were simultaneously yet unknowingly working on the same molecule and came to this realization within a short period of time allows us to paraphrase Winston Churchill: never in the history of cytokine biology has so much been known about a molecule by so many, but so few realized it.

The earliest record of cloning the molecule belongs to Weissenbach et al. (3), who identified the activity as an interferon (interferon-β_2, IFN-β_2) (4); another group (5) also described an interferon-β_2 mRNA that proved to elicit the same activity (6). These activities were derived from cytokine- or poly (I)·(C)- stimulated fibroblasts.

Similar cellular approaches led Content et al. (7) to describe a 26 kD protein of unknown function that also proved to be the same as IFN-β_2 (8). T cell-derived factors involved in B cell development and immunoglobulin synthesis were described by Teranishi et al. (9), and cloning (10) proved they were the same molecule as IFN-β_2 (11). At the same time, two groups were working on a human factor that modified the proliferation of plasmacytoma and hybridoma cells, one derived from fibroblasts (12,13) and a second from monocytes (14,15), both of which were shown to be IL-6. Similar studies had been completed in the mouse with the cytokine IL-HPI (16,17), and a further activity, PCT-GF (18,19), was shown to be identical to IL-HPl and to be homologous to human HPGF/HGF, or IL-6. Murine IL-6 was also cloned as a hematopoietic factor from stromal cells (20). Possibly the earliest description of IL-6 activity was the report of a stem cell differentiation factor, MGI-2A (21), which was later shown to be IL-6 (22). The intriguing aspect here is that Sachs (MGI-2A) and Ravel (IFN-β_2) unknowingly worked on the same molecule within the same institute for many years before they were able to show identity, a testament to the difficulties of working with factors in cell systems in the absence of cloning. The importance of IL-6 as part of the body's immediate defense or stress response came with the search for the cytokine that regulated the hepatic response in inflammation. Termed hepatocyte stimulating factor (HSF) (23,24), its identification as IL-6 indicated a most important function of IL-6 (25), that of regulating the acute-phase response.

Thus the discovery that such diverse activities were resident in one molecule brought a large amount of data together within a short period of time. The molecule was cloned by numerous groups, and recombinant material was readily available. From the first realization of shared functions to the first summary conference (26) was only 2 years. Several reviews on the cytokine have been published in the last few years (26–33).

STRUCTURE OF IL-6

Gene Structure

The IL-6 gene has been cloned from human, mouse, and rat, and is approximately 5, 7, and 10 kb in length, respectively (34–36). IL-6 is a single-copy gene located on chromosome 7p21 for human (37,38) and on chromosome 5 in the mouse (39). In all three species there are five exons and four introns and the exon/intron boundaries are conserved between the three species (36). The gene structure shares homology with murine and human granulocyte colony-stimulating factor (G-CSF) (10) and with the chicken myelomonocytic growth factor (40).

The cDNAs of the three species share reasonable homology (rat-mouse, 92%; mouse-human, 65%; and rat-human, 68%), with a slightly different comparison of predicted amino acid sequences (rat-mouse, 93%; mouse-human, 42%; and rat-human, 58%) (36).

The mRNA transcripts appear to initiate from several cap sites in the human, possibly differentially used in various cell types (34), and the rat has two possible cap sites, only one of which has been proven to be used (36). The human has two species of mRNA, each approximately 1.3 kb (Refs. 10, 41, and 42 and Gauldie, Northemann, and Fey, unpublished), using two different polyadenylation signals 78 bp apart, and the two are equally abundant in human fibroblast and macrophage. The mouse has the same two polyadenylation signals, but to date only one species of mRNA has been reported (32). The rat also has two mRNA species, one at 1.2–1.3 kb and another, using a second polyadenylation site (36), with a size of 2.4 kb occurring at about 20% abundance of the smaller species in both

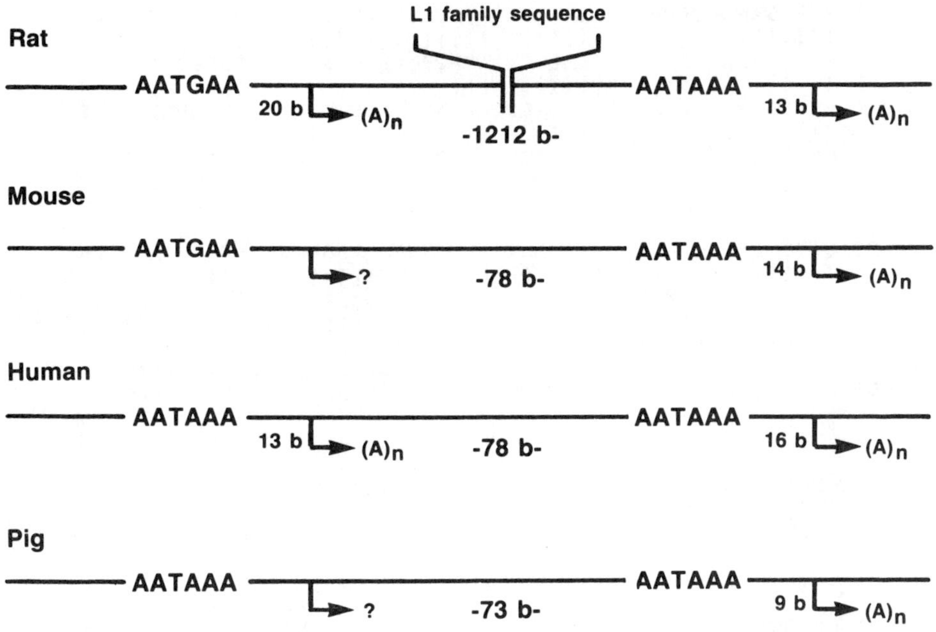

FIGURE 1 Comparison of the polyadenylation sites used in rat, mouse, human, and porcine IL-6 genes. The AATGAA polyadenylation signal for the rodent and AATAAA signal for human and porcine are shown adjacent to the polyadenylation site $(A)_n$. The position of the L1 family sequence insert (730 bp) is shown, and the distance between the two potential poly(A) sites in each gene is marked. Only the human and rat are confirmed for both RNA species.

macrophages and fibroblasts (Gauldie, Geisterfer, and Braciak, unpublished). This increased size is caused by the insertion into the rate gene of a 730 bp L1 repetitive sequence element (Fig. 1). Since the transcripts differ in their content of AUUUA sequences presumably coding for message stability (43), the longer of the human transcripts having six such sequences and the shorter four, the two messages may thus have differential stability under different conditions of stimulation, perhaps performing fine-tuning on the regulation of gene expression.

Protein Structure

The open reading frame in the gene codes for a 211 amino acid protein in mouse and rat and 212 in the human. Depending on the site of cleavage of the signal peptide, this yields a mature protein of 183–185 amino acids. Human IL-6 has two N-glycosylation sites and several O-glycosylation sites and expresses glycosyl and phosphoryl microheterogeneity (44–46) with an apparent molecular weight of 23–30 kD (13, 47–49): reviewed by Sehgal (50). Neither rat nor mouse has N-glycosylation sites, and purification of murine IL-6 from P388D$_1$ cells indicated the lack of glycosyl residues in the natural protein (51). Recently, porcine IL-6 was cloned and shows 62% homology with human IL-6 at the protein level

```
  1 MKFLSARDFQPVAF.LGLMLLTATAFPTSQVRRGDFTEDTTHNRPVYTTS  49 R
  1 MKFLSARDFHPVAF.LGLMLVTTTAFPTSQVRRGDFTEDTTPNRPVYTTS  49 M
  1 MNSFSTSAFGPVAFSLGLLLVLPAAFPAPVPPGEDSKDVAAPHRQPLTSS  50 H
  1 MNSLSTSAFSPVAFSLGLLLVMATAFPTPGRLEEDAKGDATSDKMLFTSP  50 P

 50 Q.VGGLITYVLREILEMRKELCNGNSDCMNSDDALSENNLKLPEIQRNDG  98 R
 50 Q.VGGLITHVLWEIVEMRKELCNGNSDCMNNDDALAENNLKLPEIQRNDG  98 M
 51 ERIDKQIRYILDGISALRKETCNKSNMCESSKEALAENNLNLPKMAEKDG 100 H
 51 DKTEELIKYILGKISAMRKEMCEKYEKCENSKEVLAENNLNLPKMAEKDG 100 P

 99 CFQTGYNQEICLLKICSGLLEFRFYLEFVKNNLQDNKKDKARVIQSNTET 148 R
 99 CYQTGYNQEICLLKISSGLLEYHSYLEYMKNNLKDNKKDKARVLQRDTET 148 M
101 CFQSGFNEETCLVKIITGLLEFEVYLEYLQNRFESS.EEQARAVQMSTKV 149 H
101 CFQSGFNQETCLMRITTGLVEFQIYLDYLQKEYESN.KGNVEAVQISTKA 149 P

149 LVHIFKQEIKDSYKIVLPTPTSNALLMEKLESQKEWLRTKTIQLILKALE 198 R
149 LIHIFNQEVKDLHKIVLPTPISNALLTDKLESQKEWLRTKTIQFILKSLE 198 M
150 LIQFLQKKAKNLDAITTPDPTTNASLLTKLQAQNQWLQDMTTHLILRSFK 199 H
150 LIQTLRQKGKNPDKATTPNPTTNAGLLDKLQSQNEWMKNTKIILILRSLE 199 P

199 EFLKVTMRSTRQT  211 R
199 EFLKVTLRSTRQT  211 M
200 EFLQSSLRALRQM  212 H
200 DFLQFSLRAIRIM  212 P
```

FIGURE 2 Comparison of rat (R), mouse (M), human (H), and porcine (P) IL-6 amino acid sequences showing homology between the species (dashes). The cysteine residues are marked with boxes. The rat has an additional cysteine at position 114. Gaps (.) are introduced to produce optimal alignments.

(52). Figure 2 shows homologous comparison of human, rat, mouse, and porcine IL-6 proteins. All proteins have four cysteine residues at conserved positions in the chain, and the intrachain disulfide bonds are identical in mouse (53) and human (Cys45-Cys51 and Cys74-Cys84) (54). The rat has an additional free cysteine at position 103, possibly able to form covalent structures with other proteins.

The N terminus of the molecule is not necessary for bioactivity. Residues 1–28 can be removed and the human molecule maintains activity in the hybridoma bioassay (55); removal of two residues from the C terminus causes marked loss of activity (56). It is likely that the C and N termini are held in proximity to create the active site in the intact molecule as shown by mapping studies using epitope-specific monoclonal antibodies (41).

GENE REGULATION

Expression of the gene is stimulated by a number of cytokines and growth factors and by bacterial endotoxins. The most potent stimuli in fibroblasts are IL-1 and tumor necrosis factor (TNF), with platelet-derived growth factor (PDGF) and fibroblast growth factor (FGF) also causing upregulation. In monocytes-macrophages, lipopolysaccharide (LPS) is the most potent stimulator, with phorbol ester (TPA) also being prominent. In macrophages, there is a rapid increase in IL-6 mRNA after LPS addition, with raised levels detected at 1–2 h and maximum accumulation occurring at 4–6 h (36). Inhibition of stimulated expression occurs with corticosteroid treatment. Pretreatment with 10^{-8}–10^{-6}M dexamethasone shuts off IL-6 production in vitro in most cells, and IL-1 or LPS is then not able to upregulate the expression (57,58).

Stimulation of IL-6 appears to occur through at least three different pathways of signal transduction, including cyclic AMP (59), calcium activation (60), and diacylglycerol (61). Regulation is achieved through the coordination of at least three cis-acting elements in the 5′ region of the gene. The region at −113 to −225 codes for a serum-responsive element (SRE) similar to that seen in c-*fos* oncogene expression (62). The second region at −145 to −158 has been called the NFIL-6 region (63), and the nuclear factor (NFIL-6) has recently been cloned and shows high homology to C/EPB, another important liver-specific nuclear factor (64). A third site, termed NFKB-like, at −63 to −73 has proven to be necessary for induction (65,66). With respect to the negative regulation by corticosteroids, there are several potential sites of action in the 5′ regulatory region of the gene. There are two homologous AP1 sites, but neither has as yet been shown to be functional for induction. These sites may be important for down-regulation as was recently shown for the collagenase gene, which is also stimulated by IL-1 treatment of fibroblasts (67–69). More recently, Ray et al. (70) described a steroid-sensitive negative regulatory region that appears to overlap the TATA box and the Inr element. It is possible that both regions are involved in the steroid regulation of expression.

CELLS OF ORIGIN

Most if not all nucleated cells have been shown to express and synthesize IL-6 in vitro. The most prominent source appears to be endotoxin (LPS)-stimulated monocyte-macrophages and cytokine-stimulated (IL-1 or INF) stromal cells—fibroblasts and epithelial cells as well as endothelial cells. In addition, T and B cell lines can express IL-6, as can mast cell lines, numerous tumor cell lines, and even polymorphonuclear leukocytes (32,71–74). Within the cells of the central nervous system, IL-6 can be expressed by astrocytes, microglial cells, and folliculostellate cells in vitro (30,75–77).

Although many cells can be shown to secrete IL-6 in vitro, examination of normal and inflamed tissue by northern gel analysis and in situ hybridization reveals that only a few cell types are active in pathological conditions. Thus although synoviocytes and chondrocytes can release high levels of IL-6 upon IL-1 or TNF stimulation in vitro (52) and high levels of IL-6 are found in the synovial fluid of a rheumatoid joint, only the synovial fibroblasts were seen to be active by in situ examination (78–81).

IL-6 IN PLASMA: ACTION AS A HORMONE

Among the various cytokines that have been described, there is evidence that IL-6 acts as an autocrine, paracrine, and exocrine inflammatory hormone. Its activity as a growth factor for plasmacytomas demonstrates its autocrine capability (82), as does its role in renal carcinoma (83) and in the proliferation of mesangial cells (84). This interpretation in B cell myelomas has been challenged (85,86), and a paracrine role has been suggested. Paracrine activity is also suggested by data showing Kupffer's cell activation and IL-6 release with subsequent hepatocyte response (see later) in the generation of acute-phase proteins in endotoxin-treated rats (87).

The exocrine function of IL-6 can be shown in a system in which a sterile abscess induced subcutaneously causes an increase in IL-6 in the plasma and response of the hepatocyte with acute-phase protein synthesis. Primary cultures of hepatocytes can be seen to make IL-6 in vitro (58), but at no time during the abscess challenge does the hepatocyte show IL-6 protein or message, even using sensitive polymerase chain reaction detection techniques. Thus, in this model, the signal must be derived from the distal inflamed tissue and travel through the circulation to elicit the metabolic change in the hepatocyte (88).

Under experimental conditions in animals or associated with trauma or infection in humans, IL-6 levels are shown to rise in plasma shortly after challenge (89–94). There is a temporal lag compared to plasma levels of TNF, and thus it is likely that macrophages-monocytes are the primary cell of activation, releasing their many cytokines, but predominantly IL-1 and TNF. These early alarm cytokines can recruit adjacent stromal cells (fibroblasts, smooth muscle cells, and endothelial cells) to release high levels of IL-6 and other mediators. Such a sequence was recently shown in mice treated with exogenous IL-1 and exhibiting a subsequent IL-6 response (95). This augmentation of signal is important in the generation of raised plasma levels of IL-6 suitable to cause systemic changes. Figure 3 outlines a scheme involving sequential activation and development of a cytokine cascade leading to high IL-6 levels in inflammation. Since IL-6 can induce cortisol levels (see later) and cortisol is required for the hepatic acute-phase response, IL-6 plays an inductive role in providing a second required signal to the liver (48,96). At the same time, cortisol is a potent inhibitor of IL-6 gene expression (57,58,97) and can subsequently reduce the levels of IL-6. Obviously, the timing and intensity of these hormone cascades are carefully controlled to elicit the appropriate effect needed in the correct temporal sequence to cope with the infective or traumatic challenge.

IL-6 RECEPTORS

As expected from the pleiotropic nature of its action, many diverse cells have IL-6 receptors (29,98,99) detected through binding studies. With the cloning of

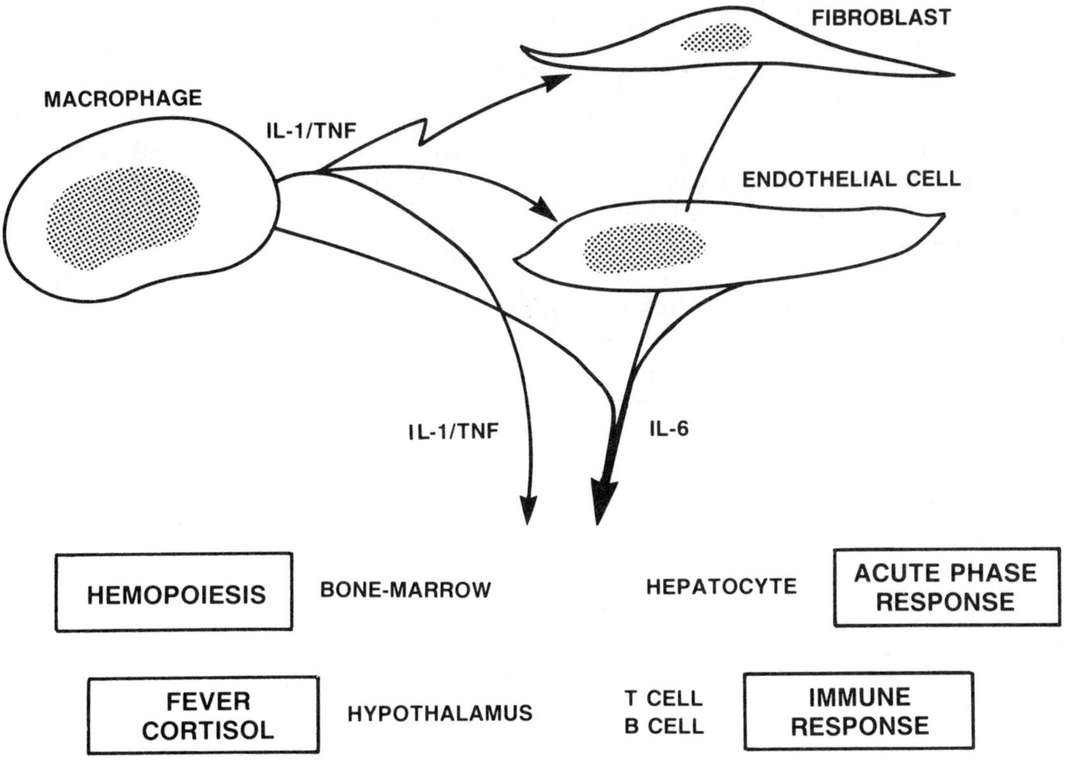

FIGURE 3 Sequence of cytokine cascades that result in the raised IL-6 levels and the multiple effects of exposure of cells and tissue to the various signls. The initial release of IL-1 and TNF result in the activation of adjacent tissue cells and further release of IL-6.

the human IL-6 binding receptor (100), the novel characteristics of IL-6-mediated signal transduction became apparent. The 80 kD receptor, a member of the Ig supergene family, is present on monocytes, hepatocytes, and T and B cells. The receptor lacks an intracellular tyrosine kinase domain and appears to require association with a second molecule, a 130 kD glycoprotein (101), for signal transduction. Thus the two-chain receptor model may explain the low- and high-affinity receptors detected on various cells (102) and is in common with the structures of many cytokine receptors (103).

The regulation of expression of the receptor has been studied in vitro in the human. Bauer et al. (104,105) reported that in monocytes, LPS and IL-6 decrease the expression of IL-6R, as does corticosteroid. Hepatoma cells seem to behave in the opposite fashion, with IL-6 and IL-1 as well as corticosteroid causing increased expression of the receptor (106). Similar positive regulation of IL-6R on epithelial cells by glucocorticoid has been reported (107). The homologous rat 80 kD receptor was recently cloned (108). Using this probe we examined the behavior of the receptor in vivo. The role of corticosteroid as an upregulator does not appear to be as dramatic in vivo, and during inflammation, the receptor expression on hepatocytes appears to be both up- and downregulated, depending on the kinetics of the inflammation (Geisterfer et al., unpublished). This area requires considerable work to clarify the regulation of the ligand binding receptor.

FUNCTION OF IL-6

B Cell Function: Antibody Production

One of the earliest identified activities of IL-6 was that of a T cell-derived signal that induced the final maturation of B lymphocytes to plasma cells (71,109,110). Using pokeweed mitogen (PWM)-stimulated peripheral blood mononuclear cells, human IL-6 caused 3- to 10-fold increases in IgG, IgM, and IgA antibody production in a dose-dependent fashion (111). Evidence that IL-6 could act directly on activated B cells includes the detection of IL-6 receptor on the surface of activated B cells (although not on resting B cells, which are not stimulated to produce Ig by IL-6), and experiments showing the requirement for IL-6 when purified B cells are cultured in the presence of irradiated T cells and mitogen.

That IL-6 is in fact an essential factor for antibody production is suggested by the finding that anti-IL-6 diminished antibody production by 90% in PWM-stimulated peripheral blood lymphocytes (PBL) (111). Because this effect was present when antibody was added even after 4 days of culture (8 days total), IL-6 likely acts a later stage of B cell differentiation.

The effect of IL-6 on immune responses in vivo has been studied using mice. Both the primary and the secondary antibody responses to sheep red blood cells were enhanced by IL-6, modifying both the intensity and the kinetics of antibody production (112).

B Cell Function: Growth

Evidence for the role of IL-6 in mediating the stimulation of proliferation of B cells is mixed. In the work by Muraguchi et al., the addition of anti-IL-6 did not alter the mitogen-induced proliferation of B cells. Alderson et al. (113) used a single hapten-specific murine B cell line to show enhancement of antibody production without proliferation in response to human IL-6. On the other hand, one of the earliest activities described for IL-6 was that of a B cell growth factor (14,114), and it is a potent growth factor for myeloma and plasmacytoma cells (18,82,86).

Epstein-Barr virus (EBV)-transformed human B cell lines have been used by a number of investigators to examine responses to IL-6. The earlier work demonstrated stimulation of Ig production by IL-6 but did not support a role for the molecule in growth promotion. In 1987, Taga et al. (98) demonstrated IL-6 receptors on EBV-transformed B cells, and later Tosato et al. (115) found IL-6 to promote the proliferation of these lines. Yokoi et al. (116) showed such lines expressed messenger RNA for IL-6 and also produced the protein. Thus IL-6 could act as an autocrine growth factor. It appears the effect is present mainly when cells are cultured at low density, and this perhaps is why the early work did not detect this activity.

That IL-6 may play a role in the development of human B cell malignancies is suggested by the finding of IL-6 receptors on freshly isolated human multiple myeloma cells (82). These cells also produce IL-6, respond to exogenous IL-6 by increased proliferation, and show inhibition of growth by anti-IL-6, all of which suggests that IL-6 can act as an autocrine factor for human myeloma cells. Whether IL-6 functions as an autocrine or paracrine hormone in this regard (85), its activity may be dependent on the expression of transferrin receptors by the myeloma cells (117).

T Cell Function

In contrast to B cells, both resting and activated T cells express receptors for IL-6, and a variety of effects on T cells at different levels of differentiation have been described. IL-6 stimulates the proliferation of both thymocytes and peripheral T cells (118–121). In addition, IL-6 promotes differentiation and proliferation (122,123), as well as augmenting the activity of natural killer (NK) cells (124). Many of these actions may be enhanced through synergy with IL-1 (125) and appear to be mediated via IL-2 and the IL-2R (42). Induction and enhancement of IL-2R expression in T cells by IL-6 has been shown (119,126). Addition of antibody to the p55 chain of IL-2R partially abrogated the proliferation of thymocytes and T cells in response to IL-6 (118,119,127), and anti-IL-2R blocked the effect of IL-6 on NK cell activity (28). A second IL-2-independent pathway of stimulation of thymocyte and T cell proliferation is suggested, since anti-IL-2R failed to inhibit IL-6 responses under different experimental conditions of low phytohemagglutin (PHA) concentrations (31,128).

In a murine system to study delayed type hypersensitivity (DTH) responses, IL-6, in addition to TNF-α, was shown to enhance DTH in a dose-dependent manner. The augmentation required the presence of T cells in the inoculum, again suggesting it is mediated by IL-2 (129). Interestingly, Scott et al. (130) failed to demonstrate significant IL-6 effects in a system examining T cell "retention," which comprises survival and proliferation, in the presence of rheumatoid synoviocyte culture medium. One might have expected to see a role for IL-6 given the activities already described on T cell proliferation. This highlights the difficulties of extrapolating from in vitro data to human diseases.

IL-6 AS A HEMATOPOIETIC FACTOR

Support for a role of IL-6 as a hematopoietic growth factor includes the finding that bone marrow stromal cells are potent sources of this cytokine (20). The myeloid growth factor known as macrophage and granulocyte inducer type 2 (MGI-2) or differentiation factor was shown to be IL-6 by Shabo et al. (22). This murine factor induces monocytic and granulocytic differentiation of normal myeloid precursor cells and some clones of murine leukemic cells. Chiu and others showed that murine IL-6 is both a growth factor for hematopoietic progenitor and leukemic cells and a differentiation factor, inducing dose-dependent monocytic development from the M1 and WEHI-3B myeloid leukemic cell lines (131). In addition to morphological evidence of differentiation, the cells showed increased expression of FcγRII mRNA and enhanced phagocytic activity within 6 h. While exhibiting differentiation, the M1 cells had markedly diminished rates of proliferation and subsequent loss of viability. Whether this represents a true antiproliferative activity of IL-6 or occurs as a result of differentiation is unclear. IL-6 can interact with IL-1, IL-3, IL-4, and the CSFs to promote colony formation by multipotential hematopoietic progenitors (132–139). Human IL-6 also stimulated murine hematopoietic colony formation (140), and Suda et al. (141) showed that human progenitors could similarly be stimulated to proliferate and differentiate in response to IL-6. Rennick et al. (138), using a model of colony formation from murine bone marrow cultures, demonstrated a synergy of action between IL-6 and IL-4 to induce granulocyte-macrophage (GM) colony formation similar to the synergy seen between IL-6 and IL-4 on T cell proliferation (128,142), and in the presence of erythropoietin IL-6 acted to increase numbers of erythroid colonies. In contrast, Ishibashi et al. (143) found no effect of IL-6 on GM colony formation from bone marrow.

Ishibashi et al. (144) reported the effect of IL-6 on megakaryocyte maturation and, later, that administration of rhIL-6 to mice induced elevated platelet levels and increased megakaryocyte diameter (143). Hill et al. (145) noted that treatment of mice with rhIL-6 [eight injections subcutaneously (SC) over 54 h] resulted in elevated platelet levels in a dose-dependent fashion, and this was accompanied by increased megakaryocyte colony-forming cells in the spleen and bone marrow. No change in hematocrit and only a modest increase in white cell count with the highest dose of IL-6 were detected in this study. When rIL-6 was given to rats as a single intravenous (IV) injection, a transient (< 24 h) increase in neutrophil and lymphocyte counts was found with subsequent bone marrow myeloid and erythroid hyperplasia (146), and in our hands, chronic administration of IL-6 for 10 days at a level adequate to induce a marked acute-phase protein response in rats (10 μg per rat per day) did not result in raised platelet counts (unpublished data). Obviously the levels required to initiate the various responses in vivo vary depending on the species and the specific response examined.

With the recent increase in interest in the potential role of colony-stimulating factors in the recovery from leukopenia associated with chemotherapy and radiotherapy, the effects of IL-6 have been studied. In mice, Okano et al. (147) reported that following bone marrow transplantation administration of IL-6 resulted in increases in white blood cell counts both in marrow and in the circulation. However, they found no effect on red blood cell or platelet counts. Furthermore, survival rates following transplantation could be increased from 20 to 90% when the transplanted material was preincubated with IL-6 and IL-3.

IL-6 AND THE ACUTE-PHASE REACTION

Injury or infection induces the acute-phase response, a coordinated homeostatic reaction that includes fever, leukocytosis, and changes in the circulating levels of particular proteins, the acute-phase proteins (APP). IL-6 is the cytokine primarily responsible for regulation of production of the acute-phase proteins by the liver. This, and regulation of B and T cell function, are likely the most important physiological roles of IL-6. The majority of these acute-phase reactants are glycoproteins, and they play a variety of roles in the homeostatic response to injury. From Table 1, we see that the proteins can both mediate the process and be consumed by it (reviewed in Refs. 96 and 148).

In 1983, Ritchie and Fuller (23) described a monocyte-derived acute-phase regulatory protein and termed it hepatocyte-stimulating factor (HSF). This molecule required the presence of corticosteroid for maximal activity. Others, including our group, confirmed that monocyte conditioned medium could regulate most of the APP genes in isolated rat hepatocytes and hepatoma cells in a co-

TABLE 1 Acute-Phase Proteins

Protein	Symbol	Species	Function
	Major changes		
C-reactive protein	CRP	Human, rabbit	Opsonin
Serum amyloid A protein	SAA	Human, mouse, rat	Apolipoprotein
Cysteine proteinase inhibitor	CPI	Rat	Antiproteinase
α_2-Macroglobulin	α2M	Rat	Antiproteinase
α_1-Acid glycoprotein	α1AGP	Most species	Transport
	Medium changes		
Fibrinogen	FBG	Most species	Coagulation
α_1-Proteinase inhibitor	α1Pi	Human, rat, mouse	Antiproteinase
α_1-Antichymotrypsin	α1ACHY	Human, rat, mouse	Antiproteinase
Haptoglobin	HPT	Most species	Binds and removes hemoglobin
Hemopexin	HPX	Most species	Binds heme
Ceruloplasmin	CER	Mouse	O_2 scavenger, transport
Complement C3	C3	Human, mouse	Opsonin
Serum amyloid P	SAP	Human, mouse	(?)
	Negative changes		
Albumin	Alb	Most species	(?)
Transferrin	Tf	Most species	Transport

ordinated manner similar to that seen in vivo. We showed that our HSF was identical to the previously cloned molecule interferon-β_2, or IL-6. Before the recognition of HSF/IL-6 and development of anti-IL-6 and rIL-6, much of the regulation of hepatocyte function was attributed to interleukin-1 and tumor necrosis factor. The evidence was derived from studies involving the in vivo administration of IL-1 or TNF, and because these cytokines are potent inducers of IL-6 the observed activities were incorrectly attributed to IL-1 and TNF. However, these agents contribute to the regulation of APP (Table 2).

The IL-6 receptor has been identified on the surface of hepatoma cells and hepatocytes (106). How the signal is transduced to the nucleus is unknown, but the response to IL-6 includes accumulation of mRNA for the AP proteins via increased transcriptional activity (44,47,48149–152). Regulation of the acute-phase protein genes by IL-6 occurs through an IL-6-responsive element (IL-6RE) in the 5′ promoter region of the genes. One such element, represented by the nucleotide sequence CTGGGAA/T, has been shown to be functional in a number of proteins from different species (153–158). A second element, with a sequence AGTGAnGnAA, may also be involved with IL-6 regulation of acute-phase protein genes (159–161). This region is similar to that described for the binding site of NFIL-6, the nuclear factor that is involved in initiating IL-6 gene transcription

Table 2 Acute-Phase Protein Genes Regulated by Inflammatory Cytokines

Induced by IL-1 and IL-6	Induced by IL-6 only
C-reactive protein (human)	Cysteine proteinase inhibitor
α_1-Acid glycoprotein	α_2-Macroglobulin
C3	Fibrinogen
Factor B	α_1-Proteinase inhibitor
SAA	Haptoglobin (human)
SAP	α_1-Antichymotrypsin
Haptoglobin (rat)	Ceruloplasmin
Hemopexin (rat)	C1 esterase inhibitor

(64). The relationship of these two elements and the IL-1 response element(s) on some genes (156) remains to be clarified.

There is in vivo evidence that supports the hypothesis that IL-6 is the principal regulator of APP production. Human rIL-6 given intraperitoneally (IP) to rats mimics the AP response seen following turpentine, but it occurs sooner and may require coadministration of corticosteroid (dexamethasone) (150,151), which likely induces IL-6R. Also the response seen in vivo parallels the in vitro response of rat hepatoma cells to IL-6. In burn patients the increase in IL-6 preceded elevations in C-reactive protein levels and correlated directly with the febrile response (93). In other clinical situations elevated IL-6 levels have been detected early in the course of infectious diseases (75,162). When rTNF was given to patients with malignancies, there was a prompt (5 minute) increase in IL-6, peaking at 3 h, followed at 4 h by elevated cortisol levels; at 8 h increased C-reactive protein was found (89). The molecular control of the hepatic acute-phase response has been recently reviewed (50,96,108,163–165).

As mentioned earlier, other elements of the response to injury include fever and leukocytosis. Endogenous pyrogen (interleukin-1) is well known to cause fever, and rhIL-6 given IV to rabbits induced fever in a dose-dependent manner, detectable at 15 minutes and peaking at 1 h (120). Furthermore, Rothwell et al. (submitted) have shown antibody to rat IL-6 inhibits the fever induced by systemic LPS treatment. As yet there is no concrete evidence that IL-6 contributes to the neutrophilia of early inflammation; however, it appears to enhance the proliferation of hematopoietic precursors (see earlier) and may activate mature neutrophils (see later). IL-6 stimulates adrenocorticotropic hormone (ACTH) release via the induction of corticotropin releasing hormone, and subsequently corticosteroid production (166), and thus may indirectly lead to neutrophilia via corticosteroid-induced demargination of neutrophils.

IL-6 AND THE NERVOUS SYSTEM

The effects of IL-6 on the neoplastic chromaffin cell line, PC12, have been studied. IL-6 maintained viability and induced differentiation accompanied by chemical and morphological changes similar to those induced by nerve growth factor (NGF)

(167). The finding of specific IL-6 receptors, distinct from NGF receptors, suggests IL-6 acts directly on the PC12 cells. This is relevant in the light of the finding that IL-6 can induce NGF secretion by astrocytes (28).

Stimulation of astrocytoma or glioblastoma cells with IL-1 induced expression of IL-6 mRNA. IL-6 was produced in a model of central nervous system CNS viral infection in mice, and later microglial cells and astrocytes were shown to produce IL-6 following infection with virus (75,76). This potential for local IL-6 production by central nervous system cells provides a mechanism for enhancing the intrathecal production of antibody in inflammatory CNS diseases, such as multiple sclerosis.

One direct action of IL-6 on the CNS in vivo is on the release of ACTH. Administration of antibody to corticotropin releasing factor (CRF) abolishes the effect, implying that IL-6 acts on the hypothalamus to release CRF, which in turn acts on the anterior pituitary to stimulate ACTH release (166).

MISCELLANEOUS

There is increasing evidence that IL-6 can modify the behavior of mature leukocytes. Although rIL-6 could not directly stimulate the respiratory burst of human neutrophils or monocytes, it primed these cells for the enhanced generation of oxygen radicals following stimulation with f-met-leu-phe-peptide (168). In addition, IL-6 was found to be a secretogog for human neutrophils, causing the release of both primary and secretory granule contents (169).

Interestingly, IL-6 may modulate the production of other cytokines by monocytes. Schindler et al. showed that IL-6 inhibited both LPS- and PHA-induced IL-1β and TNF production by human peripheral blood mononuclear cells (PBMC). Furthermore, they report the control appeared to be mediated at the level of transcription. In a system employing GM-CSF-primed human U937 histiocytic lymphoma cells, Aderka et al. (170) found that treatment with IL-6 prevented subsequent TNF production in response to LPS and also showed that IL-6 was effective in reducing TNF production in vivo in mice.

Cardiac myxoma is a rare benign tumor of the heart most often found in the atria. It is usually associated with hypergammaglobulinemia and autoantibody formation, features that disappear following removal of the tumor. Because tumor cells have been shown to express mRNA for IL-6 and release the protein in vitro, it is possible that the associated antibody abnormalities are mediated by IL-6 (10,49,171).

Overproduction of IL-6 may also contribute to the expression of Castleman's disease, a condition characterized by lymph node hyperplasia, hypergammaglobulinemia, fever, and elevated acute-phase proteins. Again, removal of affected tissue results in disappearance of the signs (28). Furthermore, Yoshizaki et al. (172) demonstrated IL-6 production by the germinal centers of such affected lymph nodes.

IL-6 may also be associated with IgM gammopathy as B cells from patients with this abnormality spontaneously differentiate to plasma cells in vitro and following differentiation these plasma cells produce IL-6 (173). This differentiation could be largely inhibited by antibodies to IL-6.

Raised levels of IL-6 have been detected in the body fluids of patients with a variety of systemic autoimmune diseases, for example the synovial fluid of rheumatoid joints (81) and the cerebrospinal fluid of systemic lupus erythematosus (SLE) associated CNS disease (174). Levels of IL-6 may fluctuate with disease activity and therapy, but whether there is a specific causal association between elevated levels of IL-6 and the various immunoglobulin abnormalities and the systemic inflammatory response seen in these conditions remains to be proven.

Similarly, the relevance of increased serum levels of IL-6 seen in severe illnesses, such as extensive burns (93), septic shock (175,176), and meningitis (75,162), remains to be determined. They may simply reflect severity of the condition: large injections of rIL-6 (50–100 μg) have little toxicity in mice or rats (176,177). Alternatively, toxic effects of IL-6 may only be seen when other processes or cytokines are also active.

Abnormal levels of IL-6 have been detected in both the serum and the urine of patients with certain renal diseases. Mesangial cells from patients with proliferative mesangial glomerulonephritis produce IL-6 in vitro. IL-6 can be detected in their urine but not in the urine of patients with other forms of glomerulonephritis, and in addition IL-6 has been shown to act as an autocrine growth factor for rat mesangial cells (178). Evidence for a direct role for IL-6 in development of disease comes from experiments using IL-6 transgenic mice, with the human IL-6 gene coupled to the human Ig heavy-chain gene enhancer (179). These mice develop a proliferative glomerulonephritis associated with marked polyclonal plasmacytosis and elevated immunoglobulins. IL-6 has been found in the serum and urine of patients following renal transplantation, prompting interest in its potential use as a marker of rejection (180).

Elevated levels of IL-6 have been reported in association with a variety of infectious processes, ranging from septic shock (46,92,175) to subclinical intrauterine infection (181). Using a preselected cutoff level, Romero et al. (181) correctly identified all 10 of 56 pregnant mothers who went into premature labor, 4 of whom had previously undetected intrauterine infection. Production of IL-6 by decidual or endometrial tissue was also demonstrated (180,182). In the case of human immunodeficiency virus (HIV) infection, increased levels of IL-6 have been found in the serum, and monocytes-macrophages from the peripheral blood of these patients spontaneously produce more IL-6 than matched controls (183). This elevation is detected even when no overt coinfection or complication is present, and it may contribute to the polyclonal B cell activation seen with HIV infection (184).

Mouse osteoblasts were recently shown to express IL-6 mRNA and produce IL-6, particularly in response to bone-resorbing agents, like IL-1, TNF, and LPS (185). IL-6 stimulates osteoclast number and activity, leading to resorption of bone either alone or in combination with other factors.

SUMMARY

Many cells have been shown to be capable of producing this important cytokine in vitro. However, only a few cell types have been proven to be directly involved in physiological responses. Much work remains to be done in detailing the expression of IL-6, and the regulation of expression of its receptor, in various clinical situations. Those functions of IL-6 that are clearly relevant in vivo include the regulation of the inflammatory response, the differentiation and maturation of hematopoietic cells, and the regulation of aspects of the immune response. It seems that although IL-6 has little or no direct toxicity, it can behave as an important cofactor in the expression of disease.

REFERENCES

1. Paul WE. Pleiotropy and redundancy: T cell derived lymphokines in the immune response. Cell 1989; 57:521–4.
2. Hotta M, Baird A. Differential effects of transforming growth factor type beta on the growth and function of adrenocortical cells in vitro. Proc Natl Acad Sci USA 1986; 83:7795–9.
3. Weissenbach J, Chernajovsky Y, Zeevi M, et al. Two interferon mRNAs in human fibroblasts: in vitro translation and *Escherichia coli* cloning studies. Proc Natl Acad Sci USA 1980; 77:7152–6.
4. Zilberstein A, Ruggieri R, Korn JH, Revel M. Structure and expression of cDNA and genes for human interferon-β2, a distinct species inducible by growth-stimulatory cytokines. EMBO J 1986; 5:2529–37.
5. Sehgal PB, Sagar AD. Heterogeneity of poly(I)·poly(C)-induced human fibroblast interferon mRNA species. Nature 1980; 288:95–7.
6. May LT, Helfgott DC, Sehgal PB. Anti-β-interferon antibodies inhibit the increased expression of HLA-B7 mRNA in tumor necrosis factor treated human fibroblasts: structural studies of the β2 interferon involved. Proc Natl Acad Sci USA 1986; 83:8957–61.
7. Content J, de Wit L, Pierard D, Derynck R, de Clercq E, Fiers W. Secretory proteins induced in human fibroblasts under conditions used for the production of interferon B. Proc Natl Acad Sci USA 1982; 79:2768–72.
8. Haegeman G, Content J, Volckaert G, Derynck R, Tavernier J, Fiers W. Structural analysis of the sequence coding for an inducible 26-kDa protein in human fibroblasts. Eur J Biochem 1986; 159:625–32.
9. Teranishi T, Hirano T, Naomichi A, Onoue K. Human helper T cell factor(s) (ThF). II. Induction of IgG production in B lymphoblastoid cell lines and identification of T cell-replacing factor-(TRF) like factor(s). J Immunol 1982; 128:193–8.
10. Hirano T, Yasukawa K, Harada H, et al. Complementary DNA for a novel human interleukin (BSF-2) that induces B lymphocytes to produce immunoglobulin. Nature 1986; 324:73–6.
11. Billiau A. BSF-2 is not just a differntiation factor. Nature 1986; 324:415.
12. van Damme J, Cayphas S, Opdenakker G, Billiau A, Van Snick J. Interleukin 1 and poly(rI)·poly(rC) induce proliferation of a hybridoma growth factor by human fibroblasts. Eur J Immunol 1987, 17:1–7.
13. van Damme J, Opdenakker G, Simpson RJ, et al. Identification of the human 26-kD protein, interferon β2, as a cell hybridoma/plasmacytoma growth factor induced by interleukin-1 and tumor necrosis factor. J Exp Med 1987, 165:914–9.
14. Aarden LA, Lansdorp PM, De Groot ER. A growth factor for B cell hybridomas produced by human monocytes. Lymphokines 1985; 10:175–85.
15. Brakenhoff JPJ, De Groot ER, Evers RF, Pannekoek H, Aarden LA. Molecular cloning and expression of hybridoma growth factor in *E. coli*. J Immunol 1987; 139:4116–21.
16. van Snick J, Cayphas S, Vink A, Uttenhoye C, Coulie P, Simpson R. Purification and NH_2-terminal amino acid sequence of a new T cell-derived lymphokine with growth factor activity for B cell hybridomas. Proc Natl Acad Sci U S A 1986; 83:9679–83.

17. van Snick J, Cayphas S, Szikora J-P, et al. cDNA cloning of murine interleukin-HP1; homology with human interleukin-6. Eur J Immunol 1988; 18:193–8.
18. Nordan R, Potter M. A macrophage-derived factor required by plasmacytomas for survival and proliferation in vitro. Science 1986; 233:566–9.
19. Nordan R, Pumphrey J, Rudikoff S. Purification and NH_2-terminal amino acid sequence of a plasmacytoma growth factor derived from the murine macrophage cell line, P388DI. J Immunol 1987; 139:813–7.
20. Chiu CP, Moulds C, Coffman RL, Rennick D, Lee F. Multiple biological activities are expressed by a mouse interleukin-6 cDNA clone isolated from bone marrow stromal cells. Proc Natl Acad Sci U S A 1988; 85:7099–103.
21. Fibach E, Sachs L. Control of normal differentiation of myeloid leukemic cells. XI. Induction of a specific requirement for cell viability and growth during the differentiation of myeloid leukemic cells. J Cell Physiol 1976; 89:259–66.
22. Shabo Y, Lotem J, Rubinstein M, et al. The myeloid blood cell differentiation inducting protein MGI-2A is interleukin-6. Blood 1988; 72:2070–3.
23. Ritchie DG, Fuller GM. Hepatocyte-stimulating factor: a monocyte-derived acute-phase regulatory protein. Ann NY Acad Sci 1983; 408:490–502.
24. Koj A, Gauldie J, Regoeczi E, Sauder DN, Sweeney GD. The acute-phase response of cultured rat hepatocytes. System characterization and the effect of human cytokines. Biochem J 1984; 224:505–14.
25. Gauldie J, Richards C, Harnish D, Lansdorp P, Baumann, H. Interferon β2/B-cell stimulatory factor type 2 shares identity with monocyte-derived hepatocyte-stimulating factor and regulates the major acute phase protein response in liver cells. Proc Natl Acad Sci U S A 1987; 84:7251–5.
26. Sehgal PB, Grieninger G, Tosato G eds. Regulation of the acute phase and immune responses: interleukin-6. Ann NY Acad Sci 1989; 557:583.
27. Wong GC, Clark SC. Multiple actions of IL-6 within a cytokine network. Immunol Today 1988; 9:137–9.
28. Kishimoto T. The biology of interleukin-6. Blood 1989; 74:1–10.
29. Kishimoto T, Taga T, Matsuda T, Hirano T. Interleukin-6 and its receptorin immune regulation. Immunol 1989; 7:633–40.
30. Hirano T, Kishimoto T. Interleukin-6 (IL-6) In: Sporn MB, Roberts AB, eds. Handbook of experimental pharmacology: peptide growth factors and their receptors. Berlin: Springer-Verlag, 1989; 633–65.
31. Le J Vilcek J. Interleukin 6: a multifunctional cytokine regulating immune reactions and the acute phase protein reponse. Lab Invest 1989; 61:588–602.
32. van Snick J. Interleukin-6: an overview. Annu Rev Immunol 1990; 8:253–78.
33. Akira S, Hirano T, Taga T, Kishimoto T. Biology of multifunctinal cytokines: IL 6 and related molecules (IL 1 and TNF). FASEB J 1990; 4:2860–7.
34. Yasukawa K, Hirano T, Watanabe Y, et al. Structure and expression of human B cell stimulatory factor-2 (BSF2/IL-6) gene. EMBO J 1987; 6:2939–45.
35. Tanabe O, Akira S, Kamiya T, Wong GG, Hirano T, Kishimoto T. Genomic structure of the murine IL-6 gene: high degree conservation of potential regulatory sequences between mouse and human. J Immunol 1988; 141:3875–81.
36. Northemann W, Braciak TA, Hattori M, Lee F, Fey GH. Structure of the rat interleukin 6 gene and its expression in macrophage-derived cells. J Biol Chem 1989; 264:16072–82.
37. Sehgal PB, Zilberstein A, Ruggieri R, et al. Human chromosome 7 carries the β2 interferon gene. Proc Natl Acad Sci U S A 1986; 83:5219–22.
38. Bowcock AM, Kidd JR, Lathrop M, et al. The human "β2 interferon/hepatocyte stimulating factor/interleukin-6" gene: DNA polymorphism studies and localization to chromosome 7p21. Genomics 1988; 3:8–16.

39. Mock BA, Nordan RP, Justice MJ et al. The murine IL-6 gene maps to the proximal region of chromosome 5. J Immunol 1989; 142:1372–6.
40. Leutz A, Damm K, Sterneck E, et al. Molecular cloning of the chicken myelomonocytic growth factor (cMGF) reveals relationship to interleukin 6 and granulocyte colony stimulating factor. EMBO J 1989; 8:175–81.
41. Brakenhoff JPJ, Hart M, de Groot ER, Di Padova F, Aarden LA. Structure-function analysis of human IL-6 Epitope mapping of neutralizing monoclonal antibodies with amino- and carboxyl-terminal deletion mutants. J Immunol 1990; 145:561–8.
42. Garman RD, Jacobs AJ, Clark SC, Raulet DH. B-cell-stimulatory factor 2 (β2 interferon) functions as a second signal for interleukin 2 production by mature murine T cells. Proc Natl Acad Sci U S A 1987; 84:7629–33.
43. Shaw G, Kamen R. A conserved AU sequence from the 3′ untranslated region of GM-CSF mRNA mediates selective mRNA degradation. Cell 1986; 46:659–67.
44. May LT, Ghrayeb J, Santhanam U, et al. Synthesis and secretion of multiple forms of "β2-interferon/B cell differentiation factor 2/hepatocyte stimulating factor" by human fibroblasts and monocytes. J Biol Chem 1988; 262:7760–6.
45. May LT, Santhanam U, Tatter SB, Bhardwaj N, Ghrayeb J, Sehgal PB. Phosphorylation of secreted forms of human β2-interferon/hepatocyte stimulating factor/interleukin-6. Biochem Biophys Res Comm 1988; 152:1144–50.
46. Helfgott DC, Tatter SB, Santhanam U et al. Multiple forms of IFN-β1/IL-6 in serum and body fluids during acute bacterial infection. J Immunol 1989; 142:948–53.
47. Baumann H, Onorato V, Gauldie J, Jahreis GP. Distinct sets of acute phase plasma proteins are stimulated by separate hepatocyte stimulating factors and monokines in rat heptoma cells. J Biol Chem 1987; 262:9756–68.
48. Baumann H, Richards C, Gauldie J. Interactions among hepatocyte stimulating factors, interleukin-1, and glucocorticoids for regulation of acute phase plasma proteins in human hepatoma (HepG2) cells. J Immunol 1987; 139:4122–8.
49. Hirano T, Taga T, Yasukawa K, et al. Human B cell differentiation factor defined by an anti-peptide antibody and its possible role in autoantibody production. Proc Natl Acad Sci U S A 1987; 84:228–31.
50. Sehgal PB. Interleukin-6: a regulator of plasma protein gene expression in hepatic and non-hepatic tissues. Mol Biol Med 1990; 7:117–30.
51. Fuller GM, Grenett HE. The structure and function of the mouse hepatocyte stimulating factor. Ann NY Acad Sci 1989; 557:31–45.
52. Richards CD, Saklatvala J. Molecular cloning and sequence of porcine IL-6 cDNA and expression of mRNA in synovial fibroblasts in vitro. (in press), 1991;
53. Simpson RJ, Moritz RL, Van Roost E, Van Snick J. Characterization of a recombinant murine interleukin-6: assignment of disulfide bonds. Biochem Biophys Res Commun 1988; 157:364–72.
54. Clogston CL, Boone TC, Crandall BC, Mendiaz EA, Lu HS. Disulfide structures of human interleukin-6 are similar to those of human granulocyte colony stimulating factor. Arch Biochem Biophys 1989; 272:144–51.
55. Brakenhoff JPJ, Hart M, Aarden LA. Analysis of human IL-6 mutants expressed in *Escherichia coli*. Biologic activities are not affected by deletion of amino acids 1-28. J Immunol 1989; 143:1175–82.
56. Kruttgen A, Rose-John S, Moller C, et al. Structure-function analysis of human IL-6: evidence for the involvement of the carboxy-terminus in function. FEBS Lett 1990; 262:323–6.
57. Kohase M, Henrickson-Destefano D, Sehgal PB, Vilcek J. Dexamethasone inhibits feedback regulation of the mitogenic activity of TNF, IL-1 and EGF in human fibroblasts. J Cell Physiol 1987; 132:271–8.

58. Baffet G, Braciak T, Gauldie J, Fey, GH, Northeman W. Autocrine activity of IL-6 secreted by hepatocarcinoma cell lines. Mol Biol Med (in press), 1991;
59. Zhang Y, Lin Y, Vilcek J. Synthesis of interleukin-6 (interferon-β2/B cell stimulatory factor 2) in human fibroblasts is triggered by an increase in intracellular cyclic AMP. J Biol Chem 1988; 263:6117–82.
60. Sehgal PB, Walther Z, May LT. Rapid enhancement of β2-interferon/B cell differentiation factor BSF-2 gene expression in human fibroblasts by diacylglycerols and the calcium ionophore A23187. Proc Natl Acad Sci U S A 1987; 84:3663–7.
61. Ray A, Tatter SB, May LT, Seghal PB. Activation of the human "β2-interferon/heptocyte stimulating factor/interleukin-6" promoter by cytokines, viruses and second messengers. Proc Natl Acad Sci U S A 1988; 85:6701–5.
62. Ray A, Sassone-Corsi P, Sehgal PB. A multiple cytokine- and second messenger-responsive element in the enhancer of the human interleukin-6 gene: similarities with *c-fos* gene regulation. Mol Cell Biol 1989; 9:5537–47.
63. Isshiki H, Akira S, Tanabe O, et al. Constitutive and interleukin-1 (IL-1)-inducible factors interact with the Il-1-responsive element in the IL-6 gene. Mol Cell Biol 1990; 10:2757–64.
64. Akira S, Isshiki H, Sugita T, et al. A nuclear factor for IL-6 expression (NF-IL-6) is a member of a C/EBP family. EMBO J 1990; 9:1897–906.
65. Shimizu H, Mitomo K, Watanabe T, Okamoto S, Yamamoto K-I. Involvement of NF-kappa B-like transcription factor in the activation of the interleukin-6 gene by inflammatory lymphokines. Mol Cell Biol 1990; 10:561–8.
66. Libermann TA, Baltimore D. Activation of interleukin-6 gene expression through the NF-kappa β transcription factor. Mol Cell Biol 1990; 10:2327–34.
67. Schule R, Rangarajan P, Kliewer S, et al. Functional antagonism between oncoprotein c-Jun and the glucocorticoid receptor. Cell 1990; 62:1217–26.
68. Yang-Yen HF, Chambard J-C, Sun Y-L, et al. Transcriptional interference between c-Jun and the glucocorticoid receptor: mutual inhibition of DNA binding due to direct protein-protein interaction. Cell 1990; 62:1205–15.
69. Jonat C, Rahmsdorf HJ, Park K-K, et al. Antitumor promotion and antiinflammation: down-modulation of AP-1 (Fos/Jun) activity by glucocorticoid hormone. Cell 1990; 62:1189–204.
70. Ray A, LaForge KS, Sehgal PB. On the mechanisms for efficient repression of the IL-6 promoter by glucocorticoids: enhancement of TATA box,and RNA start site (Inr motif) occlusion. Mol Cell Biol 1990; 10:5736–46.
71. Kishimoto T, Hirano T. Molecular regulation of B lymphocyte response. Annu Rev Immunol 1988; 6:485–512.
72. Kato K, Yokoi T, Takano N, et al. Detection by in situ hybridization and phenotypic characterization of cells expressing IL-6 mRNA in human stimulated blood. J Immunol 1990; 144:1317–22.
73. Plaut M, Pierce JH, Watson CJ, Hanley-Hyde J, Nordan RP, Paul WE. Mast cell lines produce lymphokines in response to cross-linkage of FεRI or to calcium ionophores. Nature 1989; 339:64–7.
74. Cicco NA, Lindemann A, Content J, et al. Inducible production of interleukin-6 by human polymorphonucler neutrophils: role of granulocyte-macrophage colony-stimulating factor and tumor necrosis factor-alpha. Blood 1990; 75:2049–52.
75. Frei K, Leist TP, Meager A, et al. Production of B-cell stimulatory factor-2 and interferon-gamma in the central nervous system during viral meningitis nd encephalitis. J Exp Med 1988; 168:449–53.
76. Frei K, Malipiero UV, Leist TP, Zinkernagel RM, Schwab ME, Fontana A. On the cellular source and function of interleukin 6 produced in the central nervous system in viral diseases. Eur J Immunol 1989; 19:689–94.

77. Vankelecom H, Carmeliet P, Van Damme J, Billiau A, Denef C. Production of interleukin-6 by folliculo-stellate cells of the anterior pituitary gland in a histiotypic cell aggregate culture system. Neuroendocrinology 1989; 49:102–6.
78. Firestein GS, Alvaro-Garcia JM, Maki R. Quantitative analysis of cytokine gene expression in rheumtoid arthritis. J Immunol 1990; 144:3347–53.
79. Guerne P-A, Zuraw BL, Vaughan JH, Carson DA, Lotz M. Synovium as a source of interleukin-6 in vitro. Contribution to loval and systemic manifestations of arthritis. J Clin Invest 1989; 83:585–92.
80. Guerne P-A, Carson DA, Lotz M. IL-6 production by human articular chondrocytes: modulation of its synthesis by cytokines, growth factors, and hormones in vitro. J Immunol 1990; 144:499–505.
81. Hirano T, Matsuda T, Turner M, et al. Excessive production of interleukin-6/B cell stimulatory factor-2 in rheumatoid arthritis. Eur J Immunol 1988; 18:1797–801.
82. Kawano M, Hirano T, Matsuda T, et al. Autocrine generation and requirement of BSF-2/IL-6 for human multiple myelomas. Nature 1988; 332:83–5.
83. Miki S, Iwano M, Miki Y, et al. IL-6 functions as an in vitro autocrine growth factor in renal carcinomas. FEBS Lett 1989; 250:607–10.
84. Ruef C, Budde K, Lacy J, et al. Interleukin 6 is an autocrine growth factor for mesangial cells. Kidney Int, 1990; 38:249–257.
85. Klein B, Zhang XG, Jourdan M, et al. Paracrine rather than autocrine regulation of myeloma-cell growth and differentiation by interleukin-6. Blood 1989; 73:517–26.
86. Klein B, Zhang XG, Jourdan M, et al. Interleukin-6 is the central tumor growth factor in vitro and in vivo in multiple myeloma. Eur Cytokine Net 1990; 1:193–201.
87. Podor TJ, Hirsh J, Gelehrter T, et al. Type I plasminogen activator inhibitor (PAI1) is not an acute phase reactant in rats: plasma PAI1 expression is independent of hepatocyte synthesis and elevations in plasma interleukin-6. (in press), 1991;
88. Gauldie J, Northeman W, Fey GH. IL-6 functions as an exocrine hormone in inflammation: hepatocytes undergoing acute phase responses require exogenous IL-6. J Immunol 1990; 144:3804–8.
89. Jablons DM, Mule JJ, McIntosh JK, et al. IL-6/IFN-β-2 as a circulating hormone. Induction by cytokine administration in humans. J Immunol 1989; 142:1542–7.
90. Brouckaert P, Spriggs DR, Demetri G, Kufe DW, Fiers W. Circulating interleukin-6 during a continuous infusion of tumor necrosis factor and interferon-γ. J Exp Med 1989; 169:2257–62.
91. Houssiau F, Devogelaer J-P, Van Damme J, Nagant de Deuxchaisnes C, Van Snick J. Interleukin 6 in synovial fluid and serum of patients with rheumatoid arthritis and other inflammatory arthritides. Arthritis Rheum 1988; 31:784–8.
92. Hack CE, De Groot ER, Felt-Bersma RJF, et al. Increased plasma levels of interleukin 6 in sepsis. Blood (in press), 1990;
93. Nijsten MWN, de Groot ER, ten Duis HJ, Hack CE, Aarden LA. Serum levels of interleukin-6 an acute phase responses (letter). Lancet 1987; 2:921.
94. Fong Y, Moldawer LL, Marano M, et al. Endotoxemia elicits increased circulating β2-IFN/IL-6 in man. J Immunol 1989; 142:2321–4.
95. Libert C, Brouckaert P, Shaw A, Fiers W. Induction of IL-6 by human and murine recombinant IL-1 in mice. Eur J Immunol 1990; 20:691–5.
96. Gauldie J, Baumann H. Cytokines and acute phase protein expression. In: Kimball EH, ed. Cytokines in inflammation. Telford Press, (in press), 1991:
97. Helfgott DC, May LT, Sthoerger Z, Tamm I, Sehgal PB. Bacterial lipopolysaccharide (endotoxin) enhances expression and secretion of B-2 interferon by human fibroblasts. J Exp Med 1987; 166:1300–9.

98. Taga T, Kawanishi K, Hardy RR, Hirano T, Kishimoto T. Receptors for the B cell stimulatory factor 2 (BSF-2): quantitation, specificity, distribution and regulation of the expression. J Exp Med 1987; 166:967–81.
99. Coulie PG, Vanhecke A, Van Damme J, et al. High-affinity binding sites for human 26-kDa protein (interleukin 6, B cell stimulatory factor-2, human hybridoma plasmacytoma growth factor, interferon β2), different from those of type I interferon (α, β) on lymphoblastoid cells. Eur J Immunol 1987; 17:1435–40.
100. Yamasaki K, Taga T, Hirata Y, et al. Cloning and expression of the human interleukin-6 (BSF-2/IFNβ2) receptor. Science 1988; 241:825–8.
101. Taga T, Hibi M, Hirata Y, et al. Interleukin 6 (IL-6) triggers the association of its receptor (IL-6-R) with a possible signal transducer, gp 130. Cell 1989; 58:573–81.
102. Coulie PG, Stevens M, Van Snick J. High- and low-affinity receptors for murine interleukin 6. Distinct distribution on B and T cells. Eur J Immunol 1989; 19:2107–14.
103. Arai K, Lee F, Miyajima A, Miyatake S, Arai N, Yokota T. Cytokines: coordinators of immune and inflammatory responses. Annu Rev Biochem 1990; 59:783–836.
104. Bauer J, Lengyel G, Bauer TM, Acs G, Gerok W. Regulation of interleukin-6 receptor expression in human monocytes and hepatocytes. FEBS Lett 1989; 249:270–30.
105. Bauer J, Bauer TM, Kalb T, et al. Regulation of interleukin 6 receptor expression in human monocytes and monocyte-derived macrophages. Comparison with the expression in human hepatocytes. J Exp Med 1989; 170:1537–49.
106. Rose-John S, Schooltink H, Lenz D, et al. Studies on the structure and regulation of the human hepatic interleukin-6 receptor. Eur J Biochem 1990; 190:79–83.
107. Snyers L, DeWitt L, Content J. Glucocorticoid up-regulation of high affinity IL-6 receptors on human epithelial cells. Proc Natl Acad Sci U S A 1990; 87:2838–42.
108. Baumann M, Baumann H, Fey GH. Molecular cloning, characterization and functional expression of the rat liver interleukin 6 receptor. J Biol Chem, 1990; 265:19853–19862.
109. Muraguchi A, Kishimoto T, Miki Y et al. T cell-replacing factor (TRF)-induced IgG secretion in human B blastoid cell line and demonstration of acceptors for TRF. J Immunol 1981; 127:412–6.
110. Hirano T, Taga T, Nakano N, et al. Purification to homogeneity and characterization of human B cell differentiation factor (BCDF or BSFp-2). Proc Natl Acad Sci U S A 1985; 82:5490–4.
111. Muraguchi A, Hirano T, Tang B, et al. The essential role of B-cell stimulatory factor (BSF-2/IL-6) for the terminal differentiation of B cells. J Exp Med 1988; 167:332.
112. Takatsuki F, Okano A, Suzuki C, et al. Human recombinant interleukin 6/B cell stimulatory factor 2 IIL-6/BSF-2) augments murine antigen-specific antibody responses in vitro and in vivo. J Immunol 1988; 141:3072–7.
113. Alderson AR, Pike BL. Recombinant human interleukin-6 (B cell stimulating factor 2) enhances immunoglobulin secretion by single murine hapten-specific B cells in the absence of cell division. Int Immunol 1989; 1:20–8.
114. Aarden LA, De Groot ER, Schaap OL, Lansdorp PM. Production of HGF by human monocytes. Eur J Immunol 1987; 17:1411–6.
115. Tosato G, Seamon KB, Goldman ND, et al. Monocyte-derived human B-cell growth factor identified as interferon-B2 (BSF-2, IL-6). Science 1988; 239:502–4.
116. Yokoi T, Miyawaki T, Yachie A, Kato K, Kasahara Y, Taniguchi N. Epstein-Barr virus immortalized B cells produce IL-6 as an autocrine growth factor. Immunology 1990; 70:100–5.
117. Neckers LM, Nordan RP. Regulation of murine plasmacytoma transferrin receptor

expression and G_1 traversal by plasmacytoma cell growth factor. J Cell Physiol 1988; 135:495–501.

118. Lotz M, Jirik F, Kabouridis P, et al. B cell stimulating factor/interleukin 6 is a co-stimulant for human thymocytes and T lymphocytes. J Exp Med 1988; 167:1253–8.

119. Le J, Fredrickson G, Reis LFL, et al. Interleukin 2-independent and interleukin 2 dependent pathways of regulation of thymocyte function by interleukin 6. Proc Natl Acad Sci U S A 1988; 85:8643–8647

120. Helle M, Brakenhoff J, De Groot E, Aarden L. Interleukin-6 is involved in interleukin-1-induced activities. Eur J Immunol 1988; 18:957–9.

121. Helle M, Boeije L, Aarden LA. IL-6 is an intermediate in IL-1 induced thymocyte proliferation. J Immunol 1989; 142:4335–8.

122. Takai Y, Wong GC, Clark SC, Burakoff SJ, Herrman SH. B cell stimulatory factor-2 is involved in the differentiation of cytotoxic T lymphocytes. J Immunol 1988; 140:508–12.

123. Okada M, Kitihara M, Kishimoto S, Matsuda T, Hirano T, Kishimoto T. IL-6/BSF-2 functions as a killer helper factor in the in vitro induction of cytotoxic T cells. J Immunol 1988; 141:1543–9.

124. Luger TA, Krutman J, Kirnbauer R, et al. IFN-B2/IL-6 augments the activity of human natural killer cells. J Immunol 1989; 143:1206–9.

125. Mizutani H, May LT, Sehgal PB, Kupper TS. Synergistic interactions of IL-1 and IL-6 in T-cell activation. J Immunol 1989; 143:896–901.

126. Noma T, Mizuta T, Rosen A, Hirano T, Kishimoto T, Honjo T. Enhancement of the interleukin 2 receptor expression on T cells by multiple B-lymphotropic lymphokines. Immunol Lett 1987; 15:249–53.

127. Garman RD, Raulet DH. Characterization of a novel murine T cell-activting factor. J Immunol 1987; 138:112–9.

128. Houssiau F, Coulie PG, Olive D, van Snick J. Synergistic activation of human T cells by interleukin 6. Eur J Immunol 1988; 18:653–6.

129. Jayarman S, Martin CA, Dorf ME. Enhancement of in vivo cell-mediated immune responses by three distinct cytokines. J Immunol 1990; 144:942–51.

130. Scott S, Pandolfi F, Kurnick JT. Fibroblasts mediate T cell survival: a proposed mechanism for retention of primed T cells. J Exp Med 1990; 172:1873–6.

131. Chiu CP, Lee F. IL-6 is a differentiation factor for M1 and Wehi-3B myeloid leukemic cells. J Immunol 1989; 142:1909–15.

132. Bot FJ, Eijk L, Broeders L, Aarden LA, Lowenberg B. Interleukin-6 synergizes with M-CSF in the formation of macrophage colonies from purified human marrow progenitor cells. Blood 1989; 73:435–7.

133. Caracciolo D, Clark SC, Rovera G. Human interleukin 6 supports granulocytic differentiation of hematopoietic progenitor cells and acts synergistically with GM-CSF. Blood 1989; 73:666–70.

134. Hoang T, Haman A, Gonclaves O, Wong GC, Clark SC. Interleukin-6 enhances growth factor-dependent proliferation of the blast cells of acute myeloblastic leukemia. Blood 1988; 72:823–6.

135. Ikebuchi K, Wong GC, Clark SC, Ihle JN, Hirai Y, Ogawa M. Interleukin 6 enhancement of interleukin 3-dependent proliferation of multipotential hemopoietic precursors. Proc Ntl Acad Sci U S A 1987; 84:9035–9.

136. Ikebuchi K, Ihle JN, Hirai Y, Wong GG, Clark SC, Ogawa M. Synergistic factors for stem cell proliferation: further studies of the target stem cells and the mechanism of stimulation by interleukin-1, interleukin-6, and granulocyte colony-stimulating factor. Blood 1988; 72:2007–14.

137. Leary AG, Ikebuchi K, Hirai Y, et al. Synergism between interleukin-6 and inter-

leukin-3 in supporting proliferation of human haematopoietic stem cells: comparison with interleukin-1α. Blood 1988; 71:1759–63.

138. Rennick D, Jackson J, Yang G, Wideman J, Lee F, Hudak S. Interleukin 6 interacts with interleukin 4 and other hemopoietic growth factors to selectively enhance the growth of megakaryococytic, erythroid, myeloid, and multipotential progenitor cells. Blood 1989; 73:1828–35.

139. Suzuki C, Okano A, Takatsuki F, et al. Continuous perfusion with interleukin 6 (IL-6) enhances production of hematopoietic stem cells (CFU-S). Biochem Biophys Res Commun 1989; 159:933–8.

140. Wong GC, Witek-Giannotti JS, Temple PA, et al. Stimulation of murine hemopoietic colony formation by human IL-6. J Immunol 1988; 140:3040.

141. Suda T, Yamaguchi Y, Suca J, Miura Y, Okano A, Akiyama Y. Effect of interleukin 6 (IL-6) on the differentiation and proliferation of murine and human hemopoietic progenitors. Exp Hematol 1988; 16:891.

142. Hodgkin PD, Bond MW, O'Garra A, et al. Identification of IL-6 as a T cell-derived factor that enhances the proliferative response of thymocytes to IL-4 and phorbol myristate acetate. J Immunol 1988; 141:151–7.

143. Ishibashi T, Kimura H, Shikama T, et al. Interleukin-6 is a potent thrombopoietic factor in vivo in mice. Blood 1989; 74:1241–4.

144. Ishibashi T, Kimura H, Uchida T, Kariyone S, Friese P, Burstein SA. Human interleukin-6 is a direct promoter of maturation of megakaryocytes in vitro. Proc Natl Acad Sci USA 1988; 86:5953–7.

145. Hill RJ, Warren MK, Levin J. Stimulation of thrombopoiesis in mice by human recombinant interleukin 6. J Clin Invest 1990; 85:1242–7.

146. Ulich TR, del Castilo J, Guo K. In vivo hematologic effects of recombinant interleukin 6 on hematopoiesis and circulating numbers of RBC's and WBC's. Blood 1989; 73:108–10.

147. Okano A, Suzuki C, Takatsuki F, et al. Effects of interleukin 6 on haematopoiesis in bone-marrow transplanted mice. Transplantation 1989; 47:738–40.

148. Koj A. Definition and classification of acute phase proteins in the acute phase response to injury and infection. Amsterdam: Elsevier, In: The Acute Phase Response to Injury and Infection. Gordon AH, Koj A, eds. 1985:139–232.

149. Morrone G, Ciliberto G, Oliviero S, et al. Recombinant interleukin 6 regulates the transcriptional activation of a set of human acute phase genes. J Biol Chem 1988; 263:12554–8.

150. Geiger T, Andus T, Klapproth J, Hirano T, Kishimoto T, Heinrich PC. Induction of rat acute-phase proteins by interleukin-6 in vivo. Eur J Immunol 1988; 18:717–21.

151. Marinkovic S, Jahreis GP, Wong GG, Baumann H. IL-6 modulates the synthesis of a specific set of acute phase plasma proteins in vivo. J Immunol 1989; 142:808–12.

152. Ganapathi MK, May LT, Schultz D, et al. Role of interleukin-6 in regulating synthesis of C-reactive protein and serum amyloid A in human hepatoma cell lines. Biochem Biophys Res Comm 1988; 157:271–7.

153. Tsuchiya Y, Hattori M, Hayashida K, Ishibashi H, Okubo H, Sakaki Y. Sequence analysis of the putative regulatory region of rat α_2-macroglobulin gene. Gene 1987; 57:73–80.

154. Fey GH, Hattori M, Northemann W, et al. Regulation of rat liver acute phase genes by interleukin-6 and production of hepatocyte stimulating factors by rat hepatoma cells. Ann NY Acad Sci 1989; 557:317–31.

155. Kunz D, Zimmermann R, Heisig M, Heinrich PC. Identification of the promotor

sequences involved in the interleukin-6 dependent expression of the rat α_2-macroglobulin gene. Nucleic Acids Res 1989; 17:1121.

156. Prowse KR, Baumann H. Hepatocyte-stimulating factor, β2 interferon, and interleukin-1 enhance expression of the rat α1-acid glycoprotein gene via a distal upstream regulatory region. Mol Cell Biol 1988; 8:42–51.

157. Ito T, Tanahashi H, Misumi Y,Sakaki Y. Nuclear factors interacting with an interleukin-6 responsive element of rat α_2-macroglobulin gene. Nucleic Acids Res 1989; 17:9425–35.

158. Hattori M, Abraham LJ, Northemann W, Fey GH. Acute-phase reaction induces a specific complex between hepatic nuclear proteins and the interleukin 6 response element of the rat α_2-macroglobulin gene. Proc Natl Acad Sci U S A 1990; 87:2364–8.

159. Majello B, Arcone R, Toniatti C, Ciliberto G. Constitutive and IL-6 induced nuclear factors that interact with the human C-reactive protein promoter. EMBO J 1990; 9:457–65.

160. Oliviero S, Cortese R. The human haptoglobin gene promoter: interleukin-6-responsive elements interact with a DNA-binding protein induced by interleukin-6. EMBO J 1989; 8:1145–51.

161. Poli V, Cortese R. Interleukin 6 induces a liver-specific nuclear protein that binds to the promoter of acute-phase genes. Proc Natl Acad Sci U S A 1989; 86:8202–6.

162. Houssiau FA, Bukasa K, Sindic CJM, Van Damme J, Van Snick J. Elevated levels of the 26K human hybridoma growth factor (interleukin 6) in cerebrospinal fluid of patients with acute infection of the central nervous system. Clin Exp Immunol 1988; 71:320–3.

163. Fey GH, Gauldie J. The acute phase response of the liver in inflammation. In: Popper H, Schaffner F, eds. Progress in liver diseases, Vol. 9, Chap. 7. Philadelphia: W. B. Saunders, 1990:89–116.

164. Baumann H, Gauldie J. Regulation of hepatic acute phase plasma protein genes by hepatocyte stimulating factors and other mediators of inflammation. Mol Biol Med 1990; 7:147–59.

165. Heinrich PC, Castell JV, Andus T. Interleukin-6 and the acute phase response. Biochem J 1990; 265:621–36.

166. Naitoh Y, Fukata J, Tominaga T, et al. Interleukin 6 stimulates the secretion of adrenocorticotrophic hormone in conscious, freely moving rats. Biochem Biophys Res Commun 1988; 155:1459–1463.

167. Satoh T, Nakamura S, Taga T, et al. Induction of neural differentiation in PC12 cells by B cell stimulatory factor/interleukin 6. Mol Cell Biol 1988; 8:3546.

168. Kharazmi A, Nielsen H, Rechnitzer C, Bendtzen K. Interleukin-6 primes neutrophil and monocyte oxidative burst response. Immunol Lett 1989; 21:177–84.

169. Borish L, Rosenbaum R, Albury L, Clark S. Activation of neutrophils by recombinant interleukin-6. Cell Immunol 1989; 121:280–9.

170. Aderka D, Le J, Vilcek J. IL-6 inhibits liposaccharide-induced tumor necrosis factor production in cultured human monocytes, U937 cells, and in mice. J Immunol 1989; 143:3517–23.

171. Graham SL, Sellers AL. Atrial myxoma with multiple myeloma. Arch Intern Med 1979; 139:116–7.

172. Yoshizaki K, Matsuda T, Nishimoto N, et al. Pathogenic significance of interleukin-6 (IL-6/BSF-2) in Castleman's disease. Blood 1989; 74:1360–7.

173. Levy Y, Fermand J-P, Navarro S, et al. Interleukin 6 dependence of spontaneous in vitro differentiation of B cells from patients with IgM gammapathy. Proc Natl Acad Sci U S A 1990; 87:3309–13.

174. Hirohata S, Miyamoto T. Elevated levels of interleukin-6 in cerebrospinal fluid from

patients with systemic lupus erythematosus and central nervous system involvement. Arthritis Rheum 1990; 33:644–9.

175. Waage A, Brandtzaeg P, Halstensen A, Kierulf P, Espevik T. The complex pattern of cytokines in serum from patients with meningococcal septic shock. J Exp Med 1989; 169:333–8.

176. Neta R, Vogel SN, Sipe JD, Wong GG, Nordan RP. Comparison of in vovo effects of human recombinant IL-1 and human recombinant IL6 in mice. Lymphokine Res 1988; 7:403–12.

177. Mulé JJ, McIntosh JK, Jablons DM, Rosenberg SA. Antitumor activity of recombinant interleukin 6 in mice. J Exp Med 1990; 171:629–36.

178. Horii Y, Muraguchi A, Iwano M, et al. Involvementof IL-6 in mesangial proliferative glomerulonephritis. J Immunl 1989; 143:3949–55.

179. Suematsu S, Matsuda T, Aozasa K, et al. IgG_1 plasmacytosis in interleukin 6 transgenic mice. Proc Natl Acad Sci U S A 1989; 86:7547–51.

180. van Oers MHJ, van der Heyden AAPAM, Aarden LA. Interleukin 6 (IL-6) in serum and urine of renal transplant recipients. Clin Exp Immunol 1988; 71:314–9.

181. Romero R, Avila C, Santhanam U, Sehgal PB. Amniotic fluid interleukin 6 in preterm labor. Association with infection. J Clin Invest 1990; 85:1392–400.

182. Tabibzadeh SS, Santhanam U, Sehgal PB, May LT. Cytokine-induced production of IFN-B2/IL-6 by freshly explanted human endometrial stromal cells. J Immunol 1989; 142:3134–9.

183. Breen EC, Rezai AR, Nakajima K, et al. Infection with HIV is associated with elevated IL-6 levels and production. J Immunl 1990; 144:480–4.

184. Nakajima K, Martinez-Maza O, Hirano T, et al. Induction of IL-6 (B cell stimulatory factor-2/IFN-β2) production by HIV. J Immunol 1989; 142:531–6.

185. Ishimi Y, Miyaura C, He Jin C, et al. IL-6 is produced by osteoblasts and induces bone resorption. J Immunol 1990; 145:3297–303.

186. Lansdorp PM, Aarden LA, Calafat J, Zeijlemaker WP. A growth-factor dependent B-cell hybridoma. Curr Top Microbiol Immunol 1986; 132:105–13.

187. Schindler R, Mancilla J, Ghorbani R, Clark SC, Dinarello CA. Correlations and interactions in the production of interleukin-6 (IL-6), IL-1, and tumor necrosis factor (TNF) in human blood mononuclear cells: IL-6 suppresses IL-1 and TNF. Blood 1990; 75:40–7.

CHAPTER 7

INTERLEUKIN-8 AND THE INFLAMMATORY RESPONSE

Steven L. Kunkel, Theodore J. Standiford, Stephen W. Chensue, and Robert M. Strieter

The University of Michigan Medical School
Ann Arbor, Michigan

John Westwick

Royal College of Surgeons of England
London, England

INTRODUCTION

As with many inflammatory processes, the chemotactic response is controlled by both positive and negative signals expressed in a coordinated manner. Many of the initial interactions that are important to the elicitation of individual inflammatory cells occur in the lumen of regional blood vessels. In this environment, both chemical and physical alterations in the blood may result in leukoconcentration and the generation of proximal mediators. These early inflammatory signals likely include both tumor necrosis factor α (TNF) and interleukin-1 (IL-1). Although these cytokines have been implicated in chronic immune reactions, recent experimental studies have demonstrated that these polypeptides are early response mediators and are actively involved in acute inflammation (1–3). For example, it is becoming increasingly clear that both IL-1 and TNF are key mediators that promote the adherence between inflammatory cells and the endothelium (4). The binding of inflammatory cells to endothelial cells is due, in part, to IL-1-and/or TNF-induced adherence proteins on the surface of endothelial cells. The major cytokine-induced adherence proteins that are expressed on the surface of endothelial cells are designated intercellular adhesions molecule 1 (ICAM), endothelial leukocyte adhesions molecule (ELAM), or vascular leukocyte adhesion molecule (VLAM). A number of very elegant in vitro studies have demonstrated that the induction of these surface molecules by either TNF or IL-1 is a rapid process (4). Although de novo transcription and translation are required for ICAM, ELAM, or VLAM to be expressed, the induction process and expression occur within a few hours of TNF or IL-1 treatment. An additional aspect of certain adhesion molecules is the surface expression of these proteins on cells independent of the endothelium. In particular, published reports now demonstrate that epithelial cells can express adherence molecules that can bind inflammatory cells in a specific manner (5). With regard to the induction of adherence protein or endothelial cells, both IL-1 and TNF are potent in the ng/ml concentration range. These adherence proteins appear to serve as the natural ligand for additional proteins that are expressed on the surface of inflammatory cells. The inflammatory cell-derived adherence proteins belong to the CD11/CD18 family of surface proteins and include CD11a, CD11b, and CD11c. This adherence mechanism allows a high degree of specific binding. The interactions that occur between the triumvirate of endothelial cells, cytokines, and inflammatory cells is crucial, as this proximal event is designed to initially bind inflammatory cells to a restricted area of inflammation. The adherence phenomenon is a unique interaction in that the binding must be strong enough to allow significant attachment of the inflammatory cells to the endothelium but be controlled by some mechanisms(s) that allows the adherence process to be reversible. This aspect of an inflammatory response is somewhat paradoxical in that adhesion is an absolute requirement for the recruitment process, yet this binding cannot be permanent. This proximal event of the inflammatory response is a good example of one of many highly orchestrated processes that are operative during normal inflammation.

MEDIATORS OF CHEMOTAXIS

Although the recruitment process is not unique to any particular organ, certain tissues appear to be more susceptible to inflammatory cell recruitment. This may be true of the lung, as this organ contains a large vascular bed where endothelial cells and inflammatory cells can initiate inflammation. In addition, the lungs are anatomically located to receive a number of inflammatory stimuli via the vasculature. For example, any insult to the small bowel or liver results in the generation of factors that are released into the blood and impact on the lung endothelium. Thus, the number of endothelial cells in the lung and the potential for a variety of stimuli to mediate endothelium-inflammatory cell interactions are all factors that place the lung in a unique immunoresponsive location. An additional structural aspect of the lung is the limited interstitial area. The small interstitium between the airspace and pulmonary vasculature affords only a small area for the movement of inflammatory cells.

The reversible binding of inflammatory cells to the endothelium is becoming increasingly clear, but the mechanisms responsible for the movement of peripheral circulating cells through the endothelium and basement membrane remain unknown. A number of coordinated events must occur in a timely manner to elicit the adherent cells on the lumen of the vessel to a restricted area of inflamed tissue. The chemotactic response has been an intriguing aspect of inflammation for over a century. Historically, a number of lipid, peptide, and polypeptide signals have been identified that possess potent chemotactic activity (Table 1). These inflammatory chemotaxins have a limited temporal window of in vivo activity. This group of traditional chemotactic factors include f-met-leu-phe, C5a, leukotriene B_4, and platelet-activating factor. Recent studies have now demon-

Table 1 Chemotactic Factors Comprise a Large Collection of Peptide, Polypeptide, and Lipid Mediators[a]

Chemotactic factor	Source
Leukotriene B_4	Neutrophils, macrophages
Platelet activating factor	Inflammatory cells
fMLP	Bacterial metabolism
C5a	Complement activation
Chemotactic cytokines	Immune, nonimmune cells

[a] These agents are derived from a variety of sources, yet all demonstrate potent activity for moving neutrophils.

strated that other polypeptide mediators, chemotactic cytokines, are synthesized during inflammation (6–9). These novel chemotactic cytokines include neutrophil activating peptide 1, interleukin-8 (IL-8), monocyte chemotactic protein 1 (MCP), neutrophil activating peptide 2 (NAP-2), and MGSA/GRO (10). Table 2 lists these chemotaxins and their cellular sources. Interleukin-8 is especially interesting, as this polypeptide mediator has a relatively long half-life and is stable under a number of adverse physical and chemical conditions (Table 3). In addition, IL-8 is extremely potent in vitro, as the chemotactic response of human neutro-

Table 2 Chemotactic Cytokines Represented by a Variety of Polypeptides Isolated from a Number of Sources[a]

Chemotactic cytokines	Cellular source
Interleukin-8	Phagocytes, nonimmune cells
Neutrophil activating peptide-2	Platelets
GRO/MGSA	Various cells
Monocyte chemotactic protein	Various cells

[a] Interestingly, IL-8 is a product of many cells, including mononuclear phagocytes, fibroblasts, and epithelial cells.

Table 3 Stability of IL-8 as Assessed by Treatment Under a Variety of Altered Physical and Chemical Conditions

Treatment	Conditions	% Activity remaining
Temperature	95°C/5 minutes	80
Temperature	56°C/1 h	80
pH 2.0	22°C/3 h	75
pH 10.0	22°C/3 h	90
β-ME (1.0%)[a]	22°C/3 h	30
Trypsin (100 μg/ml)	37°C/4 h	100

[a] Only B-ME (2-mercaptoethanol) was found to reduce the activity of IL-8.

phils in the Boyden chamber can be observed in the nM range. To place the biological activity of IL-8 in perspective, this chemotactic cytokine appears to be more potent in moving human neutrophils then fMLP.

Although IL-8 is more potent than other chemotactic factors, the mechanism by which this chemotactic cytokine activates human neutrophils is similar to that for other chemoattractants. Interleukin-8 can activate neutrophils by a GTP-binding protein pathway that is both calcium and protein kinase C dependent (11,12). Thus, inhibitors of protein kinase C, such as staurosporin, are inhibitors of both IL-8 and fMLP-induced neutrophil activation. Apparently a number of chemotactic factors share a common mechanism of signal transduction that may lead to cell activation.

SUPERGENE FAMILY OF CHEMOTACTIC CYTOKINES

Structurally IL-8 is quite different from other characterized chemotaxins, and this chemotactic cytokine belongs to a supergene family of immune mediators (13). Significant homology exists between IL-8 and such diverse factors as platelet factor 4, β-thromboglobulin, and MGSA (Table 4). As with IL-8, the monocyte chemotactic protein also belongs to a distinct supergene family of mediators (Table 5). Recently MCP was shown to be structurally identical to the cell competence factor JE (14,15). This finding raises a number of speculations regarding the full spectrum of biological activities for the various chemotactic cytokines. Although

Table 4 High Degree of Homology Between Isolated, Cloned, and Sequenced Proteins and IL-8[a]

β-Thromboglobulin	Platelet factor 4
GRO	Platelet basic protein
IP-10 inducible protein	9E3-U-SRC induced protein

[a] A major area of conservation in all proteins in this supergene family is the absolute position of the four cysteine residues.

Table 5 Monocyte Chemotactic Proteins Also Belong to a Supergene Family of Mediators[a]

Protein	Homology (%)
RANTES	28
TCA-3	25
JE (mouse)	55
JE (human)	100
MCP	36

[a] As shown, MCP has a high degree of homology with a variety of other proteins. IL-8 and MCP possess approximately 21% homology.

IL-8 has both neutrophil and lymphocyte chemotactic activity (16), it has been referred to in the literature by a number of different labels, all based on the neutrophil chemotactic and activating activity. The other names for IL-8 include monocyte-derived neutrophil chemotactic factor (MDNCF), neutrophil chemotactic factor (NCF), neutrophil activating peptide, monocyte-derived neutrophil activating peptide (NAP-1), and monocyte-derived neutrophil activating peptide (MONAP) (10). Interleukin-8 is classified as an inflammatory mediator because it possesses structural similarity to other inflammatory agents, it has chemotactic activity, and the synthesis of IL-8 can be induced by other well-characterized inflammatory compounds, including lipopolysaccharide (LPS), IL-1, and TNF. The last two cytokines again are crucial to the recruitment of inflammatory cells from the lumen of a vessel to an area of inflammation. Not only are IL-1 and TNF instrumental in adhering the inflammatory cells to the endothelium, but these two cytokines also induce the expression of chemotactic factors necessary to actually move the cells. Yet, neither IL-1 nor TNF is directly chemotactic. Recent studies have shown that IL-8 possesses selective activity for neutrophils in the phagocytic cell lineage, as blood monocytes are not responsive to IL-8. It must be further noted that IL-8 has been shown to induce the movement of lymphocytes (16). The elicitation of lymphocytes appears to occur at a much lower molar concentration of IL-8 compared to neutrophils. The actual roles of IL-8 in promoting the recruitment of lymphocytes in disease states must await further studies.

STIMULUS-SPECIFIC INDUCTION OF INTERLEUKIN-8 EXPRESSION

Recently, the synthesis and gene expression of both IL-8 and MCP has generated much interest in the scientific area of chemotactic mediators, as these chemotactic cytokines are expressed by a number of different cells. For example, IL-8 can be expressed by both immune and nonimmune cells. Monocytes (13), alveolar macrophages (17), fibroblasts (8), epithelial cells (18), and hepatocyte cell lines (19) have all been identified as cellular sources of IL-8. A variety of cells are a potential source of IL-8, and many exhibit stimulus specificity with regard to IL-8 gene expression and the subsequent synthesis of bioactive protein. As shown in Table 6, a number of cell types previously considered targets of an inflammatory response can synthesize IL-8 when appropriately stimulated. This aspect of stimulus specificity is clearly shown by the densitometric tracing of the northern blot analysis of IL-8 mRNA isolated from primary human fibroblasts treated with LPS, IL-1, heated IL-1, or control media (Fig. 1). LPS was not efficacious in triggering IL-8 gene expression by fibroblasts, but IL-1 was a potent stimulus. As a further control, heat-inactivated IL-1 was not effective in the induction of steady-state IL-8 mRNA. Investigations have now demonstrated that fibroblasts treated with low concentrations of TNF (20 pg/ml) can express IL-8 mRNA by 2 h and secrete biologically active IL-8 by 4 h. The peak in TNF-induced fibroblast IL-8 was shown to occur at 8 h and persist for the next 24 h. A similar kinetic pattern was observed using either IL-1α or IL-1β. Interestingly, the induction of IL-8 by fibroblasts, epithelial cells, and hepatocytes appears to be dependent upon initial host-derived cytokines. IL-1 and TNF are again the key polypeptide mediators that play a central role in the expression of IL-8. In this scenario, the

TABLE 6 Stimulus-Specific Induction of IL-8 mRNA and Active Protein[a]

Cell type	Stimulus			
	LPS	IL-1	TNF	IL-6
Alveolar macrophage	+ + + +	+ + + +	+ + +	− − −
Blood monocyte	+ + + +	+ + + +	+ + +	− − −
Endothelial cell	+ + +	+ + + +	+ + +	− − −
Epithelial cells	− − −	+ + + +	+ + +	− − −
Fibroblast	− − −	+ + + +	+ + +	− − −
Hepatocyte line	− − −	+ + + +	+ + +	− − −

[a] Alveolar macrophages, monocytes, and endothelial cells all responded to LPS, IL-1, or TNF. The noninflammatory cells (fibroblasts, epithelial cells, and hepatocytes) apparently need the host to respond to an initial challenge and generate IL-1 and/or TNF before the expression of IL-8, as LPS was not effective in the induction of IL-8 gene expression.

synthesis of IL-8 is dependent upon cytokine networking. The production of IL-8 by fibroblasts, epithelial cells, and hepatocytes is not directly influenced by LPS, but LPS-induced IL-1 and TNF are major stimuli. Thus LPS serves as the initial signal to upregulate IL-1 and TNF, which in turns induce the expression of IL-8 by the noninflammatory cells.

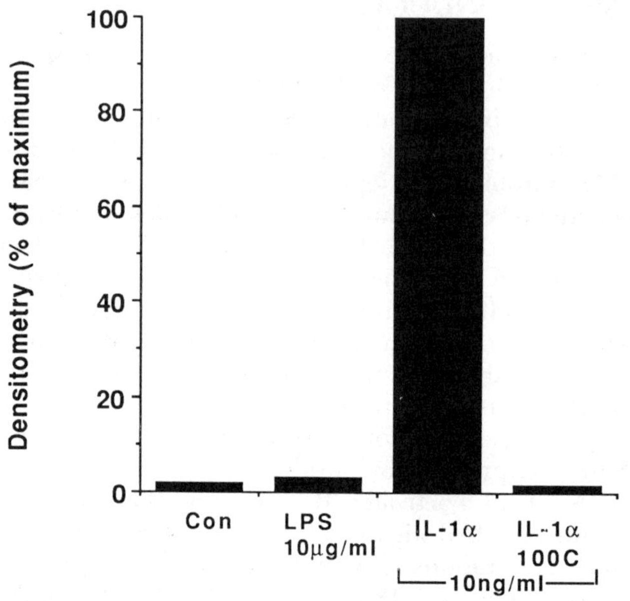

FIGURE 1 Fibroblast interleukin-8 gene expression is not dependent upon LPS but is specifically expressed by 10 ng/ml of IL-1α. As shown in the densitometry of the northern blot, fibroblast IL-8 was not induced by LPS (10 μg/ml) or heat-inactivated IL-1α, but significant expression was observed with native IL-1α. Similar expression was found using either IL-1β or TNF.

INTERLEUKIN-8 GENE EXPRESSION AND CYTOKINE NETWORKS

Our laboratory has assessed the cytokine network phenomenon for the induction of IL-8 gene expression using a coculture technique. The conditioned media from LPS-responsive cells, such as blood monocytes and alveolar macrophages, is overlaid on cells not susceptible to LPS stimulation. The latter cells are then assessed for steady-state IL-8 mRNA expression. In addition, neutralizing antibodies specific for either IL-1 or TNF are added to the macrophage-conditioned media before challenging the second cultures. As shown in Fig. 2, conditioned media generated by the addition of 100 ng/ml of LPS to human alveolar macrophages (isolated from nondiseased, nonsmoking volunteers) served as a potent stimulus for IL-8 mRNA expression by human type II-like pulmonary epithelial cells (A549 cells). Densitometry of the northern blots also demonstrated that the conditioned media contained stimulatory levels of IL-1 and TNF, as neutralizing antibodies to these cytokines were effective in reducing the activity of the conditioned media. Steady-state epithelial cell IL-8 mRNA levels induced by the alveolar macrophage-conditioned media could be suppressed by 50% when anti-IL-1β antibodies were added to the conditioned media, and an approximate 20% reduction was observed using anti-TNF antibodies. These data demonstrate that nontraditional immune cells can become active "effector" cells during an inflammatory response. An important regulatory step in the generation of IL-8 by fibroblasts and epithelial cells involves cytokine networking, as these cells are dependent upon an initial host response before the production of IL-8.

As previously discussed, the endothelium is of paramount importance for the normal recruitment of inflammatory cells. Not only are endothelial cells important in binding inflammatory cells as a proximal event of chemotaxis, but these cells can synthesize a number of inflammatory mediators when stimulated with LPS,

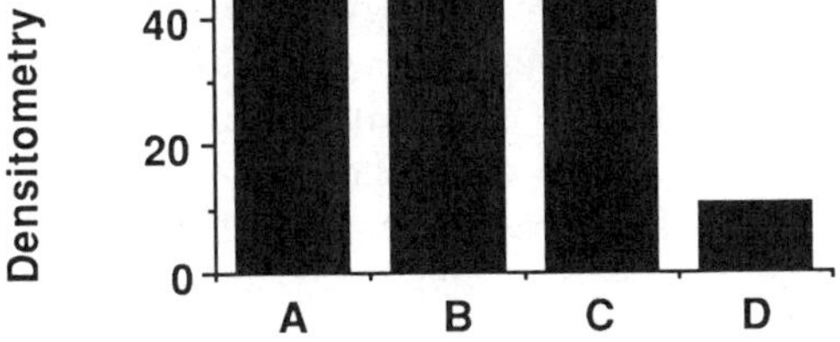

FIGURE 2 Densitometric analysis of IL-8 mRNA northern blots demonstrating cytokine networking. (A) Conditioned media from LPS-treated alveolar macrophages could induce a significant steady-state IL-8 mRNA from LPS-resistant human type II-like pulmonary epithelial cells. Pretreating the LPS-conditioned media with antihuman IL-1β (B) or antihuman TNF antibody (C), or both (D), reduced IL-8 mRNA expression by 50, 20, and 90%, respectively.

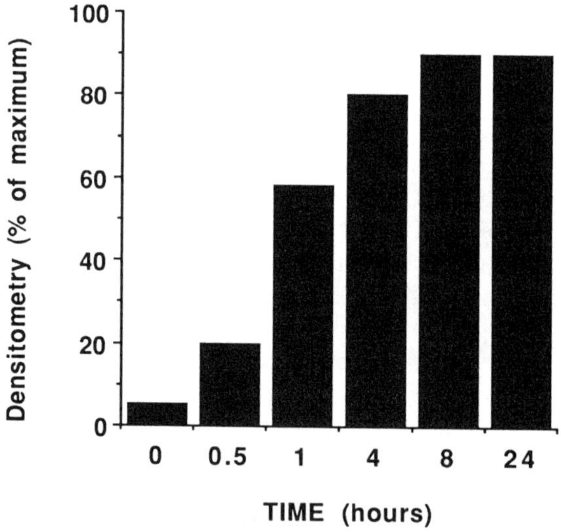

FIGURE 3 Relative densitometric analysis of steady-state IL-8 mRNA from human umbilical endothelial cells treated with TNF. The data represent a time-dependent expression of IL-8 mRNA.

IL-1, or TNF. Various studies have identified endothelial cells as a source of arachidonate metabolites (20), tissue factor (2), and numerous cytokines (3,21,22). The central role that the endothelium plays during the initial phases of inflammation is further strengthened by our studies showing that primary endothelial cell cultures can synthesize IL-8 in response to LPS, IL-1, or TNF (9). Human umbilical endothelial cells demonstrated a time-dependent expression of IL-8 mRNA in response to TNF. As shown by the densitometric scans of the northern blots in Fig. 3, IL-8 mRNA could be observed by 2 h after endothelial cell stimulation and the expression persisted for the next 24 h. The production of chemotactic activity followed a similar kinetic curve. Further studies demonstrated that IL-1-, TNF-, or LPS-challenged endothelial cells could result in a primary induction of IL-8 mRNA that was superinducible. This suggests that all three stimuli can directly induce the expression of IL-8 mRNA (an intermediate protein is not involved) and that IL-8 mRNA is regulated by intracellular repressor proteins. This observation has also been observed with other cytokines (23). Interestingly, treatment of endothelial cells with either prostaglandin E_2 or dexamethasone, two compounds known to regulate the expression of certain cytokines, did not alter steady-state IL-8 mRNA induced by LPS, TNF, or IL-1. These data further support the role of the endothelium as an important source of cytokines necessary to initial inflammatory processes.

SUMMARY

A number of recent investigations support the theory that the interactions between immune and nonimmune cells, LPS, and certain cytokines are pivotal events for the initiation and amplification of an inflammatory response. A number of infectious agents have been associated with the initiation of an inflammatory response, but only recently has the pathophysiological response been directly related to host-derived soluble cytokines. A number of theories have been provided for the maintenance of an inflammatory response, and data from our laboratories support the role of cytokine networking as a major mechanism for sustaining inflammation. Undoubtedly, further studies will continue to uncover the involvement of cytokine networks in various facets of the inflammatory response.

ACKNOWLEDGMENTS

The authors thank Peggy Otto and Suzanne Miller for excellent secretarial support. These studies were supported in part by National Institutes of Health Grants DK38149, HL319634, and HL35276. Dr. Kunkel is an Established Investigator of the American Heart Association.

REFERENCES

1. Beck G, Habict GS, Benach JL, Miller F. Interleukin-1: a common endogenous mediator of inflammation and the local Shartman reaction. Am J Pathol 1986; 125:421.
2. Bevilacqual MP, Pober JS, Majeau GR, Fiers W, Cotrain RS, Gimbrone MA. Recombinant tumor necrosis factor induces procoagulant activity in cultured human vascular endothelium. Proc Natl Acad Sci U S A 1986; 83:4533.
3. Nawroth PP, Bank I, Handley D, Cassimeris J, Chess L, Stern D. Tumor necrosis factor/cachectin interacts with endothelial cell receptors to induce release of interleukin-1. J Exp Med 1986; 163:1363.
4. Pohlman TH, Stanness KA, Beatty PG, Ochs HD, Harlan JM. An endothelial cell surface factor(s) induced in vitro by lPS, IL-1, and TNF-alpha increases neutrophil adherences by a CDW 18-dependent mechanism. J Immunol 1986; 136:4548.
5. Dustin ML, Rothlein R, Bhan AK, Dinarello CA, Springer TA. Induction by IL-1 and interferon-γ: tissue distribution, biochemistry, and function of a natural adherence molecule (ICAM-1). J Immunol 1986; 137(1):245–54.
6. Yoshimura T, Matsushima K, Oppenheim JJ, Leonard EJ. Neutrophil chemotactic factor produced by lipopolysaccharide (LPS)-stimulated human blood mononuclear leukocytes: partial characterization and separation from interleukin-1 (IL-1). J Immunol 1987; 139:788–793.
7. Matsushima K, Morishita K, Yoshimura T, et al. Molecular cloning of a human monocyte-derived neutrophil chemotactic factor (MDNCF) and the induction of MDNCF mRNA by interleukin-1 and tumor necrosis factor. J Exp Med 1988; 167:1883–93.
8. Strieter RM, Kunkel SL, Showell HR, et al. Monokine-induced neutrophil chemotactic factor gene expression in human fibroblasts. J Biol Chem 1989;264:10621–6.
9. Strieter RM, Kunkel SL, Showell HJ, et al. Endothelial cell gene expression of a neutrophil chemotactic factor by TNF-α, LPS, and IL-1β. Science 1989; 243:1467–9.
10. Matsushima K, Oppenheim JJ. Interleukin-8 and MCAF: novel inflammatory cytokine inducible by IL-1 and TNF. Cytokine 1989; 1:2–13.
11. Thelen M, Peveri P, Kernen P, on Tscharner V, Walz A, Baggiolini M. Mechanisms of neutrophil activation by NAF, a novel monocyte-derived peptide agonist. FASEB J 1988; 2:2702.
12. Simon RH, DeHart PD, Todd III RF. Neutrophil-induced injury of rat pulmonary alveolar epithelial cells. J Clin Invest 1986; 78:1375–86.

13. Yoshimura T, Matsushima K, Tanaka S, et al. Purification of a human monocyte-derived neutrophil chemotactic factor that has peptide sequence similarity to other defense cytokines. Proc Natl Acad Sci USA 1989; 84:9233.
14. Yoshimura T, Yuhki N, Moore S, Appella E, Lerman M, Leonard EJ. Human monocyte chemoattractant protein-1 (MCP-1). Full-length cDNA cloning, expression of mitogen-stimulated blood mononuclear leukocytes and sequence similarity to mouse competence gene JE. FEBS Lett 1989; 244:487–93.
15. Rollins BJ, Morrison ED, Stiles CD. Cloning and expression of JE, a gene inducible by platelet-derived growth factor and whose product has cytokine-like properties. Proc Natl Acad Sci U S A 1988; 85:3738–49.
16. Larsen CG, Anderson AO, Appella E, Oppenheim JJ, Matsushima K. Neutrophil activating protein (NAP-1) is also chemotactic for lymphocytes 1989; Science 243:1464–9.
17. Strieter RM, Chensue SW, Basha MA, et al. Human alveolar macrophage gene expression of interleukin-8 by tumor necrosis factor-α, lipopolysaccharide, and interleukin-1β. Am J Respir Cell Mol Biol 1990; 2:321–6.
18. Elner VM, Strieter RM, Elner SG, Baggiolini M, Lindley I, Kunkel SL. Neutrophil chemotactic factor (IL-8) gene expression by cytokine treated retinal pigment epithelial cells. Am J Respir Cell Mol Biol 1990; 136:745–50.
19. Thornton AJ, Strieter RM, Lindley I, Baggiolini M, Kunkel SL. Cytokine-induced gene expression of a neutrophil chemotactic factor/IL-8 in human hepatocytes. J Immunol 1990; 144:2609–13.
20. Kawakani M, Ishibashi S, Ogawa H, Murose T, Takaku F, Shibata S. Cachectin/TNF as well as interleukin-1 induces prostacyclin synthesis in cultured vascular endothelial cells. Biochem Biophys Res Comm 1986; 141:482.
21. Libby P, Ordovas JM, Auger KR, Robbins AH, Biringi LK, Dinarello DA. Endotoxin and tumor necrosis factor induce interleukin-1 gene expression in adult human vascular endothelial cell. Am J Pathol 1986; 124:179.
22. Warner SJ, Auger RK, Libby P. Recombinant human IL-1 induces IL-1 by adult human vascular endothelial cells. J Immunol 1987; 139:1911.
23. Collart MA, Belin D, Vassalli J, DeKossodo S, Vassalli P. Gamma-interferon enhances macrophage transcription of the tumor necrosis factor/cachectin, interleukin-1, and urokinase genes, which are controlled by short-lived repressors. J Exp Med 1986; 164:2113–8.

CHAPTER 8

TUMOR NECROSIS FACTOR
Structure and Function

Yoshiaki Tsuji and Frank M. Torti

Stanford University Medical Center and Palo Alto Veterans Administration Medical Center Palo Alto, California

INTRODUCTION

There have been rapid advances in our knowledge of tumor necrosis factor α (TNF, cachectin) structure and function in the past 5 years. In 1985, the TNF gene was cloned (see later); investigations of the effects of cachectin on adipocyte gene expression revealed that cachectin and TNF had the same biological functions. These were among the first demonstrations that tumor necrosis factor α had normal tissue targets. This brought together the research initiated by Dr. Old and collaborators on tumor necrosis and the newly discovered activities of TNF on cellular genes. Research in the last 5 years has extended the range of target cells and tissues responsive to this hormone to muscle cells, cells of hematopoietic lineage, endothelium, bone, cartilage, and fibroblasts, among others. This process defined not only a set of targets for TNF function but has clarified the pathogenesis a number of important acute and chronic disease states, including sepsis, chronic infections, inflammatory conditions, and cancer.

Another area of progress has been in defining the structure and function of the protein itself, as well as its receptors. This, almost of necessity, has led to investigation of signal transduction that links TNF binding to specific cell surface receptors to alterations in gene transcription. Although this is an active area of investigation for many cytokines and hormones, it is a particularly intriguing area of TNF research, due in large part to our limited understanding of what distinguishes cytotoxic signaling pathways from those pathways that effect normal tissue responses. The involvement of TNF in both the direct cytotoxicity of cells in culture and the hemorrhagic necrosis that Dr. Old and collaborators first observed will require further elucidation.

PROTEIN STRUCTURE OF TNF

TNF is a polypeptide secreted from macrophages and other immune effector cells in response to physiological stress (1). TNF has a subunit molecular weight of 17 kD by sodium dodecyl sulfate–polyacrylamide gel electrophoresis (SDS-PAGE) under both reducing and nonreducing conditions (2). The cDNA and genomic sequences of TNF derived from human (3–6), mouse (7), and rabbit (8,9) indicated that TNF is highly conserved among these species. TNF is produced as a precursor molecule with a presequence consisting of 79 amino acids (human), 76 amino acids (mouse), and 80 amino acids (rabbit) followed by a mature TNF sequence of 157, 156, and 154 amino acids, respectively (3,7,8). The isoelectric point of TNF is 5.3 (human), 3.9 (mouse), and 4.0 (rabbit). Amino acid sequences of the TNF precursors are highly homologous among these species (9); for example, there is 79% identity between the mouse and human TNF precursors (7). Further, a 26 amino acid hydrophobic stretch in the TNF presequence is highly conserved, suggesting an important role in TNF secretion or processing. The unusually long leader sequence of TNF is thought to function as a transmembrane domain. Decker et al. suggested the existence of membrane-associated TNF in activated macrophages (10), and Kriegler et al. identified a transmembrane form of 26 kD precursor TNF, which displayed cytotoxicity against L929 cells (11).

TNF has two cysteine residues conserved at positions 69 and 101, which are involved in a single intramolecular disulfide bond (2,7,8). Analysis by site-directed mutagenesis of the TNF protein has shown that the absence of a disulfide bond decreases such diverse biological activities as cytotoxicity, macrophage activation, and inhibition of lipogenesis by severalfold with no apparent secondary and tertiary conformational changes (12).

The amino acid sequence of mouse TNF has one N-glycosylation site at positions 7–9 (*Asn*-Ser-Ser) (7). In contrast, there is no glycosylation site in either human or rabbit TNF. This is consistent with the observation that natural TNF purified from mouse serum is able to bind concanavalin A (ConA) (13). However, the function of glycosylation in mouse TNF is still unknown, since recombinant mouse TNF produced in *Escherichia coli* displays an equivalent biological activity (7,13).

The elution profile of TNF activity following gel-filtration chromatography indicated that active conformation of TNF consists of dimer, trimer, or higher oligomers (2,5,6,14–16). The variation in the native TNF conformation has been attributed to differences in species or purification procedures. However, recent reports have shown that recombinant human TNF forms noncovalently associated trimers (17) and that the trimer form of natural and recombinant human and mouse TNF preferentially bind to cellular receptors and elicit cytotoxic activity (18). Furthermore, x-ray crystallography visualized a trimeric structure of the TNF molecule, which has shown that each subunit with antiparallel β-sandwich structure forms a trimeric molecule through an edge-to-face packing (19).

GENOMIC STRUCTURE OF TNF AND GENE REGULATION

TNF is a single-copy gene consisting of four exons and spans approximately 3 kilobases (6,9,20). The human TNF gene has been mapped to the short arm of chromosome 6 (between 6p23 and 6q12 segment) by analysis of human-mouse somatic cell hybrids (20). Chromosome *in situ* hybridization further defined the locus between 6p21.1 and 6p22 (21). The mouse TNF gene has been mapped to chromosome 17 (22). Genomic analysis demonstrated that TNF gene is closely linked to the lymphotoxin gene (TNF-β) (20), which is located approximately 1 kilobase upstream of TNF gene (22,23). Lymphotoxin is a structurally related cytokine with many similar biological activities to TNF (24). The homology of amino acid sequence between human TNF and human lymphotoxin was initially reported to be 28% and later increased to 35% by refining the gaps in the amino acid sequence comparisons (2,20). Human lymphotoxin is a glycosylated protein consisting of 171 amino acids. The leader sequence of the human lymphotoxin precursor is 34 amino acids long, 18 longer than TNF. Lymphotoxin does not have an intramolecular disulfide bond. The human TNF and human lymphotoxin genes share 56% homology in the fourth exon, which encodes 89 and 80% of mature protein, respectively, suggesting the fourth exon of TNF and lymphotoxin was derived from a common ancestral gene (20). Both TNF and lymphotoxin genes lie in similar orientations and are linked in the locus of major histocompatibility complex (MHC) to HLA-B and HLA-C, to the class III genes in human (21,25), and to H-2D in mouse (23,26). These observations are consistent with the finding that the human MHC is located between 6p21.1 and 6p21.3 (27).

Bacterial lipopolysaccharide (LPS), as well as some cytokines, activate macrophages to induce tumoricidal activity through the induction of TNF (28–31). The induction of TNF by LPS is regulated both at the transcriptional and the posttranscriptional levels (32). Interferon-γ increases TNF mRNA and TNF protein in LPS-stimulated macrophages (33,34) through the enhancement of transcription of the TNF gene (35). Expression of the TNF gene appears in part to be controlled by short-lived repressor proteins, since the inhibition of protein synthesis by cycloheximide alone induces the transcription of the TNF gene (35). TNF mRNA, as well as mRNAs of some other inflammatory mediators, has a common nucleotide sequence (UUAUUUAU) in the 3′-untranslated regions (36) that may be partly involved in the regulation of TNF gene expression, either at a transcriptional level or at a posttranscriptional level through the formation of complexes with AUUUA-specific mRNA binding protein (37). Jongeneel et al. recently characterized the regulatory elements of 5′ promoter and enhancer regions involved in the transcriptional regulation of TNF gene expression. It was demonstrated that (a) the TNF gene and the lymphotoxin gene are under the independent control of their own promoters, (b) the lymphotoxin promoter is silent in macrophages, and (c) more than one κB-type enhancer participates in the LPS-induced activation of the TNF promoter (38,39). Another group has identified a phorbol ester-responsive region in the TNF gene. This region is proximal to the TATAA box and does not include kB-type sequences (40), suggesting the existence of inducer-specific multiple regulatory mechanisms.

TNF RECEPTOR

The action of polypeptide hormones, including various cytokines, is initiated by binding to their specific receptors; not surprisingly, binding of TNF to its receptor(s) is also the initial step in the biological activities of TNF. Subsequent signal transduction pathways activated by TNF-receptor interaction are involved in the expression of multiple TNF biological activities; this is consistent with a report that microinjection of TNF into the cells does not produce TNF activity (41) and also that some of monoclonal antibodies to TNF receptor can mimic such biological effects of TNF as cytotoxic activity in U937 cells and growth-stimulating activity in FS4 fibroblasts (42). However, a contrasting result demonstrating cytotoxicity of microinjected TNF has recently been reported (43), perhaps due to cell type specificity.

Extensive characterization of TNF receptor has been carried out comparing TNF-sensitive and TNF-resistant cells to clarify the mechanism of selective cytotoxic activity of TNF. This approach has demonstrated the cell surface expression of a single class of high-affinity TNF receptors in both types of cells. TNF binding sites per cell ranged from 10^3 to 10^4, with a dissociation constant of between 10^{-9} and 10^{-10} M. However, there was a poor correlation between the number of TNF binding sites per cell, affinity for TNF, and susceptibility to TNF cytotoxic activity (44–46). Additionally, the internalization and subsequent degradation of the TNF receptor complex occurred similarly in both TNF-sensitive and TNF-resistant cells (45). These results suggest that the cell surface expression of TNF receptor is necessary but not sufficient for target cells to be susceptible to TNF cytotoxic activity. The measurement of molecular mass for the TNF receptor by cross-linking the receptor to ^{125}I-TNF has been carried out by several groups and indicated the presence of multiple TNF-receptor peptide complexes of 95 and 75 kD (44), 100 kD (47–49), and 138, 90, 75, and 54 kD (50). The size discrepancies among investigators may come from diversity of TNF oligomer forms and/or differences in the cell lines and cross-linkers used. Furthermore, it has been demonstrated that the TNF receptor is associated with a cell surface component with a molecular weight of 200 kD (Fas antigen) that is involved in mediating the cytotoxic signal of TNF (51).

The level of TNF receptor expression can be regulated by certain immune modulators. TNF binding capacity is enhanced by interferon-γ by increasing the receptor number without changing binding affinity (52–54). The expression of Fas antigen is also increased by interferon γ (51). Interleukin-1 (IL-1) does not compete with TNF binding to TNF receptor in 3T3-L1 adipocytes (55), or vice versa in B lymphocytes (56). However, IL-1 as well as protein kinase C activators, such as phorbol ester, downmodulate TNF receptor in human fibroblasts (57,58). An additional complexity arises because TNF and lymphotoxin share a common receptor (52).

The interaction of TNF and its receptor is not clearly defined. However the N-terminal region of TNF appears to be in part involved in TNF receptor binding, since specific antibodies against amino acid positions between 1 and 15 of TNF blocked TNF binding to its receptor (59); mutant TNF lacking the 10 N-terminal amino acids showed decreased binding ability to TNF receptor and a concomitant decrease in cytotoxic activity (60,61).

Characterization of the TNF receptor has recently moved forward with the isolation of cDNAs for a human 55 kD TNF receptor by two groups (62,63). Loetscher et al. initially prepared several monoclonal antibodies against human TNF receptor and demonstrated the existence of two distinct TNF receptors with molecular weights of 55 and 75 kD (42,64). They purified the 55 kD protein, thought to be a functional TNF receptor (42), and determined the partial amino acid sequence of this receptor protein. Oligo screening of a cDNA library led to the isolation of the 55 kD TNF receptor cDNA. Using another approach, Schall et al. purified a TNF binding protein from the serum of cancer patients, determined the amino acid sequence, and also identified the cDNA for this binding protein as a 55 kD TNF receptor (63). The rationale for this approach was derived from the observations of Seckinger et al. and Engelmann et al., who demonstrated the existence of TNF binding proteins in human urine (65–67) and indicated that the TNF binding proteins are soluble forms of two types of TNF receptors (68). The N-terminal amino acid sequence in one of their TNF binding proteins (Asp-Ser-Val-Cys-Pro) is identical to Schall's material.

The cDNA for the 55 kD human TNF receptor has an open reading frame encoding a 455 amino acid peptide with a 28 amino acid leader sequence and a single transmembrane domain in the middle of the mature receptor protein. The discrepancy between an apparent molecular weight of 55 kD on SDS-PAGE and the calculated molecular weight of mature protein of 47.5–50.5 kD could be explained by a posttranscriptional modification, such as N-glycosylation (three N-glycosylation sites in mature protein). Southern and northern blot analyses indicate that the 55 kD TNF receptor gene is a single gene consisting of at least three exons and a single mRNA species of about 3 kb (62,63). The extracellular domain of the receptor protein has a cysteine-rich sequence and significant homology to both the nerve growth factor receptor and B cell activation molecule Bp50 (62,63). It is likely that the TNF binding protein found in urine and in serum, corresponding to the 55 kD TNF receptor, is secreted after proteolytic cleavage between Arg and Asp [at position 11 and 12 (62); at position −1 and 1 (63,67,68)]. Soluble forms of other cytokine receptors, such as interleukin and interferon receptors, have also been reported (69–72), suggesting that the soluble form of these cytokine receptors may regulate ligand biological activity and ligand stability.*

BIOLOGICAL ACTIVITIES OF TNF

Effects on Adipocytes and Muscle: Roles in Cachexia and in Endotoxic Shock

Certain chronic infections and neoplastic diseases are associated with a condition termed cachexia, a syndrome of weight loss, profound wasting, anorexia, and muscle weakness. In a trypanosome-infected animal model, cachexia accompanied hypertriglycemia and a systemic suppression of lipoprotein lipase (LPL) (73). Subsequent studies demonstrated an activity that causes adipocyte LPL suppression (74–77) and animal weight loss (78) in the cultured supernatant of

* During preparation of this manuscript, another TNF receptor cDNA that encodes second TNF binding protein with a (Val-Ala-Phe-Thr-Pro) N-terminal amino acid sequence (67) was cloned by two groups. One used direct expression screening (Smith et al. Science 1990; 248:1019–23), the other a polymerase chain reaction (Heller et al. Proc Natl Acad Sci USA 1990; 87:6151–5). This TNF receptor also has a cysteine-rich extracellular domain and similarity to nerve growth factor receptor. These data indicate that there exist two types of TNF receptors in the cell surface and that both these TNF receptors have a secreted form in serum and urine with TNF binding activity.

endotoxin-stimulated macrophages. This mediator produced by activated macrophages was termed cachectin, in view of its presumed involvement in the pathogenesis of cachexia. Beutler et al. further purified cachectin and identified this molecule as TNF, based on the similarities of N-terminal amino acid sequences and biological activity (1,79). Torti et al. demonstrated that both cachectin and TNF inhibit adipocyte-specific gene expression at the transcriptional level (80). It has also been reported that purified TNF suppresses LPL activity and stimulates lipolysis in cultured adipocytes (81,82) and that both the chronic administration of human TNF in rats (83) and implantation of tumors secreting TNF in mice (84) induce a syndrome of cachexia.

TNF also appears to be involved in the pathogenesis of endotoxic shock. Infusion of human TNF into rats evokes a syndrome of endotoxemia, including hypotension and histopathological changes in a number of organs, as well as cachexia (85). Passive immunization against TNF protected animals from the lethal effects of endotoxin and bacteremia (86,87).

TNF is a potent modulator of cellular metabolism and gene expression. At higher concentrations in vitro, TNF alters glucose metabolism in cultured myotubes by increasing glucose uptake and glycogen breakdown (88) and muscle plasma membrane potential (89). At lower concentrations of TNF, Miller et al. reported that TNF specifically inhibits myoblast differentiation by suppressing muscle-specific gene expression. This effect was demonstrated to be differentiation stage specific by the lack of inhibition on fully differentiated myotubes (90). In adipocytes, TNF not only inhibits the differentiation process of preadipocytes but at least partially reverses differentiated adipocytes to a preadipocyte morphology and pattern of adipocyte gene expression (91). Torti et al. demonstrated that TNF induces the expression of ferritin heavy chain, a subunit of the iron storage protein ferritin, in muscle and adipocytes (90,92). This observation suggests that TNF [as well as IL-1 (93,94)] plays a regulatory role in cellular iron metabolism. The effects of TNF on ferritin regulation are different from those of cellular iron concentration (95). This is consistent with the observation that infectious and immunological insults, including those in which endotoxin is administered to animal models, are often accompanied by a disorder of iron homeostasis, causing an increase in serum ferritin and a decrease in serum iron (96).

Effects on Endothelium, Bone, and Cartilage

Endothelial cells participate in the development of immune and inflammatory responses as well as coagulation. TNF affects the expression of cell surface molecules of endothelial cells, stimulates the adhesion of neutrophils, and alters chemotaxis and procoagulant neutrophil activity. TNF was found to enhance the adherence of neutrophils to umbilical vein endothelial cells *in vitro* by acting on both the neutrophil and the endothelial cell (97). It was demonstrated that TNF increases the cell surface expression of neutrophil antigens required for optimum adherence and for complement component C3bi receptor function. Another experiment, showing that the TNF- (and IL-1) induced adherence of neutrophils to endothelium was inhibited by anti-CDw18 complex antibody, indicated the involvement of CDw18 complex on the endothelial cell surface in cytokine-mediated neutrophil adherence (98). Endothelial cell surface expression of inducible molecules in response to TNF and other cytokines was also characterized by immunological analysis using monoclonal antibodies to endothelial cell surface antigens, which demonstrated that TNF induces intercellular adhesion molecule 1 (ICAM-1) and class I major histocompatibility antigens (99,100). TNF induces the mRNAs for class I MHC antigens in human vascular endothelial cells and dermal fibroblasts *in vitro* in a manner dependent on the synthesis of an intermediate protein (101). This intermediate protein was suggested to be IL-6 (interferon-β_2) by antibody blocking experiments (102). The IL-6 gene has also been shown to be TNF inducible (103). Production of neutrophil chemotactic factor was also induced in human endothelial cells by TNF (104). This factor is similar to monocyte-derived neutrophil chemotactic factor produced in response to TNF and IL-1 (105). This neutrophil chemotactic factor was further characterized and renamed IL-8 (106).

TNF enhances endothelial procoagulant activity by inducing tissue factor, a cofactor initiating coagulation, and concomitant suppression of anticoagulant protein C pathway (107). Induction of procoagulant activity was observed not only with TNF but also with IL-1, and it was dependent on *de novo* protein and RNA synthesis (108). This effect of promoting clot formation may be important in the hemorrhagic tumor necrotizing activity of TNF and in the pathogenesis of coagulopathy associated with inflammatory and malignant disorders. TNF stimulates the release of platelet-derived growth factor (PDGF) (109) and IL-1 (110) from cultured endothelial cells. IL-1 is known to induce the synthesis of plasminogen activator inhibitor in endothelial cells (111). Plasminogen activator inhibitor is also inducible by TNF (112), indicating that TNF can initiate a cascade of inflammatory events on the endothelial cell surface both directly and through the stimulation of IL-1 production. Additionally, TNF promotes angiogenesis (113,114), which is consistent with the observation that inflammatory stimuli, especially infiltration of macrophages into inflammatory sites and wound repair, triggers angiogenesis.

Inflammation, immunological disorders, and malignant diseases are frequently associated with osteoclastic bone destruction and hypercalcemia. Osteoclast activating factor was initially purified from conditioned media of peripheral blood leukocytes and was found to be identical to IL-1β (115). It was found that TNF and lymphotoxin also stimulate bone resorption in fetal rat long bone culture through osteoclast activation. This effect was completely inhibited by salmon calcitonin, a specific inhibitor of osteoclast activity. Histological observation showed increased osteoclast number and decreased mineralized bone matrix following TNF treatment (116). TNF and lymphotoxin inhibit bone collagen synthesis and decrease the content of alkaline phosphatase, a marker enzyme of new bone formation, in cells with the osteoblast phenotype (116). TNF also stimulates cartilage resorption, release of proteoglycan from cartilage by a limited proteolytic degradation, and inhibition of proteoglycan synthesis (117). These phenomena may in part be promoted by the activities of collagenase and prostaglandin E_2. Collagenase and prostaglandin E_2 are produced by TNF-stimulated fibroblasts and macrophages (118–120) and are involved in the destruction of collagen matrix and stimulation of intracellular protease production responsible for tissue remodeling, respectively.

Effects on Fibroblasts and Gene Regulation

TNF was initially identified in the serum of mice treated with bacillus Calmette-Guerin (BCG), followed by an endotoxin challenge (121). It was shown to be capable of inducing hemorrhagic necrosis of transplanted tumors. Later experiments demonstrated that TNF showed preferential cytostatic and cytolytic activities on some tumor cell lines *in vitro* (122). As described earlier, TNF receptor analysis indicated poor correlation between receptor number or affinity for TNF and the susceptibility of cells to TNF cytotoxicity (44–46). In contrast to cytotoxicity on sensitive tumor cells, TNF was found to stimulate the growth of normal diploid fibroblasts (46,123). Vilcek et al. further demonstrated that the growth stimulatory activity of TNF is enhanced in the presence of an appropriate concentration of serum as well as insulin in culture media (123). TNF also induces the expression of epidermal growth factor receptor (124) and c-*fos* and c-*myc* mRNAs (125) in human diploid fibroblasts, which may be functionally related to the mitogenic action of TNF.

TNF was found to induce multiple cytokines in human diploid fibroblasts, including membrane-associated IL-1 (126), IL-6 (IFN-β_2) (103), and granulocyte-monocyte colony-stimulating factor (GM-CSF) (127). TNF-mediated induction of IL-6 appears to be important in the antiviral activity of TNF. It may also participate in an autocrine loop to control cell growth stimulated by TNF (103,128). TNF-induced antiviral activity was studied by several groups (129–132). These studies were not entirely consistent and indicated the probable existence of complex mechanisms in TNF-mediated antiviral activity. The antiviral activity of TNF was induced in some but not all cell types (129,130). Mestan et al. demonstrated that antibodies against IFN-β, but not against IFN-α or IFN-γ, partially blocked TNF-induced antiviral activity (129). Van Damme et al. and Rubin et al. found the participation of IFN-β_1 in TNF-induced antiviral activity (131,132). Wong and Goeddel indicated that the antiviral activity induced by TNF, as well as lymphotoxin, was not due to the induction of interferons by showing (a) absence of antiviral activity in conditioned medium from cells pretreated with TNF, (b) lack of adsorption of TNF-induced antiviral activity by anti-IFN antibodies (α, β, and γ), and (c) poor correlation between antiviral activity of TNF and the induction of IFN mRNAs (130). They further showed that virus infection induced cellular TNF production and susceptibility of killing by TNF. Induction of TNF synthesis by virus infection is also reported in monocytes (133). Although further work is necessary to clarify the entire mechanism of TNF-induced antiviral activity, that TNF induces antiviral activity in certain cells suggests the importance of TNF in the host defense system against viral infection.

The mechanism by which TNF activates IL-6 gene expression has been studied by several groups. Zhang et al. demonstrated in human diploid fibroblasts that TNF increases intracellular cAMP level, which can trigger IL-6 gene activation (134,135). The enhancer elements responsible for the activation of IL-6 gene expression by TNF have been identified: one is a 23 bp oligonucleotide sequence (designated AR1) containing a AP-1-like sequence (136,137); the other is a NF-κB binding site (138). TNF-induced IL-6 gene expression may likely be complex and cooperatively regulated by these enhancer elements, since TNF increases AP-1 activity in the stimulation of the collagenase gene expression (139) and increases NF-kB-like activity in the stimulation of IL-2 receptor α chain (140) or MHC class I gene (141). It has also been reported that TNF induces expression of human immunodeficiency virus (HIV) in chronically infected T cells (142,143) through activation of NF-kB (144), an observation that has implications for the pathogenesis of HIV disease.

In addition to the characterization of specific cellular proteins stimulated by TNF (145,146) and phosphorylation of proteins induced by TNF (147,148), further characterization of recently isolated TNF-induced genes by differential screening (149) may help elucidate the mechanism of TNF signal transduction and gene regulation.

Cytotoxic Action of TNF

The killing of neoplastic cells mediated by monocytes-macrophages is an important part of the host immune surveillance system. In addition to the initial finding of tumor necrosis activity in the sera of BCG-primed, endotoxin-treated mice (121), subsequent studies have revealed that TNF is principally derived from monocytes-macrophages (150,151) and also a mediator of cell killing by monocytes (29,30,152,153). Although the recent finding of a membrane-associated form of TNF presented a new insight into the direct cytotoxicity of macrophages on target cells through cell-to-cell contact (10,11), the molecular mechanisms by which TNF exerts cytotoxic activity to certain tumor cells remains unclear. The susceptibility of target cells to TNF cytotoxic activity likely relates to specific cellular responses after TNF binding to its receptor(s). The possibility that multiple components of TNF receptor determine the specificity and multiplicity of the TNF activities also cannot be excluded.

Metabolic inhibitors, such as actinomycin D and cycloheximide, and higher incubation temperatures are known to potentiate TNF cytotoxic activity in various cell types (154,155), and in some cases, treatment with these inhibitors renders TNF-resistant cells susceptible to lysis by TNF (145) (164). This suggests that newly synthesized RNA or protein is not necessary in TNF-induced cytotoxic pathways. However, the use of cycloheximide often complicates the interpretation by independently inducing cellular genes. Interferon-γ also enhances cytotoxic activity of TNF (46), which may be in part due to the induction of TNF receptor expression (54).

In contrast, pretreatment with TNF or IL-1 protects cells susceptible to TNF cytotoxicity from subsequent challenge with TNF plus cycloheximide (145,155) (164). It has been demonstrated that TNF induces TNF production and that TNF-resistant cells constituitively express TNF mRNA and protein, which resulted in an apparent decrease in the TNF receptor level (156–158). However, it seems to be difficult to explain the protective effect of TNF or IL-1 pretreatment simply through the downregulation of TNF receptor, since TNF and IL-1 are structurally unrelated and bind to different cell surface receptors (55,56). It is rather likely that, in TNF-sensitive cells, certain molecules induced by pretreatment of TNF or IL-1 may be involved in a cellular protection mechanism against TNF cytotoxicity. The idea of cellular protection mechanisms against TNF cytotoxicity has been supported by the finding that the TNF-resistant phenotype is dominant after formation of TNF-sensitive and TNF-resistant heterokaryons

(159). Several potential pathways have been implicated. Defilippi et al. demonstrated a correlation between IL-6 (IFN-β_2) mRNA expression and the resistance of cells to the cytotoxic effect of TNF (160). Heat shock also induces TNF resistance in WEHI-164 cells, which suggests the involvement of heat-shock protein (hsp68) in acquired resistance to the cytotoxic effects of TNF (161). Wong et al. demonstrated that manganous superoxide dismutase (MnSOD), a mitochondrial enzyme involved in the scavenging of superoxide radicals (O_2^-), is inducible by TNF or IL-1 and is involved in moderating the sensitivity to the cytotoxic action of TNF (162,163). As they pointed out, however, the protective effect of MnSOD overproduction on TNF cytotoxicity is not complete (163), suggesting that the cellular protection mechanism consists of a complex of several effector molecules or another unique cellular function specific to TNF-resistant cells. Ferritin heavy chain, one subunit of cellular iron binding protein ferritin, could be another candidate for a protection molecule against TNF cytotoxicity since it is inducible by TNF or IL-1 in TNF-resistant cells, such as preadipocytes, muscle, and normal diploid fibroblasts (90,92,93), and the level of intracellular iron affects TNF cytotoxicity, that is, augmentation and moderation of TNF cytotoxicity by iron and iron chelator, respectively (164).

Other effects of TNF also seem to be partly involved in regulating TNF cytotoxicity. These include endonuclease-induced DNA fragmentation (165,166), activation of phospholipase A_2 (167,168), and the activities of specific proteases (169,170). Glucocorticoids are known to protect target cells from TNF cytotoxicity (171–174) through the possible induction of a specific phospholipase A_2 inhibitor, lipocortin.

The effects of oncogene expression in target cells has been assessed with respect to cellular sensitivity to the cytotoxic action of TNF. Amplified expression of the HER2 (human epidermal growth factor 2) induces resistance to TNF in NIH3T3 cells (175) through alterations in the binding of TNF to its receptor. Expression of adenovirus E3 product also induces resistance to TNF (176). In contrast, adenovirus E1A oncogene expression induces cellular susceptibility to lysis by natural killer (NK) cells and activated macrophages (177,178) and to TNF cytotoxicity (179,180) (Torti et al., unpublished), although the E1A cellular targets responsible for TNF sensitivity remain unknown.

CONCLUSION

Although progress in understanding the functions and activities of tumor necrosis factor has been substantive, large areas of ignorance remain. We still do not understand the role of tumor necrosis factor in normal physiological functions, or how those functions relate to pathological processes that appear to be mediated by tumor necrosis factor. Furthermore, we are just beginning to understand the complex interrelationships among cytokines, growth factors, and hormones in health and disease.

ACKNOWLEDGMENTS

We are grateful to Doctors A. Taylor and S. Torti for suggestions and for reviewing the manuscript. We also thank J. Lozada and L. Stroschein for their excellent secretarial assistance.

REFERENCES

1. Beutler B, Cerami A. Cachectin and tumor necrosis factor as two sides of the same biological coin. Nature 1986; 320:584–8.
2. Aggarwal BB, Kohr WJ, Hass PE, et al. Human tumor necrosis factor: production, purification and characterization. J Biol Chem 1985; 260(4):2345–54.
3. Pennica D, Nedwin GE, Hayflick JS, et al. Human tumor necrosis factor: precursor structure, expression and homology to lymphotoxin. Nature 1984; 312:724–9.
4. Wang AM, Creasey AA, Ladner MB, et al. Molecular cloning of the complementary DNA for human tumor necrosis factor. Science 1985; 228:149–54.
5. Marmenout A, Fransen L, Tavernier J, et al. Molecular cloning and expression of human tumor necrosis factor and comparison with mouse tumor necrosis factor. Eur J Biochem 1985; 152:515–22.
6. Shirai T, Yamaguchi H, Ito H, Todd CW, Wallace RB. Cloning and expression in *Escherichia coli* of the gene for human tumor necrosis factor. Nature 1985; 313:803–6.
7. Pennica D, Hayflick JS, Bringman TS, Palladino MA, Goeddel DV. Cloning and expression in *Escherichia coli* of the cDNA for murine tumor necrosis factor. Proc Natl Acad Sci U S A 1985; 82:6060–4.
8. Ito H, Yamamoto S, Kuroda S, et al. Molecular cloning and expression in *Escherichia coli* of the cDNA coding for rabbit tumor necrosis factor. DNA 1986; 5:149–56.
9. Ito H, Shirai T, Yamamoto S, et al. Molecular cloning of the gene encoding rabbit tumor necrosis factor. DNA 1986; 5:157–65.
10. Decker T, Lohmann-Matthes M-L, Gifford GE. Cell-associated tumor necrosis factor (TNF) as a killing mechanism of activated cytotoxic macrophages. J Immunol 1987; 138(3):957–62.
11. Kriegler M, Perez C, DeFay K, Albert I, Lu SD. A novel form of TNF/cachectin is a cell surface cytotoxic transmembrane protein: ramifications for the complex physiology of TNF. Cell 1988; 53:45–53.
12. Narachi MA, Davis JM, Hsu Y-R, Arakawa T. Role of single disulfide in recombinant human tumor necrosis factor-alpha. J Biol Chem 1987; 262(27):13107–10.
13. Haranaka K, Carswell EA, Williamson BD, Prendergast JS, Satomi N, Old LJ. Purification, characterization, and antitumor activity of nonrecombinant mouse tumor necrosis factor. Proc Natl Acad Sci U S A 1986; 83:3949–53.
14. Beutler B, Mahoney J, Le Trang N, Pekala P, Cerami A. Purification of cachectin, a lipoprotein lipase-suppressing hormone secreted by endotoxin-induced raw 264.7 cells. J Exp Med 1985; 161:984–95.
15. Kull FC, Cuatrecasas P. Necrosin: purification and properties of a cytotoxin derived from a murine macrophage-like cell line. Proc Natl Acad Sci U S A 1984; 81:7932–6.
16. Haranaka K, Satomi N, Sakurai A, Nariuchi H. Purification and partial amino acid sequence of rabbit tumor necrosis factor. Int J Cancer 1985; 36:395–400.
17. Arakawa T, Yphantis DA. Molecular weight of recombinant human tumor necrosis factor-α. J Biol Chem 1987; 262(16):7484–5.
18. Smith RA, Baglioni C. The active form of tumor necrosis factor is a trimer. J Biol Chem 1987; 262(15):6951–4.
19. Jones EY, Stuart DI, Walker NPC. Structure of tumor necrosis factor. Nature 1989; 338:225–8.
20. Nedwin GE, Naylor SL, Sakaguchi AY, et al. Human lymphotoxin and tumor necrosis factor genes: structure, homology, and chromosomal localization. Nucleic Acids Res 1985; 13:6361–73.
21. Spies T, Morton CC, Nedospasov SA, Fiers W, Pious D, Strominger JL. Genes for

the tumor necrosis factors α and β are linked to the human major histocompatibility complex. Proc Natl Acad Sci U S A 1986; 83:8699–702.
22. Nedospasov SA, Hirt B, Shakhov AN, et al. The genes for tumor necrosis factor (TNF-alpha) and lymphotoxin (TNF-beta) are tandemly arranged on chromosome 17 of the mouse. Nucleic Acids Res 1986; 14:7713–25.
23. Gardner SM, Mock BA, Hilgers J, Huppi KE, Roeder WD. Mouse lymphotoxin and tumor necrosis factor: structural analysis of the cloned genes, physical linkage, and chromosomal position. J Immunol 1987; 139(2):476–83.
24. Gray PW, Aggarwal BB, Benton CV, et al. Cloning and expression of cDNA for human lymphotoxin, a lymphokine with tumor necrosis activity. Nature 1984; 312:721–4.
25. Carroll MC, Katzman P, Alicot EM, et al. Linkage map of the human major histocompatibility complex including the tumor necrosis factor genes. Proc Natl Acad Sci U S A 1987; 84:8535–9.
26. Muller U, Jongeneel CV, Nedospasov SA, Lindahl KF, Steinmetz M. Tumor necrosis factor and lymphotoxin genes map close to H-2D in the mouse major histocompatibility complex. Nature 1987; 325:265–7.
27. Morton CC, Kirsch IR, Nance WE, Evans GA, Korman AJ, Strominger JL. Orientation of loci within the human major histocompatibility complex by chromosomal *in situ* hybridization. Proc Natl Acad Sci U S A 1984; 81:2816–20.
28. Zacharchuk CM, Drysdale B-E, Mayer MM, Shin HS. Macrophage-mediated cytotoxicity: role of a soluble macrophage cytotoxic factor similar to lymphotoxin and tumor necrosis factor. Proc Natl Acad Sci U S A 1983; 80:6341–5.
29. Philip R, Epstein LB. Tumor necrosis factor as immunomodulator and mediator of monocyte cytotoxicity induced by itself, γ-interferon and interleukin-1. Nature 1986; 323:86–9.
30. Urban JL, Shepard HM, Rothstein JL, Sugarman BJ, Schreiber H. Tumor necrosis factor: a potent effector molecule for tumor cell killing by activated macrophages. Proc Natl Acad Sci U S A 1986; 83:5233–7.
31. Kornbluth RS, Edgington TS. Tumor necrosis factor production by human monocytes is a regulated event: induction of TNF-α-mediated cellular cytotoxicity by endotoxin. J Immunol 1986; 137(8):2585–91.
32. Beutler B, Krochin N, Milsark IW, Luedke C, Cerami A. Control of cachectin (tumor necrosis factor) synthesis: mechanisms of endotoxin resistance. Science 1986; 232:977–80.
33. Beutler B, Tkacenko V, Milsark I, Krochin N, Cerami A. Effect of γ interferon on cachectin expression by mononuclear phagocytes: Reversal of the $1ps^d$ (endotoxin resistance) phenotype. J Exp Med 1986; 164:1791–6.
34. Koerner TJ, Adams DO, Hamilton TA. Regulation of tumor necrosis factor (TNF) expression: interferon-γ enhances the accumulation of mRNA for TNF induced by lipopolysaccharide in murine peritoneal macrophages. Cell Immunol 1987; 109:437–43.
35. Collart MA, Belin D, Vassalli J-D, de Kossodo S, Vassalli P. γ Interferon enhances macrophage transcription of the tumor necrosis factor/cachectin, interleukin 1, and urokinase genes, which are controlled by short-lived repressors. J Exp Med 1986; 164:2113–8.
36. Caput D, Beutler B, Hartog K, Thayer R, Brown-Shimer S, Cerami A. Identification of a common nucleotide sequence in the 3'-untranslated region of mRNA molecules specifying inflammatory mediators. Proc Natl Acad Sci U S A 1986; 83:1670–4.
37. Malter JS. Identification of an AUUUA-specific messenger RNA binding protein. Science 1989; 246:664–6.
38. Jongeneel CV, Shakhov AN, Nedospasov SA, Cerottini J-C. Molecular control of

tissue-specific expression at the mouse TNF locus. Eur J Immunol 1989; 19:549–52.

39. Shakhov AN, Collart MA, Vassalli P, Nedospasov SA, Jongeneel CV. kB-type enhancers are involved in lipopolysaccharide-mediated transcriptional activation of the tumor necrosis factor α gene in primary macrophages. J Exp Med 1990; 171:35–47.
40. Economou JS, Rhoades K, Essner R, McBride WH, Gasson JC, Morton DL. Genetic analysis of the human tumor necrosis factor α/cachectin promoter region in a macrophage cell line. J Exp Med 1989; 170:321–6.
41. Niitsu Y, Watanabe N, Sone H, Neda H, Yamauchi N, Urushizaki I. Mechanism of the cytotoxic effect of tumor necrosis factor. Jpn J Cancer Res 1985; 76: 1193–7.
42. Espevik T, Brockhaus M, Loetscher H, Nonstad U, Shalaby R. Characterization of binding and biological effects of monoclonal antibodies against a human tumor necrosis factor receptor. J Exp Med 1990; 171:415–26.
43. Smith MR, Munger WE, Kung H-F, Takacs L, Durum SK. Direct evidence for an intracellular role for tumor necrosis factor-α: microinjection of tumor necrosis factor kills target cells. J Immunol 1990; 144(1):162–9.
44. Kull FC, Jacobs S, Cuatrecasas P. Cellular receptor for ^{125}I-labeled tumor necrosis factor: specific binding, affinity labeling, and relationship to sensitivity. Proc Natl Acad Sci U S A 1985; 82:5756–60.
45. Tsujimoto M, Yip YK, Vilcek J. Tumor necrosis factor: specific binding and internalization in sensitive and resistant cells. Proc Natl Acad Sci U S A 1985; 82:7626–30.
46. Sugarman BJ, Aggarwal BB, Hass PE, Figari IS, Palladino MA, Shepard HM. Recombinant human tumor necrosis factor-α: effects on proliferation of normal and transformed cells *in vitro*. Science 1985; 230:943–5.
47. Tsujimoto M, Feinman R, Kohase M, Vilcek J. Characterization and affinity crosslinking of receptors for tumor necrosis factor on human cells. Arch Biochem Biophys 1986; 249(2):563–8.
48. Stauber GB, Aiyer RA, Aggarwal BB. Human tumor necrosis factor-α receptor. Purification by immunoaffinity chromatography and initial characterization. J Biol Chem 1988; 263(35):19098–104.
49. Stauber GB, Aggarwal BB. Characterization and affinity cross-linking of receptors for human recombinant lymphotoxin (tumor necrosis factor-β) on a human histiocytic lymphoma cell line, U-937. J Biol Chem 1989; 264(6):3573–6.
50. Creasey AA, Yamamoto R, Vitt CR. A high molecular weight component of the human tumor necrosis factor receptor is associated with cytotoxicity. Proc Natl Acad Sci U S A 1987; 84:3293–7.
51. Yonehara S, Ishii A, Yonehara M. A cell-killing monoclonal antibody (ANTI-Fas) to a cell surface antigen co-downregulated with the receptor of tumor necrosis factor. J Exp Med 1989; 169:1747–56.
52. Aggarwal BB, Eessalu TE, Hass PE. Characterization of receptors for human tumor necrosis factor and their regulation by γ-interferon. Nature 1985; 318:665–7.
53. Tsujimoto M, Yip YK, Vilcek J. Interferon-γ enhances expression of cellular receptors for tumor necrosis factor. J Immunol 1986; 136(7):2441–4.
54. Ruggiero V, Tavernier J, Fiers W, Baglioni C. Induction of the synthesis of tumor necrosis factor receptors by interferon-γ. J Immunol 1986; 136(7):2445–50.
55. Beutler BA, Cerami A. Recombinant interleukin 1 suppresses lipoprotein lipase activity in 3T3-L1 cells. J Immunol 1985; 135(6):3969–71.
56. Matsushima K, Akahoshi T, Yamada M, Furutani Y, Oppenheim JJ. Properties of a specific interleukin 1 (IL-1) receptor on human Epstein-Barr virus-transformed

B lymphocytes: identity of the receptor for IL 1-α and IL 1-β. J Immunol 1986; 136(12):4496–502.
57. Holtmann H, Wallach D. Down regulation of the receptors for tumor necrosis factor by interleukin 1 and 4β-phorbol-12-myristate-13-acetate. J Immunol 1987; 139(4):1161–7.
58. Unglaub R, Maxeiner B, Thoma B, Pfizenmaier K, Scheurich P. Downregulation of tumor necrosis factor (TNF) sensitivity via modulation of TNF binding capacity by protein kinase C activators. J Exp Med 1987; 166:1788–97.
59. Socher SH, Riemen MW, Martinez D, et al. Antibodies against amino acids 1-15 of tumor necrosis factor block its binding to cell-surface receptor. Proc Natl Acad Sci U S A 1987; 84:8829–33.
60. Creasey AA, Doyle LV, Reynolds T, Jung T, Lin LS, Vitt CR. Biological effects of recombinant human tumor necrosis factor and its novel muteins on tumor and normal cell lines. Cancer Res 1987; 47:145–9.
61. Carlino JA, Lin LS, Creasey AA. Use of a sensitive receptor binding assay to discriminate between full-length and truncated human recombinant tumor necrosis factor proteins. J Biol Chem 1987; 262(3):958–61.
62. Loetscher H, Pan Y-CE, Lahm H-W, et al. Molecular cloning and expression of the human 55 kd tumor necrosis factor receptor. Cell 1990; 61:351–9.
63. Schall TJ, Lewis M, Koller KJ, et al. Molecular cloning and expression of a receptor for human tumor necrosis factor. Cell 1990; 61:361–70.
64. Brockhaus M, Schoenfeld H-J, Schlaeger E-J, Hunziker W, Lesslauer W, Loetscher H. Identification of two types of tumor necrosis factor receptors on human cell lines by monoclonal antibodies. Proc Natl Acad Sci U S A 1990; 87:3127–31.
65. Seckinger P, Isaaz S, Dayer J-M. A human inhibitor of tumor necrosis factor α. J Exp Med 1988; 167:1511–6.
66. Seckinger P, Isaaz S, Dayer J-M. Purification and biologic characterization of a specific tumor necrosis factor α inhibitor. J Biol Chem 1989; 264(20):11966–73.
67. Engelmann H, Novick D, Wallach D. Two tumor necrosis factor-binding proteins purified from human urine. Evidence for immunological cross-reactivity with cell surface tumor necrosis factor receptors. J Biol Chem 1990; 265(3):1531–6.
68. Engelmann H, Aderka D, Rubinstein M, Rotman D, Wallach D. A tumor necrosis factor-binding protein purified to homogeneity from human urine protects cells from tumor necrosis factor toxicity. J Biol Chem 1989; 264(20):11974–80.
69. Rubin LA, Kurman CC, Fritz ME, et al. Soluble interleukin 2 receptors are released from activated human lymphoid cells *in vitro*. J Immunol 1985; 135(5):3172–7.
70. Marcon L, Fritz ME, Kurman CC, Jensen JC, Nelson DL. Soluble Tac peptide is present in the urine of normal individuals and at elevated levels in patients with adult T cell leukemia (ATL). Clin Exp Immunol 1988; 73:29–33.
71. Novick D, Engelmann H, Wallach D, Rubinstein M. Soluble cytokine receptors are present in normal human urine. J Exp Med 1989; 170:1409–14.
72. Mosley B, Beckmann MP, March CJ, et al. The murine interleukin-4 receptor: molecular cloning and characterization of secreted and membrane bound forms. Cell 1989; 59:335–48.
73. Rouzer CA, Cerami A. Hypertriglyceridemia associated with *Trypanosoma brucei brucei* infection in rabbits: role of defective triglyceride removal. Mol Biochem Parasitol 1980; 2:31–8.
74. Kawakami M, Cerami A. Studies of endotoxin-induced decrease in lipoprotein lipase activity. J Exp Med 1981; 154:631–9.
75. Kawakami M, Pekala PH, Lane MD, Cerami A. Lipoprotein lipase suppression in 3T3-L1 cells by an endotoxin-induced mediator from exudate cells. Proc Natl Acad Sci U S A 1982; 79:912–6.

76. Pekala P, Kawakami M, Vine W, Lane MD, Cerami A. Studies of insulin resistance in adipocytes induced by macrophage mediator. J Exp Med 1983; 157:1360–5.
77. Mahoney JR, Beutler BA, Le Trang N, et al. Lipopolysaccharide-treated raw 264.7 cells produce a mediator that inhibits lipoprotein lipase in 3T3-L1 cells. J Immunol 1985; 134(3):1673–5.
78. Cerami A, Ikeda Y, Le Trang N, Hotez PJ, Beutler B. Weight loss associated with an endotoxin-induced mediator from peritoneal macrophages: The role of cachectin (tumor necrosis factor). Immunol Lett 1985; 11:173–7.
79. Beutler B, Greenwald D, Hulmes JD, et al. Identity of tumor necrosis factor and the macrophage-secreted factor cachectin. Nature 1985; 316:552–4.
80. Torti FM, Dieckmann B, Beutler B, Cerami A, Ringold GM. A macrophage factor inhibits adipocyte gene expression: an *in vitro* model of cachexia. Science 1985; 229:867–71.
81. Semb H, Peterson J, Tavernier J, Olivecrona T. Multiple effects of tumor necrosis factor on lipoprotein lipase *in vivo*. J Biol Chem 1987; 262(17):8390–4.
82. Kawakami M, Murase T, Ogawa H, et al. Human recombinant TNF suppresses lipoprotein lipase activity and stimulates lipolysis in 3T3-L1 cells. J Biochem 1987; 101:331–8.
83. Tracey KJ, Wei H, Manogue KR, et al. Cachectin/tumor necrosis factor induces cachexia, anemia, and inflammation. J Exp Med 1988; 167:1211–27.
84. Oliff A, Defeo-Jones D, Boyer M, et al. Tumors secreting human TNF/cachectin induce cachexia in mice. Cell 1987; 50:555–63.
85. Tracey KJ, Beutler B, Lowry SF, et al. Shock and tissue injury induced by recombinant human cachectin. Science 1986; 234:470–4.
86. Beutler B, Milsark IW, Cerami AC. Passive immunization against cachectin/tumor necrosis factor protects mice from lethal effect of endotoxin. Science 1985; 229:869–71.
87. Tracey KJ, Fong Y, Hesse DG, et al. Anti-cachectin/TNF monoclonal antibodies prevent septic shock during lethal bacteraemia. Nature 1987; 330:662–4.
88. Lee MD, Zentella A, Pekala PH, Cerami A. Effect of endotoxin-induced monokines on glucose metabolism in the muscle cell line L6. Proc Natl Acad Sci U S A 1987; 84:2590–4.
89. Tracey KJ, Lowry SF, Beutler B, Cerami A, Albert JD, Shires GT. Cachectin/tumor necrosis factor mediates changes of skeletal muscle plasma membrane potential. J Exp Med 1986; 164:1368–73.
90. Miller SC, Ito H, Blau HM, Torti FM. Tumor necrosis factor inhibits human myogenesis *in vitro*. Mol Cell Biol 1988; 8(6):2295–301.
91. Torti FM, Torti SV, Larrick JW, Ringold GM. Modulation of adipocyte differentiation by tumor necrosis factor and transforming growth factor beta. J Cell Biol 1989; 108:1105–13.
92. Torti SV, Kwak EL, Miller SC, et al. The molecular cloning and characterization of murine ferritin heavy chain, a tumor necrosis factor-inducible gene. J Biol Chem 1988; 263(25):12638–44.
93. Wei Y, Miller SC, Tsuji Y, Torti SV, Torti FM. Interleukin 1 induces ferritin heavy chain in human muscle cells. Biochem Biophys Res Commun 1990; 196(1):289–96.
94. Rogers JT, Bridges KR, Durmowicz GP, Glass J, Auron PE, Munro HN. Translational control during the acute phase response. J Biol Chem 1990; 265(24):14572–8.
95. Miller LL, Miller SC, Torti SV, Tsuji Y, Torti FM. Iron-independent induction of ferritin H chain by tumor necrosis factor alpha. Proc Natl Acad Sci U S A 1991; 88:4946–4950.

96. Roeser HP. Iron in biochemistry and medicine, Vol. II. New York: Academic Press, 1980:605–40.
97. Gamble JR, Harlan JM, Klebanoff SJ, Vadas MA. Stimulation of the adherence of neutrophils to umbilical vein endothelium by human recombinant tumor necrosis factor. Proc Natl Acad Sci U S A 1985; 82:8667–71.
98. Pohlman TH, Stanness KA, Beatty PG, Ochs HD, Harlan JM. An endothelial cell surface factor(s) induced *in vitro* by lipopolysaccharide, interleukin 1, and tumor necrosis factor-α increases neutrophil adherence by a CDw18-dependent mechanism. J Immunol 1986; 136(12):4548–53.
99. Pober JS, Bevilacqua MP, Mendrick DL, Lapierre LA, Fiers W, Gimbrone MA. Two distinct monokines, interleukin 1 and tumor necrosis factor, each independently induce biosynthesis and transient expression of the same antigen on the surface of cultured human vascular endothelial cells. J Immunol 1986; 136(5):1680–7.
100. Pober JS, Gimbrone MA, Lapierre LA, et al. Overlapping patterns of activation of human endothelial cells by interleukin 1, tumor necrosis factor, and immune interferon. J Immunol 1986; 137(6):1893–6.
101. Collins T, Lapierre LA, Fiers W, Strominger JL, Pober JS. Recombinant human tumor necrosis factor increases mRNA levels and surface expression of HLA-A,B antigens in vascular endothelial cells and dermal fibroblasts *in vitro*. Proc Natl Acad Sci U S A 1986; 83:446–50.
102. May LT, Helfgott DC, Sehgal PB. Anti-β-interferon antibodies inhibit the increased expression of HLA-B7 mRNA in tumor necrosis factor-treated human fibroblasts: Structural studies of the β_2 interferon involved. Proc Natl Acad Sci U S A 1986; 83:8957–61.
103. Kohase M, Henriksen-DeStefano D, May LT, Vilcek J, Sehgal PB. Induction of β_2-interferon by tumor necrosis factor: a homeostatic mechanism in the control of cell proliferation. Cell 1986; 45:659–66.
104. Strieter RM, Kunkel SL, Showell HJ, et al. Endothelial cell gene expression of a neutrophil chemotactic factor by TNF-α, LPS, and IL-1β. Science 1989; 243:1467–9.
105. Matsushima K, Morishita K, Yoshimura T, et al. Molecular cloning of a human monocyte-derived neutrophil chemotactic factor (MDNCF) and the induction of MDNCF mRNA by interleukin 1 and tumor necrosis factor. J Exp Med 1988; 167:1883–93.
106. Larsen CG, Anderson AO, Appella E, Oppenheim JJ, Matsushima K. The neutrophil-activating protein (NAP-1) is also chemotactic for T lymphocytes. Science 1989; 243:1464–6.
107. Nawroth PP, Stern DM. Modulation of endothelial cell hemostatic properties by tumor necrosis factor. J Exp Med 1986; 163:740–5.
108. Bevilacqua MP, Pober JS, Majeau GR, Fiers W, Cotran RS, Gimbrone MA. Recombinant tumor necrosis factor induces procoagulant activity in cultured human vascular endothelium: characterization and comparison with the actions of interleukin 1. Proc Natl Acad Sci U S A 1986; 83:4533–7.
109. Hajjar KA, Hajjar DP, Silverstein RL, Nachman RL. Tumor necrosis factor-mediated release of platelet-derived growth factor from cultured endothelial cells. J Exp Med 1987; 166:235–45.
110. Nawroth PP, Bank I, Handley D, Cassimeris J, Chess L, Stern D. Tumor necrosis factor/cachectin interacts with endothelial cell receptors to induce release of interleukin 1. J Exp Med 1986; 163:1363–75.
111. Nachman RL, Hajjar KA, Silverstein RL, Dinarello CA. Interleukin 1 induces endothelial cell synthesis of plasminogen activator inhibitor. J Exp Med 1986; 163:1595–600.
112. Medcalf RL, Kruithof EKO, Schleuning W-D. Plasminogen activator inhibitor 1

and 2 are tumor necrosis factor/cachectin-responsive genes. J Exp Med 1988; 168:751–9.

113. Leibovich SJ, Polverini PJ, Shepard HM, Wiseman DM, Shively V, Nuseir N. Macrophage-induced angiogenesis is mediated by tumor necrosis factor-α. Nature 1987; 239:630–2.

114. Frater-Schroder M, Risau W, Hallmann R, Gautschi P, Bohlen P. Tumor necrosis factor type α, a potent inhibitor of endothelial cell growth *in vitro,* is angiogenic *in vivo.* Proc Natl Acad Sci U S A 1987; 84:5277–81.

115. Dewhirst FE, Stashenko PP, Mole JE, Tsurumachi T. Purification and partial sequence of human osteoclast-activating factor: Identity with interleukin 1 β. J Immunol 1985; 135(4):2562–8.

116. Bertolini DR, Nedwin GE, Bringman TS, Smith DD, Mundy GR. Stimulation of bone resorption and inhibition of bone formation *in vitro* by human tumor necrosis factor. Nature 1986; 319:516–8.

117. Saklatvala J. Tumor necrosis factor α stimulates resorption and inhibits synthesis of proteoglycan in cartilage. Nature 1986; 322:547–9.

118. Dayer J-M, Beutler B, Cerami A. Cachectin/tumor necrosis factor stimulates collagenase and prostaglandin E_2 production by human synovial cells and dermal fibroblasts. J Exp Med 1985; 162:2163–8.

119. Bachwich PR, Chensue SW, Larrick JW, Kunkel SL. Tumor necrosis factor stimulates interleukin-1 and prostaglandin E_2 production in resting macrophages. Biochem Biophys Res Commun 1986; 136(1):94–101.

120. Elias JA, Gustilo K, Baeder W, Freundlich B. Synergistic stimulation of fibroblast prostaglandin production by recombinant interleukin 1 and tumor necrosis factor. J Immunol 1987; 138(11):3812–6.

121. Carswell EA, Old LJ, Kassel RL, Green S, Fiore N, Williamson B. An endotoxin-induced serum factor that causes necrosis of tumors. Proc Nat Acad Sci U S A 1975; 72(9):3666–70.

122. Old LJ. Tumor necrosis factor (TNF). Science 1985; 230:630–2.

123. Vilcek J, Palombella VJ, Henriksen-DeStefano D, et al. Fibroblast growth enhancing activity of tumor necrosis factor and its relationship to other polypeptide growth factors. J Exp Med 1986; 163:632–43.

124. Palombella VJ, Yamashiro DJ, Maxfield FR, Decker SJ, Vilcek J. Tumor necrosis factor increases the number of epidermal growth factor receptors on human fibroblasts. J Biol Chem 1987; 262(5):1950–4.

125. Lin J-X, Vilcek J. Tumor necrosis factor and interleukin-1 cause a rapid and transient stimulation of c-*fos* and c-*myc* mRNA levels in human fibroblasts. J Biol Chem 1987; 262(25):11908–11.

126. Le J, Weinstein D, Gubler U, Vilcek J. Induction of membrane-associated interleukin 1 by tumor necrosis factor in human fibroblasts. J Immunol 1987; 138(7):2137–42.

127. Munker R, Gasson J, Ogawa M, Koeffler HP. Recombinant human TNF induces production of granulocyte-monocyte colony-stimulating factor. Nature 1986; 323:79–82.

128. Kohase M, May LT, Tamm I, Vilcek J, Sehgal PB. A cytokine network in human diploid fibroblasts: interactions of β-interferons, tumor necrosis factor, platelet-derived growth factor, and interleukin-1. Mol Cell Biol 1987; 7(1):273–80.

129. Mestan J, Digel W, Mittnacht S, et al. Antiviral effects of recombinant tumor necrosis factor *in vitro.* Nature 1986; 323:816–9.

130. Wong GHW, Goeddel DV. Tumor necrosis factors α and β inhibit virus replication and synergize with interferons. Nature 1986; 323:819–22.

131. VanDamme J, De Ley M, Van Snick J, Dinarello CA, Billiau A. The role of interferon-

β_1 and the 26-kDa protein (interferon-β_2) as mediators of the antiviral effect of interleukin 1 and tumor necrosis factor. J Immunol 1987; 139(6):1867–72.

132. Rubin BY, Anderson SL, Lunn RM, et al. Tumor necrosis factor and IFN induce a common set of proteins. J Immunol 1988; 141(4):1180–4.
133. Aderka D, Holtmann H, Toker L, Hahn T, Wallach D. Tumor necrosis factor induction by sendai virus. J Immunol 1986; 136(8):2938–42.
134. Zhang Y, Lin J-X, Yip YK, Vilcek J. Enhancement of cAMP levels and of protein kinase activity by tumor necrosis factor and interleukin 1 in human fibroblasts: role in the induction of interleukin 6. Proc Natl Acad Sci U S A 1988; 85:6802–5.
135. Zhang Y, Lin J-X, Vilcek J. Synthesis of interleukin 6 (interferon-β_2/B cell stimulatory factor 2) in human fibroblasts is triggered by an increase in intracellular cyclic AMP. J Biol Chem 1988; 263(13):6177–82.
136. Ray A, Tatter SB, May LT, Sehgal PB. Activation of the human "β_2-interferon/hepatocyte-stimulating factor/interleukin 6" promoter by cytokines, viruses, and second messenger agonists. Proc Natl Acad Sci U S A 1988; 85:6701–5.
137. Ray A, Sassone-Corsi P, Sehgal PB. A multiple cytokine- and second messenger-responsive element in the enhancer of the human interleukin-6 gene: similarities with c-*fos* gene regulation. Mol Cell Biol 1989; 9(12):5537–47.
138. Libermann TA, Baltimore D. Activation of interleukin-6 gene expression through the NF-kB transcription factor. Mol Cell Biol 1990; 10(5):2327–34.
139. Brenner DA, O'Hara M, Angel P, Chojkier M, Karin M. Prolonged activation of *jun* and collagenase genes by tumor necrosis factor-α. Nature 1989; 337:661–3.
140. Lowenthal JW, Ballard DW, Bohnlein E, Greene WC. Tumor necrosis factor α induces proteins that bind specifically to kB-like enhancer elements and regulate interleukin 2 receptor α-chain gene expression in primary human T lymphocytes. Proc Natl Acad Sci U S A 1989; 86:2331–5.
141. Israel A, Le Bail O, Hatat D, et al. TNF stimulates expression of mouse MHC class I genes by inducing an NFkB-like enhancer binding activity which displaces constitutive factors. EMBO J 1989; 8(12):3793–800.
142. Folks TM, Clouse KA, Justement J, et al. Tumor necrosis factor α induces expression of human immunodeficiency virus in a chronically infected T-cell clone. Proc Natl Acad Sci U S A 1989; 86:2365–8.
143. Matsuyama T, Hamamoto Y, Soma G-I, Mizuno D'I, Yamamoto N, Kobayashi N. Cytocidal effect of tumor necrosis factor on cells chronically infected with human immunodeficiency virus (HIV): enhancement of HIV replication. J Virol 1989; 63(6):2504–9.
144. Osborn L, Kunkel S, Nabel GJ. Tumor necrosis factor α and interleukin 1 stimulate the human immunodeficiency virus enhancer by activation of the nuclear factor kB. Proc Natl Acad Sci U S A 1989; 86:2336–40.
145. Kirstein M, Baglioni C. Tumor necrosis factor induces synthesis of two proteins in human fibroblasts. J Biol Chem 1986; 261(21):9565–7.
146. Beresini MH, Lempert MJ, Epstein LB. Overlapping polypeptide induction in human fibroblasts in response to treatment with interferon-α, interferon-γ, interleukin 1α, interleukin 1β, and tumor necrosis factor. J Immunol 1988; 140(2):485–93.
147. Schutze S, Scheurich P, Pfizenmaier K, Kronke M. Tumor necrosis factor signal transduction. Tissue-specific serine phosphorylation of a 26-kDa cytosolic protein. J Biol Chem 1989; 264:3562–7.
148. Marino MW, Pfeffer LM, Guidon PT, Donner DB. Tumor necrosis factor induces phosphorylation of a 28-kDa mRNA cap-binding protein in human cervical carcinoma cells. Proc Natl Acad Sci U S A 1989; 86:8417–21.
149. Lee TH, Lee GW, Ziff EB, Vilcek J. Isolation and characterization of eight tumor

necrosis factor-induced gene sequences from human fibroblasts. Mol Cell Biol 1990; 10(5):1982–8.

150. Mannel DN, Moore RN, Mergenhagen SE. Macrophages as a source of tumoricidal activity (tumor necrotizing factor). Infect Immun 1980; 30(2):523–30.
151. Kelker HC, Oppenheim JD, Stone-Wolff D, et al. Characterization of human tumor necrosis factor produced by peripheral blood monocytes and its separation from lymphotoxin. Int J Cancer 1985; 36:69–73.
152. Kornbluth RS, Edgington TS. Tumor necrosis factor production by human monocytes is a regulated event: induction of TNF-α-mediated cellular cytotoxicity by endotoxin. J Immunol 1986; 137(8):2585–91.
153. Feinman R, Henriksen-DeStefano D, Tsujimoto M, Vilcek J. Tumor necrosis factor is an important mediator of tumor cell killing by human monocytes. J Immunol 1987; 138(2):635–40.
154. Kull FC Jr, Cuatrecasas P. Possible requirement of internalization in the mechanism of *in vitro* cytotoxicity in tumor necrosis serum. Cancer Res 1981; 41:4885–90.
155. Hahn T, Toker L, Budilovsky S, Aderka D, Eshhar Z, Wallach D. Use of monoclonal antibodies to a human cytotoxin for its isolation and for examining the self-induction of resistance to this protein. Proc Natl Acad Sci U S A 1985; 82:3814–8.
156. Rubin BY, Anderson SL, Sullivan SA, Williamson BD, Carswell EA, Old LJ. Nonhematopoietic cells selected for resistance to tumor necrosis factor produce tumor necrosis factor. J Exp Med 1986; 164:1350–5.
157. Spriggs D, Imamura K, Rodriguez C, Horiguchi J, Kufe DW. Induction of tumor necrosis factor expression and resistance in a human breast tumor cell line. Proc Natl Acad Sci U S A 1987; 84:6563–6.
158. Niitsu Y, Watanabe N, Neda H, et al. Induction of synthesis of tumor necrosis factor in human and murine cell lines by exogenous recombinant human tumor necrosis factor. Cancer Res 1988; 48:5407–10.
159. Nophar Y, Holtmann H, Ber R, Wallach D. Dominance of resistance to the cytocidal effect of tumor necrosis factor in heterokaryons formed by fusion of resistant and sensitive cells. J Immunol 1988; 140(10):3456–60.
160. Defilippi P, Poupart P, Tavernier J, Fiers W, Content J. Induction and regulation of mRNA encoding 26-kDa protein in human cell lines treated with recombinant human tumor necrosis factor. Proc Natl Acad Sci U S A 1987; 84:4557–61.
161. Jaattela M, Saksela K, Saksela E. Heat shock protects WEHI-164 target cells from the cytolysis by tumor necrosis factor α and β. Eur J Immunol 1989; 19:1413–7.
162. Wong GHW, Goeddel DV. Induction of manganous superoxide dismutase by tumor necrosis factor: possible protective mechanism. Science 1988; 242:941–4.
163. Wong GHW, Elwell JH, Oberley LW, Goeddel DV. Manganous superoxide dismutase is essential for cellular resistance to cytotoxicity of tumor necrosis factor. Cell 1989; 58:923–31.
164. Warren S, Miller SC, Torti SV, Tsuji Y, Torti FM. The role of iron in the cytotoxicity of tumor necrosis factor, submitted.
165. Rubin BY, Smith LJ, Hellermann GR, Lunn RM, Richardson NK, Anderson SL. Correlation between the anticellular and DNA fragmenting activities of tumor necrosis factor. Cancer Res 1988; 48:6006–10.
166. Laster SM, Wood JG, Gooding LR. Tumor necrosis factor can induce both apoptic and necrotic forms of cell lysis. J Immunol 1988; 141(8):2629–34.
167. Suffys P, Beyaert R, Van Roy F, Fiers W. Reduced tumor necrosis factor-induced cytotoxicity by inhibitors of the arachidonic acid metabolism. Biochem Biophys Res Commun 1987; 149(2):735–43.
168. Bayaert R, Vanhaesebroeck B, Suffys P, Van Roy F, Fiers W. Lithium chloride

potentiates tumor necrosis factor-mediated cytotoxicity *in vitro* and *in vivo*. Proc Natl Acad Sci U S A 1989; 86:9494–8.

169. Ruggiero V, Johnson SE, Baglioni C. Protection from tumor necrosis factor cytotoxicity by protease inhibitors. Cell Immunol 1987; 107:317–25.
170. Suffys P, Beyaert R, Van Roy F, Fiers W. Involvement of a serine protese in tumor-necrosis-factor-mediated cytotoxicity. Eur J Biochem 1988; 178:257–65.
171. Hepburn A, Boeynaems J-M, Fiers W, Dumont JE. Modulation of tumor necrosis factor-α cytotoxicity in L929 cells by bacterial toxins, hydrocortisone and inhibitors of arachidonic acid metabolism. Biochem Biophys Res Commun 1987; 149(2):815–22.
172. Tsujimoto M, Okamura N, Adachi H. Dexamethasone inhibits the cytotoxic activity of tumor necrosis factor. Biochem Biophys Res Commun 1988; 153(1):109–15.
173. Reid TR, Torti FM, Ringold GM. Evidence for two mechanisms by which tumor necrosis factor kills cells. J Biol Chem 1989; 264(8)4583–9.
174. Abe S, Yamamoto T, Iihara S, Yamazaki M, Mizuno D. A possible role of glucocorticoids: an intrinsic inhibitor of the cytotoxic activity of tumor necrosis factor. Jpn J Cancer Res 1988; 79:305–8.
175. Hudziak RM, Lewis GD, Shalaby MR, et al. Amplified expression of the HER2/ERBB2 oncogene induces resistance to tumor necrosis factor α in NIH 3T3 cells. Proc Natl Acad Sci U S A 1988; 85:5102–6.
176. Gooding LR, Elmore LW, Tollefson AE, Brady HA, Wold WSM. A 14,700 MW protein from the E3 region of adenovirus inhibits cytolysis by tumor necrosis factor. Cell 1988; 53:341–6.
177. Cook JL, Walker TA, Lewis Jr AM, Ruley HE, Graham FL, Pilder SH. Expression of the adenovirus E1A oncogene during cell transformation is sufficient to induce susceptibility to lysis by host inflammatory cells. Proc Natl Acad Sci U S A 1986; 83:6965–9.
178. Cook JL, May DL, Lewis Jr AM, Walker TA. Adenovirus E1A gene induction of susceptibility to lysis by natural killer cells and activated macrophages in infected rodent cells. J Virol 1987; 61(11):3510–20.
179. Chen M-J, Holskin B, Strickler J, et al. Induction by E1A oncogene expression of cellular susceptibility to lysis by TNF. Nature 1987; 330:581–3.
180. Cook JL, May DL, Wilson BA, et al. Role of tumor necrosis fctor-α in E1A oncogene-induced susceptibility of neoplastic cells to lysis by natural killer cells and activated macrophages. J Immunol 1989; 142(12):4527–34.

CHAPTER 9

TUMOR NECROSIS FACTOR, INTERLEUKIN-1, INTERLEUKIN-6, INTERLEUKIN-8, AND INTERFERON-γ IN SEPTIC SHOCK

Anders Waage, Refaat Shalaby,* and Terje Espevik

Institute of Cancer Research
University of Trondheim
Trondheim, Norway

INTRODUCTION

Septic shock is a serious pathophysiological derangement characterized by circulatory failure and often leading to multiorgan failure, adult respiratory distress syndrome, and death (1). Monocytes, neutrophils, and endothelial cells appear to be particularly important in the pathogenesis of the syndrome, which often affects the lungs, kidneys, brain, and heart. At the cellular level the syndrome is associated with hypermetabolism and energy deficit leading to cellular injury. The systemic circulation is affected by decreased vascular tonus, hypotension, and compensatory tachycardia. The composition and distribution of the body fluids are changed, including hyperglycemia, electrolyte abnormalities, and fluid retention. The coagulation and fibrinolytic system is frequently imbalanced. In the initial phase hypercoagulation occurs with widespread deposition of fibrin; later increased fibrinolysis occurs, often leading to a marked tendency to hemmorhage.

The syndrome is associated with Gram-negative bacteremia, although it may also occur during Gram-positive, viral, and fungal infections. It is now recognized that endotoxin initiates a complex cascade of reactions involving host-derived mediators, and among these, the cytokines, in particular tumor necrosis factor (TNF), have attracted considerable attention.

The availability of recombinant cytokines has facilitated several types of studies

---

* *Current affiliation:* Genentech, Inc., South San Francisco, California

that have greatly expanded our knowledge about the biological significance of cytokines in septic shock. The multitude of studies in this area can be divided into the following categories: (a) detection of cytokines in serum from septic shock patients, (b) observation of pathophysiological and histopathological changes after injection of cytokines into experimental animals, (c) observation of the effects of injection of combinations of cytokines, (d) observation of the effects of injection of specific antibodies into experimental animals, (e) demonstration of the relevant in vitro effects of cytokines, and (f) demonstration of the kinetics of production and elimination of cytokines in humans and experimental animals. On the basis of the array of studies in the field, in this chapter we discuss the roles of TNF, interleukins IL-1, IL-6, and IL-8, and interferon-γ (IFN-γ) in septic shock.

INDUCTION OF CYTOKINES

In the early phase of septic shock, the main pathophysiological events take place in the systemic circulation, and within this compartment monocytes (2,3) and endothelial cells (4–7) appear to be major cellular sources of cytokines, although lymphocytes (8) may also contribute. Endotoxin derived from the invading Gram-negative bacteria is a powerful stimulator to the release of the cytokines TNF, IL-1, IL-6, and IL-8 from monocytes and endothelial cells. In part there may also be a stepwise secretion by one secreted substance stimulating the production of the next. Figure 1 depicts the complex induction of cytokines with relevance to release into the systemic circulation.

ROLE OF CYTOKINES IN SEPTIC SHOCK

TNF

For almost 100 years it has been well known that Gram-negative bacterial products may induce tumor necrosis activity (9), and the possible application of this prin-

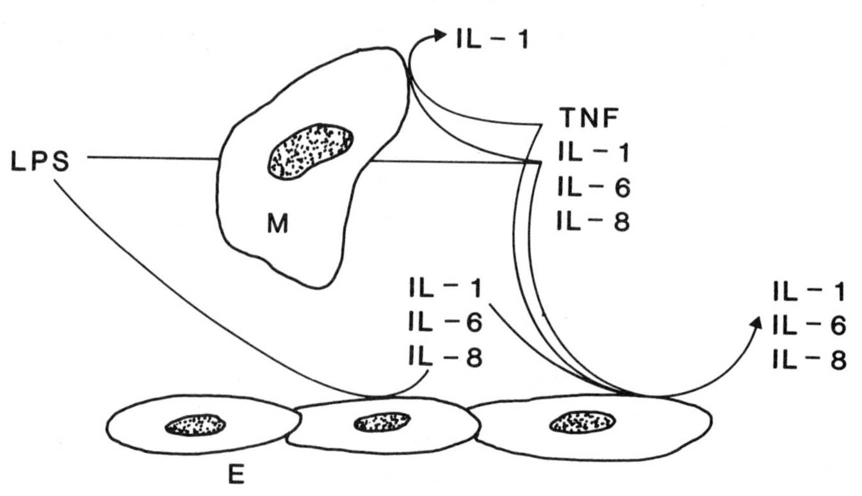

FIGURE 1 The complex induction of cytokines from monocytes (M) and endothelial cells (E).

ciple to the treatment of cancer patients has fascinated scientists. However, it is surprising that the significance of TNF in the pathophysiological states induced by endotoxinemia was not thoroughly investigated earlier. In fact, it was not until 1985 that Beutler and Tracey in Cerami's group, in a series of elegant studies, provided convincing evidence for the role of TNF as a mediator in septic shock. They showed that bacterial endotoxin can be lethal to mice and that the lethality was significantly reduced when the mice were pretreated with antiserum to TNF (10). Furthermore, this observation was supported by studies in baboons infected with lethal doses of *Escherichia coli* (11). Antibodies to TNF completely prevented the lethality in these animals.

A second category of studies with contributions from several research groups (12–14) showed that the histopathological and pathophysological changes induced by TNF were similar to those induced by endotoxin. These changes include hemorrhagic and ischemic necrosis of the gastrointestinal tract, hemorrhages and leukocyte infiltration in the lungs, acute tubular necrosis of the kidneys, metabolic acidosis, hypermetabolism, hypotension, and increased pituitary and stress hormone elaboration.

A third group of data supporting the view that TNF is a mediator in septic shock comes from patients with meningococcal disease (15). In a study of 79 patients with meningococcal disease, we found that 10 of 11 patients who died had TNF in serum, whereas only 8 of 68 patients who survived had TNF in serum. Moreover, there appeared to be a critical concentration of TNF above which all patients died. Essentially, this study demonstrated that TNF in serum was strongly associated with septic shock and fatal outcome. This observation was later supported by other studies on patients with septic shock of various bacterial etiologies, although the association is not so strong as in meningococcal disease (16). It should be emphasized that assays employed in various studies may reflect different properties of the TNF molecule, and the results are not directly comparable.

TNF has a number of in vitro effects that are relevant to the manifestations observed in septic shock. In particular, there is evidence that TNF may contribute to the hypercoagulability frequently occurring in the initial phase. For instance, TNF has a marked procoagulant effect on endothelial cells (17,18). It also induces the production of IL-1 from endothelial cells (4), and this cytokine has a procoagulant activity similar to that of TNF (17,19). This effect is further increased by the induction of plasminogen activator inhibitor by IL-1 (20). It should also be mentioned that TNF and IL-1 may also induce anticoagulant activity via the induction of prostacyclin (21), but altogether the effect of TNF clearly favors a procoagulant state.

Also, TNF induces the production of platelet-activating factor from endothelial cells, granulocytes, and monocytes (22), and there is evidence that this may be an important sequence of mediators in the development of shock.

TNF induces the activation of granulocytes, including the production of superoxide (23,24). This may be a mechanism by which tissue damage is mediated in the course of septic shock, in particular in late complications like the adult respiratory distress syndrome.

These in vitro studies give support to the role of TNF as a mediator in septic shock. However, they also indicate that TNF is involved in manifestations frequently observed in septic shock but not directly related to the pathogenesis of the shock.

The four groups of data together meet the classic requirements of Koch's postulates (25) and must together be regarded as convincing evidence for a causative relationship between TNF in the circulation and the development of septic shock.

Interleukin-1

TNF and IL-1 share a number biological activities, and apparently they play similar roles in many physiological and pathophysiological reactions (26). The role of IL-1 in septic shock has been elaborated, although not to the same extent as for TNF. In rabbits, IL-1 induces hypotension and histopathological changes similar to those of TNF (27,28). On the other hand, we did not observe acute toxic effects when IL-1 was given to mice (29). However, when IL-1 was given together with TNF, it markedly potentiated the lethal effect of TNF (29), as shown in Fig. 2. The effect was present at low concentrations of IL-1, and apparently IL-1 becomes a very potent molecule in combination with TNF.

IL-1 was detected in the serum in 3 of 20 patients with meningococcal disease (30). Interestingly, these 3 patients had severe septic shock and the most rapid

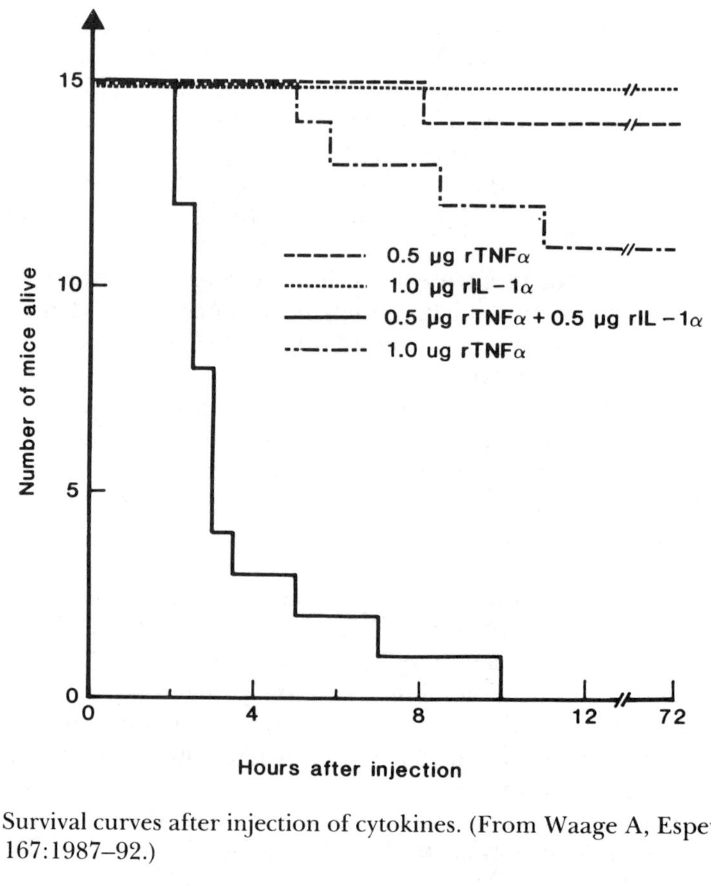

FIGURE 2 Survival curves after injection of cytokines. (From Waage A, Espevik T. J Exp Med 1988; 167:1987–92.)

fatal outcome of all the patients studied. These patients also had TNF in serum, and this observation is consistent with the TNF-potentiating effect of IL-1 in mice. Altogether, IL-1 alone probably has a weaker effect than TNF with respect to the induction of shock. However, its impact in human septic shock may be the marked potentiating effect on TNF activities.

Interferon-γ

Similarly to TNF, high levels of IFN-γ are associated with severe shock and fatal outcome in patients with meningococcal disease (31). Experimental studies indicate that IFN-γ has negligible acute toxicity in mice (32). However, it potentiates the lethal effect of TNF when these cytokines are given together (32). The effect of IFN-γ is thus very similar to that of IL-1 with regard to synergistic effects of TNF, and these cytokines may both influence the development of septic shock by potentiating TNF activities.

Interleukin-6

IL-6 was detected in almost all serum samples from patients with meningococcal meningitis, bacteremia, septic shock, or combinations of these (30). However, patients with septic shock had about 1000 times higher concentrations as patients with other manifestations. This suggests a role for IL-6 in septic shock, and this possibility has been further elaborated in experimental studies. In animals, IL-6 has by itself no acute toxic effects but possibly a slight potentiating effect on the lethal effect of TNF (Waage et al., unpublished results). However, others found no potentiating effect of IL-6 in animals treated with TNF. In summary, IL-6 appears to be a peripheral molecule in the pathogenesis of septic shock. It has even been proposed that IL-6 may have a protective role in this syndrome. IL-6 has been demonstrated to induce the production of acute-phase proteins (33) and to induce fever (34) and biphasic neutrophilia (35). It may thus contribute to many of the manifestations that are not directly involved in the pathogenesis of septic shock. Altogether, the exact role of IL-6 in septic shock remains to be clarified.

Interleukin-8

The term IL-8 was suggested by Larsen and colleagues (36) to describe a neutrophil activating protein produced by monocytes following stimulation with endotoxin. The gene for human IL-8 was cloned and expressed in *E. coli* by Matsushima and colleagues (37) and by others as well (38). The IL-8 molecule, also called monocyte-derived neutrophil chemotactic factor, consists of 72 amino acids, has a molecular mass of approximately 8 kD, and contains no N-glycosylation sites. A major biological function of IL-8 is to act as a chemotactic factor of neutrophils and for T lymphocytes (36). Because endotoxin and TNF can induce IL-8 production from monocytes and endothelial cells (7,37), one may anticipate the presence of elevated levels of IL-8 in patients with septic shock, especially following the attainment of the serum TNF peak. In fact, immunoreactive IL-8 can be detected in plasma in baboons with experimental sepsis (H. Redl, personal communication). Whether IL-8 contributes to the pathogenesis of the shock is

Table 1 Cytokine Involvement in the Pathogenesis of Septic Shock[a]

Cytokines	Alone	Together with TNF
TNF	+ + +	− − −
IL-1	+	+ + +
IL-6	0	(+)
IFN-γ	0	+ + +
IL-8	0	0

[a] Based on effects leading to hypotension or lethality, whereas effects like chemotaxis or pyrogenicity are not considered pathogenetic in a strict meaning of the term.

not yet known, but it is reasonable to suggest that it may participate as a mediator in the development of local inflammatory lesions associated with bacterial infections and in late complications to septic shock like adult respiratory distress syndrome. This view is supported by the demonstrated ability of IL-8 to induce the accumulation of neutrophils and to stimulate them for the production of phlogistic substances, such as superoxide anion, leukotrienes, and lysozomal enzymes (39). An abundance of stimulated neutrophils can aggravate both the inflammatory reaction and the adult respiratory distress syndrome.

Table 1 summarizes the involvement of the various cytokines in the pathogenesis of septic shock. It should be stressed that in vivo, many of the cytokines coexist in the systemic circulation together with a number of other factors. There are many possibilities for synergistic and antagonistic effects in this system, and the net result of a mixture of many factors is hard to predict.

KINETICS OF PRODUCTION AND ELIMINATION OF CYTOKINES

Septic shock is a dynamic process with rapidly changing serum levels of factors, and knowledge about the sequence of reactions at the cytokine level is essential.

Tumor Necrosis Factor

When endotoxin is injected into human volunteers, the TNF levels markedly rise within 1 h and thereafter decline to base levels after 3 h (40). The same release pattern has been demonstrated in all animals investigated and seems to be universal (41–43). The burst release of TNF is thus an early event in endotoxinemia.

In patients with meningococcal septic shock we analyzed consecutively drawn serum samples for the presence of TNF (30). The first sample was taken on admission, and this was later than the peak concentration. TNF was eliminated at a constant rate in half of the patients. The half-life of TNF was calculated as 72 minutes in these patients. In the other half of the patients there was a constant elimination of TNF after admission, but additional release occurred at a later stage. In all patients, TNF was completely eliminated within 16 h. The release and elimination pattern in meningococcal patients is thus similar to that in experimental animals, although other release mechanisms may be responsible for the late release of TNF.

Tolerance to LPS

After the initial burst release of TNF, the cells producing TNF become resistant to the TNF-inducing effect of liposaccharide (LPS). This can be demonstrated in experimental animals in several ways. For instance, the same release pattern is observed in rats whether a bolus injection of endotoxin is given or persisting high levels of endotoxin are maintained (43). Also, by giving two consecutive bolus injections of endotoxin, it can be shown that the peak concentration after the second injection is only about 15% of the peak concentration after the first injection (Fig. 3) (43). This tolerance to LPS lasts for at least 3 days.

Furthermore, it has been found that alveolar macrophages isolated from normal donors produce TNF upon LPS stimulation, whereas macrophages from patients with septicemia do not (44). This may be explained by exposure to endotoxin of the macrophages in the early phase of septicemia and development of resistance to the TNF-inducing effect of endotoxin.

IL-1 and IL-6

IL-1 is difficult to assay in serum because of the presence of inhibitory activity (45), and the exact point of time of release of IL-1 after LPS injection is thus uncertain. In other compartments of the organism, however, like the subarach-

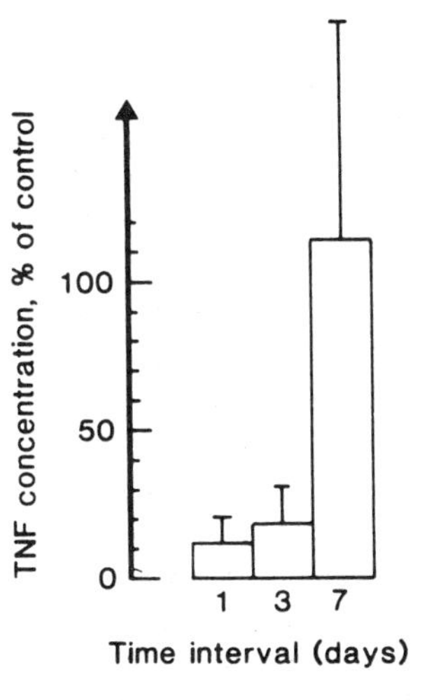

FIGURE 3 TNF in rat serum after sequential doses of LPS. A group of 18 rats were injected with LPS (0.2 μg/g) on day 0, and the same dose was repeated in groups of 6 rats on days 1, 3, and 7, respectively. The concentration of TNF in serum 1 h after the second LPS injection was calculated as a percentage of the concentration after the first injection in each rat. The columns represent the means of the percentage values ± standard error of the mean (SEM). (From Waage A. Clin Immunol Immunopathol 1987; 45:348–55.)

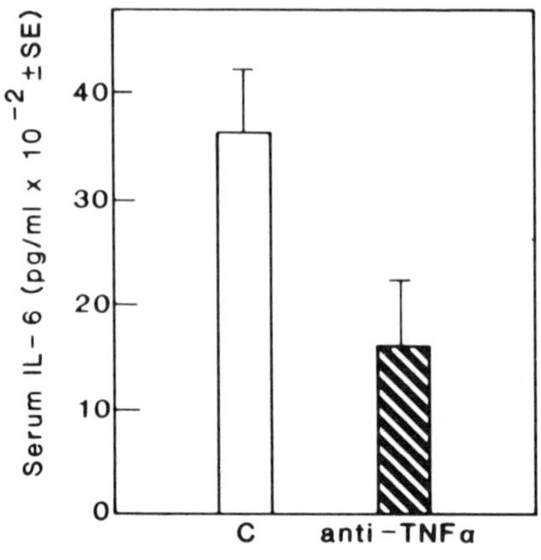

FIGURE 4 LPS induction of IL-6 following administration of antiserum against mur-TNF-α; six mice were injected with either 0.5 μg LPS + 50 μl normal rabbit serum (C) or 0.5 μg LPS + 50 μl rabbit antiserum to rMuTNF-α (anti-TNF-α). Serum samples were collected and tested for IL-6 activity 2 h later. TNF-α activity was present in serum of control group (590 ± 139 pg/ml) but not in serum of anti-TNF-α-treated mice monitored 1 h after LPS injection. (From Shalaby R, Waage A, Aaarden L, Espevik T. Clin Immunol Immunopathol 1989; 53:488–9.)

noid space, IL-1 is clearly released later than TNF (46), and it is reasonable to believe that the same occurs in the systemic circulation as well.

The peak of IL-6 occurs about 2 h after injection of endotoxin in human volunteers (47). The same time relation is found in mice (48). This cytokine is thus released after TNF under experimental condition. This time relation between the release of TNF and IL-6 was also obvious when we examined consecutively drawn serum samples from meningococcal septic shock patients (30).

IL-6 is also induced by TNF and IL-1 in mice, and the peak concentration occurs 1 h after cytokine injection (48). This observation, coupled with the finding that IL-6 peaks 2 h after LPS injection, suggests that LPS induces TNF and IL-1, which in turn induce IL-6. We obtained evidence for this cascade of reactions in an experiment involving the treatment of mice with antiserum to TNF concomitant with injection of LPS (48). The results (Fig. 4) show a significant reduction in the IL-6 peak level among antiserum-treated mice, indicating that IL-6 is at least in part induced by intermediate mediators like TNF.

In summary, the following initial reactions are likely to occur in septic shock (Fig. 5). Gram-negative bacteria invade the organism and multiply in the circulation, resulting in a rise in the serum endotoxin concentration. When a certain level of endotoxin is attained, the induction mechanism of TNF in the monocytes is triggered and TNF is released into the circulation as a burst 1–2 h later. IL-6 is released in a similar manner 30–60 minutes after the TNF burst, partly caused by TNF and IL-1 stimulation of monocytes and endothelial cells. The release of IL-1 in serum probably occurs between those of TNF and IL-6. Studies indicate that IL-8 is released at about the same time as IL-6 in baboons (H. Redl, personal communication).

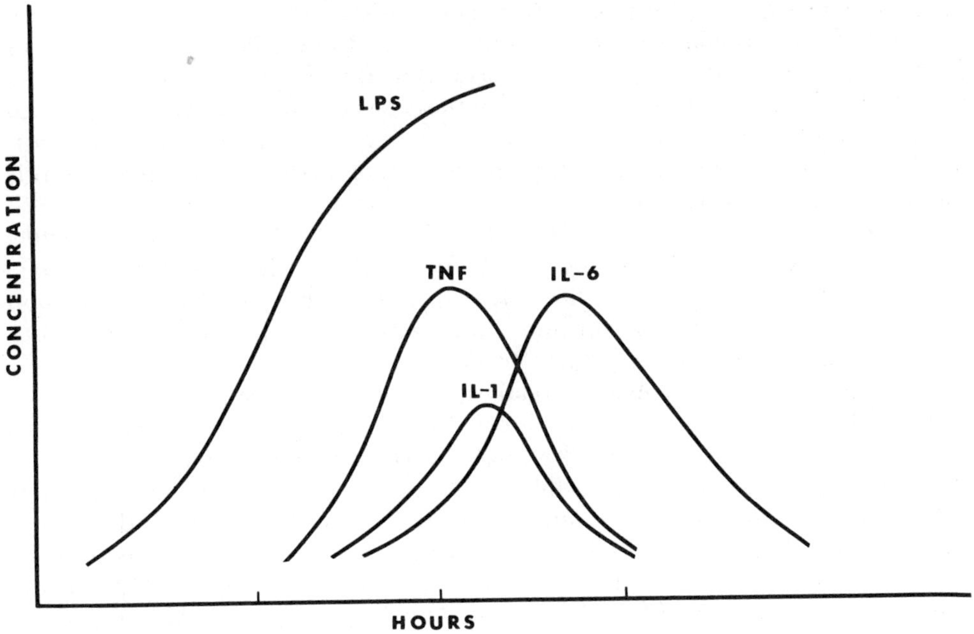

FIGURE 5 Sequential appearance of TNF, IL-1, and IL-6 in the systemic circulation in the initial phase of septic shock.

PROTECTIVE ROLE OF CYTOKINES

A fascinating aspect of TNF biology emerged after the finding that low doses of TNF can protect against the toxicity of TNF itself and may be useful in the prevention of the lethality associated with sepsis. In one study, mice pretreated with TNF and challenged 12–24 h later with TNF, in conjunction with actinomycin D, tolerated the toxicity significantly better than control animals (49). Pretreatment with TNF or IL-1 also protected bacillus Calmette-Guerin (BCG)-sensitized mice from the lethality of endotoxin injected 12 h later. In another study, a cecal ligation and puncture model that produces septic shocklike changes, was utilized to show that pretreatment with TNF conferred protection against the lethal effects of cecal ligation or endotoxin (50). Importantly, protection against sepsis lethality did not occur when TNF was administered 24 h after the insult. The mechanisms responsible for the protective actions of TNF are not known. It has been suggested that, besides downregulation of TNF receptors, TNF treatment may also induce the production of protective or repair proteins as has been demonstrated recently (51). Another view states that TNF administration may induce tolerance or tachyphylaxis to the lethality of endogenous TNF (49).

MODULATION OF CYTOKINE EFFECTS

An exciting area of research involves efforts for the development of antagonists or analogs to block the interaction of the natural molecule with its targets without themselves provoking a response. Such antagonists and analogs may be useful adjuvants for the management of septic shock and other immune disorders or disease states associated with the hyperproduction of inflammatory cytokines (11,52,53). Septic shock is a serious complication to infections and is often associated with surgery, burns, and cancer. It is a worldwide health problem, affecting a great number of patients. Identification of TNF as a mediator in septic shock is therefore important.

As mentioned earlier, neutralization of TNF by antibodies can completely prevent the development of shock (10,11). Interestingly, there may also be some protection when the antibodies are given up to half an hour after the infusion of the bacteria. With this background, multicenter clinical trials have been undertaken, but the results are yet not known.

Glucocorticoids are involved at many levels of the regulation of TNF, IL-1, and IL-6. It has been shown that the glucocorticoid analog dexamethasone inhibits the production of TNF at both the mRNA level and the protein level (54,55). Dexamethasone also effectively inhibits TNF production when it is given to rats (43). However, dexamethasone must be given at least 3 h before endotoxin to have an effect. Furthermore, it has been shown that dexamethasone reduces the cytotoxicity of TNF in cell culture systems (56). Similarly to TNF, the production of IL-1 (57) and IL-6 (58,59) is also inhibited by dexamethasone. Although there is good evidence that glucocorticoids downregulate the expression of TNF, IL-1, and IL-6, it is difficult to show that treatment of patients with septic shock with dexamethasone provides any benefit. At least three clinical trials have recently demonstrated that glucocorticoids administered to patients with septic shock have no effect on the case fatality rate associated with this syndrome (60–62).

CONCLUDING REMARKS

In this chapter we have focused on the cytokines and discussed their role and early appearance in septic shock. Thus far, TNF is the most important of the cytokines, and it is consequently the main target for efforts aiming to block the cascade reactions. One should bear in mind, however, the complex pattern of cytokines and other mediators in this syndrome. Although the development of septic shock can be blocked by anti-TNF under optimal experimental conditions, a similar monotherapy approach may be too optimistic in a clinical setting. The greatly expanded understanding of the underlying cytokine cascades in septic shock during the latest 5 years will, it is hoped, enable the development of more efficient treatment of this serious syndrome.

NOTES ADDED IN PRESS

While this book was in publication, more information about the role of cytokines in septic shock was produced, and this is briefly reviewed here.

The role of IL-1 has been further elaborated by experiments using IL-1 receptor antagonist in septic shock in rabbits (63). Administration of the antagonist increased survival from 20 to 90% and markedly reduced bleeding, transudation, and cellular infiltration in the lungs. The effect of IL-1 receptor antagonist was dose dependent, and interestingly, it could be given at least 2 h after endotoxin and retain its effect.

The rapidly expanding information about soluble TNF receptors is important for understanding the role of TNF in septic shock. The two types of TNF receptors are shed and can be detected in serum and urine during infection (Liabakk et al., submitted). They create an endogenously produced neutralizing system that may counteract the TNF effect during infection.

The association between TNF levels in serum and the severity of septic shock has now been supported by a number of studies (64–66). Various enzyme-linked immunosorbent assays as well as bioassays sensitive to different properties of the TNF molecule have been used, strengthening this conclusion. Elevated levels of IL-1 have been found in severe septic shock in two studies (31,64), but another study found no such correlation (65). IL-6 (67,68) and IL-8 (69, 70, Waage et al., in preparation) can be detected in serum in septic shock, and the levels correlate with the severity of the shock.

Finally, it should be emphazised that septic shock is not a single entity. The cytokine cascade as described in this chapter is probably characteristic of septic shock in an organism not previously influenced by immunological or other kinds of stress. In septic shock in patients with multitrauma, surgery, and burns, the cytokine cascade and its pathogenetic significance may have other causes.

REFERENCES

1. Shoemaker WC. Pathophysiology, monitoring, outcome, prediction, and therapy of shock states. Crit Care Clinics 1987; 3:307–57.
2. Nathan CF. Secretory products of macrophages. J Clin Invest 1987; 79:319–26.
3. Bauer J, Ganter U, Geiger T, et al. Regulation of interleukin-6 expression in cultured human blood monocytes and monocyte-derived macrophages. Blood 1988; 72:1134–40.
4. Libby P, Ordovas JM, Auger KR, Robbins AH, Birinyi LK, Dinarello CA. Endotoxin and tumor necrosis factor induce interleukin-1 gene expression in adult human vascular endothelial cells. Am J Pathol 1986; 124:179–85.
5. Shalaby MR, Waage A, Espevik T. Cytokine regulation of interleukin 6 production by human endothelial cells. Cell Immunol 1989; 121:372–82.
6. Warner SJC, Auger KR, Libby P. Interleukin 1 induces interleukin 1. II. Recombinant human interleukin 1 induces interleukin 1 production by adult human vascular endothelial cells. J Immunol 1987; 139:1911–7.
7. Strieter RM, Kunkel SL, Showell HJ, et al. Endothelial cell gene expression of a neutrophil chemotactic factor by TNF-α, LPS, and IL-1β. Science 1989; 243:1467–9.
8. Espevik T, Waage A, Faxvaag A, Shalaby R. Regulation of interleukin-2 and interleukin-6 production from T cells: involvement of interleukin-1 beta and transforming growth factor-beta. Cell Immunol, in press 1990.
9. Coley WB. The treatment of malignant tumors by repeated inoculations of erysipelas: with a report of ten original cases. Am J Med Sci 1893; 105:487–511.
10. Beutler B, Milsark IW, Cerami AC. Passive immunization against cachectin/tumor necrosis factor protects mice from lethal effect of endotoxin. Science 1985; 229:869–71.
11. Tracey KJ, Fong Y, Hesse DG, et al. Anti cachectin/TNF antibodies prevent septic shock during lethal bacteremia. Nature 1987; 330:662–4.

12. Tracey KJ, Beutler B, Lowry SF, et al. Shock and tissue injury induced by recombinant human cachectin. Science 1986; 234:470–4.
13. Remick DG, Kunkel RG, Larrick JW, Kunkel SL. Acute in vivo effects of human recombinant tumor necrosis factor. Lab Invest 1987; 56:583–90.
14. Bauss F, Droge W, Männel DN. Tumor necrosis factor mediates endotoxic effects in mice. Infect Immun 1987; 55:1622–5.
15. Waage A, Halstensen A, Espevik T. Association between tumour necrosis factor in serum and fatal outcome in patients with meningococcal disease. Lancet 1987; 1:355–7.
16. Debets JMH, Kampmeijer R, van der Linden MPMH, Buurman WA, van der Linden CJ. Plasma tumor necrosis factor and mortality in critically ill septic patients. Crit Care Med 1989; 17:489–94.
17. Bevilacqua MP, Pober JS, Majeau GR, Fiers W, Cotran RS, Gombrone MA Jr. Recombinant tumor necrosis factor induces procoagulant activity in cultured human vascular endothelium: characterization and comparison with the actions of interleukin 1. Proc Natl Acad Sci U S A 1986; 83:4533–7.
18. Nawroth PP, Stern DM. Modulation of endothelial cell hemostatic properties by tumor necrosis factor. J Exp Med 1986; 163:740–5.
19. Bevilacqua MP, Pober JS, Majeau GR, Cotran RS, Gimbrone MA Jr. Interleukin 1 (IL-1) induces biosynthesis and cell surface expression of procuagulant activity in human vascular endothelial cells. J Exp Med 1984; 160:618–23.
20. Dejana E, Brevario F, Erroi A, et al. Modulation of endothelial cell function by different molecular species of interleukin-1. Blood 1987; 69:695–9.
21. Kawakami M, Ishibashi S, Ogawa H, Murase T, Takaku F, Shibata S. Cachectin/TNF as well as interleukin-1 induces prostacyclin synthesis in cultured vascular endothelial cells. Biochem Biophys Res Commun 1986; 141:482–7.
22. Camussi G, Bussolini F, Salvidio G, Baglioni C. Tumor necrosis factor/cachectin stimulates peritoneal macrophages, polymorphonuclear neutrophils, and vascular endothelial cells to synthesize and release platelet-activating factor. J Exp Med 1987; 166:1390–404.
23. Shalaby MR, Aggarwal BB, Rinderknecht E, Svedersky LP, Finkle BS, Palladino MA Jr. Activation of human polymorphonuclear neutrophil functions by interferon-gamma and tumor necrosis factors. J Immunol 1985; 135:2069–73.
24. Klebanoff SJ, Vadas MA, Harlan JM, et al. Stimulation of neutrophils by tumor necrosis factor. J Immunol 1986; 136:4220–5.
25. Burrows W. Textbook of microbiology. New York: W. B. Saunders, 1985:318–9.
26. Le J, Vilcek J. Biology of disease. Tumor necrosis factor and interleukin-1: cytokines with multiple overlapping biological activities. Lab Invest 1987; 56:234–48.
27. Okusawa S, Gelfand JA, Ikejima T, Conolly RJ, Dinarello CA. Interleukin 1 induces a shock-like state in rabbits. Synergism with tumor necrosis factor and the effect of cyclooxygenase inhibition. J Clin Invest 1988; 81:1162–72.
28. Weinberg JR, Wright DJM, Guz A. Interleukin-1 and tumour necrosis factor cause hypotension in the conscious rabbit. Clin Sci 1988; 75:251–5.
29. Waage A, Espevik T. Interleukin 1 potentiates the lethal effect of tumor necrosis factor-α/cachectin in mice. J Exp Med 1988; 167:1987–92.
30. Waage A, Brandtzaeg P, Halstensen A, Kierulf P, Espevik T. The complex pattern of cytokines in serum from patients with meningococcal septic shock. J Exp Med 1989; 169:333–8.
31. Girardin E, Grau GE, Dayer J-M, Roux-Lombard P, Lambert P-H. Tumor necrosis factor and interleukin-1 in the serum of children with severe infectious purpura. N Engl J Med 1988; 319:397–400.
32. Talmadge JE, Bowersox O, Tribble H, Lee SH, Shepard HM, Liggit D. Toxicity of

tumor necrosis is synergistic with γ-interferon and can be reduced with cyclooxygenase inhibitors. Am J Pathol 1987; 128:410–25.

33. Gauldie J, Richards C, Harnish D, Lansdorp P, Baumann H. Interferon-β_2/B-cell stimulatory factor type 2 shares identity with monocyte-derived hepatocyte-stimulating factor and regulates the major acute phase protein response in liver cells. Proc Natl Acad Sci U S A 1987; 84:7251–5.
34. Helle M, Brakenhoff JPJ, de Groot E, Aarden LA. Interleukin 6 is involved in interleukin 1-induced activities. Eur J Immunol 1988; 18:957–9.
35. Ulich TR, del Castillo J, Guo K. In vivo hemtologic effects of recombinant interleukin-6 on hematopoiesis and circulating numbers of RBCs and WBCs. Blood 1989; 73:108–10.
36. Larsen CG, Anderson AO, Appella E, et al. The neutrophil-activating protein (NAP-1) is also chemotactic for T lymphocytes. Science 1989; 243:1464–6.
37. Matsushima K, Morishita K, Yoshimura T, et al. Molecular cloning of a human monocyte-derived neutrophil chemotactic factor (MDNCF) and the induction of MDNCF mRNA by interleukin-1 and tumor necrosis factor. J Exp Med 1988; 167:1883–93.
38. Westwick J, Li SW, Camp RD. Novel neutrophil-stimulating peptides. Immunol Today 1989; 10:146–7.
39. Schröder JM. The monocyte-derived neutrophil activating peptide (NAP/interleukin 8) stimulates human neutrophil arachidonate-5-lipoxygenase, but not the release of cellular arachidonate. J Exp Med 1989; 170:847–63.
40. Michie HR, Manogue KR, Spriggs DR, et al. Detection of circulating tumor necrosis factor after endotoxin administration. N Engl J Med 1988; 318:1481–6.
41. Beutler BA, Milsark IW, Cerami A. Cachectin/tumor necrosis factor: production, distribution, and metabolic fate in vivo. J Immunol 1985; 135:3972–7.
42. Flick DA, Gifford GE. Production of tumor necrosis factor in unprimed mice: mechanism of endotoxin-mediated tumor necrosis. Immunobiology 1986; 171:320–8.
43. Waage A. Production and clearance of tumor necrosis factor in rats exposed to endotoxin and dexamethasone. Clin Immunol Immunopathol 1987; 45:348–55.
44. Simpson SQ, Casey LC. Role of tumor necrosis factor in sepsis and acute lung injury. Crit Care Clin 1989; 5:27–47.
45. Larrick JW. Native interleukin 1 inhibitors. Immunol Today 1989; 10:61–6.
46. Waage A, Halstensen A, Shalaby R, Brandtzæg P, Kierulf P, Espevik T. Local production of tumor necrosis factor-α, interleukin 1, and interleukin 6 in meningococcal meningitis. Relation to the inflammatory response. J Exp Med 1989; 170:1859–67.
47. van Deventer SHJ, Buller HR, Tencate JW, Aarden L, Hack E, Sturk A. Endotoxin-induced biological effect: the role of cytokines. In: Thesis, van Deventer SHJ. Endotoxins in the pathogenesis of gram-negative septicemia. University of Amsterdam, 1988:113–27.
48. Shalaby R, Waage A, Aarden L, Espevik T. Endotoxin, tumor necrosis factor-alpha/cachectin and interleukin 1 induce interleukin 6 production in vivo. Clin Immunol Immunopathol 1989; 53:488–98.
49. Wallach D, Holtmann H, Engelmann H, Nophar Y. Sensitization and desensitization to lethal effects of tumor necrosis factor and IL-1. J Immunol 1988; 140:2994–9.
50. Sheppard BC, Fraker DL, Norton JA. Prevention and treatment of endotoxin and sepsis lethality with recombinant human tumor necrosis factor. Surgery 1989; 106:156–62.
51. Wong GHW, Goeddel DV. Induction of manganous superoxide dismutase by tumor necrosis factor: possible protective mechanism. Science 1988; 242:941–3.
52. Grau GE, Kindler V, Piguet PF, et al. Prevention of experimental cerebral malaria by anticytokine antibodies. J Exp Med 1988; 168:1499–504.

53. Shalaby MR, Fendly B, Sheehan KC, et al. Prevention of the graft-versus-host reaction in newborn mice by antibodies to tumor necrosis factor-alpha. Transplantation 1989; 47:1057–61.
54. Beutler B, Krochin N, Milsark IW, Luedke C, Cerami A. Control of cachectin (tumor necrosis factor) synthesis: mechanisms of endotoxin resistance. Science 1986; 232:977–80.
55. Waage A, Bakke O. Glucocorticoids suppress the production of tumour necrosis factor by lipopolysaccharide-stimulated human monocytes. Immunology 1988; 63:299–302.
56. Tsujimoto M, Okamura N, Adachi H. Dexamethasone inhibits the cytotoxic activity of tumor necrosis factor. Biochem Biophys Res Commun 1988; 153:109–15.
57. Snyder DS, Unanue ER. Corticosteroids inhibit murine macrophages la expression and interleukin 1 production. J Immunol 1982; 129:1803–5.
58. Waage A, Slupphaug G, Shalaby R. Glucocorticoids inhibit the production of IL 6 from monocytes, endothelial cells and fibroblasts. Eur J Immunol 1990; 20:2439–43.
59. Ray A, LaForge KS, Sehgal PB. On the mechanism for efficient repression of the interleukin-6 promoter by glucocorticoids: enhancer, TATA box, and RNA start site (inr motif) occlusion. Mol Cell Biol 1990; 10:5736–46.
60. Bone RC, Fisher CJ, Clemmer TP, et al. A controlled clinical trial of high-dose methylprednisolone in the treatment of sepsis and septic shock. N Engl J Med 1987; 317:653–8.
61. Sprung CL, Caralis PV, Marcial EH, et al. The effect of high-dose corticosteroids in patients with septic shock: a prospective controlled study. N Engl J Med 1984; 311:1137–43.
62. Veterans Administration systemic sepsis cooperative study group. Effect of high-dose glucocorticoid therapy on mortality in patients with clinical signs of systemic sepsis. N Engl J Med 1987; 317:659–65.
63. Ohlsson K, Björk P, Bergenfeldt M, Hageman R, Thompson RC. Interleukin-1 receptor antagonist reduces mortality from endotoxin shock. Nature 1990; 348:550–2.
64. Calandra T, Baumgartner J-D, Grau GE, et al. Prognostic values of tumor necrosis factor/cachectin, interleukin-1, interferon-α, and interferon-γ in the serum of patients with septic shock. J Infect Dis 1990; 161:982–7.
65. Damas P, Reuter A, Gysen P, Demonty J, Lamy M, Franchimont P. Tumor necrosis factor and interleukin-1 serum levels during severe sepsis in humans. Crit Care Med 1989; 17:975–8.
66. Marano MA, Fong Y, Moldawer LL, et al. Serum cachectin/tumor necrosis factor in critically ill patients with burns correlates with infection and mortality. Surg Gynecol Obstet 1990; 170:32–8.
67. Hack CE, De Groot ER, Felt-Bersma RJ, et al. Increased plasma levels of interleukin-6 in sepsis. Blood 1989; 74:1704–10.
68. Holfgott DC, Tatter SB, Santhanam U, Clarick RH, Bhardwaj N, May LT, Sehgal PB. Multiple forms of IFN-β_2/IL-α in serum and body fluids during acute bacterial infection. J Immunol 1989; 142:948–53.
69. Redl H, Schlag G, Bahrami S, Schade V, Ceska M, Stütz P. Plasma neutrophil-activating peptide-1/interleukin 8 and neutrophil elastase in a primate bacteremia model. J Infect Dis 1991; 164:383–8.
70. van Zee KJ, de Forge LA, Fischer E, et al. IL-8 in septic shock, endotoxemia, and after IL-1 administration. J Immunol 1991; 146:3478–82.

CHAPTER 10

CYTOKINES AND BACTERIAL INFECTION

Jon S. Friedland and George E. Griffin

St. George's Hospital Medical School
London, England

INTRODUCTION

The systemic effects of infection have been recognized for many centuries and were initially attributed to pathogenic organisms themselves. However, in recent years the discovery of cytokines and the subsequent evolution of knowledge concerning their immunophysiology and molecular biology have provided new insights into the role of the host in the mediation of such systemic effects as fever, anorexia, and cachexia. In addition, cytokines have been shown to be pivotal in host defense mechanisms and are of central importance in the response to bacterial infection. The acute-phase response represents the final common pathophysiological consequence of bacterial infection and is now known to be the result of a cascade of cytokines.

Knowledge of cytokines in infection is principally derived from animal models with clearly defined onset following a controlled stimulus. Under these circumstances it is relatively simple to define patterns of cytokine release related to such physiological parameters as fever, anorexia, and changes in blood pressure. Great advances have been made in the understanding of the physiological and molecular control of the host response to infection using such model systems, which range from administration of endotoxin to the injection of live bacteria either intravenously or directly into tissues. The situation in naturally occuring human infection is less well understood, principally because patients tend to present relatively late in the course of infection when early events in cytokine activation are likely to have been initiated. Model systems using endotoxin infusion into the human have suggested the existence of patterns of cytokine activation similar to those described in animals. In studying the modulation of cytokines in human infections there are practical and ethical problems in obtaining relevant clinical specimens from patients. Consequently, plasma concentrations of cytokines have been the principal source of human data but are only a distant, indirect reflection of the local inflammatory response to infection.

Tumor necrosis factor (TNF) was first described as a lipoprotein lipase suppressing hormone produced by cells stimulated with *Escherichia coli* lipopolysaccharide (LPS) (1,2). Since then it has become clear that numerous cytokines are involved in modulating bacterial infections. Particularly important are TNF, interleukin-1 (IL-1), interleukin-6 (IL-6), and the powerful chemoattractant interleukin-8 (IL-8), and polypeptides such as interferon have so far been principally associated with the response to viral infection. The purpose of this chapter is to review current knowledge of cytokines involved in human infections in the light of information from both animal models of infection and the cellular studies. The response to mycobacteria and the effect of a second concurrent pathogen, such as the human immunodeficiency virus (HIV), are discussed. On the basis of such information the possibilities for rational therapeutic interventions in the cytokine pathways are also discussed.

MODELS OF BACTERIAL INFECTION

Animal Endotoxin Studies

There are many animal models of bacterial infection, and several have been studied to elucidate cytokine pathophysiology. The simplest such model involves the administration of a sublethal dose of endotoxin (LPS). Under these conditions a typical physiological and biochemical acute-phase response is seen. However, the phenomenon of tachyphylaxis (resistance) to endotoxin emerged and remained unexplained before the development of an understanding of cytokine generation. Using a lapin model the pattern of TNF release into plasma was shown to be pulsatile, dependent upon dose of LPS administered, and of short duration (3). Plasma TNF concentration increased within 15 minutes, peaked at 100 minutes, and was no longer detectable at 200 minutes. Repeated exposure to LPS did not elicit additional TNF release. Changes in messenger RNA (mRNA) in elicited peritoneal macrophages following stimulation by LPS closely parallel the kinetics of TNF concentration in plasma (4).

There is strong evidence that the generation of TNF is a principal mediator of the profound pathophysiological changes observed in vivo following the administration of LPS. Recombinant TNF given to rats by intravenous infusion over 5 minutes at a dose of 3.6 mg/kg causes hypotension, metabolic acidosis, hemoconcentration, hyperglycemia, and hyperkalemia and is uniformly fatal. Postmortem findings reveal widespread lung and gut hemorrhage and acute tubular damage in the kidneys. However, lower doses of TNF are compatible with survival (5). Monoclonal antibodies to TNF are protective against potentially lethal doses of endotoxin (6), emphasizing the pivotal role of this cytokine. However, such antibody treatment does not abolish all the pathophysiological changes seen in LPS-treated animals.

Current evidence strongly suggests that bacterial endotoxin exerts its effects by initiating a cascade of cytokines commencing with TNF followed rapidly by

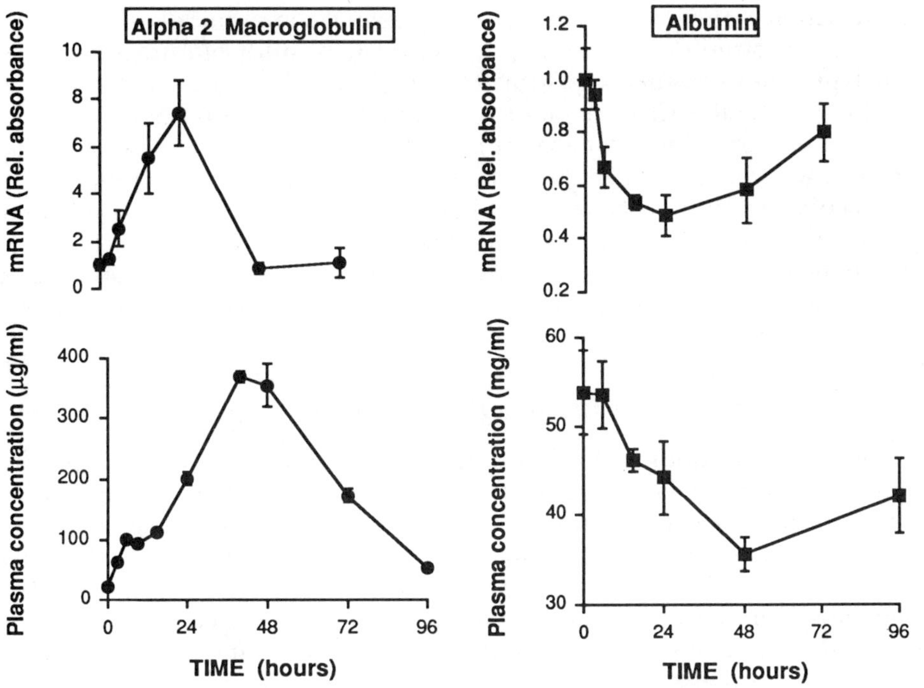

FIGURE 1 Time course of changes in hepatic mRNA (measured by densitometry of northern blots) and plasma concentrations of α_2-macroglobulin and albumin in rats receiving a bolus intraperitoneal injection of *E. coli* o127:B8 at time zero. (From Sharma et al. Am J Physiol, in press.)

a sequence of interleukins. The relatively short half-life of mRNA species for TNF-α and IL-1 are indicative of a probable site of prime importance in the fine control of pathophysiological changes. IL-6 is important in mediating the acute-phase response (synthesis of acute-phase proteins and pyrexia) (7) and in activation of B cells (8), natural killer (NK) cells (9), and T cells and thymocytes (10). This cytokine is thought to be important in dampening the inflammatory process and in repair mechanisms. Work in our laboratory has shown that IL-6 is released in a pulsatile fashion a short time after TNF in response to a single injection of LPS into a rat. However, the rise in mRNA for hepatic acute-phase proteins in vivo in rats is evident for up to at least 24 h, long after IL-6 has disappeared from plasma, and there is a similar time course for the depression of albumin mRNA (Fig. 1). The plasma levels of these two proteins closely reflect the relative changes in the mRNA species. These data possibly suggest the involvement of other cytokines in the acute-phase response in vivo or a sustained hepatic response resulting from the pulse of IL-6 release.

IL-8 is synthesized in response to LPS, TNF, and IL-1β in macrophages and other cells, including endothelial cells (11,12) and fibroblasts (13), and appears to be of central importance in bacterial infection. There is little documentation of the importance of this powerful neutrophil chemoattractant cytokine in animal models, although there is preliminary evidence suggesting that IL-8 is released into the circulation in a pulsatile fashion (personal communication, D. Remick).

The administration of endotoxin and subsequent study of cytokine release in animals provides a useful model with a clearly defined onset of a well-characterized stimulus. Clearly the actual situation in bacterial sepsis is more complicated, with activation of a broad immunological response including the release of multiple cytokines acting both locally and systemically. Hence, more recent models have been focused on the consequences of injecting known concentrations of specific live bacteria rather than only LPS into animals. Initially these models involved the production of lethal bacteremia with a syndrome resembling septic shock. The role of cytokines in the pathophysiological response to more subtle, sublethal infections is currently being evaluated.

Human Endotoxin Studies

The use of intravenous endotoxin infusion in human volunteers has provided important evidence concerning regulation of cytokines in vivo and the associated clinical symptomatology. Although this is a highly artificial model, it provides very important detail concerning the cytokine cascade in the human, which helps in interpretation of the complex data obtained from infected patients. The effects of endotoxin on the human are profound and include increased cardiac index, decreased peripheral resistance, and poor response to volume overload (14). The extent to which these changes are due to the release of cytokines is as yet not fully documented. Infusion of *E. coli* endotoxin into human volunteers resulted in a rise in plasma TNF concentration associated with fever, tachycardia, and increased plasma epinephrine and adrenocorticotropic hormone levels (15). In contrast, there was no change in plasma IL-1β concentration following the LPS. Other human experiments confirmed the rise in TNF following LPS and also demonstrated a pulsatile increase in IL-6, peaking 3 h after the bolus intravenous injection of endotoxin (16). Confirmation of the important role of TNF in mediating the systemic effects of infection comes from the intravenous infusion of TNF directly into human volunteers, which results in constitutional disturbance, including severe headache, fevers, and vomiting (17). However, since TNF has autocrine and paracrine effects it is possible that in vivo TNF may act indirectly through the release of other cytokines.

Animal Bacterial Studies

Gram-Negative Pathogens

The use of a baboon model of bacteremia has provided important information for our understanding of the in vivo cytokine cascade in primates during severe infection. In this model intravenous injection of live *E. coli* resulted in a peak plasma TNF concentration of 20,500 ± 9,890 pg/ml at 1 h and a peak plasma IL-1 concentration of 14.2 ± 10.1 units/ml at 3 h after injection (18). Pretreatment of baboons with a monoclonal antibody against TNF before injection of *E. coli* reduced lethality (99). In a separate series of experiments in the same model, plasma IL-1β concentration peaked at 3–4 h following injection of *E. coli* and plasma IL-6 concentration increased throughout the 8 h study period (20). Anti-TNF monoclonal antibody reduced the magnitude of the increase in plasma concentration of both interleukins, although the bacteremia remained fatal in these experiments.

Parallel studies, with a rodent bacteremic model in which neutropenic mice were injected with *Pseudomonas aeruginosa*, monoclonal antibody to TNF decreased mortality (21). In another rodent model in which intraperitoneal injection of *Salmonella typhimurium* causes death, the administration of granulocyte-monocyte-colony-stimulating factor (GM-CSF) into A/J mice was shown to augment survival (22). The mechanism of such protection is unknown but nevertheless indicates that cytokines may exert a beneficial effect in the response to bacterial infection.

These animal models suggest that TNF is pivotal in severe bacterial infection. However, more recent experiments indicate that although TNF is important other major factors are involved in host defense. Antibodies directed against IL-6 increase survival in a mouse bacteremic model (23). In a similar bacteremic rodent model protection against mortality due to *E. coli* was effected by antibody against endotoxin core. Measurement of TNF and IL-6 plasma concentrations in this model showed that protection was independent of measured plasma concentrations of both cytokines (24). The relative contribution of the different cytokines known to pathophysiology is currently unclear and is likely to be complex.

These primate and rodent models, although extremely important in providing knowledge of the cytokine cascade, represent very aggressive infection acquired artificially. The study of naturally acquired infections principally through mucosal routes has received relatively little attention in animal models, although this clearly represents the natural pathophysiological situation. The study of such models is crucial to developing an understanding of the role of the cytokine cascade in vivo. For example, TNF has recently been shown to be of pivotal importance in the evolution of the host response to *Salmonella* infection acquired via the intestinal mucosa. In these experiments the humoral response to an orally administered attenuated strain of *S. typhimurium* was completely ablated by pretreatment of mice with monoclonal antibody against TNF (25).

Gram-Positive Pathogens

In contrast to our understanding of the importance of LPS as a stimulus for the immune response in Gram-negative bacteremia, little is known about the biochemical nature of factors involved in the etiology of the response to Gram-positive organisms. Since the pathophysiological events in Gram-positive and Gram-negative bacteremia are similar, however, it is reasonable to suppose that the same cytokines are involved in both, perhaps through different signaling mechanisms.

In a lapin model of Gram-positive meningitis, intracisternal injection of heat-killed *Streptococcus pneumoniae* results in an intracerebral inflammatory response with cerebrospinal fluid (CSF) leukocytosis, raised CSF protein concentration, and brain edema (26). CSF leukocytosis was reduced by prior administration of either anti-TNF or anti-IL-1 antibodies. Another inflammatory cytokine studied in this series of experiments was macrophage inflammatory protein (MIP) (27). Anti-MIP-1 and anti-MIP-2 reduced the magnitude of rise in CSF protein but had no effect on CSF leukocytosis. In contrast, CSF leukocytosis and brain edema were induced by intracisternal injection of either TNF or IL-1α and also by injection of MIP-1 or MIP-2. Clearly, these models are highly contrived but will provide important information on cytokine pathophysiology in central nervous system infections.

In contrast to the adverse physiological responses induced by massive cytokine release as found in severe bacteremia, the protective effects of cytokines are becoming apparent. This is illustrated in a mouse model of *Listeria monocytogenes* infection in which administration of pure murine rTNF protects mice against a normally lethal intravenous *Listeria* challenge given 1–24 h later. In addition, anti-TNF administered during the first 3 days of infection, when peak numbers of bacteria are present in liver and spleen, resulted in increased mortality (28). The same phenomenon was observed in athymic nude mice, demonstrating that resistance to infection in this model does not depend on T cell immune responses. Histological studies in such animals showed that the organism was present within hepatocytes of anti-TNF-treated mice but absent from hepatocytes of control mice, indicating that a TNF-dependent mechanism is involved in the termination of intra-cellular infection.

Intracellular Pathogens

Mycobacteria Mycobacteria are important intracellular pathogens; however, relatively little is known about the role of cytokines in the in vivo response to infection. Mycobacterial infections are often chronic and are characterized by anorexia, weight loss, and fever, all of which have been associated with the production of cytokines (29,30). Activation of the cellular immune system in these infections is central to the host defense mechanism, and cytokines are likely to be of central importance.

It is clear that phagocytosis of mycobacteria by macrophages and their subsequent intracellular location is a stimulus for cytokine release. Live virulent *Mycobacterium tuberculosis* has been shown to result in TNF and interferon-γ release from cultured human monocytes (31), although the cytokine kinetics described for control endotoxin experiments in this series were atypical. Little is currently known about the pattern of cytokine production and release in chronically infected macrophages in contrast to our knowledge of the brief pulsatile nature of the response to LPS and the subsequent relatively long refractory period. Experiments carried out in our own laboratory, using monocyte and macrophage cell lines and a whole-blood model (32) stimulated by phagocytosis of live virulent *M. tuberculosis*, show that messenger RNA levels for TNF-α follow pulsatile kinetics similar to the pattern induced by LPS.

Several cytokines (interferon-γ, TNF, IL-4, and IL-6) have been shown to enhance macrophage antimycobacterial mechanisms (33–35), suggesting an important protective role against mycobacterial infection. This concept is directly supported by in vivo work in a mouse model of hepatic granuloma formation in response to BCG (bacillus Camette-Guerin) (36) in which anti-TNF treatment 1–2 weeks after BCG infection dramatically interferes with granuloma formation. In addition, fully developed BCG granulomas regressed rapidly after anti-TNF treatment, indicating the importance of sustained TNF release in the maintenance of the granulomatous response. Similar data concerning rodent granuloma formation were obtained from a model of pulmonary fibrosis induced by silica particles (37).

Nonmycobacterial The relationship between intracellular infection and cytokine activation and function has been shown to be important in nonmycobacterial intracellular infection and has been studied in models involving *Leishmania* and *Toxoplasma* infections. Such work may aid understanding of other bacterial intracellular pathogens. Further evidence for a protecting role of TNF comes from a mouse model of *Toxoplasma gondii* infection in which treatment with recombinant murine TNF or recombinant human IL-1 protected against death. Treatment with TNF antibodies blocked the anti-toxoplasmic effect of interferon-γ, suggesting the effect of this cytokine may depend partly on the production of TNF (38).

Insight into the mechanism by which TNF may result in intracellular killing comes from a mouse model of *Leishmania major*. TNF-activated murine macrophages kill the organism and anti-TNF treatment results in larger pathological lesions (39). These effects appear to be mediated via nitric oxide derived from L-arginine as the specific inhibitor L-N^G-monomethylarginine blocks the killing action of TNF (40).

HUMAN BACTERIAL INFECTION

Animal models and controlled injections of endotoxin into human volunteers have provided a large amount of information concerning the pathophysiology of cytokines in bacterial infection. However, the situation in human disease is more complex both because the patient is not normally seen at the onset of infection and because cytokines may not behave in an exactly analogous fashion in humans and other animals (41).

Bacteremia

In human septic shock (discussed in a previous chapter), massively elevated levels of TNF have been detected that appear to be a poor prognostic index (42,43). However, it is clear that the degree of elevation of plasma TNF concentration is not the sole determinant of survival since endotoxin infusion into humans resulted in peak TNF levels five times higher than those measured in patients with septicemia (30). A relationship has been demonstrated between TNF plasma concentrations and prognosis in meningococcal meningitis (44). In this condition raised TNF levels were detected in only 18 of 79 patients, of whom 10 died from infection. However, there was still 1 death among the 69 patients with undetectable levels of TNF. Further research on the serum of patients with meningococcal disease showed a complex pattern of cytokines in septic shock and that the release of IL-6 and IL-1 as well as TNF is associated with fatal outcome (45). Other studies have not demonstrated any relationship between plasma IL-1 concentration and mortality in septic shock (30,42). In septic meliodosis due to *Pseudomonas pseudomallei* bacteremia, death was also associated with raised plasma TNF concentration (personal communication, N.J. White). However, in septicemic patients neither plasma TNF nor plasma IL-1 concentrations were as good as prognostic markers as the more traditional indicators of severity, such as age of patient, documented bacteremia, urine output, and arterial pH when analyzed by stepwise logistic regression (46).

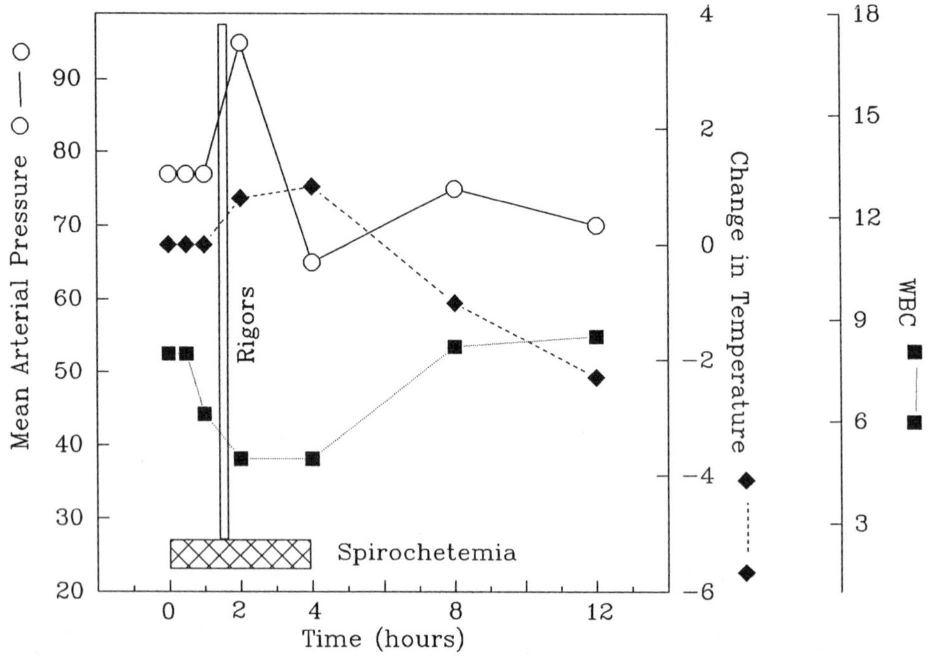

FIGURE 2 Clinical time course of the Jarisch-Herxheimer reaction in louse-borne relapsing fever (*Borrelia reurrentis*) following treatment with intravenous penicillin at time zero.

Recent evidence has implicated a cytokine cascade involving TNF, IL-6, and IL-8 in the etiology of the Jarisch-Herxheimer reaction (JHR) seen following treatment with penicillin of louse-borne relapsing fever due to *Borrelia recurrentis*. The JHR is a violent clinical syndrome of fever, rigors, and worsening of symptoms occurring with a very predictable time course following antibiotic treatment (Fig. 2). A peak of TNF activity (up to 470 pg/ml) was detected in association with a rise in temperature and briefly preceded coincidental pulsatile peaks of IL-6 (up to 28,447 pg/ml) and IL-8 (up to 70,000 pg/ml). The cytokine cascade in this condition coincides with removal of the organism from the bloodstream. The JHR of louse-borne relapsing fever demonstrates a predictable pattern of cytokine release for the first time in a human clinical situation. Although this particular JHR is clinically extremely violent in its manifestations, it has been known for many years that the treatment of a variety of bacterial infections with antibiotics may cause worsening of symptoms before cure (47,48). It is possible that the evolution of a cytokine cascade similar to that in the JHR may well explain this phenomenon. A parallel situation was demonstrated in the lapin model of *Hemophilus influenzae* meningitis in which antibiotic therapy resulted in increased TNF concentration in the cerebrospinal fluid (49).

Intracellular Pathogens

Mycobacterial disease is a major killer on a global scale, and the importance of both *M. tuberculosis* and rarer species, such as *M. avium intracellulare*, is increasing because of the acquired immunodeficiency syndrome (AIDS) pandemic. Tuberculosis is the classic wasting disease and historically was called consumption. Macrophages within granulomata may be a persistent source of cytokines, in particular TNF, and the cause of such cachexia. TNF has been shown to decrease albumin gene expression (50) and produce skeletal muscle wasting (51), both of which are classic features of chronic infection.

Little is known about cytokine levels in vivo in human tuberculosis, and they may well vary depend upon the organ affected. One study of tuberculous pleuritis examined local production of TNF and Interferon-γ by measuring the cytokine concentrations in pleural fluid and examined pleural tissue biopsies for messenger RNA for these cytokines (52). Both TNF and interferon-γ were selectively concentrated in pleural fluid compared to plasma, and messenger RNA for both cytokines was detected in pleural tissue. In addition, serum levels of IL-1 have been shown to be raised in patients with active tuberculosis (53) and monocyte stimulation by mycobacterial protein antigens (PPD, purified protein derivative) results in IL-1 release (54). Mycobacteria can survive in macrophages and in other nonprofessional phagocytic cells and so must be able to resist the cell killing that should result from the induction of manganese superoxide dismutase occurring in response to TNF production (55). High plasma levels of TNF have been demonstrated in patients with active lepromatous leprosy (56).

Cytokines, Bacteria, and HIV Transcription

There is strong evidence implicating cytokines in the transcriptional control of HIV. In particular, TNF has been shown to upregulate HIV transcription in many cells in vitro (57). For example, the transcription of HIV in infected or transfected monocyte cell lines is known to be augmented by TNF (58). Such stimulation may be of crucial importance in the clinical progression of HIV infection during episodes of secondary infection.

Bacterial infections are known to be of great importance in HIV disease and include *Pneumococcus* and *Salmonella* infections (59) and *M. tuberculosis* (60). In addition, LPS has been shown to be a potent stimulus for HIV transcription in vitro (61). Recent unpublished work from our own laboratory shows that phagocytosis of *M. tuberculosis* by monocytes transfected with HIV promotor gene (LTR)-reporter gene (CAT) complex increases HIV transcription. This work strongly supports the hypothesis that intracellular pathogens phagocytosed by HIV-infected monocytes may induce viral replication and hence disease progression. Coincidentally, these experiments confirm the importance of nuclear factor-κB in the control of HIV transcription already suggested by work on mononuclear cell lines (58).

The question remains of whether the regulation of cytokine production in HIV-infected monocytes is the same as that reported in uninfected cells. HIV infection of mononuclear cells in vitro is associated with production of TNF and interferon-γ (62). In addition, constitutively raised levels of TNF and IL-6 have been reported in vivo (63,64), providing a potential explanation for some of the constitutional features of HIV infection and the polyclonal gammopathy. It has been shown that HIV-infected human mononuclear cells stimulated by endotoxin have the same pattern of cytokine release in terms of TNF, IL-1β, IL-6, and GM-

CSF as noninfected cells (65,66). Conversely, LPS stimulation of peripheral blood monocytes taken from patients with the acquired immunodeficiency syndrome resulted in an augmented release of TNF that was thought to be due to an increased half-life of the transcript for TNF (67). Similarly IL-1 production in response to *Neisseria meningitidis* is increased in monocytes in AIDS patients (68).

TREATMENT OF BACTERIAL INFECTIONS USING ANTICYTOKINE AGENTS

Increased knowledge of the cytokine cascade derived from both animal models and studies in human infection has progressed to the point that therapeutic measures aimed at reducing mortality from bacterial infection by influencing cytokine action and release have been undertaken. Such trials in humans and animals (described earlier) have principally involved severe sepsis, and a significant decrease in mortality has been recorded in the short term. The accumulating evidence that low concentrations of cytokines have an important protective effect in host resistance (28,37) suggests that selection of patients for anticytokine therapy may be important to avoid potentially harmful immunosuppressive effects.

Immunotherapy

The use of human polyvalent sera directed against LPS moieties was initially investigated in patients with Gram-negative septic shock (69). This study suggested a beneficial effect, although this was not seen in all patients. However, a more detailed prospective trial using human IgG antibody to *E. coli* J5 did not show any benefit compared to a nonspecific pooled immunoglobulin preparation (70). Further clinical trials are currently in progress involving monoclonal antibodies directed against TNF-α or LPS and the results are awaited. The fundamental therapeutic problem remains that most patients with overwhelming sepsis present clinically at a time following activation of the cytokine cascade when irreversible damage may already have occurred.

Drug Therapy

Glucocorticoids

The use of corticosteroids in the clinical management of profound sepsis has been the subject of much debate. Major studies on the use of steroids in septic patients have shown little (71) or no beneficial effect on mortality (72,73). One trial in children with bacterial meningitis demonstrated reduced morbidity, in particular decreased sensorineural hearing loss (74).

There is evidence that steroids can inhibit TNF production both in vitro (75,76) and in animal models (4) and that they also affect IL-1 generation (77). In both these situations the timing of glucocorticoid administration is critical in that it must be given before or shortly after the stimulus for cytokine release. Thus it is not surprising that the clinical use of glucocorticoids does not have major beneficial effects in severe infection since activation of the cytokine cascade may be complete before the initiation of therapy.

Nonsteroidal Antiinflammatory Drugs (NSAIDs)

There is evidence that NSAIDs can affect cytokine production in vitro (75,78). Ibuprofen abrogates the clinical manifestations that follow the intravenous injection of endotoxin into human volunteers, although the rise in plasma TNF concentration is not altered by this treatment (15). A more detailed recent study of ibuprofen treatment of human volunteers receiving LPS has confirmed that this NSAID blunts clinical response to intravenous endotoxin but paradoxically augments both circulating TNF-α and IL-6 concentrations (79), suggesting that other mediators may be involved. The dual problems of timing of therapy and the potential reduction of the protective effects of cytokines are potential problems in the use of NSAIDs in bacterial infection.

Oxypentifylline

Oxypentifylline has been shown to decrease TNF production in vitro (80). The effects of this drug, which has been used safely for many years in the management of peripheral vascular disease (81), are now being reinvestigated because of its properties in modifying cytokine production. Such investigations are providing important understanding of the complex regulatory mechanisms of cytokine regulation and activity. Oxypentifylline has been known for some years to have beneficial pharmacological effects in animal models of respiratory distress syndrome, multiorgan failure, and shock (82). It has recently been shown in human volunteers to inhibit the rise in plasma TNF-α concentrations in response to intravenous endotoxin, while not inhibiting IL-6 production, fever, myalgia, or cortisol release due to endotoxin (16). There is the potential for using oxypentifylline for therapy, and it is possible that dual therapy with glucocorticoids and oxpentifylline may be useful because the former appears to affect messenger RNA for TNF via a translation control mechanism and the latter via a transcription control mechanism (83).

CONCLUSIONS

It is now clear that the many clinical manifestations of bacterial infections are mediated by a complex pattern of cytokines. Knowledge of these mechanisms is currently in a rapid phase of evolution, and information obtained from defined animal and human models of infection is providing a firm basis from which to understand the complicated human situation in naturally acquired infections. The use of such information is being tested clinically in the form of immunotherapy directed against specific cytokines. In addition, our understanding of the control mechanisms of signaling and release have opened pathways for the use of specific drugs. Other possible targets in the cytokine signaling effector pathway are yet to be explored. For example, the use of specific cytokine receptor blockers or antagonists directed against receptors known to be involved in cytokine signaling, such as ICAM-1 (84). Problems remain in the modulation of the cytokine cascade in human infection in terms of a narrow therapeutic window and the danger of dampening protective mechanisms.

ACKNOWLEDGMENTS

Friedland is a Medical Research Council (UK) Training Fellow. Griffin acknowledges support from the Welcome Trust.

REFERENCES

1. Kawakami M, Cerami A. Studies of endotoxin-induced decrease in lipoprotein lipase activity. J Exp Med 1981; 154:631–9.
2. Beutler B, Mahoney J, Le Trang N, Pekala P, Cerami A. Purification of cachectin, a lipoprotein lipase-suppressing hormone secreted by endotoxin-induced RAW 264.7 cells. J Exp Med 1985; 161:984–95.
3. Mathison J, Wolfson E, Ulevitch J. Participation of tumor necrosis factor in the mediation of Gram-negative bacterial lipopolysaccharide-induced injury in rabbits. J Clin Invest 1988; 81:1925–37.
4. Remick D, Strieter R, Lynch J, Nguyen D, Eskandari M, Kunkel S. In vivo dynamics of murine tumor necrosis factor-alpha gene expression: kinetics of dexamethasone-induced suppression. Lab Invest 1989; 60(6):766–71.
5. Tracey K, Beutler B, Lowry S, et al. Shock and tissue injury induced by recombinant human cachectin. Science 1986; 234:470–4.
6. Bagby G, Plessala K, Wilson L, Thompson J, Nelson S. Divergent efficacy of antibody to tumor necrosis factor-α in intravascular and peritonitis models of sepsis. J Infect Dis 1990; 163:83–8.
7. Gauldie J, Richards C, Harnish D, Lansdorf P, Baumann H. Interferon β2/B-cell stimulatory factor type 2 shares identity with monocyte-derived hepatocyte-stimulating factor and regulates the major acute phase protein response in liver cells. Proc Natl Acad Sci 1990; 84:7251–5.
8. Hirano T, Yasukawa K, Harada H, et al. Complementary DNA for a novel human interleukin (BSF-2) that induces B lymphocytes to produce immunoglobulin. Nature 1986; 324:73–6.
9. Luger T, Krutmann J, Kirnbauer R, et al. IFN-β2/IL-6 augments the activity of human natural killer cells. J Immunol 1989; 143(4):1206–9.
10. Lotz M, Jirik F, Kabouridis P, et al. B cell stimulating factor 2/interleukin 6 is a co-stimulant for human thymocytes and T lymphocytes. J Exp Med 1988; 167:1253–8.
11. Sica A, Matsushima K, van Damme J, et al. IL-1 transcriptionally activates the neutrophil chemotactic factor/IL-8 gene in endothelial cells. Immunology 1990; 69:548–53.
12. Strieter R, Kunkel S, Showell H, et al. Endothelial cell gene expression of a neutrophil chemotactic factor by TNF-alpha, LPS and IL-1 beta. Science 1989; 243:1467–9.
13. Strieter R, Phan S, Showell H, et al. Monokine-induced neutrophil chemotactic factor gene expression in human fibroblasts. J Biol Chem 1989; 264(18):10621–6.
14. Suffredini A, Fromm R, Parker M, et al. The cardiovascular response of normal humans to the administration of endotoxin. N Engl J Med 1989; 321(5):280–7.
15. Michie H, Manogue K, Spriggs D, et al. Detection of circulating tumour necrosis factor after endotoxin administration. N Engl J Med 1988; 318(23):1481–6.
16. Zabel P, Wolter D, Schonharting M, Schade U. Oxypentifylline in endotoxaemia. Lancet 1989; 1474–7.
17. van der Poll T, Buller H, ten Cate H, et al. Activation of coagulation after administration of tumor necrosis factor to normal subjects. N Engl J Med 1990; 322(23):1622–7.
18. Hesse D, Tracey K, Fong Y, et al. Cytokine appearance in human endotoxemia and primate bacteremia. Surg Gynecol Obstet 1988; 166:149–53.
19. Tracey K, Fong Y, Hesse D, et al. Anti-cachectin/TNF monoclonal antibodies prevent septic shock during lethal bacteraemia. Nature 1987; 330:662–4.
20. Fong Y, Tracey K, Moldawer L, et al. Antibodies to cachectin/tumour necrosis factor reduce interleukin 1 β and interleukin 6 appearance during lethal bacteraemia. J Exp Med 1989; 170:1627–33.

21. Opal S, Cross A, Kelly N, et al. Efficacy of a monoclonal antibody directed against tumor necrosis factor in protecting neutropenic rats from lethal infection with *Pseudomonas aeruginosa*. J Infect Dis 1990; 161:1148–52.
22. Morrissey P, Charrier K. GM-CSF administration augments the survival of ity-resistant A/J mice, but not ity-susceptible C57BL/6 mice, to a lethal challenge with *Salmonella typhimurium*. J Immunol 1990; 144(2):557–61.
23. Starnes H, Pearce M, Tewari A, Yim J, Zou J-C, Abrams J. Anti-IL-6 monoclonal antibodies protect against lethal *Escherichia coli* infection and lethal tumor necrosis factor-α challenge in mice. J Immunol 1990; 1455(12):4185–91.
24. Silva A, Appelmelk B, Buurman W, Bayston K, Cohen J. Monoclonal antibody to endotoxin core protects mice from *Escherichia coli* sepsis by a mechanism independent of tumor necrosis factor and interleukin-6. J Infect Dis 1990; 162:454–9.
25. Tite J, Dougan G, Chatfield S. The involvement of tumor necrosis factor in immunity to *Salmonella* infection. J Immunol In press.
26. Saukkonen K, Sande S, Choffe C, et al. The role of cytokines in the generation of inflammation and tissue damage in experimental Gram-positive meningitis. J Exp Med 1990; 171:439–48.
27. Davatelis G, Wolpe S, Sherry B, Dayer J-M, Chicheportiche R, Cerami A. Macrophage Inflammatory protein-1: a prostaglandin-independent endogenous pyrogen. Science 1988; 243:1066–8.
28. Havell E. Evidence that tumor necrosis factor has an important role in antibacterial resistance. J Immunol 1989; 143(9):2894–9.
29. Tracey K, Morgello S, Koplin B, et al. Metabolic effects of cachectin/tumor necrosis factor are modified by site of production. J Clin Invest 1990; 86:2014–24.
30. Cannon J, Tompkins R, Gelfand J, et al. Circulating interleukin-1 and tumor necrosis factor in septic shock and experimental endotoxin fever. J Infect Dis 1990; 161:79–84.
31. Rook G, Taverne J, Leverton C, Steele J. The role of gamma-interferon, vitamin D_3, metabolites and tumour necrosis factor in the pathogenesis of tuberculosis. Immunology 1987; 62:229–34.
32. Strieter R, Remick D, Ham J, Colletti L, Lynch J, Kunkel S. Tumor necrosis factor-alpha gene expression in human whole blood. J Leukoc Biol 1990;
33. Flesch I, Kaufmann S. Mycobacterial growth inhibition by interferon-γ-activated bone marrow macrophages and differential susceptibility among strains of *Mycobacterium tuberculosis*. J Immunol 1987; 138(12):4408–13.
34. Flesch I, Kaufmann S. Stimulation of antibacterial macrophage activities by B-cell stimulatory factor 2 (interleukin-6). Infect Immun 1990; 58(1):269–71.
35. Flesch I, Kaufmann S. Activation of tuberculostatic macrophage functions by gamma interfereon, interleukin-4 and tumor necrosis factor. Infect Immun 1990; 58(8): 2675–7.
36. Kindler V, Sappino A, Grau G, Piguet P, Vassalli P. The inducing role of tumour necrosis factor in the development of bactericidal granulomas during BCG infection. Cell 1989; 56:731–40.
37. Piguet P, Collart M, Grau G, Sappino A-P, Vassalli P. Requirement of tumour necrosis factor for development of silica-induced pulmonary fibrosis. Nature 1990; 344:245–7.
38. Chang H, Grau G, Pechere J. Role of TNF and IL-1 in infections with *Toxoplasma gondii*. Immunology 1990; 69:33–7.
39. Liew F, Parkinson C, Millott S, Severn A, Carrier M. Tumour necrosis factor alpha in leishmaniasis: TNFα mediates host protection against cutaneous leishmaniasis. Immunology 1990; 69:570–3.
40. Liew F, Li Y, Millott S. Tumour necrosis factor (TNF-α) in leishmaniasis. II.

TNF-α induced macrophage leishmanicidal activity is mediated by nitric oxide from L-arginine. Immunology 1990; 71:556–9.

41. Callard R, Turner M. Cytokines and Ig switching: evolutionary divergence between mice and humans. Immunol Today 1990; 11(6):200–3.
42. Damas P, Reuter A, Gysen P, Demonty J, Lamy M, Franchimont P. Tumor necrosis factor and interleukin-1 serum levels during sepsis in humans. Crit Care Med 1989; 17(10):975–8.
43. Debets J, Kampmeijer R, van der Linden P, Buurman W, van der Linden C. Plasma tumour necrosis factor and mortality in critically ill septic patients. Crit Care Med 1989; 17(6):489–94.
44. Waage A, Haalstensen A, Espevik T. Association between tumour necrosis factor in serum and fatal outcome in patients with meningococcal disease. Lancet 1987; 1:355–7.
45. Waage A, Brandtzaeg P, Halstensen A, Kierulf P, Espevik T. The complex pattern of cytokines in serum from patients with meningococcal septic shock: association between interleukin 6, interleukin 1 and fatal outcome. J Exp Med 1990; 169:333–8.
46. Calandra T, Baumgartner J-D, Grau G, et al. Prognostic value of tumor necrosis factor/cachectin, interleukin-1, interferon-α and interferon-γ in the serum of patients with septic shock. J Infect Dis 1990; 161:982–7.
47. Jarisch A. Therapeutische Varsuche bei Syphylis. Wein Med Wochenschr 1895; 45:721–4.
48. Friedland JS, Warrell DA. The Jarisch-Herxheimer reaction in leptospirosis: review of the literature and possible pathogenesis. Rev Infect Dis In press.
49. Mustafa M, Ramilo o, Mertsola J, et al. Modulation of inflammation and cachectin activity in relation to treatment of experimental *Haemophilus influenzae* type b meningitis. J Infect Dis 1989; 160(5):818–25.
50. Brenner D, Buck M, Feitelberg S, Chojkier M. Tumor necrosis factor-alpha inhibits albumen gene expression in a murine model of cachexia. J Clin Invest 1990; 85:248–55.
51. Flores E, Bistrian B, Pomposelli J, Dinarello C, Blackburn G, Istfan N. Infusion of tumour necrosis factor/cachectin promotes muscle catabolism in the rat: a synergistic effect with interleukin 1. J Clin invest 1989; 83:1614–22.
52. Barnes P, Fong S, Brennan P, Twomey P, Mazumder A, Moldin R. Local production of tumor necrosis factor and IFN-γ in tuberculous pleuritis. J Immunol 1990; 145(1):149–54.
53. Chensue S, Davey M, Remick D, Kunkel S. Release of interleukin-1 by peripheral blood mononuclear cells in patients with tuberculosis and active inflammation. Infect Immun 1986; 52(1):341–3.
54. Wallis R, Fujiwara H, Ellner J. Direct stimulation of monocyte release of interleukin-1 by mycobacterial protein antigens. J Immunol 1986; 136(1):193–6.
55. Wong G, Goeddel D. Induction of manganous superoxide dismutase by tumor necrosis factor: possible protective mechanism. Science 1988; 242:941–4.
56. Pisa P, Gennene M, Soder O, Ottenhoff T, Hansson M, Kiessling R. Serum tumor necrosis factor levels and disease dissemination in leprosy and leishmaniasis. J Infect Dis 1990; 161:988–91.
57. Osborn L, Kunkel S, Nabel G. Tumor necrosis factor α and interleukin 1 stimulate the human immunodeficiency virus enhancer by activation of the nuclear factor κB. Proc Natl Acad Sci U S A 1989; 86:2336–40.
58. Griffin G, Leung K, Folks T, Kunkel S, Nabel G. Activation of HIV gene expression during monocyte differentiation by induction of NF-kB. Nature 1989; 339:70–3.

59. Gilks C, Brindle R, Otieno L, et al. Life-threatening bacteraemia in HIV-1 seropositive adults admitted to hospital in Nairobi, Kenya. Lancet 1990; 336:545–9.
60. Nunn P, Odhiambo J, Elliott A. Tubeculosis and HIV infection. Br Med J 1990; 300:1044.
61. Pomerantz R, Feinberg M, Trono D, Baltimore D. Lipopolysaccharide is a potent monocyte/macrophage-specific stimulator of human immunodeficiency virus type 1 expression. J Exp Med 1990; 172:253–61.
62. Vyakarnum A, McKeating J, Meager A, Beverley P. Tumour necrosis factors induced by HIV-1 in peripheral blood mononuclear cells potentiate virus replication. AIDS 1990; 4:21–7.
63. Lahdevirta J, Maury C, Teppo A, Repo H. Elevated levels of circulating cachectin/tumour necrosis factor in patients with acquired immunodeficiency syndrome. Am J Med 1988; 85:289–91.
64. Breen E, Rezai A, Nakajima K, et al. Infection with HIV is associated with elevated IL-6 levels and production. J Immunol 1990; 144(2):480–4.
65. Molina J-M, Schindler R, Ferriani R, et al. Production of cytokines by peripheral blood monocytes/macrophages infected with human immunodeficiency virus type1 (HIV-1). J Infect Dis 1990; 161:888–93.
66. Munis J, Richman D, Kornbluth R. Human Immunodeficiency virus-1 infection of macrophages in vitro neither induces tumor necrosis factor (TNF)/cachectin gene expression nor alters TNF/cachectin induction by lipopolysaccharide. J Clin Invest 1990; 85:591–6.
67. Voth R, Rossol S, Klein K, et al. Differential gene expression of IFN-α and tumor necrosis factor-α in peripheral blood mononuclear cells from patients with AIDS related complex and AIDS. J Immunol 1990; 144(3):970–5.
68. Weiss L, Haeffner-Cavaillon N, Laude M, Gilquin J, Kazatchkine M. HIV infection is associated with the spontaneous production of interleukin-1 (IL-1) in vivo and with an abnormal release of IL-1α in vitro. AIDS 1989; 3:695–9.
69. Ziegler E, McCutchen J, Fierer J, et al. Treatment of Gram-negative bacteremia and shock with human antiserum to a mutant *Escherichia coli*. N Engl J Med 1982; 307:125–30.
70. Calandra T, Glauser M, Schellekens J, Verhoef J, Group. S-DJIS. Treatment of Gram-negative septic shock with human IgG antibody to *Escherichia coli* J5: a prospective, double-blind, randomised trial. J Infect Dis 1988; 158:312–9.
71. Sprung C, Caralis P, Marcial E, et al. The effects of high-dose corticosteroids in patients with septic shock: a prospective controlled study. N Engl J Med 1984; 311(18):1137–43.
72. Bone R, Fisher C, Clemmer T, et al. A controlled clinical trial of high-dose methylprednisolone in the treatment of severe sepsis and septic shock. N Engl J Med 1987; 317(11):653–8.
73. Veterans administration systemic sepsis cooperative study group. Effect of high-dose glucocorticoid therapy on mortality in patients with clinical signs of systemic sepsis. N Engl J Med 1987; 317(11):659–65.
74. Lebel M, Freij B, Syrogiannopoulos G, et al. Dexamethasone therapy for bacterial meningitis: results of two double-blind placebo controlled trials. N Engl J Med 1988; 319:964–71.
75. Kunkel S, Spengler M, Kwon G, May M, Remick D. Production and regulation of tumour necrosis factor alpha: a cellular and molecular analysis. Methods Achiev Exp Pathol 1988; 13:240–59.
76. Strieter R, Remick D, Lynch J, et al. Differential regulation of tumour necrosis factor-alpha in human macrophages and peripheral blood monocytes: a cellular and molecular analysis. Am J Respir Cell Mol Biol 1989; 1:57–63.

77. Scales W, Chensue S, Otterness I, Kunkel S. Regulation of monokine gene expression: prostaglandin E_2 suppresses tumour necrosis factor but not interleukin-1 or β-mRNA and cell-associated bioactivity. J Leuk Biol 1989; 45:416–21.
78. Spengler R, Spengler M, Strieter R, Remick D, Larrick J, Kunkel S. Modulation of tumour necrosis factor-alpha gene expression: desensitisation of prostaglandin E_2-induced suppression. J Immunol 1989; 142(12):4346–50.
79. Spinas G, Bloesch D, Keller U, Zimmerli W, Cammisuli S. Pretreatment with ibuprofen augments circulating tumor necrosis factor-a, interleukin-6, elastase during acute endotoxinemia. J Infect Dis 1991; 163:89–95.
80. Strieter R, Remick D, Ward P, et al. Cellular and molecular regulation of tumor necrosis factor-alpha production by pentoxyfylline. Biochem Biophys Res Commun 1988; 155(3):1230–6.
81. Porter J, Cutler B, Lee B, et al. Pentoxifylline efficacy in the tretment of intermittent claudication: multicentre controlled double-blind trial with objective assessment of chronic occlusive arterial disease patients. Am Heart J 1982; 104:66–72.
82. Ward A, Clissold S. Pentoxyfylline: a review of its pharmacodynamic and pharmacokinetic properties, and its therapeutic efficacy. Drugs 1987; 34:50–97.
83. Han J, Thompson P, Beutler B. Dexamethasone and pentoxifylline inhibit endotoxin-induced cachectin/tumor necrosis factor synthesis at separate points in the signalling pathway. J Exp Med 1990; 172:391–4.
84. Geissler D, Gaggl S, Most J, Griel R, Herold M, Dierich M. A monoclonal antibody directed against the human intercellulaar adhesion molecule (ICAM-1) modulates the release of tumor necrosis factor-α, interferon-γ and interleukin 1. Eur J Immunol 1990; 20:2591–6.

CHAPTER 11

CYTOKINE MODULATION OF VIRAL INFECTIONS

James W. Larrick and Susan C. Wright

Palo Alto Institute for Molecular Medicine
Stanford, California

INTRODUCTION

The survival of a host challenged by viral infection depends on many factors. Some are specific, such as antiviral T cell and B cell responses. Others are nonspecific, such as intrinsic cellular resistance, macrophage activation, and activation of humoral protective mechanisms (e.g., complement and coagulation). Cytokines are important mediators and regulators of both types of host response. Furthermore, orchestration of specific humoral and cellular immune responses requires the participation of many cytokines. Details of the complex and overlapping roles of cytokines in specific immune responses is beyond the scope of this chapter. Instead, this chapter we focus on the nonspecific antiviral effects of cytokines.

CYTOKINE RELEASE BY VIRUS-INFECTED CELLS

Interferon-α (IFN-α), interferon-β (IFN-β), interferon-γ (IFN-γ), interleukin-1 (IL-1), and tumor necrosis factor (TNF) are cytokines released by cells in response to a variety of stimuli, among them viruses (for review see Refs. 1 and 2). The interferons are produced primarily by lymphocytes and fibroblasts, whereas IL-1 and TNF are produced primarily by mononuclear phagocytes as well as many other cell types. These molecules apparently do not share primary or secondary structure and bind to distinct receptors. Each of these cytokines has pleiotropic effects, including antiviral activities and antiproliferative activities. All these cytokines enhance monocyte cytotoxicity for tumor cell targets (3) and nonspecific host resistance to bacterial and viral infections.

Several laboratories have shown that different viruses stimulate TNF-α release, (4–7). Berent et al. (8) showed that Sendai virus induced human peripheral blood leukocytes to produce high levels (0.6% of total mRNA) of TNF mRNA that peaked 2 h before the peak in IFN-α. In this system comparable levels of mRNA for both cytokines were induced, but the amount of bioactive TNF protein was 2 log less than that of IFN-α protein. This is of interest because TNF has a 74 amino acid N-terminal extension that is probably processed posttranscriptionally (9). It is likely that control is exerted on the release of bioactive TNF at this level; however, at the present time little is known about this process (i.e., the TNF protease). The maximal peak in TNF mRNA was at 3 h after induction. Interestingly, endotoxin and Sendai virus were equally effective inducers of TNF mRNA. Midulla et al. demonstrated that adult blood monocytes, cord blood monocytes, and alveolar macrophages are permissive for infection by respiratory syncytial virus (10). Both IFN-γ and TNF-α prevented infection of these target cells.

IFN is the most notable cytokine produced during viral infections, but other cytokines can be synthesized in abundance during viral stimulation. For example, Van Damme et al. (11) compared the ability of different viruses to induce IL-6 from several human and animal cell types. Laboratory strains of Sendai, mengo, and Newcastle disease viruses dose dependently stimulated IL-6 production in diploid fibroblasts and endothelial cells. Wild-type measles and rubella virus induced IL-6, IFN-β, and granulocyte-macrophage colony-stimulating factor (GM-CSF). Measles virus induced high titers of IL-6 in vitro, comparable to levels found in acute viral infection of the central nervous system (12,13), and Vacheron et al. demonstrated that mice infected with influenza A virus by aerosol produce IL-1 and TNF in brochoalveolar lavage fluid (14).

Goldfeld and Maniatis (15) demonstrated that several stimulators, including phorbol ester, viral RNA, or synthetic double-stranded (ds) RNA [i.e., poly (I)• poly (C)] induced TNF-α and IFN-β in B cells and monocytes. Virus was the most potent inducer of both cytokines, and this induction was blocked by the kinase inhibitor 2-aminopurine. Inhibition of protein synthesis blocked viral induction of both genes in B cell lines but not in U937 monoblasts. In the JY B lymphoblastoid cell line cycloheximide blocked viral induction of the IFN-β but not the TNF-α gene. Thus there are complex overlapping but distinct pathways of induction of cytokine genes by viruses depending upon the cell type studied.

Enzyme Activities Induced by Interferons

IFN induces many proteins (16), some of which have been identified. Among the enzyme activities identified are tissue transglutaminase (17), guanylate cyclase (18), a phosphodiesterase (19), indoleamine-2,3-dioxygenase (20), xanthine oxidase (21), a polyamine-dependent protein kinase (22), a platelet protein kinase (23), 2',5'-oligoisoadenylate synthetase (24), and a dsRNA-dependent protein kinase (25).

One of the most extensive studies of cytokine-induced genes (26), utilized computer-based two-dimensional gels. In human fibroblasts IFN-α induced 12 polypeptides, IFN-γ induced 28 polypeptides, IL-1α and IL-1β induced an identical set of 7 polypeptides, and TNF-α induced 7 polypeptides. Despite that many

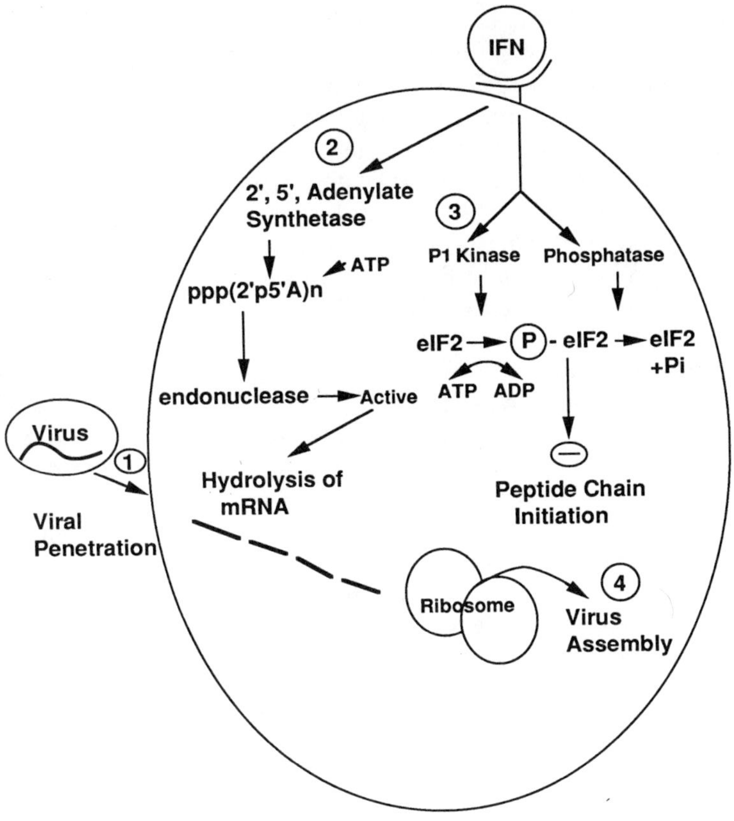

FIGURE 1 Interferon induction of the antiviral state showing intracellular sites of action of interferons. (1) Changes in membrane fluidity affect viral penetration. (2) The 2',5'-adenylate synthetase pathway results in ribonuclease activation. (3) The P1 kinase/phosphatase pathway results in inhibiton of peptide chain initiation. (4) Changes in membrane function also affect virus assembly, maturation, and relese from the cell surface.

of these proteins were induced in common, at the present time most of them remain unidentified and their role in viral protection is not known.

How Do IFNs Inhibit Viral Replication?

Interferons do not directly inactivate viruses; rather they must interact with specific cell surface receptors to induce an antiviral state (see Fig. 1) (27,28). The α and β interferons share a single receptor encoded on chromosome 21, but IFN-γ binds to a separate receptor encoded on chromosome 6 (29). Apparently the induction of the antiviral state does not require internalization of IFN. The development of an antiviral state begins within a few minutes of IFN binding and becomes maximal after 4–7 h (30).

The precise mechanisms underlying the ability of IFNs to inhibit viral replication are not known in detail, but two IFN-inducible pathways have been described (see fig. 1) (31). The IFN-induced synthesis of 2′,5′-adenylate synthetase

(32) is thought to be a key component in the establishment of the antiviral state. This enzyme is activated by double-stranded RNA and catalyzes the synthesis of oligomers of adenylate, linked 2′ to 5′ from ATP. These oligoadenylates, especially the trimer and tetramer forms, activate a latent cytoplasmic ribonuclease, called RNase L or F. Double-stranded RNA is also required for activation of the RNase activity. The half-life of the 2′,5′-adenylate oligomers is determined by a 2′,5′-adenylate phosphodiesterase. The antiviral state results from RNase L/F cleavage of viral mRNAs and cellular ribosomal RNAs. A second IFN-inducible enzyme is a 68 kD protein kinase called P1. P1 is regulated by phosphorylation, and its kinase activity is also activated by dsRNA. P1 phosphorylates eukaryotic initiation factor-2α (eIF-2α), which causes a block in initiation of translation. Presumably this blocks viral protein synthesis and thus limits viral spread. Several other mechanisms are known to help establish the antiviral state in cells exposed to IFN (33). IFN can modulate the fluidity of the cell membrane. It is possible that altered membrane function accounts for the defective envelope structures of enveloped viruses and problems these viruses have with maturation and release from the cell surface. Some viruses replicating in IFN-treated cells fail to methylate the cap site and thus fail to associate with ribosomes.

Viruses have developed several strategies to overcome the IFN-induced antiviral state. DNA viruses are less sensitive to IFN than RNA viruses, at least in part because of the paucity of dsRNA present during the infectious cycle. In addition, DNA viruses have developed several unique anti-IFN strategies. For example, herpes simplex virus-infected cells synthesize 2′,5′-A oligomeric dimers and trimers that bind to the endonuclease but do not activate it (34). Simian virus 40 (SV-40)-infected, IFN-treated CV-1 monkey kidney cells were shown to contain analogs of 2′,5′-A oligomers that lacked the terminal phosphoryl group, resulting in a reduced cleavage of mRNA (35). Paez and Esteban (36) have suggested that vaccinia viral ATPase and phosphatase activities account for the altered forms of 2′,5′-A oligomers found in vaccinia virus-infected cells. At least one RNA virus (EMCV) is known to replicate in HeLa cells having high levels of 2′,5′-A synthetase activity. Apparently the virus is able to directly inactivate the endonuclease induced by IFN.

Several mechanisms have been devised by viruses to evade the P1 kinase pathway. The genome of adenovirus type 5 encodes several small RNA molecules called VA1 RNAs that are required for efficient translation of viral and cellular genes late in infection. VA1 RNA may exist as a partially double-stranded form, and Katze et al. (37,38) showed that VA1 RNA binds to the P1 kinase and blocks autophosphorylation. Another adenovirus gene, E1A, was shown by Reich et al. (39) to encode proteins that specifically inhibit the transcription of a group of IFN-responsive genes.

Several laboratories have identified specific inhibitors of the P1 kinase in vaccinia virus-infected cells (40,41). This inhibitor appears to be a protein that binds reversibly to the P1 kinase (42). Apparently poliovirus-infected HeLa cells contain an activity that can inhibit the P1 kinase activity.

OTHER CYTOKINES THAT INDUCE AN ANTIVIRAL STATE

Although interferons have been studied for many years as prototypical antiviral cytokines, more recently several other factors have been shown to contribute to the antiviral state. TNF-α and lymphotoxin TNF-β were initially described as tumoricidal proteins produced by activated macrophages and lymphocytes, respectively. Several studies have shown that both TNF-α and TNF-β have antiviral activity and synergize with interferons in the induction of resistance to both RNA, [as for encephalomyocarditis virus (EMCV) and vesicular stomatitits virus (VSV)], and DNA virus, [as for adenovirus-2 (AD-2) and herpes simplex virus type II (HSV-2)], infection in diverse cell types in vitro. The antiviral effects of TNFs are observed with some but not all cell types. Virus-infected cells are selectively killed by TNFs, and this activity is accelerated by IFN-γ. Ruggiero et al. (43) studied the antiviral activity of TNF-α, TNF-β, and IL-1 on human WISH cells. All cytokines induced protection from vesicular stomatitis virus and Sindbis virus infection; however, on a molar basis IL-1 was about 1 log less active. Both TNF-α and TNF-β caused a dramatic inhibition of viral protein synthesis and augmented synthesis of 2′,5′A synthetase activity. In this system, antibodies against IFN-β_1 (but not IL-6, i.e., IFN-β_2) inhibited the antiviral state induced by TNF-α, TNF-β, and IL-1. In contrast, Kohase et al. reported that although IL-1 and TNF can inhibit virus replication in certain cell lines in vitro, in other cell lines (e.g., FS-4 human fibroblasts) IL-1 did not induce an antiviral state and in fact was able to block the antiviral state induced by TNF or IFN-β_1 (44).

Mechanism of Antiviral Protection

The mechanism of the antiviral effect mediated by TNF is controversial. Wong and Goeddel of Genentech, Inc., suggest that the antiviral state induced by TNFs are not due to the induction of IFN synthesis, whereas others using specific antibodies suggest that most of the antiviral state induced by TNF is secondary to induction of IL6. For example, Hughes et al. (45) demonstrated that most but not all of the synergistic antiviral activity of TNF and IFN-γ was neutralized by anti-IL-6 antibodies. This report is in agreement with the results Mestan et al. (46,47) and is consistent with findings that IL-6 is induced by TNF in vitro (48).

TNF-Induced Genes

TNF is known to induce transcription of a variety of genes in different cell types (see Table 1). However, it is unclear which of these gene products are involved in TNF-induced viral resistance. The finding that TNF lyses cells even in the presence of inhibitors of transcription or translation suggests that new gene expression is not required for cytotoxicity. In addition, it is not clear whether the intracellular pathway leading to TNF cytolysis overlaps those signals leading to viral protection. Of interest in this regard is the recent report that activated macrophages may use different cytolytic mechanisms to lyse virally infected versus tumor target cells (49). Reduction of glucose with inhibition of hexose monophosphate shunt activity and reactive oxygen intermediates and anti-TNF antibody blocked the lysis of VSV-infected 3T3 cells but not the lysis of P815 tumor cells.

Under physiological conditions the outcome of a race between induced protective genes and the deleterious consequences of TNF might determine whether a response is cytotoxic. What are the postulated protective genes, and how do they function? It is known that TNF induces mitochondrial superoxide dismutase

TABLE 1 Tumor Necrosis Factor—Inducible Genes

Upregulated
Manganese superoxide dismutase
Metallothionine
2′,5′oligo A synthetase
CD11/CD18
ICAM1
ELAM
Tissue factor
Plasminogen activator inhibitor I and II
Interleukin-6
Interleukin-8
Cytochrome P_{245}, heavy chain
Ferritin light chain
gro oncogene
Collagenase
c-*fos*
c-*myc*
c-*jun*
Heat-shock proteins
Downregulated
Protein S
Protein C
Thrombomodulin

(SOD) and ferritin heavy chain (50), both of which could function to counteract TNF-induced free-radical damage.

Heat-shock Proteins

Pretreatment of target cells at 42°C confers partial resistance to subsequent lysis by TNF (51), which correlates with synthesis of heat-shock protein 68 (HSP68); for a review of HSPs see Ref. 52). Resistance can be blocked by cycloheximide and actinomycin D, suggesting a requirement for de novo protein synthesis. Various stress stimuli, such as heat shock, or cytokines, such as interferon-γ, render cells resistant to cytolysis by natural killer cells and lymphokine-activated killer cells (53,54). However, the mechanism by which HSPs function to counteract TNF or other cytolytic processes remains unclear. The genes encoding HSP70 have been mapped to the human major histocompatibility complex (MHC) between the loci for TNF and complement components (53). Members of the HSP70 family facilitate refolding of proteins, assembly of multimeric complexes, and protein translocation. Recent evidence suggests that HSP70 cognates direct cytosolic proteins destined for lysosomal degradation into this organelle (55). Thus, one possible theory is that HSPs mediate the safe disposal of intracellular TNF via lysosomal degradation.

Virus infection of eukaryotic cells induces some heat-shock proteins. Adenovirus, herpes simplex virus type I, Newcastle disease virus, Sindbis virus, simian viruses 5 and 40, polyomaviruses, Sendai virus, paramyxovirus, and papovaviruses have all been reported to induce heat-shock proteins (56). Interestingly, viral development may require one or more heat-shock proteins, and without this induction viral growth does not proceed (57). It is possible that this is one mechanism by which viral infection can reverse the cytokine-induced antiviral state (58).

Nuclear Regulatory Factors

Studies of the regulatory enhancer regions of κ light chains have revealed several sites that bind trans-activating DNA binding proteins. One of these factors, NF-κB, was originally defined as B cell specific (59). Subsequently, it was shown that NF-κB binding sites are present in other viral and cellular genes. In B cells expression of NF-κB is constitutive. In other cells, the NF-κB is found in the cytoplasm in an inactive form bound to an inhibitor, I-κB, that prevents its translocation to the nucleus and hence its DNA binding activity (60). A variety of signals, such as lipopolysaccharide (LPS), phorbol esters, IL-1, cAMP, and TNF-α, can induce NF-κB activity in diverse cell types (61). At least two different kinases can enhance the activity of NF-κB, protein kinase C and cAMP-dependent protein kinase. Currently it is thought that phosphorylation of I-κB bound to NF-κB dissociates the complex with subsequent translocation of NF-κB to the nucleus to carry out its DNA binding and regulatory functions. Although it is known that TNF can activate NF-κB in sensitive tumor cells (62), it is not clear whether this is essential for target cell lysis to proceed. That TNF cytolysis proceeds in the presence of inhibitors of RNA and protein synthesis argues against a requirement for NF-κB-induced gene expression. In fact, the data are most consistent with a model in which NF-κB may induce TNF protective genes, such as MnSOD. However, it is not at present known whether MnSOD or other potentially protective genes are regulated by NF-κB.

The adenovirus early region 1A (E1A) encodes proteins that induce susceptibility to TNF cytotoxicity (63). The mechanism by which E1A proteins regulate transcription of viral and cellular genes (64) is not yet understood. However, E1A gene products do not directly bind to DNA, and E1A-responsive enhancers and promoters lack a consensus sequence. Transfection of NIH-3T3 cells with an adenovirus E1A cDNA induced susceptibility to lysis by natural killer cells or by activated macrophages (65). Antibodies to TNF blocked the macrophage cytolysis but not the NK cytolysis. The observation that adenovirus E1A products can activate the Ig κ-chain enhancer via the NF-κB binding site (66) suggests possible mechanisms for induction of TNF sensitivity. If activation of NF-κB is essential for TNF cytolysis, then it is possible that E1A activates a cellular kinase that can enhance the activation of NF-κB like molecules. Alternatively, the E1A protein may activate a cellular kinase that increases cytoplasmic calcium, or it may act directly in the nucleus. It is possible that these mechanisms are involved in the induction of susceptibility to TNF by viral infections in normal cells and that E1A-like proteins (67,68) regulate tumor cell sensitivity to TNF.

TNF Shares Structural Homologies With Viruses

The three-dimensional structure of TNF reveals that the monomer forms an elongated, antiparallel β-pleated sheet sandwhich with a "jelly roll" topology. Three monomers associate to form a trimer that has structural homology to viral coat proteins, such as satellite tobacco necrosis virus (69). Likewise, the TNF receptor shares structural homology with certain receptors. The cysteine-rich extracellular domain (22 conserved cysteines) of the human TNF receptor (70) shares sequence homology with T2, an open reading frame found in the Shope fibroma virus, human DC40, a B cell antigen, the nerve growth factor receptor, and a cytolytic T cell clone cDNA designated 4-1BB encoding a putative cell surface receptor with unknown ligand. More information about the structure of pathogenic viruses and cytokines and their receptors may shed light on how these molecules have coevolved.

ALTERNATE CYTOKINE ACTIVITIES THAT AID THE HOST RESPONSE

All the cytokines described earlier can initiate local microvascular inflammation characterized by activation of endothelial cells and adhesion of leukocytes. In addition, these cytokines (i.e., TNF, IL-1, and IFN) and direct viral infection augment the activation of IL-8 (71) and related genes (72,73). The precise role of these 8 kD family of cytokines is not known, although they have been shown to be chemotactic for lymphocytes (IL-8), granulocytes (NAF1 and NAF2), and macrophages (MCP1). Members of this gene family are produced by many cell types, including mononuclear phagocytes, lymphocytes, endothelial cells, fibroblasts, hepatocytes, epithelial cells, and keratinocytes. These cytokines provide a first line of defense to contain foreign microbial invasion and may account for the microvascular and coagulopathic pathology associated with many virus infections.

Other chapters in this volume describe the complex interactions of cytokine networks. Some examples of interactions that may affect the outcome of viral infections are given here. IFN-γ is known to inhibit the proliferation of B cells and favors the isotype switch of B cells to the IgG_{2a} isotype (74). IFN-γ also suppresses the growth of murine Th2 cells in response to their autocrine growth factor IL-4 (75) and blocks the IL-5-induced proliferation of BCL-1 cells (76). Lohoff et al. showed that IL-4 antagonizes the protective effects of IFN-α, IFN-β, and IFN-γ on murine fibroblasts infected with vesicular stomatitis virus (76). This antagonism must have biological relevance. For example, IL-4 and IL-3 may block the ability of IFN-γ to induce killing of intracellular leishmania parasites by macrophages (77). The preferential expansion of cells producing IL-4 may influence the capacity of IFNs to mediate their antiviral and antiintracellular pathogenic effects.

INHIBITORS AND VIRAL INHIBITION OF THE IMMUNE RESPONSE

Virus infections have long been associated with suppression of the immune response to alternative stimuli (78): influenza is a classic example (79). On the other hand, such infections as respiratory syncytial virus (RSV) are known to recur despite the development of an immune state. McCarthy et al. (80) demonstrated that exposure of purified human monocytes or peripheral blood leukocytes to respiratory syncytial virus induced the expression of an IL-1 inhibitor. Direct addition of RSV or influenza virus to cultures of human mononuclear cells markedly depressed mitogen-induced proliferation. Interestingly, these cultures contain both IL-1 and IL-1 inhibitory activity. In the case of RSV net inhibitory activity predominates, whereas with influenza net IL-1 activity predominates (81). This is of general medical interest because recurrent infections with RSV are common. It appears that the development of immunity to RSV is incomplete relative to immunity to other viruses, including influenza virus. It is likely that RSV preferentially stimulates the expression of the recently described IL-1 receptor antagonist (82,83). Recently, Nain et al. (84) demonstrated that TNF release was potentiated by lipopolysaccharide. This may account for the serious complications frequently observed when patients acquire combined influenza A virus and bacterial infections.

Activation of the immune system in response to systemic viral infections, such as measles (85), requires clonal proliferation of T cells and B cells, with differentiation of cytotoxic T cells to eliminate virus from tissue and differentiation of B cells to produce antibodies to eliminate virus from body fluid and provide long-term immunity. Measles is accompanied by secondary bacterial infections causing pneumonia and diarrhea (86) and by postmeasles encephalomyelitis, an autoimmune demyelinating disease (87). Both types of complications result from the immunological abnormalities that accompany acute measles. These types of abnormalities include reduced lymphocyte mitogenesis, reduced delayed-type hypersensitivity, and augmented cytokine production (88,89). The dysfunctional release of cytokines during viral infection may be responsible for the suppression of the immune response that accompanies many viral infections.

IN VIVO STUDIES

Studies with antiinterferon antisera demonstrated the protective activity of these cytokines in vivo (90). Despite these studies and many others unequivocally demonstrating protective actions of interferons in vivo, other studies suggest that cytokines contribute to the pathogenesis of viral infection. For example, treatment of mice infected with influenza with anti-IFN-α or anti-IFN-β antibodies ameloriated the disease and reduced mortality (91). In addition, although picornaviruses induce a poor IFN response in vitro, they rapidly induce IFN in vivo (92).

Iida et al. (93) carried out antiviral studies of cytokines in vivo. IFN-γ gave protection when administered intranasally but not intravenously (IV) several days before infection of mice with HSV. Intranasal administration of GM-CSF 1–3 days before infection was the most effective route. IL1-β could be given 1 day before Sendai virus infection. When each of the cytokines was given subcutaneously four times daily to cyclophosphamide-treated mice before administration of HSV, only GM-CSF afforded protection.

HSV causes recurring self-limited mucocutaneous infections in normal hosts. In contrast, infection in neonatal animals or humans is usually quite severe. The susceptibility of neonates is due to defects in both the early containment phase (i.e., macrophage and natural killer function) and the later specific cure phase (i.e., antibody production, elaboration of IFN-γ, and ADCC effector function) (94). Kohl showed that 1-week-old mice could be protected against lethal HSV infection by adoptive transfer of human mononuclear cells activated with IFN-γ or IL-2 (95). The cell type conferring protection was a CD4-positive macrophage driven by IFN-γ. Poor protection was afforded by untreated cells from neonatal humans (96). However, adoptive transfer of human mononuclear cells treated in vitro with human IL-2 or human IFN-γ was able to reconstitute the effector cell and antibody production defects and afforded protection of neonatal mice infected with HSV.

Cytokines have had limited success in the treatment of viral infections. A review of clinical results in beyond the scope of this chapter. However, the best results have been obtained in treatment of papovavirus and hepadnavirus infections (97,98). Prophylactic use in rhinovirus infections appear promising if side effects can be attenuated.

SUMMARY AND CONCLUSIONS

Successful immune responses to viral infection involve a complex cascade of events that include presentation of viral antigens to the immune system, proliferation of antigen-specific lymphocytes, and enumeration of a diverse array of cytokines. Viral infection of target cells causes the release of cytokines, such as the interferons, TNF, and IL-1. Cytokines acting directly (e.g., IFNs) or indirectly (e.g., TNF, IL-1) can induce a viral resistant state. Viral infection also induces molecules that participate in local inflammation to limit viral spread. In some cases cytokines potentiate viral pathogenesis and are deleterious to host. Although some of the intracellular protective mechanisms are known in some detail (e.g., 2′,5′-adenylate synthetase and P1 kinase pathways), most of this process is a "black box." A more detailed understanding of cytokine pathways at the cellular and subcellular levels will yield important pathogenetic as well as therapeutic insights.

ACKNOWLEDGMENTS

This work was supported in part by CA47669 awarded by the National Cancer Institute. High-quality secretarial help was provided by Wolfgang A. Scatman.

REFERENCES

1. Arai K, Lee F, Miyajima A, et al. Cytokines: coordinators of immune and inflammatory responses. Annu Rev Biochem 1990; 59:783.
2. Larrick JW, Kunkel SL. The role of tumor necrosis factor and interleukin 1 in the immunoinflammatory response. Pharm Res 1988; 5:129.
3. Philip R, Epstein LB. Tumor necrosis factor as immunodulator and mediator of monocyte cytotoxicity induced by itself, gamma-interferon and interleukin-1. Nature 1986; 323:86.
4. Aderka D, Holtmann H, Toker L, et al. Tumor necrosis factor induction by Sendai virus. J Immunol 136:2938.
5. Wright SC, Jewett A, Mitsuyasu R, Bonavida B. Spontaneous cytotoxicity and tumor necrosis factor production by peripheral blood monocytes from AIDS patients. J Immunol 1988; 141:99.
6. Dudding L, Haskill S, Clark BD, et al. Cytomegalovirus infection stimulates expression of monocyte-associated mediator genes. J Immunol 143:3343.
7. Molina J, Scadden T, Bryn R, et al. Production of TNFα and IL1β by monocytic cells infected with HIV. J Clin Invest 1989; 84:733.

8. Berent SL, Torczynski RM, Bollon AP. Sendai virus induces high levels of tumor necrosis factor mRNA in human peripheral blood leukocytes. Nucleic Acids Res 1986; 14:8997.
9. Kreigler M, Perez C, Defay K, et al. a novel form of TNF/cachectin is a cell surface cytotoxic transmembrane protein: ramifications for the complex physiology of TNF. Cell 1988; 53:45.
10. Midulla F, Huang YT, Gilbert IA, et al. Respiratory syncytial virus infection of human cord and adult blood monocytes and alveolar macrophages. Am Rev Respir Dis 1989; 10:771.
11. Van Damme J, Schaafsma MR, Fibbe WE, et al. Simultaneous production of interleukin 6, interferon-β and colony-stimulating activity by fibroblasts after viral and bacterial infection. Eur J Immunol 1989; 19:163.
12. Houssiau FA, Bukasa K, Sindic CJM, et al. Elevated levels of 26kd human hybridoma growth factor (IL6) in CSF of patients with infections of the CNS. Clin Exp Immunol 1988; 71:320.
13. Frei K, Leist TP, Meager A, et al. Production of B cell stimulatory factor-2 and interferon gamma in the CNS during viral meningitis and encepalitis. Evaluation in a murine model infection and in patients. J Exp Med 1988; 168:49.
14. Vacheron R, Rudent A, Perin S, et al. Production of interleukin 1 and tumour necrosis factor activities in bronchoalveolar washings following infection of mice by influenza virus. J Gen Virol 1990; 71:477.
15. Goldfeld AE, Maniatis T. Coordinate viral induction of tumor necrosis factor alpha and interferon beta in human B cells and monocytes. Proc Natl Acad Sci U S A 1989; 86:1490.
16. Taylor JL, Grossberg SE. Recent progress in interferon research: molecular mechanisms of regulation, action, and virus circumvention. Virus Res 1990; 15:1.
17. Mehta K, Lopex-Bernstein G, Moore WT, et al. Interferon-gamma requires serum retinoids to promote the expression of tissue transglutaminase in cultured human blood monocytes. J Immunol 1985; 134:2053.
18. Vesely DL, Cantell K. Human interferon enhances guanylate cyclase activity. Biochem Biophys Res Commun 1980; 96:574.
19. Schmidt A, Chernajovsky Y, Shulman L, et al. An interferon-induced phosphodiesterase degrading (2'-5') oligoisoadenylate and the C-C-A terminus of tRNA. Proc Natl Acad Sci U S A 1979; 76:4788.
20. Pfefferkorn ER, Rebhun S, Eckel M. Characterization of an indoleamine 2,3-dioxygenase induced by gamma-interferon in cultured human fibroblasts. J Interferon Res 1986; 6:267.
21. Ghezzi P, Bianchi M, Mantovani A, et al. Enhanced xanthine oxidase activity in mice treated with interferon and interferon inducers. Biochem Biophys Res Commun 1984; 119:144.
22. Chapekar MS, Glazer RI. Effects of human immune interferon on cell viability. (2'5') Oligoadenylate synthesis, and polyamine-dependent protein phosphorylation in human colon carcinoma cells *in vitro*. Cancer Res 1984; 44:2144.
23. Krust B, Galabru J, Hovanessian AG. Phosphorylation of the alpha-chain of fibrogen by a platelet kinase activity enhanced by interferon. Biochem Biophys Res Commun 1983; 117:350.
24. Chebath J, Benech P, Hovanessian A, et al. Four different forms of interferon-induced 2', 5' -oligo(A) synthetase identified by immunoblotting in human cells. J Biol Chem 1987; 262:3852.
25. West DK, Baglioni C. Induction by interferon in HeLa cells of a protein kinase activated by double-stranded RNA. Eur J Biochem 1979; 101:461.
26. Beresini MH, Lempert MJ, Epstein LB. Overlapping polypeptide induction in human

fibroblasts in response to treatment with interferon-alpha, interferon-gamma, interleukin 1 alpha, interleukin 1 beta, and tumor necrosis factor. J Immunol 1988; 140:485.

27. Issacs A, Lindenmann J. Virus interference. I. The interferon. Proc R Soc Lond [Biol] 1957; 147:258.
28. Petska S, Langer JA, Zoon KC, et al. Interferons and their action. Annu Rev Biochem 1987; 56:727.
29. Branca AA, Baglioni C. Evidence that type I and II interferons have different receptors. Nature 1981; 294:768.
30. Dianzani F, Baron S. Unexpectedly rapid action of human interferon in physiological conditions. Nature 1975; 257:682.
31. Samuel EC. Mechanism of interferon action: phosphorylation of protein synthesis inhibition factor eIF-2 interferon treated human cells by a ribosome-associated protein kinase possessing site specificity inhibition to heming-regulated rabbit reticulocyte kinase. Proc Natl Acad Sci U S A 1979; 76:600.
32. Baglioni C, Maroney PA. Mechanism of action of human interferons: induction of 2', 5'-oligo(A) polymerase. J Biol Chem 1980; 255:8390.
33. Joklik WK. Interferons. In: Fields BN, et al., eds. Virology. New York: Raven Press, 1985:281.
34. Cayley PJ, Davies JA, McCullagh KG, et al. Activation of the ppp(A2'p)$_n$A system in interferon-treated, herpes simplex virus-infected cells and evidence for novel inhibitors of the ppp(A2'p)$_n$A-dependent RNase. Eur J Biochem 1984;143:165.
35. Hersh CL, Brown RE, Roberts WK, et al. Simian virus 40-infected, interferon-treated cells contain 2'5'-oligoadenylates which do not activate cleavage of RNA. J Biol Chem 1984; 259:1731.
36. Paez E, Esteban M. Nature and mode of action of vaccinia virus products that block activation of the interferon mediated ppp(A2'p)$_n$A synthetase. Virology 1984; 134:29.
37. Katze MG, Detjen BM, Safer B, et al. Translational control by influenza virus: suppression of the kinase that phosphorylates the alpha subunit of initiation factor eIF-2 and selective translation of influenza viral messenger RNAs. Mol Cell Biol 1980; 6:1741.
38. Katze MG, Tomita J, Balck T, et al. Influenza virus regulates protein synthesis during infection by repressing autophosphorylation and activity of the cellular 68,000-M_r protein kinase. J Virol 1988; 62:3710.
39. Reich N, Pine R, Levy D, et al. Transcription of interferon-stimulated genes is induced by adenovirus particles but is suppressed by E1A gene products. J Virol 1988; 62:114.
40. Rice AP, Kerr IM. Interferon-mediated, double-stranded RNA-dependent protein kinase is inhibited in extracts from vaccinia virus-infected cells. J Virol 1984; 50:229.
41. Rice AP, Kerr SM, Roberts WK, et al. Novel 2'-5' oligoadenylates synthesized in interferon-treated vaccinia virus-infected cells. J Virol 1985; 56:1041.
42. Whitaker-Dowling P, Youngner JS. Characterization of a specific kinase inhibitory factor produced by vaccinia virus which inhibits the interferon-induced protein kinase. Virology 1984; 137:171.
43. Ruggiero V, Antonelli G, Gentile M, et al. Comparative study on the antiviral activity of tumor necrosis factor (TNF)-alpha, lymphotoxin/TNF-beta, and IL-1 in WISH cells. Immunl Lett 1989; 21:165.
44. Kohase M, Zhang YH, Lin JK, et al. Interleukin-1 can inhibit interferon-beta synthesis and its antiviral action: comparison with tumor necrosis factor. J Interferon Res 1988; 8:559.
45. Hughes TK, Kaspar TA, Coppenhaver DH. Synergy of antiviral actions of TNF and IFN-gamma: evidence for a major role of TNF-induced IFN-beta. Antivirual Res 1988; 10:1.

46. Mestan J, Digel W, Mittnacht S, et al. Antiviral effect of recombinant tumor necrosis factor in vitro. Nature 1986; 323:816.
47. Mestan J, Brockhaus M, Kirchner H, et al. Antiviral activity of tumor necrosis factor. Synergism with interferons and induction of oligo-2′,5′-adenylate synthetase. J Gen Virol 1988; 69:3113.
48. Kohase MD, Henrikson-Stefano D, May LT, et al. Induction of B_2-interferon by tumor necrosis factor: a homeostatic mechanism in the control of cell proliferation. Cell 1986; 45:659.
49. LeBlanc PA, Heath LS, Um H-D. Activated macrophages use different cytolytic mechanisms to lyse a virally infected or tumor target. J Leuk Biol 1990; 48:1.
50. Torti SV, Kwak EL, Miller SC, et al. The molecular cloning and characterization of murine ferritin heavy chain, a tumor necrosis factor-inducible gene. J Biol Chem 1988; 263:12638.
51. Jaattela M, Saksela K, Saksela E. Heat shock protects WEHI-164 target cells from cytolysis by tumor necrosis factors alpha and beta. Eur J Immunol 1989; 19:1413.
52. Kaufmann SHE. Heat shck proteins and the immune reponse. Immunol Today 1990; 11:129.
53. Renkonen R, Ristimaki A, Hayry P. Interferon-gamma protects human endothelial cells from lypmphokine-activated killer cell mediated lysis. Eur J Immunol 18:1839.
54. Gromkowski SH, Yagu J, Janeway CA. Elevated temperature regulates tumor necrosis factor-mediated immune killing. Eur J Immunol 1989; 19:1709.
55. Chiang HL, Terlecky SR, Plant CP, et al. A role for a 70-kilodalton heat shock protein in lysosomal degradation of intracellular proteins. Science 1989; 346:382.
56. Neidhart FC, et al. The genetics and regulation of heat-shock proteins. Annu Rev Genet 1984; 18:295.
57. Imperiale MJ, Kao HT, Feldman LT, et al. Cell-specific regulation of gene expression: common control of the heat shock gen and the early adenovirus genes. Mol Cell Biol 1982; 4:875.
58. Feduchi E, Carrasco L. Adenovirus infection reverses the antiviral state induced by human interferon. FEBS Lett 1987; 214:153.
59. Sen R, Baltimore D. Multiple nuclear factors interact with the immunoglobulin enhancer sequences. Cell 1984; 46:705.
60. Bauerle PA, Baltimore D. IkB: a specific inhibitor of the NF-kB transcription factor. Science 1988; 242:540.
61. Lowenthal JW, Ballard DW, Bohnlein E, et al. Tumor necrosis factor induces proteins that bind specifically to kB-like enhancer elements and regulate interleukin 2 receptor alpha-chain gene expression in primary human T lymphocytes. Proc Natl Acad Sci U S A 1989; 86:2331.
62. Osborn L, Kunkel S, Nabel GJ. Tumor necrosis factor and interleukin 1 stimulate the human immunodeficiency virus enhancer by activation of the nuclear factor kB. Proc Natl Acad Sci U S A 86:2336.
63. Chen M-J, Holskin B, Strickler J, et al. Induction of E1A oncogene expression of cellular susceptibility to lysis by TNF. Nature 1987; 330:581.
64. Berk AJ. Adenovirus promoters and E1A trans-activation. Annu Rev Genet 1986; 20:45.
65. Cook JL, May DL, Wilson BA, et al. Role of tumor necrosis factor-alpha in E1A oncogene-induced susceptibility of neoplastic cells to lysis by natural killer cells and activated macrophages. J Immunol 1989; 142:4527.
66. Shurman L, Sen R, Bergman Y. Adenovirus E1A products activate the Ig k-chain enhancer in fibroblasts: a possible involvement of the NF-kB site. J Immunol 1989; 143:3806.
67. Braithwaite AW, Diver WP, Jeune SL, et al. Human cellular sequences detectable

with adenovirus probes. I. Evidence for novel repeat sequences and a possible E1a-like cellular "gene" Chromosoma 1986; 93:537.

68. Imperiale MJ, Kao H-T, Feldman LT, et al. Common control of the heat shock gene and early adenovirus genes: evidence for a cellular E1A-like activity. Mol Cell Biol 1984; 4:867.
69. Eck MJ, Sprang SR. The structure of tumor necrosis factor-α at 2.6 Å resolution. J Biol Chem 1989; 264:17595.
70. Smith CA, Davis T, Anderson D, et al. A receptor for tumor necrosis factor defines an unusual family of cellular viral proteins. Science 1990; 248:1019.
71. Leonard EJ, Yoshimura T. Neutrophil attractant/activation protein-1 (NAP-1[interleukin-8]). Am J Respir Cell Mol Biol. 2:479.
72. Goetschy JF, Zeller H, Content J, et al. Regulation of the interferon-inducible IFI-78K gene, the human equivalent of the murine *Mx* gene, by interferons, double-stranded RNA, certain cytokines, and viruses. J Virol 1989; 63:2616.
73. Farber JM. A macrophage mRNA selectively induced by γ interferon encodes a member of the platelet factor 4 family of cytokines. Proc Natl Acad Sci U S A 1990; 87:5238.
74. Snapper CM, Paul WE. Interferon-gamma and B cell stimulatory factor-1 reciprocally regulate Ig isotype production. Science 1987; 236:9.
75. Gajewski TF, Fitch FW. Antiproliferative effects of IFN-gamma in immune regulation. I. IFN-gamma inhibits the proliferation of Th2 but not Th1 murine HTL clones. J Immunol 12:4245.
76. Lohoff M, Sommer F, Rollinghoff M. Suppressive effect of interferon gamma on the BCL-1 cell-dependent IL5 bioassay. Eur J Immunol 1989; 19:1327.
77. Liew FY, Millott S, Li Y, et al. Macrophage activation by interferon gamma from host-protective T cells is inhibited by IL3 and IL4 produced by disease promoting T cells in leishmaniasis. Eur J Immunol 1989; 19:1227.
78. Roberts NJ Jr, Domurat F. Virus-induced immunosuppression: influenza virus. In: Spector S, Bendinelli M, Friedman H, eds. Virus-induced immunosuppression. New York: Plenum, 1989:303.
79. Del Gobbo V, Balestra E, Marini S, et al. Influenza virus infection reduces cellular immunity functions. Adv Exp Med Biol 1989; 257:247.
80. McCarthy DO, Domurat FM, Nichols JE, et al. Interleukin-1 inhibitor production by human mononuclear leukocytes and leukocyte subpopulations exposed to respiratory syncytial virus: analysis and comparison with the response to influenza virus. J Leuk Biol 1989; 46:189.
81. Roberts NJ Jr, Prill AH, Mann TH. Interleukin 1 and interleukin 1 inhibitor production by human macrophages exposed to influenza virus or respiratory syncytial virus. RSV is a potent inducer of inhibitor activity. J Exp Med 1986; 163:511.
82. Hannum CH, Wilcox CJ, Arend WP, et al. Interleukin 1 receptor antagonist activity of a human interleukin-1 inhibitor. Nature 1990; 343:336.
83. Eisenberg RJ, Evans WP, Arend WP, et al. Primary structure and functional expression from complementary DNA of a human interleukin-1 receptor antagonist. Nature 1990; 343:341.
84. Nain M, Hinder F, Gong J-H, et al. Tumor necrosis factor-α production of influenza A virus-infected macrophages and potentiating effect of lipopolysaccharides. J Immunol 1990; 145:1921.
85. Griffin DE, Ward BJ, Jauregui E, et al. Immune activation in measles. N Engl J Med 1989; 320:1667.
86. Morley D. Severe measles in the tropics. Br Med J 1969; 1:297.
87. Johnson RT, Griffin DE, Hirsch RL, et al. Measles encephalomyelitis—clinical and immunologica studies. N Engl J Med 1984; 310:137.

88. Hirsch RL, Griffin DE, Johnson RT, et al. Cellular immune responses during complicated and uncomplicated measles virus infections of man. Clin Immunol Immunopathol 1984; 31:1.
89. Tamashiro VG, Perez HH, Griffin DE. Prospective study of the magnitude and duration of changes in tuberculin reactivity during uncomplicated and complicated measles. Pediatr Infect Dis J 1987; 6:51.
90. Gresser I, Tovey MG, Bandu MT, et al. Role of interferon in the pathogenesis of virus disease in mice as demonstrated by the use of anti-interferon serum. J Exp Med 1976; 144:1305.
91. Wabuke-Bunoti MAN, Bennick JR, Plotkin SA. Influenza virus-induced encepalopathy in mice: interferon production and natural killer cell activity during acute infection. J Virol 1986; 60:1062.
92. Dianzani F, Capobianchi MR, Matteucci D, et al. The role of interferon in picornavirus infections. Coxsackieviruses—a general update. New York: Plenum Press, 1988.
93. Iida J, Saiki I, Ishiara C, Azuma I. Protective activity of recombinant cytokines against Sendai virus and herpes simplex (HSV) infections in mice. Vaccine 1989; 7:229.
94. Taylor S, Bryson YJ. Impaired production of gamma interferon by newborn cells in vitro is due to a functionally immature macrophage. J Immunol 1980; 134:1493.
95. Kohl S. Protection against murine neonatal herpes simplex virus infection by lymphokine-treated human leukocytes. J Immunol 1990; 144:307.
96. Kohl S, Bigelow RH, Loo LS. Ontogeny of protection of neonatal mice from lethal herpes simplex virus infection by human leukocytes, antiviral antibody, and recombinant alpha-interferon. Pediatr Res 1984; 18:1164.
97. Rizzetto M, Actis GC, Barbara L. Interferon use during hepatitis virus infections, In: Baron S, Dianzani F, Stanton GJ, Fleischmann Jr WR, eds. The interferon system: a current review to 1987 Austin: University of Texas Medical Branch, p 439.
98. Billiau A. Interferon therapy: pharmacokinetic and pharmacological aspects. Arch Virol 1981; 67:121.

CHAPTER 12

CYTOKINES AND MALARIA
Duality of Effects in Pathology and Protection

Georges E. Grau, Pierre-François Piguet, and Pascal Pointaire

University of Geneva
Geneva, Switzerland

Dominique Mazier

INSERM Unité
Paris, France

INTRODUCTION

The involvement of soluble mediators in malaria has long been suspected. Their possible role was first recognized in the pathogenesis of complications observed in severe forms of the disease by Maegraith, who noted similarities between endotoxicosis, meningococcemia, and severe malaria (1–3). The implication of cytokines in protection against malaria was then envisaged following observations that plasmodia could induce tumor necrosis factor (TNF) (4) and that this molecule had antiparasitic effects (5). The ability of malaria infection to cause the release of other cytokines, such as interferons, was also described (6–10). In this chapter we review various effects of cytokines responsible for the pathological expression of malaria complications and those able to mediate protective immunity to the disease.

PATHOGENIC ROLE OF CYTOKINES IN MALARIA

Cerebral Malaria

Cerebral malaria (CM) is the most common clinical presentation and cause of death in severe malaria: more than 1 million children die annually in sub-Saharan Africa (11). In some reports CM accounts for up to 10% of all cases of falciparum malaria admitted to hospital and for 80% of fatal cases. This condition is invariably fatal if untreated and is associated with a 20% mortality in treated patients. The pathogenesis of cerebral malaria has been the object of considerable interest and has remained incompletely understood. In primates or rodents, infection with various strains of plasmodia can also lead to encephalopathy.

Experimental

To analyze the pathogenesis of CM, we developed an experimental model in the mouse and studied it with particular attention to the role of TNF overproduction and T cell-derived cytokines (12–14). Experimental models in animals cannot reproduce all the features of human diseases, and this is particularly true in the case of cerebral malaria. However, CM is a syndrome in which it appears that the same altered cell (the endothelial cell) has a pivotal role in human and experimental lesions; in addition, the similarities existing between defined malarial antigens in rodent and human parasites and between pathways of immune responses in mouse and human justify the use of a model. The concepts defined in experimental conditions may direct further investigations in humans. Our experimental model for cerebral malaria is the neurovascular pathology induced by the infection with *Plasmodium berghei* ANKA asexual blood stages in genetically susceptible CBA/Ca mice (15). This is a neurological syndrome occurring 6–14 days after infection and leading to a cumulative mortality of about 90%. Parasitemia at the time of death is consistently low. The neurological manifestations include paralysis (mono-, hemi-, para-, or tetraplegia), deviation of the head, ataxia, and convulsions. The remaining 10% of infected CM-susceptible mice eventually die during the third or fourth week of infection with severe anemia and hyperparasitemia but without neurological signs. Mice that are genetically resistant to CM, such as Balb/c mice, also die at that time in the same context of extremely severe anemia (less than 10^6 red blood cells per μl) and hyperparasitemia (more than 60% parasitized red blood cells).

In both human and mouse, numerous petechial hemorrhages are evident on macroscopic examination; they can be seen in the meninges, the white matter of the cerebrum, the brain stem, and the cerebellum. On histological sections in human CM, "ring hemorrhages" are a key feature. They surround medium-sized vessels, venules, and even arterioles. The vessel wall is necrotic, and the lumen is packed mostly with parasitized red blood cells; leukocytes and fibrin are occasionally observed. In the mouse model, sequestration of parasitized red blood cells is consistently absent, and the hemorrhages, apparently due to a rupture of venulae, are constantly associated with sequestration of leukocytes. Comparison between various parameters (non-immunological, immunological, and histopathological) of experimental and human CM has been reviewed (16). The only major difference between human and experimental CM is the nature of the cells that are sequestered in brain vessels. In malaria-infected mice, the focal arrest of leukocytes, monocytes-macrophages, and lymphocytes is the dominant picture in brain vessels. Such vascular plugging by mononuclear cells is also seen in lungs from patients with severe falciparum malaria (17).

The first indication that CM is the result of T cell-dependent immunopathological reactions came from the observation that athymic nude mice do not develop this neurological syndrome, although their susceptibility to *P. berghei* ANKA infection was identical to that of euthymic mice. Upon further analysis of T cells in CM, we demonstrated that $CD4^+$ T lymphocytes play a significant role in the development of murine cerebral malaria, since specific depletion by use of monoclonal antibodies prevented CM (15).

We then analyzed the role of cytokines in the pathogenesis of CM. A role for endotoxin-induced, macrophage-derived mediators was suggested earlier by Clark and colleagues (18). TNF is a hormone with a wide range of biological activities produced principally by activated macrophages (19). That TNF is a crucial mediator of acute inflammation and of septic shock (20–22) and the observation that numerous macrophages are present in lymphoid organs and at the site of neurovascular lesions in malaria-infected mice, as well as the powerful effects of TNF on endothelial cells (23,24), led us to explore the role of this molecule in CM.

Several lines of evidence indicate that TNF has a central role in the pathogenesis of murine CM. This contention is supported by the following evidence (12,25). First, there is a marked elevation of serum TNF levels only at the time of neurological syndrome. For instance, the depletion in $CD4^+$ T cells, which prevents CM, also inhibited the rise in serum TNF levels. Second, passive immunization with anti-TNF antibody of *P. berghei*-infected mice of a CM-susceptible strain significantly protected against CM and the associated early mortality. This treatment prevented all pathological abnormalities, including hemorrhages and the focal arrest of monocytes and other circulating leukocytes within brain capillaries and venules. In addition, the conspicuous macrophage accumulation in lymphoid organs was also suppressed by anti-TNF antibody treatment, suggesting that amplification loops of TNF on its own synthesis and on macrophage recruitment have been interrupted by the antibody treatment. This treatment, however, had no effect on the course of infection itself. Third, continuous perfusion of recombinant murine TNF to *P. berghei*-infected mice of a CM-resistant strain induced a lethal neurological syndrome in these mice.

In an attempt to explore the role of the immune response in TNF overproduction, our attention was focused on interleukin 3 (IL-3), granulocyte-macrophage colony-stimulating factor (GM-CSF), and interferon-γ (IFN-γ), three cytokines produced by activated $CD4^+$ T lymphocytes. We investigated the possible role of these molecules in CM lesions by injecting in vivo antibodies directed against recombinant IL-3 (rIL-3), GM-CSF (rGM-CSF), and IFN-γ (rIFN-γ). Interleukin 3 (IL-3) and GM-CSF are able to expand in vitro and in vivo the growth of granulocyte and macrophage precursors. Continuous in vivo infusion of recombinant mouse IL-3 and GM-CSF was shown by others to induce a marked leukocytosis and to increase the TNF mRNA level within tissue (Piguet et al., unpublished observations). It was found that although anti-IL3, anti-GM-CSF antibodies, or normal rabbit immunoglobulins administered alone had no effect, the combined treatment with anti-rIL-3 and anti-rGM-CSF antibodies dramatically prevented the development of the neurological syndrome (13). Also, TNF was not detectable in the serum of mice treated with both antibodies and protected against CM. Interestingly, the accumulation of macrophages in lymphoid organs, such as spleen red pulp and lymph nodes, which is consistently observed in mice developing CM, was significantly reduced, but not prevented, upon treatment with both anti-IL-3 and anti-rGM-CSF antibodies. As a consequence of CM prevention, the survival of mice receiving the dual treatment with anti-IL-3 and GM-CSF was significantly prolonged: these mice died around the third week of infection, with severe anemia and overwhelming parasitemia but without CM (13). The involvement of IFN-γ in the pathogenesis of CM is supported by observations that CM and its TNF overproduction can be prevented by treatment of *P. berghei*-

infected mice with either polyclonal or monoclonal anti-IFN-γ antibodies (14). In contrast to what was seen with anti-IL-3 and anti-GM-CSF antibodies, this treatment did not affect macrophage accumulation within lymphoid organs.

To explain the excessive production of TNF in CM, one may hypothesize the following (reviewed in Ref. 25). The requirement of $CD4^+$ T cells for CM to develop involves the release of at least three T cell-derived cytokines, IL-3, GM-CSF, and IFN-γ, since neutralization of these cytokines prevents markedly elevated blood TNF levels, which lead to cerebral vascular lesions. On the one hand, IL-3 and GM-CSF act by enlarging the pool of mononuclear phagocytes, which is manifested by the accumulation of these cells in lymphoid organs, and on the other hand, IFN-γ is responsible for their activation, further stimulating the synthesis and release of excessive amounts of TNF. A synergy between IFN-γ and TNF, particularly with respect to effects on endothelial cells, can also be envisaged. In addition, TNF has an upregulating effect on its own synthesis (26), as well as on the increase in TNF mRNA level triggered by IFN-γ, probably by increasing the number of IFN-γ receptors on cell surfaces. At some critical point, this cytokine cascade leads to a rapid autoamplification of TNF overproduction that ends in the cerebral vascular lesions of CM.

Recent in vitro studies of cytokine production by spleen and lymph node cells from mice of CM-susceptible and CM-resistant strains indicate that susceptibility to CM might be associated with a higher *P. berghei*-specific IFN-γ release (27). These preliminary data suggest that the triggering of CM might be a Th1-dependent pathological reaction.

Murine cerebral malaria is thus mediated by immune mechanisms. It is worth emphasizing that the lesions observed in CM do not correspond to well-recognized types of either cell-mediated (i.e., lympholysis or delayed-type hypersensitivity reaction) or humoral immunopathological reactions, in either murine or human CM (28). This has been taken as an argument against immune mechanisms in CM. However, the analysis of several other experimental models indicates that in various conditions the activation of the immune system leads to an elevation in TNF production and to various types of tissue damage (29–32). The autoaggravating effects of TNF release, due in part to the capacity of TNF to stimulate the growth and differentiation of macrophages, leading to a further TNF release, has been observed in other immunopathological conditions, which present a very different clinical course and type of lesions, such as the bacillus Calmette-Guerin (BCG) granulomas (26). This is strikingly apparent in the prevention of CM by anti-TNF antibodies, since it is not only the brain vascular lesions that are prevented by the neutralization of TNF, but the conspicuous macrophage accumulation in lymphoid organs as well. These observations allow one to envisage an unexplored type of immunopathological reaction in which T cell-dependent macrophage activation leads to the release of a number of cytokines, including TNF.

Human

The significance of tumor necrosis factor in the pathology of human CM has been evaluated by measuring serum concentrations of TNF in 65 Malawian children with severe *Plasmodium falciparum* malaria (33). The disease was associated with varying degrees of neurological involvement as assessed by coma score evaluated by a modified Glasgow coma scale. Although there was considerable overlap, the mean ± standard error of the mean (SEM) admission serum level of TNF was significantly higher in the 10 patients who died (709 ± 312 pg/ml) than in the 55 who survived (184 ± 31.5 pg/ml, $p < 0.02$). The mortality rate increased with the concentration of TNF: at a level of less than 100 pg/ml, 1 of 24 patients died; between 100 and 500 pg/ml, 6 of 34 patients; and at more than 500 pg/ml, 3 of 7 patients. The 10 patients who were hypoglycemic on admission to hospital had a higher mean serum TNF concentration (796 ± 319 pg/ml) than normoglycemic patients (168 ± 170 pg/ml, $p < 0.02$). High serum TNF concentrations were also associated with hyperparasitemia ($p < 0.002$), young age (<3 years $p < 0.009$), and severity of illness as measured by a prognostic index ($p < 0.0005$). The highest TNF concentrations were found in the serum of patients with profound coma. There was no significant elevation in cerebrospinal fluid TNF levels.

In the 55 survivors, the mean serum TNF level at the time of admission to hospital (148 ± 24.6 pg/ml, mean ± SEM) was significantly higher than in convalescence (15.7 ± 3.0 pg/ml, $p < 0.005$). Thus, TNF may be an important component in the pathogenesis of severe falciparum malaria, in particular in the cerebral syndrome and the hypoglycemia that can complicate this disease (33). This association between high serum levels and severity of falciparum infection was also noted in children from Gabon (Richard-Lenoble and Grau, in preparation) and Zaire (34). We found that plasma TNF concentrations were higher in 61 Zairian children with *P. falciparum* infection than in 26 severely ill, aparasitemic children ($p = 0.0003$). Among all parasitemic children, TNF levels increased with increasing levels of parasitemia ($p = 0.001$). On univariate analysis, elevated TNF levels were associated with hyperparasitemia, severe anemia, hypoglycemia, and young age but not with cerebral malaria, human immunodeficiency virus type 1 (HIV-1) seropositivity, or fatal outcome. In this series, however, mortality rate was low (7%). TNF levels were elevated equally in children with cerebral malaria and in those with other signs of severe malaria. With multiple linear regression, TNF levels were found to be elevated independently in children with hyperparasitemia ($p = 0.001$) and severe anemia ($p = 0.04$). From this study, we concluded that high TNF levels are associated with several manifestations of severe falciparum malaria and are not specific to cerebral malaria (34). In a series of European adults nonimmune to malaria (35), TNF (median 172 pg/ml, peak 896 pg/ml) and IL-6 (median 16 U/ml; peak 1000 U/ml) levels were markedly elevated in 18 patients with complicated clinical course. A highly significant correlation between serum TNF and IL-6 levels ($n = 40$, $p = 0.0002$) suggests coordinate production of these two cytokines. Thus, elevated serum levels of TNF, but also of IL-6, are associated with the occurrence of organ injury, in particular of cerebral malaria. Such a correlation was also observed in children from The Gambia (D. Kwiatkowski, personal communication).

One of the possible pathogenic links between TNF and the pathology of human CM is the potential role of this cytokine in the sequestration of parasitized erythrocytes (36), as previously hypothesized (37). Elegant studies by Berendt and colleagues demonstrated that intercellular adhesion molecule 1 (ICAM 1) is one of the molecules involved in cytoadherence of *P. falciparum*-infected erythrocytes, at least in vitro (38). Since TNF, among other cytokines, is known to upregulate the surface expression of (ICAM 1) on endothelial cells (39), it is likely that the markedly high TNF levels observed in patients with CM (33,35) lead to sequestration of parasitized erythrocytes via this pathway. Such a role for surface adhesion molecules is consistent with the recent finding that in vivo treatment with monoclonal antibodies directed against LFA1, the ligand of ICAM1, prevents murine CM (27).

Other Pathological Features of Severe Malaria

Several other pathological features of malaria depend upon an excessive release of TNF, as proposed earlier (40). Clark and colleagues injected recombinant human TNF into normal and *Plasmodium P vinckei*-infected mice with low levels of parasitemia (41): they observed that the latter develop, 4–12 h after TNF administration, a series of pathological changes that are characteristic of highly parasitized mice: increased plasma lactate level, liver midzonal necrosis, pulmonary lesions [an adult respiratory distress syndrome, ARDS-like pattern, characterized by accumulation of polymorphonuclear leukocytes, PMNs, in alveolar vessels, which is also seen in humans with falciparum infection (17)], and hypoglycemia [which is also seen in severe falciparum infection (33,42)]. In contrast, normal mice injected with the same amount of TNF had no such changes. The multiple aspects of malarial pathology are thus best understood if considered the result of a single cytokine with pleiomorphic activities.

In addition, TNF may also play an important role in malaria-induced abortion. High doses (50 μg) of recombinant human TNF do not affect normal pregnant mice, but small doses (1.5–5.0 μg) of this cytokine given intravenously caused fetal death and abortion in 16 day pregnant mice with low levels of *P. vinckei* parasitemia (43). Also, plasma TNF levels were elevated in malarial pregnant mice when, on day 17, parasitemia was high and the first signs of impending abortion were evident, but TNF was undetectable in plasma of low parasitemia animals, pregnant or not, and in the plasma of uninfected mice at day 17 of pregnancy. An important feature for this aspect of TNF toxicity appears to be the preexisting level of macrophage activation: it has indeed been shown that a small dose of TNF causes fetal death in 16 day pregnant mice that received an intravenous injection of *Coxiella burneti* extract 9–10 days earlier. Thus, TNF-induced abortion may occur in a range of infections in which systemic macrophage activation occurs and a trigger for TNF release is present (43).

Bone Marrow Changes: Anemia and Dyserythropoiesis

It has been proposed that TNF and other cytokines, such as IL-1 and IFN-α/β, are released during the acute phase of malaria infection and have a role in bone marrow depression (44). That TNF indeed makes an important contribution to the anemia in malaria has been demonstrated (45) in a study that showed that intravenous injection of recombinant human TNF into *P. vinckei*-infected mice leads to dramatic bone marrow changes: erythrophagocytosis, involving erythroblasts as well as mature red cells, and dyserythropoiesis, involving irregularly shaped nuclei and karyorrhexis. This has been confirmed in *P. berghei*-infected mice, which upon TNF infusion show a reduction in pluripotent stem cells in the bone marrow and a concomitant increase in the spleen, a reduction in erythroid progenitor cells, and a reduced incorporation of ^{59}Fe into erythrocytes. Furthermore, when *P. berghei*-infected mice were given an antiserum to recombinant murine TNF, erythropoiesis was partially restored (46,47). Whether TNF acts directly or indirectly to inhibit erythropoiesis deserves further study. Other bone marrow functions are known to be altered during malaria infection, such as granulopoiesis. It has been shown that lethal *P. berghei* infection is associated with a transient increase in production of colony-stimulating activity followed by a general recruitment of GM-CFCs in all hematopoietic organs (48). The respective roles of colony-stimulating factors and other cytokines in these granulocytic and macrophagic lineage changes remain to be clarified.

Hypergammaglobulinemia

Hypergammaglobulinemia is another aspect of malaria that involves cytokines, particularly IL-6, as suggested by recent observations in the murine model of CM (49). IL-6 is present in the serum of mice with *P. berghei* ANKA infection, the highest concentrations being observed in mice with full-blown neurological syndrome. High IL-6 levels were also observed, however, in the absence of pathology in nonlethal malaria infection. Our data suggest that IL-6 is produced in large amounts during malaria infection but does not play a major role in the pathogenesis of CM. A modulation of IL-6 production in CM was achieved by in vivo treatment with other anticytokine antibodies able to prevent CM: antibodies to IFN-γ or to TNF abolished the rise of IL-6, although anti-IL-3 and anti-GM-CSF antibodies only partially prevented this rise, suggesting that the two cytokines, TNF and IFN-γ, are important intermediates in IL-6 production. Passive immunization against IL-6 did not prevent CM but significantly reduced serum IgG levels in malaria-infected mice. Since anti-IL-6 monoclonal antibody (MAb) prevents hypergammaglobulinemia without reducing the antimalarial humoral response, one must hypothesize that cytokines other than IL-6 (such as IL-2 and IL-4) are more instrumental in specific antibody responses. Thus, IL-6 is possibly involved in malarially induced hypergammaglobulinemia and the associated complications, such as immune complex diseases and glomerulonephritis. In addition, overexpression of IL-6 has been suggested in the development of B cell lymphomas. In malaria, IL-6 production may contribute to the increased incidence of Burkitt's lymphomas, which have been associated with plasmodium infections in epidemiological studies. The significance of IL-6 production in malaria may thus go beyond the cerebral syndrome (49).

Fever

Serum TNF has been detected in falciparum-infected patients without CM (50), with particular attention to fever (51,52). Kwiatkowski and colleagues found that plasma levels of over 39 pg/ml are detected in 59% of Gambian children with acute malaria, 17% of convalescents, 9% of children with mild infections other than malaria, and 7% of healthy Gambian adults (53). In addition, TNF production was studied in vitro. Mononuclear cells from acute malaria patients, when stimulated with endotoxin in vitro, secreted twice as much TNF as did those of convalescent individuals and three times as much that of healthy adult controls. Also, *P. falciparum*-infected erythrocytes induced mononuclear cells from normal subjects to secrete TNF, and a sharp rise in the rate of secretion occurred shortly after schizont rupture. These data suggest that malaria fever is mediated, at least in part, through paroxysmal TNF release associated with schizont rupture (53). In Malawian children, blood levels of TNF and IFN-γ, but not of IL-1, were found to correlate with body temperature (27).

In view of the multiple roles of TNF in the pathology of malaria, it is of interest to determine which constituent of the parasite is responsible for the induction of TNF secretion. That plasmodium can induce TNF per se (i.e., in the absence of any contaminant endotoxin) has been demonstrated (4,54). Furthermore, soluble antigens released by malaria parasites appear to be major TNF inducers (54–57). These soluble antigens from rodent plasmodia are heat-stable molecules, distinguishable from lipopolysaccharide (LPS), that trigger TNF release in vitro and in vivo and that can kill mice made hypersensitive to TNF by D-galactosamine treatment. Medium from cultures of *P. falciparum* contain similar soluble antigens that induce TNF release from both human and mouse macrophages. Most importantly, these soluble antigens induce T cell-independent antibodies that specifically block their own ability, but not that of endotoxin, to cause the secretion of TNF. This work has two potentially very important practical consequences: first, murine macrophages, whether derived from the peritoneal cavity or from a cell line, can be used to screen potentially toxic human malaria antigens. Second, the mouse can be used not only to examine cross-reactions between toxic antigens and to study antigenic variation, but also to screen antigens in vaccination experiments as potential candidates for disease-preventing vaccines in humans. These data led Playfair and his colleagues to the concept of an antidisease vaccine (58).

PROTECTIVE ROLE OF CYTOKINES IN MALARIA

Cytokines and Blood Stages

Taverne and colleagues observed that when *Plasmodium yoelii*- or *P. berghei*-infected mice are given endotoxin, their serum contains mediators able to kill both species of parasites and tumor cells in vitro (59). This serum resembled "tumor necrosis serum" (TNS) obtained from mice given macrophage-activating agents, such as *Plasmodium acnes* or bacillus Calmette-Guerin (BCG) and then endotoxin (60). When recombinant cytokines became available, it was found than recombinant TNF is able to kill malaria parasites in vivo but not in vitro (61–63). It was found later that important components explaining the parasiticidal effect of TNS are lipid peroxidation products: when TNS was depleted of lipoproteins, no parasiticidal activity remained, and when it was separated by ultracentrifugation, more than 70% of the parasiticidal activity was found in the lipoprotein fraction (64). Other investigators have confirmed that administration of recombinant human TNF protects mice against blood stage malaria of *Plasmodium chabaudi* (65,66). Thus, the protective effect of TNF in malaria is indirect: this cytokine certainly enhances resistance to malaria in vivo but is not cytotoxic to the intraerythrocytic parasites in vitro. It has been hypothesized that nonspecific macrophage activation could be involved (67). Alternatively, it has recently been shown that TNF is able to activate neutrophils to kill *P. falciparum* in vitro (68).

These data could explain the discrepancy between in vitro and in vivo effects of TNF on erythrocytic stages of malaria.

In human malaria as well, a recent study suggests a possible protective role for TNF. In a longitudinal survey of 84 subjects living in an endemic area of malaria, the plasma TNF was found at its highest level during the malaria transmission peak and became normal again during the dry season. Children having suffered from malarial attack keep low TNF levels compared to adults and asymptomatic children. These results suggest that TNF could be associated with development of resistance against malaria (69).

Cytokines other than TNF can play an important role in the defense against malaria. Interferon has long been recognized to have antiparasitic effects on different stages of development of *P. berghei* (70). This protective effect was further demonstrated by in vivo administration of antiserum directed against interferon (71). However, in lethal *P. berghei* ANKA infection, monoclonal antibodies to recombinant murine IFN-γ had no effect on the course of parasitemia, but prevented TNF overproduction and CM (14). In the human, elevated levels of α [6] and γ (8,10) interferons have been described during *P. falciparum* infection. When recombinant molecules became available, it was shown that IFN-γ is able to induce crisis forms in *P. falciparum* cultures and that parasite killing correlated with the magnitude of the oxidative response (72). The major role played by IFN-γ in the defense against malaria was then demonstrated in vivo by suppressing *P. chabaudi adami* infection upon daily administration of recombinant murine IFN-γ (65). Using another model, Shear and colleagues were able to correlate endogenous IFN-γ production and resistance to malaria (73). When comparing susceptible and resistant murine hosts infected with lethal and nonlethal variants of *P. yoelii*, they found that resistant mice developed a burst of IFN-γ production in response to both types of parasites, whereas susceptible mice responded only to the nonlethal variant. Again, in these conditions, the kinetics of H_2O_2 response corresponded to that of IFN-γ. In addition, in vivo administration of recombinant murine IFN-γ resulted in a dose-dependent protection of mice from the lethal variant but had no significant effect on the course of the infection induced by the nonlethal *P. yoelii.* Other studies of frequencies of IFN-γ-producing cell precursors confirmed the view that IFN-γ plays an important role in the development of protective immunity against blood stages of malaria (74,75).

In the human, a possible protective role of IFN-γ is suggested by previous studies that showed that lymphocytes from malaria-immune subjects produce IFN-γ when stimulated by malarial antigens (mAg), in contrast to lymphocytes from subjects without previous exposure to malaria (76–78). This has been interpreted as evidence for antibody-independent cellular immunity (78). More recently, mAg antigen-induced IFN-γ production has been further studied with particular attention to the history of exposure to malaria (79). We found that although lymphocytes from subjects with single or few past malaria infections were able to produce high levels of IFN-γ in response to mAg, lymphocytes from adult native residents exposed since birth to malaria infection demonstrated poor proliferation and IFN-γ production. The low response in these subjects was mAg specific, since mitogens induced high levels of IFN-γ in all subjects tested. These observations raise questions about the relation between clinical immunity to malaria and IFN-γ production in vitro. Results from studies on purified $CD4^+$ and

$CD8^+$ T lymphocyte subsets indicated that the IFN-γ was produced by $CD4^+$ T cells and argued against a suppression by $CD8^+$ cells (79). An intrinsic defect of mAg-specific $CD4^+$ T cells appears to be the most likely explanation for these findings, but the precise mechanism(s) involved in low IFN-γ production remains to be defined. Interestingly, $CD4^+$ T cells from immune subjects with high proliferative responses produced lower amounts of IFN-γ than did $CD4^+$ T cells from nonimmune individuals with similar proliferative responses. If one draws a parallel between human and mouse $CD4^+$ T cells functionally subdivided into "inflammatory" Th1 and "helper" Th2 subsets, one may hypothesize that differences in the $CD4^+$ subset activated by mAg in immune versus nonimmune subjects could partially explain these findings. Also, it is tempting to speculate that IFN-γ production in the human could have adverse rather than beneficial effects: a reduced IFN-γ production could be beneficial to avoid or decrease immunopathological reactions, particularly TNF overproduction, as discussed for the experimental model of CM (14). However, low responses reflecting an impairment of the immune system would explain the difficulty in reaching sterile immunity in *P. falciparum* infection.

Last, IL-1 appears to be another potent cytokine with antimalarial effect. Curfs and colleagues recently showed that administration of recombinant human IL-1 daily from days 0 to 5 of infection reduced parasitemia and hence the cerebral syndrome in *P. berghei berghei*-infected C57BL mice (80).

Cytokines in Preerythrocytic Stages

After infatuation with antibodies, the current trend is now to attribute an essential role to cellular mechanisms in protection against the preerythrocytic stage. A number of cytokines interfere with the plasmodium during its hepatic course, both directly and/or in the context of complex cytokine interactions, with the participation of various cells including the hepatocyte itself.

It has been shown that several interferon inducers, such as Newcastle disease virus, protect mice against *P.* berghei infection and that this protection is far greater against sporozoite-induced infections than against the blood form-induced infection (81). Administration of mouse or rat IFN-γ a few hours before sporozoite challenge inhibited in a dose-dependent manner the development of exoerythrocytic forms in the liver of mice and rats infected with *P. berghei* sporozoites. The effect was less pronounced if IFN-γ was given 18 h before or a few hours after sporozoites (82). Similarly, human IFN-γ diminished the parasitemia in chimpanzees infected with *P.* falciparum sporozoites. These observations suggested that immunologically induced IFN-γ may be involved in controlling malarial infection under natural conditions. The mechanisms of action of IFN-γ were analyzed *in vitro*. Using the highly differentiated human hepatoma cell line HepG2, it was found that IFN-γ acts directly on the hepatocyte and exerts its antimalarial activity by binding to surface receptors on hepatocytes (approximately 44,000 per cell) and inducing intracellular changes unfavorable for parasite development (83). The same results were obtained using fresh human hepatocytes infected with *P. falciparum* sporozoites (84). The critical role of IFN-γ in protective immunity to irradiated sporozoites was demonstrated by further experiments in immune mice. Treatment with antimurine IFN-γ monoclonal antibody or depletion of $CD8^+$ T cells both reversed sterile immunity to sporozoite challenge by allowing the growth of exoerythrocytic forms and thus the development of parasitemia. Adoptive transfer experiments also showed that immunity to sporozoite challenge requires the neutralization of sporozoites by antibodies and the inhibition of exoerythrocytic form development by IFN-γ with the participation of $CD8^+$ T cells (85). The inhibitory effect of IFN-γ was also reported in a simian model: prophylactic treatment with recombinant human IFN-γ completely suppressed infection of rhesus monkeys with *Plasmodium cynomolgi* sporozoites but, again, had no effect on trophozoite-induced infection (86). As discussed, IFN-γ secretion can be induced not only by the sporozoite stage but also by erythrocytic stages: longitudinal studies indicate that circulating IFN-γ is present several days after human infestation. Endogenous IFN-γ production may therefore be important in protecting against malarial reinfection during the months following an acute attack, when serum IFN-γ is present. Moreover, it should be emphasized that IFN-γ has not only a parasitostatic effect but probably also a postassembly mode of action since addition of IFN-γ to developed liver stages induces lysis of a significant number of plasmodia (84). This result may have some relevance to cytotoxicity against liver stages of malaria parasites.

As previously pointed out, recombinant human or mouse interleukin-1 α (IL-1) protects against the preerythrocytic stages of *P. falciparum* malaria (84). It has been postulated that this effect of IL-1 may be mediated in part by the C-reactive protein (CRP), an acute-phase protein synthetized by IL-1-stimulated hepatocytes. Evidence for this was obtained with both in vitro and in vivo models of *P.* yoelii infection (87,88). It was recently demonstrated that hepatic IL-1 activity is mediated by secretion of IL-6 in the liver (89). We now have evidence that the effect of IL-1 on the hepatic development of *P. falciparum* or *P. yoelii* sporozoites is in part mediated by IL-6 activity, since anti-IL-6 antibodies neutralize the effect of IL-1 (Pied et al., in preparation). However, in addition to an effect on the release of acute-phase reactants, IL-6 has a direct effect on sporozoite penetration and development. As IL-6 has been found to be produced in large amounts during erythrocytic phase of malaria infection (49), this cytokine may play a role in the resistance to further challenge with sporozoites.

The effects of TNF on preerythrocytic forms of malaria have also been studied. Although a previous report indicates that TNF efficiently reduced the development of *P. berghei* in Hep G2 hepatoma cell line (90), our data using fresh hepatocytes did not provide evidence for an effect of this cytokine at the hepatocyte level, whatever the dose and the schedule of administration and whatever the strain of mice. We found nonetheless that in vivo administration of TNF prevents the appearance of *P. yoelii* erythrocytic stages. We recently attempted to clarify the role, at the hepatic level, of TNF on sporozoite-induced malaria. To this end we addressed the reasons for the discrepancies between data obtained using hepatoma cell lines and fresh hepatocytes, on the one hand, and between in vivo and in vitro results, on the other hand.

That TNF induces different acute-phase proteins (APPs) in tumor cell lines and in normal rat hepatocytes (91,92) may explain the differences observed in these two experimental models. Indeed, APP secreted after cytokine stimulation were shown to inhibit parasite development in vitro and in vivo (87,88). Since TNF clearly protects in vivo but has no effect on hepatocytes in vitro, we questioned the relevance of our in vitro hepatocyte model.

It was found that a crucial element in the effect of TNF is the presence of nonparenchymal cells (NPC). The addition of NPC to hepatocytes indeed restored the capacity of TNF to modulate parasite hepatic stage development in vitro. In our coculture assay, NPCs essentially consist of pit cells (large granular lymphocytes or natural killer cells), Kupffers cells, T cells, endothelial cells, epithelial cells, fibroblasts, and Ito cells. Some of these cells are known to produce various cytokines, such as IL-1, IFN-γ, and IL-6 (93,94), whose inhibitory effects on the hepatic stages have been established (84,95) (Pied et al., in preparation).

In this coculture model, supernatants were found to contain markedly elevated IL-6 concentrations upon addition of TNF, whereas IL-1 and IFN-γ remained undetectable. To confirm that IL-6 was involved in the TNF-induced parasite inhibition, anti-IL-6 MAb was added to mono- and cocultures of hepatocytes. Anti-IL-6 MAb dramatically decreased the TNF-induced inhibition when added 24 h before sporozoite inoculation (96). These results strongly suggest that IL-6 is a crucial mediator in the observed TNF effect. In addition, TNF has been demonstrated to be involved in the L-arginine-dependent cytotoxic effector mechanisms in macrophages (97). The potential participation of this metabolic pathway in the parasiticidal effect induced by TNF is under current investigation.

The production of various cytokines, particularly IFN-γ, TNF, and IL-6, whose production is increased during blood stage malaria (9,33,35,49,75,98), may thus modulate the preerythrocytic stage of the infection. Taken together, these data further illustrate the interdependence of different stages of development of malaria parasites.

Cytokines and Sexual Stages

The relationship between cytokine release and gametocyte production had not been studied until recently. Particular attention was paid to the period of transient loss of infectivity of the parasite to the mosquitoes. Infectivity of malarial infections to mosquitoes is due to the presence of circulating gametocytes, the sexual stages, which fertilize in the midgut of a blood-fed mosquito. In several malaria host-parasite systems, it has been noted that peaks of parasitemia are associated with "crisis," characterized by the appearance of morphologically abnormal intraerythrocytic parasites. This peculiar event is synchronous with the reduction or loss of infectivity of the parasite to the mosquito, which persists for 4–6 days. Neither of these phenomena has been explained.

In the model of *P. cynomolgi* infection in its natural host, the toque monkey (*Macaca sinica*), it was recently shown by Mendis and colleagues that the loss of infectivity at crisis is due to the death of circulating intraerythrocytic gametocytes mediated by crisis serum (99). In addition, we showed that this killing effect in the crisis serum is due to the presence of both TNF and IFN-γ. Indeed, simultaneous addition of rabbit antihuman TNF and antihuman IFN-γ-immunoglobulins completely reversed the killing effect of the crisis serum observed in vitro. In contrast, the addition of antibodies to either cytokine alone or normal rabbit immunoglobulin had no effect. Conversely, the effects of recombinant human

TNF and IFN-γ were assessed on the viability of healthy infectious gametocytes of *P. cynomolgi* in vitro. Neither cytokine when tested individually, nor a combination of both cytokines, affected the infectivity of the gametocytes to mosquitoes. However, when either cytokine was added to crisis serum previously depleted of TNF and IFN-γ, the killing effect of the crisis serum was totally restored. These results indicate that TNF and IFN-γ each mediate gametocyte killing independently of the other, but they demonstrate that each cytokine requires the presence of an unknown factor in the crisis serum to mediate this effect.

Further evidence for a role of TNF in gametocyte killing was recently obtained. When studying *Plasmodium vivax*-infected subjects, we found that soon after a paroxysm (an episode of fever with chills and rigors that coincides with the rupture of erythrocytic schizonts), the serum of malaria-nonimmune patients mediated killing of blood stage parasites (asexual erythrocytic stages and gametocytes). These sera taken 1 h after paroxysm contained elevated TNF concentrations. This in vitro killing effect of human paroxysm sera was completely abrogated by the addition of anti-TNF antibodies and was restored by the addition of recombinant human TNF. When added to normal serum, however, recombinant TNF had no parasite killing effects, indicating, as we found for monkey crisis serum, that a complementary factor(s) present in paroxysm serum, but not in normal serum, was necessary for TNF to kill blood stage parasites.

The elevated serum TNF levels and gametocyte-killing effects of human serum taken 1 h after paroxysm were transient: 4 h following a paroxysm, serum TNF levels had fallen in most patients and the loss of killing effect was dramatic in all patients. Even when recombinant TNF was added to serum taken 4 h after a paroxysm, it failed to kill gametocytes, demonstrating the very transient presence of complementary factor(s) needed for cytokine-mediated killing of blood stage parasites (100). Our observation of parasite killing effects in human paroxysm serum was done in nonimmune individuals with no previous history of malaria, who contracted the disease on a visit to an endemic region in Sri Lanka. These individuals had no clinical immunity and consequently suffered severe clinical symptoms. In contrast, semiimmune individuals resident in a malaria-endemic region of Sri Lanka, who experienced relatively mild symptoms during an infection, had low serum TNF levels and hardly any parasite killing effect in serum. These observations corroborate the view that cytokines, including complementary factor(s), may mediate the clinical symptoms of malaria.

CONCLUSIONS

During malarial infection, it appears that immunopathological reactions, in addition to complement-induced disease processes and disorders caused by immune complexes, also manifest themselves via the excessive release of cytokines. Alternatively, cytokines are actively involved in the defense mechanisms against malaria infection. The exceedingly complex picture of malaria therefore illustrates the duality of effects of cytokines, particularly TNF. The data presented here outline the importance of a balance in the cytokine network to achieve protective immunity: eventual effects will depend on the amount of cytokine released and the rate, time, and site of production. Since cytokines are harmful only when produced in inappropriately high amounts and during limited periods of time [as observed in human CM (49)], they may represent a target for therapeutic intervention. Within the network of cytokines there are probably many opportunities for therapeutic intervention. As stated recently (101), new approaches in the treatment of severe falciparum malaria, particularly CM, are needed. The data discussed here highlight the desirability to develop potent and clinically compatible antagonists of cytokines. The main cytokine that should be neutralized, in view of its potent cytotoxic effect, is TNF. Neutralization of this cytokine, or its receptor, when technically feasible, is one of the possible therapeutic approaches in acute complications of various infectious diseases, including severe malaria. In view of the correlation between serum TNF concentrations and severity in human CM (25), administration of monoclonal anti-TNF antibodies should be considered in addition to conventional treatment of severe falciparum malaria.

REFERENCES

1. Maegraith B. Pathological processes in malaria and blackwater fever. Oxford: Blackwell, 1948.
2. Maegraith B, Fletcher A. The pathogenesis of mammalian malaria. Adv Parasitol 1972; 10:49–72.
3. Maegraith B. Other pathological processes in malaria. Bull WHO 1974; 50:193–7.
4. Hotez PJ, LeTrang N, Fairlamb AH, Cerami A. Lipoprotein lipase suppression in 3T3-L1 cells by a haemoprotozoan-induced mediator from peritoneal exudate cells. Parasite Immunol 1984; 6:303–9.
5. Playfair JHL, Taverne J. Antiparasitic effects of tumor necrosis factor in vivo and in vitro. Ciba Found Symp 1987; 131:192–205.
6. Ojo Amaize EA, Salimonu LS, Williams AI, et al. Positive correlation between degree of parasitemia, interferon titers, and natural killer cell activity in *Plasmodium falciparum*-infected children. J Immunol 1981; 127:2296–2300.
7. Fribourg Blanc A, Druilhe P, Brasseur P, Rhodes Feuillette A, Tharavanij S. Immunological evaluation of cell-mediated and humoral immunity in Thai patients with cerebral and non cerebral *Plasmodium falciparum* malaria. II. Evolution of serum levels of immunoglobulins, antimalarial antibodies, complement fractions and alpha interferon. Southeast Asian J Trop Med Public Health 1985; 16:307–13.
8. Druilhe P, Rhodes Feuillette A, Canivet M, Boulland P, Peries J, Gentilini M. Production of circulating interferon in human malaria. Bull Soc Pathol Exot Filiales 1983; 76:34–42.
9. Rhodes Feuillette A, Jaureguiberry G, Ballet JJ, et al. The interfern compartment of the immune response in human malaria. I. Interferon inducers in *Plasmodium falciparum* cultures. J Interferon Res 1985; 5:159–68.
10. Rhodes Feuillette A, Bellosguardo M, Druilhe P, et al. The interferon compartment of the immune response in human malaria. II. Presence of serum interferon gamma following the acute attack. J Interferon Res 1985; 5:169–78.
11. Greenwood BM, Bradley AK, Greenwood AM, et al. Mortality and morbidity from malaria among children in a rural area of the Gambia, West Africa. Trans R Soc Trop Med Hyg 1987; 81:478–86.
12. Grau GE, Fajardo LF, Piguet PF, Allet B, Lambert PH, Vassalli P. Tumor necrosis factor (cachectin) as an essential mediator in murine cerebral malaria. Science 1987; 237:1210–2.
13. Grau GE, Kindler V, Piguet PF, Lambert PH, Vassalli P. Prevention of experimental

cerebral malaria by anticytokine antibodies. IL-3 and GM-CSF are intermediates in increased TNF production and macrophage accumulation. J Exp Med 1988; 168:1499–504.

14. Grau GE, Heremans H, Piguet PF, et al. Monoclonal antibody against interferon-gamma can prevent experimental cerebral malaria and its associated overproduction of tumor necrosis factor. Proc Natl Acad Sci U S A 1989; 86:5572–4.
15. Grau GE, Piguet PF, Engers HD, Louis JA, Vassalli P, Lambert PH. L3T4$^+$ T lymphocytes play a major role in the pathogenesis of murine cerebral malaria. J Immunol 1986; 137:2348–54.
16. Lambert PH, Grau GE. Cerebral malaria. In: McAdam KPWJ, ed. New strategies in parasitology. Frontiers in infectious diseases. Edinburgh: Churchill Livingstone, 1989:51–73.
17. Duarte MIS, Corbett CEP, Boulos M, Amto Neto V. Ultrastructure of the lung in falciparum malaria. Am J Trop Med Hyg 1985; 34:31–5.
18. Clark IA. Monokines and lymphokines in malarial pathology. Ann Trop Med Parasitol 1987; 577–85.
19. Beutler B, Cerami A. Cachectin: more than a tumor necrosis factor. N Engl J Med 1987; 316:379–85.
20. Tracey KJ, Beutler B, Lowry SF, et al. Shock and tissue injury induced by recombinant human cachectin. Science 1986; 234:470–4.
21. Beutler B, Milsark IW, Cerami AC. Passive Immunization against cachectin/tumor necrosis factor protects mice from lethal effect of endotoxin. Science 1985; 229:869–71.
22. Tracey KJ, Fong Y, Hesse DG, et al. Anticachectin/TNF monoclonal antibodies prevent septic shock during lethal bacteraemia. Nature 1987; 330:662–4.
23. Pober JS. Warner-Lambert/Parke-Davis award lecture. Cytokine-mediated activation of vascular endothelium. Physiology and pathology. Am J Pathol 1988; 133:426–33.
24. Cotran RS, Pober JS. Effects of cytokines on vascular endothelium: their role in vascular and immune injury. Kidney Int 1989; 35:969–75.
25. Grau GE, Piguet PF, Vassalli P, Lambert PH. Tumor necrosis factor and other cytokines in cerebral malaria: experimental and clinical data. Immunol Rev 1989; 112:49–70.
26. Kindler V, Sappino AP, Grau GE, Piguet PF, Vassalli P. The inducing role of tumor necrosis factor in the development of bactericidal granulomas during BCG infection. Cell 1989; 56:731–40.
27. Grau GE, Bieler G, Pointaire P, et al. Significance of cytokine production and adhesion molecules in malarial immunopathology. Immunol Lett 1990; in press.
28. MacPherson GG, Warrell MJ, White NJ, Looareesuwan S, Warrell DA. Human cerebral malaria. A quantitative ultrastructural analysis of parasitized erythrocyte sequestration. Am J Pathol 1985; 119:385–401.
29. Piguet PF, Grau GE, Allet B, Vassalli P. Tumor necrosis factor is an effector of skin and gut lesions of the acute phase of graft-versus-host disease. J Exp Med 1987; 166:1280–9.
30. Piguet PF, Grau GE, Collart MA, Vassalli P, Kapanci Y. Pneumopathies of the graft-versus-host reaction. Lab Invest 1989; 61:37–45.
31. Piguet PF, Collart MA, Grau GE, Kapanci Y, Vassalli P. Tumor necrosis factor cachectin plays a key role in bleomycin-induced pneumopathy and fibrosis. J Exp Med 1989; 170:655–63.
32. Piguet PF, Collart MA, Grau GE, Sappino AP, Vassalli P. Requirement of tumour necrosis factor for development of silica-induced pulmonary fibrosis. Nature 1990; 344:245–7.

33. Grau GE, Taylor TE, Molyneux ME, et al. Tumor necrosis factor and disease severity in children with falciparum malaria. N Engl J Med 1989; 320:1586–91.
34. Schaffer N, Grau GE, Hedberg K, et al. Tumor necrosis factor and severe malaria. J Infect Dis 1991; 163:96–101.
35. Kern P, Hemmer CJ, Vandamme J, Gruss HJ, Dietrich M. Elevated tumor necrosis factor-alpha and interleukin-6 serum levels as markers for complicated *Plasmodium falciparum* malaria. Am J Med 1989; 87:139–43.
36. Miller LH. Malaria—binding of infected red cells. Nature 1989; 341:18–18.
37. Grau GE, Piguet PF, Vassalli P, Lambert PH. Involvement of tumour necrosis factor and other cytokines in immune-mediated vascular pathology. Int Arch Allergy Appl Immunol 1989; 88:34–9.
38. Berendt AR, Simmons DL, Tansey J, Newbold CI, Marsh K. Intercellular adhesion molecule-1 is an endothelial cell adhesion receptor for *Plasmodium falciparum*. Nature 1989; 341:57–9.
39. Rothlein R, Czajkowski M, O'Neill MM, Marlin SD, Mainolfi E, Merluzzi VJ. Induction of intercellular adhesion molecule 1 on primary and continuous cell lines by proinflammatory cytokines. J Immunol 1988; 137:245–50.
40. Clark IA. Suggested importance of monokines in pathophysiology of endotoxin shock and malaria. Klin Wochenschr 1982; 60:756–8.
41. Clark IA, Cowden WB, Butcher GA, Hunt NH. Possible roles of tumor necrosis factor in the pathology of malaria. Am J Pathol 1987; 129:192–9.
42. Taylor TE, Molyneux ME, Wirima JJ, Fletcher KA, Morris K. Blood glucose levels in Malawian children before and during the administration of intravenous quinine for severe falciparum malaria. N Engl J Med 1988; 319:1040–7.
43. Clark IA, Chaudhri G. Tumor necrosis factor in malaria-induced abortion. Am J Trop Med Hyg 1988; 39:246–9.
44. Clark IA, Virelizier JL, Carswell EA, Wood PR. Possible importance of macrophage-derived mediators in acute malaria. Infect Immun 1981; 32:1058–66.
45. Clark IA, Chaudhri G. Tumour necrosis factor may contribute to the anaemia of malaria by causing dyserythropoiesis and erythrophagocytosis. Br J Haematol 1988; 70:99–103.
46. Miller KL, Silverman PH, Kullgren B, Mahlmann LJ. Tumor necrosis factor alpha and the anemia associated with murine malaria. Infect Immun 1989; 57:1542–6.
47. Miller KL, Schooley JC, Smith KL, Kullgren B, Mahlmann LJ, Silverman PH. Inhibition of erythropoiesis by a soluble factor in murine malaria. Exp Hematol 1989; 17:379–85.
48. Mungyer G, Poels LG, Jerusalem C, Jerusalem P. *Plasmosdium berghei*: influence on granulopoiesis and macrophage production in BALB/c mice. Exp Parasitol 1983; 56:266–76.
49. Grau GE, Frei K, Piguet PF, et al. Interleukin 6 production in experimental cerebral malaria. Modulation by anti-cytokine antibodies and possible role in hypergammaglobulinemia. J Exp Med 1990; 172:1505–1508.
50. Scuderi P, Lam KS, Ryan KJ, et al. Raised serum levels of tumor necrosis factor in parasitic infections. Lancet 1986; 2:1364–5.
51. Van der Meer JWM, Endres S, Lonnemann G, et al. Concentrations of immunoreactive human tumor necrosis factor alpha produced by human mononuclear cells in vitro. J Leukoc Biol 1988; 43:216–23.
52. Kwiatkowski D. Febrile temperatures can synchronize the growth of *Plasmodium falciparum* in vitro. J Exp Med 1989; 169:357–61.
53. Kwiatkowski D, Cannon JG, Manogue KR, Cerami A, Dinarello CA, Greenwood BM. Tumour necrosis factor production in falciparum malaria and its association with schizont rupture. Clin Exp Immunol 1989; 77:361–6.

54. Bate CA, Taverne J, Playfair JH. Malarial parasites induce TNF production by macrophages. Immunology 1988; 64:227–31.
55. Bate CAW, Taverne J, Playfair JHL. Soluble malarial antigens are toxic and induce the production of tumour necrosis factor in vivo. Immunology 1989; 66:600–5.
56. Taverne J, Bate CAW, Playfair JHL. Induction of TNF in vitro as a model for the identification of toxic malaria antigens. Lymphokine Res 1989; 8:317–22.
57. Taverne J, Bate CAW, Sarkar DA, Meager A, Rook GAW, Playfair JHL. Human and murine macrophages produce TNF in response to soluble antigens of *Plasmodium falciparum*. Parasite Immunol 1990; 12:33–43.
58. Playfair JHL, Taverne J, Bate CAW, Desouza JB. The malaria vaccine—anti-parasite or anti-disease. Immunol Today 1990; 11:25–7.
59. Taverne J, Depledge P, Playfair JH. Differential sensitivity in vivo of lethal and nonlethal malarial parasites to endotoxin-induced serum factor. Infect Immun 1982; 37:927–34.
60. Carswell EA, Old LJ, Kassel RL, Green S, Fiore N, Williamson B. An endotoxin-induced serum factor that causes necrosis of tumors. Proc Natl Acad Sci U S A 1975; 72:3666–70.
61. Taverne J, Tavernier J, Fiers W, Playfair JHL. Recombinant tumor necrosis factor inhibits malaria parasites in vivo but not in vitro. Clin Exp Immunol 1987; 67:1–4.
62. Jensen JB, Vande Waa JA, Karadesh AJ. Tumor necrosis factor does not induce *Plasmodium falciparum* crisis forms. Infect Immun 1987; 55:1722–4.
63. Hviid L, Reimert CM, Theander TG, Jepsen S, Bendtzen K. Recombinant human tumor necrosis factor is not inhibitory to *Plasmodium falciparum* in vitro. Trans R Soc Trop Med Hyg 1988; 82:48–9.
64. Rockett KA, Targett GA, Playfair JHL. Killing of blood-stage *Plasmodium falciparum* by lipid peroxides from tumor necrosis serum. Infect Immun 1988; 56:3180–3.
65. Clark IA, Hunt NH, Butcher GA, Cowden WB. Inhibition of murine malaria (*Plasmodium chabaudi*) in vivo by recombinant interferon-gamma or tumor necrosis factor, and its enhancement by butylated hydroxyanisole. J Immunl 1987; 139:3493–6.
66. Stevenson MM, Ghadirian E. Human recombinant tumor necrosis factor alpha protects susceptible A/J mice against lethal *Plasmodium chabaudi* as infection. Infect Immun 1989; 57:3936–9.
67. Ockenhouse CF, Shear HL. Malaria-induced lymphokines: stimulation of macrophages for enhanced phagocytosis. Infect Immun 1983; 42:733–9.
68. Kumaratilake LM, Ferrante A, Rzepczyk CM. Tumor necrosis factor enhances neutrophil-mediated killing of *Plasmodium falciparum*. Infect Immun 1990; 58:788–93.
69. Peyron F, Vuillez JP, Barbe G, et al. Plasma levels of tumor necrosis factor during a longitudinal survey in an endemic area of malaria. Acta Trop (Basel) 1990; 47:47–51.
70. Jahiel RI, Nussenweig RS, Vanderberg J, Vilcek J. Antimalaria effect of interferon inducers at different stages of development of *Plasmodium berghei* in the mouse. Nature 1968; 220:710–2.
71. Sauvager F, Fauconnier B. The protective effect of endogenous interferon in mouse malaria, as demonstrated by the use of anti-interferon globulins. Biomedicine 1978; 29:184–7.
72. Ockenhouse CF, Schulman S, Shear HL. Induction of crisis forms in the human malaria parasite *Plasmodium falciparum* by gamma-interferon-activated monocyte-derived macrophages. J Immunol 1984; 133:1601–8.
73. Shear HL, Srinivasan R, Nolan T, Ng C. Role of IFN-gamma in lethal and nonlethal malaria in susceptible and resistant murine hosts. J Immunol 1989; 143:2038–44.

74. Langhorne J, Simon B. Limiting dilution analysis of the T-cell response to *Plasmodium chabaudi chabaudi* in mice. Parasite Immunol 1989; 11:545–59.
75. Langhorne J, Meding SJ, Eichmann K, Gillard SS. The response of CD4$^+$ T-cells to *Plasmodium chabaudi chabaudi*. Immunol Rev 1989; 112:71–94.
76. Troye Blomberg M, Andersson G, Stoczkowska M, et al. Production of IL 2 and IFN-gamma by T cells from malaria patients in response to *Plasmodium falciparum* or erythrocyte antigens in vitro. J Immunol 1985; 135:3498–504.
77. Riley EM, Jepsen S, Andersson G, Otoo LN, Greenwood BM. Cell-mediated immune responses to *Plasmodium falciparum* antigens in adult Gambians. Clin Exp Immunol 1988; 71:377–82.
78. Kabilan L, Troye Blomberg M, Perlmann H, et al. T-cell epitopes in Pf155/RESA, a major candidate for a *Plasmodium falciparum* malaria vaccine. Proc Natl Acad Sci U S A 1988; 85:5659–63.
79. Chizzolini C, Grau GE, Geinoz A, Schrijvers D. lymphocyte-T interferon-gamma production induced by *Plasmodium falciparum* antigen is high in recently infected non-immune and low in immune subjects. Clin Exp Immunol 1990; 79:95–9.
80. Curfs JHAJ, Van der Meer JWM, Sauerwein R, Eling WMC. Low dose interleukin 1 protects mice from lethal cerebral malaria (abstract). 4th European Congress of Clinical Microbiology 1990.
81. Jahiel RI, Vilcek J, Nussenweig RS. Exogenous interferon protects mice against *Plasmodium berghei* malaria. Nature 1970; 227:1350–1.
82. Ferreira A, Schofield L, Enea V, et al. Inhibition of development of exoerythrocytic forms of malaria parasites of gamma-interferon. Science 1986; 232:881–4.
83. Schofield L, Ferreira A, Altszuler R, Nussenzweig V, Nussenzweig RS. Interferon-gamma inhibits the intrahepatocytic development of malaria parasites in vitro. J Immunol 1987; 139:2020–5.
84. Mellouk S, Maheshwari RK, Rhodes-Feuillette A, et al. Inhibitory activity of interferons and interleukin 1 on the development of *Plasmodium falciparum* in human hepatocyte cultures. J Immunol 1987; 139:4192–5.
85. Schofield L, Villaquiran J, Ferreira A, Schellekens H, Nussenzweig R, Nussenzweig V. Gamma interferon, CD8$^+$ T cells and antibodies required for immunity to malaria sporozoites. Nature 1987; 330:664–6.
86. Mahehswari RK, Czarniecki CW, Dutta GP, Puri SK, Dhawan BN, Friedman RM. Recombinant human gamma-interferon inhibits simian malaria. Infect Immun 1986; 53:628–30.
87. Pied S, Nussler A, Pontet M, et al. C-reactive protein protects against pre-erythrocytic stages of malaria. Infect Immun 1989; 57:278–82.
88. Nussier A, Pied S, Pontet M, et al. Inflammatory status and the pre-erythrocytic stages of malaria. Role of the C-reactive protein. Exp Parasitol 1990; in press.
89. Helle M, Brakenhoff JP, De Groot ER, Aarden LA. Interleukin 6 is involved in interleukin 1 induced activities. Eur J Immunol 1988; 18:957–9.
90. Schofield L, Nussenzweig RS, Nussenzweig V. CD8$^+$ T-cells and gamma-interferon required for immunity to sporozoite challenge. Report of the tenth meeting of the scientific working group on the immunology of Malaria. Geneva: WHO 1988: 17–9.
91. Andus T, Heinrich PC, Bauer J, et al. Discrimination of hepatocyte-stimulating activity from human recombinant tumor necrosis factor alpha. Eur J Immunol 1987; 17:1193–7.
92. Perlmutter DH, Dinarello CA, Punsel PI, Colten HR. Cachectin/tumor necrosis factor regulates hepatic acute-phase gene expression. J Clin Invest 1986; 78:1378.
93. Lotze M, Jirik F, Kabouridis P, et al. B cell stimulating factor 2/interleukin 6 is a costimulant for human thymocytes and T lymphocytes. J Exp Med 1988; 167:1253.

94. Katz Y, Strunk RC. Similarities and differences in stimulation of expression of alternative pathway of complement and IFN-beta2/IL-6 genes in human fibroblasts. J Immunol 1989; 142:3862–7.
95. Mazier D, Goma J, Pied S, et al. Hepatic phase of malaria. A crucial role as "go-between" with other stages. In: Pre-erythrocytic stage malaria vaccine development: current status and future prospects. Bulletin of the World Health Organization 1990, in press.
96. Nussier A, Goma J, Miltgen F, et al. TNF inhibits malaria hepatic stages via IL-6 liver synthesis. Submitted 1990.
97. Drapier JC, Wietzerbin J, Hibbs JB. Interferon gamma and tumor necrosis factor induce the L-arginine-dependent cytotoxic effector mechanism in murine macrophages. Eur J Immunol 1988; 18:1587–92.
98. Kwiatkowski D, et al. Immunol Lett 1990, in press.
99. Naotunne TDS, Karunaweera ND, DelGiudice G, et al. Malaria infection crisis: sexual parasites killed by cytokines and complementary factors. Submitted 1990.
100. Mendis KN, Naotune TDS, Karunaweera N, DelGiudice G, Grau GE, Carter R. Anti-parasite effects of cytokines in malaria. Immunol Lett 1990 in press.
101. Wyler DJ. Steroids are out in the treatment of cerebral malaria: what's next. J Infect Dis 1988; 158:320–4.

CHAPTER 13

THE BENEFICIAL ROLE OF CYTOKINES, PARTICULARLY INTERLEUKIN-1, IN THE HOST RESPONSE TO INJURY, INFECTION, AND INFLAMMATION

Lyle L. Moldawer

Cornell University Medical Center
New York, New York

METABOLIC RESPONSE TO INFECTION AND INJURY A BENEFICIAL HOST RESPONSE

Recent studies have emphasized the dual nature of cytokines in the physiological and pathophysiological responses to inflammation (1–3). Other chapters of this book deal extensively with the role of cytokines, particularly interleukin-1 (IL-1), tumor necrosis factor α (TNF-α), and IL-6, in the pathogenesis of a variety of specific disease processes. Yet the role that cytokines play in the normal host response to bacterial and viral infections, injury, and even neoplasia is often overlooked.

This review focuses principally on the metabolic response to inflammatory disease that has been defined historically as nonspecific host responses, or nonspecific host immunity. Although "nonspecific host immunity" is a misnomer, it describes a reproducible, well-defined panoply of nonimmune tissue responses that occur during disparate inflammatory stimuli, including trauma, surgical injury, infection, chemical inflammation, many autoimmune diseases, and cancer. These nonspecific host responses include fever, granulocytosis, trace mineral redistribution, hepatic acute-phase protein synthesis, altered sleep patterns, increased stress hormone levels (corticosteroids, glucagon, and catecholamines), anorexia, and a redistribution of body protein and fuel substrates (2,4–6). Despite the wasting diathesis that follows an inflammatory insult, this overall host nonspecific response to injury and infection is beneficial and is aimed at reducing tissue damage and the likelihood of a secondary bacterial infection. The similarity of the host response to dissimilar exogenous stimuli have led to the conclusion that it is the local and systemic release of cytokines by circulating blood monocytes and tissue macrophages of the reticuloendothelial system that is responsible for initiating and regulating this normal physiological response. Administration of the cytokines IL-1, TNF-α, and to a lesser extent IL-6 can replicate most if not all of the host nonspecific responses to inflammation (4–6).

Although the killing and removal of a localized bacterial, fungal, or protozoal infection is ultimately T cell dependent, activation of host nonspecific immune functions by cytokines in the immediate postinfection period is critical to an early concerted effort to reduce microbial virulence, decrease tissue damage, and limit the risk of secondary opportunistic infections. The induction fever, decreased iron and zinc availability, increased synthesis and release of a variety of acute-phase proteins from the liver, anorexia, accelerated amino acid release from skeletal muscle protein and connective tissue, release of mature and immature neutrophils from bone marrow, and activation and recruitment of neutrophils and phagocytic mononuclear cells, which all occur in the minutes to hours immediately following a bacterial challenge or injury, contribute to the induction of an antimicrobial state.

Although the importance of individual components of the host nonspecific immune response to infection has been reviewed extensively by others (7–9), it is important to note that although each component of this response in itself is inadequate to eliminate bacterial infestation, all facilitate the inhibition of bacterial overgrowth and reduce the degree of tissue damage. Initial studies conducted over a half-century ago demonstrated that when small quantities of bacterial endotoxins were administered to healthy rodents to induce a nonspecific host immune response, the animals exhibited enhanced resistance to antigenically unrelated pathogens (10). Unlike the pathogen-specific T cell response, these protective effects were clearly pathogen unspecific. Since then, efforts have been made to identify the endogenous mediator or mediators responsible for induction of host nonspecific immunity (11), and it is clear that the endogenous release of interleukin-1, among other cytokines, contributes to a heightened antimicrobial response.

Induction of host nonspecific immune resistance places energetic and substrate burdens on the host and necessitates a redistribution of tissue reserves to maintain protein and energy homeostasis. It is when these acute responses are either overly exaggerated, as during shock, are localized to closed tissue compartments, as in rheumatoid arthritis, become chronic in nature, as during repeated gastroenteric or pulmonary infections in undeveloped countries, or occur in patients without adequate reserves, as in protein-calorie malnutrition, that the response itself can be pathophysiological. The challenge is to determine when cytokine-mediated host nonspecific responses are inadequate to meet the acute needs of the host and require supplementation or when the responses are either exaggerated or chronic in nature and require inhibition.

BENEFICIAL NONSPECIFIC HOST RESPONSES MEDIATED BY CYTOKINES

The original isolation of endogenous mediators of the inflammatory response has been inextricably linked to the production of fever. In early reports, fever induction in rabbits and mice was the sole means of determining the presence of cytokines in leukocyte exudates (11). Similarly, fever has been historically linked to both the beneficial and the pathological responses to inflammation (7,9–12).

Several in vitro studies demonstrate that febrile temperatures decrease the replication rate of many pathogenic bacteria and increase both monocyte and neutrophil antimicrobial activity (7,12,13). Duff and Durum reported that when T lymphocytes were incubated in the presence of mitogen at febrile temperatures, their blastogenic response was significantly enhanced (14). Humoral immune response are also enhanced at febrile temperatures (15).

Some investigators have shown that blocking a febrile response in vivo often causes a nonlethal infection to become lethal. This has been most convincingly shown in poikilotherms by Kluger and Rothenburg, who demonstrated in lizards given a nonlethal *Streptococcus* infection that the inability of these animals to warm themselves resulted in increased lethality (7).

Like most of the host nonspecific responses to inflammation, induction of a febrile state is associated with significant metabolic costs to the host. A 1°C increase in core temperature requires a 7–12% increase in energy production, and this often occurs during a period of reduced food intake. This energy deficit is usually met by increased oxidation of endogenous fuels, primarily lipid from adipose tissue and protein from skeletal muscle and connective tissue.

Superficially, it appears unlikely that anorexia, which can be mediated to a large extent by cytokines (4,5), is a beneficial host response to inflammation. After all, anorexia leads to losses of lean tissue, and the development of malnutrition has been shown to be associated with increased incidence of bacterial infection and increased morbidity and mortality following infection (16,17). However, several studies have shown that acute periods of anorexia, per se, are important to the successful nonspecific immune response to bacterial infection. Murray et al. reported that mice force fed normal amounts of food during a Gram-negative bacteremia expired at a much greater rate than animals allowed to regulate their own food intake spontaneously (18). We showed that rats fed 130% of the normal spontaneous food intake by continuous enteral feeding expired twice as frequently to an intravenous challenge with live *Pseudomonas* as rats fed only 80% of the estimated spontaneous intake (19). The mechanism by which anorexia promotes survival is unclear, although excess micronutrient availability, postprandial changes in the hormonal substrate milieu, and gastrointestinal function have all been implicated.

Despite the anorexia that follows inflammation, total hepatic synthesis of secretory proteins is increased. The contribution of the liver to whole-body protein synthesis and energy expenditure is often not appreciated: approximately 25% of whole-body protein synthesis and 25% of resting energy expenditure occur in the liver (20). Of this, approximately 50% of total hepatic protein synthesis is secreted, and albumin represents the principal secretory product in healthy humans. During inflammation, plasma albumin concentrations decline as a result of decreases in its synthetic rate and increases in degradation and loss into extravascular compartments. The decline in albumin synthesis by the liver is offset by the increased synthesis of a variety of glycoproteins, which have been classified as acute-phase reactants. Total hepatic protein synthesis may increase by up to 50% following infection. These proteins, many of whose functions are still not fully known, are presumed to play a beneficial role in the inflammatory response

Table 1 Beneficial Aspects of Acute-Phase Proteins

Host function	Acute-phase protein[a]
Protease and free-radical inhibitors	α_2-Macroglobulin, α_1-antitrypsin (α_1-protease inhibitor), α_2-chymotrypsin, haptoglobin, inter α-trypsin inhibitor, metallothionein, superoxide dismutase
Trace metal binding and of biologically active compounds	Haptoglobin, hemopexin, ceruloplasmin, α_1-acid transport glycoprotein, α_2-macroglobulin, metallothionein, *albumin, transferrin, prealbumin*
Directly modulates the immune response	CRP, C3 (complement), haptoglobin, α_1-acid glycoprotein, fibrinogen
Antiinflammatory proteins	Protease inhibitors, haptoglobin, ceruloplasmin, fibrinogen degradation products
Binding or removal of foreign material	CRP, amyloid (A and P), C3 (complement), fibrinogen
Blood clotting and fibrinolysis	Fibrinogen, α_2-antiplasmin, C1-esterase inactivator, α_1-acid glycoprotein, amyloid P, CRP

[a] Italics refer to proteins whose concentrations decline during inflammation.
Source: Adapted from Ref. 21.

(Table 1) (21). Many of these proteins are protease inhibitors or free-radical scavengers [α_2-macroglobulin, α_1-antitrypsin (α_1-protease inhibitor), α_2-chymotrypsin, haptoglobin, and inter α-trypsin inhibitor], others may serve as opsonins or scavengers of foreign proteins [C-reactive protein (CRP), amyloid (A and P), C3 (complement), and fibrinogen], some may be involved in the transport of biologically active mediators or compounds (α_2-macroglobulin, haptoglobin, hemopexin, ceruloplasmin, and α_1-acid glycoprotein), and some may be directly active on immunological tissues [CRP, C3 (complement), haptoglobin, α_1-acid glycoprotein, and fibrinogen]. The protease inhibitors and free-radical scavengers are presumed to reduce the magnitude of tissue damage associated with the release of toxic compounds and oxygen free radicals from activated blood neutrophils and tissue macrophages. α_2-Macroglobulin is thought to serve as a binding protein for several cytokines, such as TNF-α, IL-1, IL-6, and transforming growth factor β (TGF-β), and cytokine–α_2-macroglobulin complexes are presumed to modulate the biological activity of these mediators. Other acute-phase proteins reduce trace mineral availability for pathogenic bacteria, and some act directly to facilitate phagocytosis of microbial pathogens.

The loss of body weight and lean tissue and the catabolic wasting secondary to acute and chronic inflammatory disease have often been used as the paradigm for pathophysiological responses mediated by the cytokines. Losses of skeletal muscle and connective tissue protein can be quite large in hospitalized patients with sepsis, long bone fractures, and thermal injury, often exceeding 200 g/day of lean tissue (22). Recent studies by several groups have emphasized that cytokines play at least a facilitative role (23–25) and perhaps even directly mediate the increased catabolism that occurs following inflammatory disease (26). Although continued losses of skeletal muscle protein can have significant pathological effects, such as reduced cardiac and smooth muscle function, delayed recovery, and general fatigue, accelerated skeletal muscle proteolysis is essential to the mobilization of endogenous substrates (principally amino acids) required for increased amino acid requirements by anabolic hepatic and inflammatory tissues, as well as for gluconeogenesis.

The healthy adult breaks down and resynthesizes approximately 250 g/day of protein; approximately 25% (65 g) comes from skeletal muscle (27). During sepsis, extensive long bone fracture, and thermal injury, protein turnover can increase to as much as 400 g/day (28). Because of the release of cytokines and their effects on counterregulatory hormones, such as cortisol, catecholamines, and glucagon, skeletal muscle protein becomes net catabolic and can release as much as 100 g/day of free amino acids from net protein catabolism (27). This free amino nitrogen is not entirely lost from the body but serves as amino acid precursors for increased hepatic and immune system protein synthesis. Wannemacher estimated that the amount of protein required to produce and sustain a leukocytosis of 15,000 cells per mm^3 is approximately 20 g/day and the amount of protein employed to support an hepatic acute-phase protein response is another 25 g/day (29). Since the free amino acid pool of adult humans consists of only approximately 7 g of amino acids, during periods of inflammation-associated anorexia, increased proteolysis of somatic tissues is essential to sustain an hepatic and immunological anabolic response.

Although increased urea production is a common occurrence during inflammatory disease, utilization of carbon fragments from gluconeogenic amino acids released by somatic tissues is an essential component of the cytokine-mediated redistribution of lean tissue during inflammation. Because of the associated anorexia and limited glycogen stores, obligate glucose-utilizing tissues, such as brain, erythrocytes, granulating tissue, and many inflammatory cells, depend on hepatic gluconeogenesis for adequate provision of fuel. Cytokines released during inflammation play a significant role in assuring the availability of gluconeogenic precursors by (1) stimulating the release of catecholamines and glucagon, which accelerate hepatic glycogenolysis (30,31), (2) promoting, either directly or through the neuroendocrine axis, the release of gluconeogenic precursors from skeletal muscle and connective tissue, and (3) stimulating uptake of gluconeogenic amino acids into the hepatocyte and induction of gluconeogenic enzyme pathways (32,33).

Acutely, induction of these pathways provides the substrates required by the anorectic host to meet the energy and protein requirements of the inflammatory response. However, the cost in lean tissue wasting to the host can be significant, especially when the cytokine-mediated stimulus is excessive or chronic in nature. Survey studies have shown that when losses of skeletal muscle protein exceed 15–20%, as measured by anthropometrics, increased morbidity and mortality may occur (16). This generally is not observed during less than a week of inflammation, as in patients with bacteremia, urosepsis, pneumonia, or other significant microbial infections. Under such conditions in previously healthy and well-nourished individuals, most investigators do not recommend invasive efforts to reduce skeletal muscle protein wasting with parenteral nutrition support because reserves are adequate and efforts to blunt this redistribution of protein may actually impair host immune responses. If the infected individual is protein depleted, however, or the infection has lasted for longer than 1 week, efforts to reduce cytokine- and neuroendocrine-mediated skeletal muscle protein wasting may be beneficial. Under these circumstances, the adverse effects of skeletal muscle protein depletion, such as cardiac cachexia and decreased respiratory work capacity, may outweigh the beneficial effects of this redistribution.

CONTRIBUTIONS MADE BY INDIVIDUAL CYTOKINES TO THE HOST NONSPECIFIC RESPONSE

During the 1970s, when many of the initial studies were conducted into the role of leukocyte products on host nonspecific immune responses, cytokines were known simply by the functional monikers as leukocytic or endogenous pyrogen, leukocyte endogenous mediator, or hepatocyte stimulating factor. It is now recognized that these functional characteristics are not limited to a single peptide or peptide family but represent an entire class of pleiotropic cytokines with overlapping and distinct biological properties. To date, at least three cytokines, interleukin-1α and β (also known as lymphocyte activating factor), tumor necrosis factor (also known as cachectin), and interleukin-6 (also known as interferon-β_2, hepatocyte stimulating factor, 24 kD protein, and hybridoma growth factor), meet the criteria as leukocyte endogenous mediators or inducers of the host nonspecific immune response. Several other cytokines, including interleukin-8, GRO, MIP-1, and MIP-2, may also be included. All these cytokines meet the criteria of being possible endogenous mediators of host nonspecific immune responses in that they are produced within hours of an inflammatory stimuli and are pleiotropic in nature.

Summarized in Table 2 are some of the overlapping biological responses known to be mediated by IL-1, TNF-α, and IL-6. Distinctions among the three cytokines in terms of their presumed unique capabilities to stimulate T cell proliferation (a presumed IL-1 function), tumor cytolysis and host cachexia (a presumed TNF-α function), and hepatic acute-phase stimulation (a presumed IL-6 function) have blurred considerably.

Efforts to identify which host responses are mediated by individual cytokines have been complicated by the apparent redundancy in biological actions as well as the capacity of individual cytokines to induce the synthesis of each other. For example, it is now known that IL-1, TNF-α, IL-6, interferon-α, and MIP-1 are all endogenous pyrogens (34–37). In addition, the induction of specific components of the hepatic acute-phase protein response to inflammation appears to be dependent upon one or more of these cytokines. For example, TNF-α, IL-1, and IL-6 all decrease the synthesis of albumin, the principal negative hepatic acute-phase response protein (38–40), whereas IL-6 and to a much lesser extent, IL-1, but not TNF-α, is responsible for the induction of fibrinogen and α_1-antitrypsin biosynthesis (41,42).

In other cases, individual cytokines strongly potentiate the actions of one another. The anorectic effects of IL-1 and TNF-α are greatly exaggerated when the cytokines are administered together. In addition, many components of the hepatic acute-phase protein response, particularly amyloid (P and A component) and complement (C_3) production, are markedly increased when IL-1 and IL-6 are administered simultaneously (41,42).

The capacity to produce shock and irreversible tissue damage appears to be

TABLE 2 Biological Responses and Tissue Sources of IL-1, TNF-α, and IL-6

	IL-1 (α and β)	TNF-α	IL-6
Tissue sources	Blood monocytes, tissue macrophages, keratinocytes, Kupffer's cells, LGLs, B lymphocytes, neutrophils, fibroblasts, astrocytes, endothelial cells	Blood monocytes, macrophages, keratinocytes, Kupffer's cells, astrocytes, microglial cells, fibroblasts, endothelial cells	Blood monocytes macrophages, T lymphocytes, fibroblasts, keratinocytes, Kupffer's cells
Biological responses			
Fever	Yes	Yes	Yes
Shock	Limited yes (synergizes with TNF-α)	Yes	Maybe
Leukocyte margination	Yes at high doses	Yes	No
Stimulation of hematopoietic growth and differentiation	Yes	Yes	Yes
Acute-phase induction	Yes	Yes (but not as strong as IL-1 or IL-6)	Yes (very strong)
Endothelial cell activation, increased procoagulant activity	Yes (with TNF-α)	Yes	Weak
Trace metal distribution	Yes	Yes	Yes
Anorexia, weight loss	Yes	Yes	Weak
Skeletal muscle proteolysis	Yes	Yes	Unknown
Prostaglandin synthesis	Yes	Yes	Weak
Osteoclast activation	Yes	Yes	Unknown
Induction of CSFs	Yes	Yes	Yes
Adrenocorticotropic hormone (ACTH) synthesis	Yes (as well as direct adrenal effect)	Yes	Yes
Islet cell toxicity	Yes (synergizes with TNF-α)	Yes	Unknown
Induction of cytokine biosynthesis	Yes for IL-6, very weak for TNF-α	Yes for IL-1 and IL-6	Suppresses TNF-α

the one principal function of TNF-α that is not shared by the three cytokines. However, recent studies have shown that whereas IL-1 administration cannot readily produce irreversible tissue damage (43), IL-1 administration produces hypotension and tachycardia. Furthermore, very small amounts of TNF-α greatly potentiate the hemodynamic effects of IL-1 and, when TNF-α and IL-1 are administered simultaneously in combinations that when administered individually are not lethal, produces irreversible shock and tissue damage (44,45). At present, there is no direct evidence that IL-6 has any of the hemodynamic and shock-producing characteristics of IL-1 or TNF-α, although the appropriate studies have not been completed.

In addition, it is now recognized that TNF-α can induce the synthesis of IL-1 (34), and both TNF-α and IL-1 can induce the synthesis of IL-6 (46,47). More importantly, Fong and colleagues showed that passive immunization against TNF-α can attenuate the subsequent IL-1β and IL-6 responses to a lethal bacteremia in primates (48). Similarly, Gershenwald et al. observed that passive immunization of mice with an antibody against the IL-1 receptor blocked the IL-6 response to a turpentine abscess (49). Such findings raise the important question of whether the inhibition produced by cytokine blockade can be attributed to that cytokine being blocked or merely to the disruption of the cytokine cascade and the block downstream of secondary cytokines or mediators. This is especially relevant with shock and tissue damage produced by overwhelming Gram-negative infections and endotoxemia. Whereas earlier studies clearly showed that TNF-α blockade prevented death to endotoxin or *Escherichia coli* bacteremia, such treatment also blocks the endogenous IL-1β and IL-6 response. Recent studies by Ohlssen and Thompson (50) and Dinarello (51) showed that IL-1 receptor blockade also prevents death to *E. coli* bacteremia, suggesting that in addition to TNF-α, a normal endogenous IL-1 response is critical to mortality from overwhelming Gram-negative infections. In addition, in a very preliminary report, Starnes *et al.* reported that passive immunization of mice with antibodies against IL-6 can prevent shock and mortality secondary to endotoxemia (52). These findings suggest that IL-6, like IL-1, may play a facilitative role in the TNF-α-mediated tissue damage secondary to endotoxin and Gram-negative bacteria. Taken together with the observations that (1) TNF-α administration, but not IL-1 or IL-6, causes shock and tissue damage to healthy animals, (2) TNF-α is a strong in vivo inducer of IL-1 and IL-6, whereas IL-1 (53) and IL-6 are weak in vivo inducers of TNF-α, and (3) TNF-α, IL-1, or IL-6 blockade prevents irreversible tissue damage secondary to endotoxin or Gram-negative bacteria, one can conclude that endogenous TNF-α, IL-1, and IL-6 responses are all required for induction of shock and tissue damage. The toxicity of TNF-α in vivo, relative to that of IL-1 and IL-6, may then be explained by the inability of IL-1 and IL-6 to induce sufficient endogenous TNF-α versus the ability of TNF-α to induce endogenous IL-1 and IL-6.

Recently, antibodies to individual cytokines were employed to resolve the relative contribution of IL-1 and TNF-α to other components of the nonspecific host response to inflammation. For example, Gershenwald et al. demonstrated that IL-1 receptor blockade could attenuate almost 50% of the anorexia associated with a sterile turpentine abscess (49). In contrast, TNF-α blockade was without effect, suggesting that at least in this model of inflammation, the anorexia was dependent at least in part upon an endogenous IL-1, but not TNF-α, response. Similar results were seen with the murine hepatic acute-phase protein, amyloid P. However, because IL-1 blockade also attenuated the IL-6 response, it is still unresolved whether the effects could be directly attributed to IL-1 or are the result of IL-1 inhibition of other cytokines.

Kluger and colleagues also explored the role of individual cytokines in the febrile response to endotoxin (54). Not unexpectedly, IL-1β blockade attenuated the febrile response to endotoxin, whereas TNF-α blockade actually increased the febrile response. The underlying mechanism of this increased febrile response to TNF-α blockade remains unclear.

THERAPEUTIC USE OF IL-1 AS A HOST NONSPECIFIC IMMUNE STIMULANT

Our interest in the beneficial components of the host response to infection came initially from observations of malnutrition in underdeveloped nations. It was there that several investigators, principally Scrimshaw and colleagues, observed that protein-malnourished individuals, when infected, often do not manifest a normal metabolic response (55). Malnourished individuals suffering repeated gastrointestinal infections often did not become febrile or leukocytotic and had a markedly reduced catabolic response. Furthermore, Gordon and Scrimshaw observed that those individuals who failed to develop a normal febrile or leukocytotic response had a significantly higher morbidity and mortality than individuals who became febrile and leukocytotic when infected (56).

The first indication that an abnormal cytokine response may be involved in the increased pathogenesis of malnutrition were studies performed by Hoffman-Goetz et al. (57). Earlier studies by Kluger and Rothenburg (7) emphasized the importance of fever in the survival response to Gram-positive infections. In their ongoing studies, these investigators demonstrated that protein-depleted rabbits did not develop a febrile response or a normal hypoferremia when infected with *Pasteurellosis* (58). However, these same protein-depleted rabbits developed a normal febrile response when injected with glucan-activated macrophage products (leukocytic pyrogen) obtained from healthy rabbits, demonstrating that such protein-depleted rabbits were capable of generating a fever when administered an endogenous pyrogen. The failure to respond to *Pasteurellosis* could be attributed to the inability of blood monocytes-macrophages to synthesize these cytokines in response to the bacteria. In addition, we demonstrated that protein-malnourished guinea pigs with deficient IL-1 production had a normal febrile and trace mineral response when administered partially purified IL-1 preparations (59). However, acute-phase protein synthesis and the catabolic muscle protein response to IL-1 were still attenuated when exogenous cytokines were administered (60). Later studies showed that protein malnutrition also decreases the capacity of blood monocytes and macrophages to synthesize IL-1 in hospitalized patients suffering protein-calorie malnutrition (61). For example, approximately 50% of blood mononuclear cells harvested from critically ill patients had deficient in vitro IL-1 production, and these patients had a significantly greater mortality than similar patients whose leukocytes were capable of generating IL-1 in vitro.

These studies led to the hypothesis that the increased morbidity and mortality associated with protein malnutrition could be explained at least in part by a deficient in vivo IL-1 production (62). When protein-malnourished guinea pigs were pretreated with partially purified IL-1, their ability to clear a lethal intravenous bacterial challenge was significantly enhanced and survival improved.

Since this hypothesis was advanced in early 1982, a greater appreciation for IL-1 as a generalized nonspecific host immune stimulant in healthy and otherwise immune-suppressed animals has developed. IL-1 pretreatment can increase bacterial resistance to *Pseudomonas* in animals immunosuppressed by splenectomy and/or portocaval anastomosis (63). In recent years, a great interest has developed regarding the capability of IL-1 to protect normal and neutropenic animals from infection with *Klebsiella*, *Pseudomonas*, *Listeria*, *Candida*, and *Staphylococcus* (3).

The rationale behind the use of IL-1 in neutropenic animals has rested principally with its capability to facilitate proliferation of hematopoietic precursors (64). Although IL-1 alone appears incapable of inducing hematopoietic progenitors to proliferate and differentiate, IL-1 induces the synthesis of several colony stimulating factors (CSFs) (65,66) and can potentiate the effect of other growth factors to induce primitive progenitor cells to become responsive to CSFs (64). Unlike several other growth factors, IL-1 appears to act very early in the proliferation and differentiation of hematopoietic progenitors.

Patients with neoplastic disease often have bone marrow suppression secondary to a variety of radiation and chemotherapy regimens. The associated hematological deficiencies, including anemia, leukopenia, and thrombocytopenia, lead to increased risk of bacterial infections and often limit the quantities of antineoplastic therapies that can be administered. Preliminary results have been obtained with IL-1 in phase I clinical trials in patients with chemotherapy-induced myelosuppression (68). Results suggest that IL-1 may have a usefulness in restoring more normal numbers of granulocytes and thrombocytes in patients simultaneously receiving doxorubicin. The theoretical advantage of IL-1 therapy in such patients is not solely limited to stimulation of hematopoietic recovery, however, but includes the previously described ability of IL-1 to activate reticuloendothelial system function and host nonspecific immune responses. In this latter regard, IL-1 offers a distinct advantage over other hematopoietic growth factors, such as granulocyte-macrophage colony-stimulating factor (GM-CSF) and G-CSF, which are also in clinical trials in cancer patients with chemotherapy-associated myelosuppression. The pleiotropic nature of IL-1, relative to the CSFs, offers the advantage of simultaneously inducing several antimicrobial pathways that cannot be replicated by any other single cytokine.

This last point is shown most graphically by the studies of the Campanile (69), van der Meer (70–72), Czuprinski (73–76) and others (73,74) in normal and neutropenic mice. Van der Meer et al. demonstrated that a single low-dose injection of human IL-1β (400 ng/kg body weight) prevented death against a lethal *Pseudomonas* or *Candida* infection in neutropenic mice (70) and induced survival against a lethal *Listeria* or *Klebsiella* infection in nonneutropenic mice (71,72). Similar effects were not observed with pretreatments with either TNF-α or IL-6. IL-1-induced protection in neutropenic mice could not be explained by any single mechanism. For example, van der Meer et al. were unable to demonstrate any significant improvement in the antibacterial action of granulocytes or increased hematopoietic recovery in neutropenic mice treated with IL-1 (70). In contrast, the Czuprinski (72,73), Kurtz (76), McIntyre (77), Kurlander (78), Nakai (79), and Hamawy (63) groups were all able to show evidence for increased bactericidal activity in animals pretreated with IL-1 and exposed to a variety of lethal Gram-negative and Gram-positive infections.

Summarized in Table 3 is a list of putative mechanisms by which IL-1 may confer survival benefit to healthy as well as immunocompromised animals. As observed, the antibacterial effects of IL-1 are diverse, acting on all leukocyte cell populations as well as on somatic tissues for induction of host nonspecific immunity. Based on these actions, it is not surprising that IL-1 therapies are most beneficial when administered before the infectious challenge. For example, several investigators, including ourselves, demonstrated that maximal antibacterial resistance was achieved when IL-1 was administered 12–24 h before the infectious challenge (63,69–79). Only limited beneficial effects were seen when IL-1 was given simultaneously with or after a bacterial infection.

Although such a requirement for pretreatment clearly limits the patient populations that might benefit from IL-1 therapies, large groups of hospitalized patients exist in whom a 24 h pretreatment period would be advantageous in reducing subsequent risks of infection. In addition to myelosuppressed cancer patients in danger of developing opportunistic bacterial infections, individuals with extensive thermal injury are commonly immunosuppressed and routinely develop bacterial infections. Such patients may benefit from a short course (less than 5 days) of IL-1 as a means to prevent thermal injury-associated leukopenia as well as reduce the likelihood of subsequent Gram-negative infections.

Protein malnutrition is also a common occurrence in hospitalized patients, and such patients have increased susceptibility to bacterial infections following surgical injury, as well as increased morbidity to infectious insults. In some estimates, as many as 50% of all surgical patients have some degree of moderate protein-calorie malnutrition (80,81). Protein-malnourished patients have less successful surgical outcomes and increased incidence of pulmonary infections, wound dehiscence and infection, and urosepsis than their well-nourished counterparts. A 24 h preoperative course of IL-1 therapy in such patients might reduce the risk of operative infection, wound dehiscence, and secondary pulmonary or urinary tract infection.

Given the pleiotropic nature of IL-1, it is not surprising that undesirable host responses have been observed frequently. The nature of IL-1 toxicity can be divided into those side effects seen after acute IL-1 administration and those that manifest themselves only with chronic IL-1 administration (Table 4). Since IL-1 is now in phase I clinical trials, considerable toxicity and safety data have accumulated (63,82). As expected, fever, nausea, myalgia, changes in sleeping patterns, and hypoglycemia have all been observed in humans and nonhuman primates receiving IL-1. Symptoms appear to be dose related and occur more frequently with administrations of greater than 100 ng/kg body weight. Rather unexpectedly, however, dose-limiting toxicity in both humans and nonhuman primates is due to hypotension and in some cases has been life-threatening. Studies we conducted in baboons showed that significant drops in mean arterial blood pressure and tachycardia were seen with doses as low as 100 ng/kg body weight, and doses as high as 100 μg/kg body weight produced 40% declines in mean

TABLE 3 Beneficial Effects of IL-1 on Nonimmune and Immune Tissues

Tissue	Response
Liver	Acute-phase protein induction
	Trace mineral uptake
	Kupffer's cell activation of phagocytosis
	Cytochrome P-$_{450}$ induction
	Induction of gluconeogenesis
	Increased energy expenditure
	Extramedullary nematopoiesis
Brain	Fever
	Induction of neuroendocrine axis (ACTH and CRH 41)
	Altered pain sensation
	Anorexia
	Stimulation of somatostatin biosynthesis
Skeletal muscle	Release of amino acids for new protein synthesis and gluconeogenesis
	Myalgia
Kidneys	Decreases renal sodium resorption
Pancreas	Increased glucagon and decreased insulin release promoting redistribution of endogenous substrates
Endothelial cells	Stimulation of fibrinolysis
	Induction of leukocyte adhesion molecules
	Promotes transendothelial migration of leukocyte populations into wounds
	Induction of procoagulant activity
	Induction of plasminogen activator inhibitor
	Induction of other cytokines, including IL-6, IL-8
Bone marrow	Induction of other cytokines including CSFs, IL-2, IL-6, IL-8
	Synergy with CSFs
	Hematopoietin I activity
	Release of neutrophils
	Induction of increased numbers of thrombocytes
	Induction of radioresistance
Reticuloendothelial system	Enhanced phagocytosis
	Increased antimicrobial actions
Other immunological responses	Induction of cytotoxic T cells, natural killer cells
	Induction of other cytokines, including IL-2, CSFs, TNF-α, IL-6, IL-8
	Induction of monocyte antitumor and bactericidal activity
	Adjuvant in vivo
Wound microenvironment	Promotes tissue remodeling by increasing collagenase activity
	Stimulates production of chemotactic cytokines by macrophages and fibroblasts
	Induction of osteoclast activity for bone remodeling

TABLE 4 Adverse Side Effects of Acute and Chronic IL-1 Administration

Acute		Chronic
Hypotension[a]	Fever[a]	TNFα appearance
Nausea	Rigors[a]	Decreased number of myeloid precursors
Lacticacidemia	Lymphopenia adrenal cortex hemorrhage	Anemia
Thrombocytopenia (transitory)[a]	Malaise[a]	Lymphopenia
Tachycardia[a]	Hypoglycemia[a]	
Myalgia[a]	Hyperglycemia[a]	
Hypothyroidemia		

[a] Obtained from phase I clinical trials.

arterial blood pressure requiring fluid support (83). In addition, in preclinical trials with baboons, IL-1 administration produces a sustained lactic acidemia. The etiology of the lactic acidemia did not appear to be due to enhanced production of lactate by skeletal muscle resulting from inadequate perfusion and oxygenation. Rather, the increased lactic acidemia appeared to result from reduced hepatic gluconeogenesis, as lactate release from the hindlimb was unaffected by IL-1 treatment. The hypoglycemia was transitory in nature and was only seen with doses exceeding 1 μg/kg body weight.

In addition, there have been additional adverse responses to chronic IL-1 treatment. Moore and colleagues demonstrated in cynomologus monkeys that chronic administration of therapeutic quantities of IL-1β for periods exceeding 7 days resulted in decreased numbers of bone marrow myeloid progenitors that coincided with the appearance of TNF-α in the circulation (84). Although recently Ikejima et al. reported the appearance of TNF-α-like bioactivities in the serum of rabbits following a single administration of human IL-1β (53), there was no evidence of a systemic TNF-α response in our preclinical trials in baboons with IL-1α administration. Similarly, Moore et al. were unable to detect circulating TNF-α in their phase I clinical trials with IL-1α administration exceeding 3 weeks (82).

Nevertheless, there have been other reported side effects with chronic IL-1 administration, and many of them relate to changes in myelopoiesis. Anemia has been infrequently reported (85), and the IL-1-mediated defect appears to be at the stage of terminal erythroid differentiation. Similarly, a transient thrombocytopenia has been observed in the first week of chronic IL-1 administration, although more chronic administration is frequently associated with thrombocytophilia (68). Gasparetto observed in primates made neutropenic by 5-fluorouracil treatment that 14 days of continuous IL-1β treatment actually delayed neutrophil recovery, whereas a shorter course (2 or 7 days) of IL-1β abbreviated the period of neutropenia (84).

SUMMARY

The metabolic response to infection, trauma, and surgical injury is mediated in part through the release of a variety of cytokines, including interleukin-1, tumor necrosis factor α, and interleukin-6. Although considerable research has focused on the pathophysiological changes produced by excessive or chronic release of cytokines—such as that during shock, rheumatoid arthritis, many autoimmune diseases, and such chronic inflammatory diseases as cancer, renal, and cardiac disease—recent studies have demonstrated that an orchestrated cytokine response is essential for maintenance of normal immune function following bacterial infections and acute surgical injury. In certain patient populations, such as individuals with protein-calorie malnutrition, cancer cachexia, or chemotherapy induced myelosuppression, treatment with exogenous IL-1 may restore deficient antimicrobial functions and confer a survival benefit against secondary bacterial infections. Furthermore, recent studies suggest that pretreatment of healthy animals with IL-1 or TNF-α can induce an antimicrobial state and confer survival to otherwise subsequent lethal Gram-negative or Gram-positive infections. Maximum effectiveness of these therapies is achieved when cytokines are administered systemically before the infectious insult, so that the beneficial metabolic responses to cytokine administration are operative before the infectious insult. Furthermore, it appears that such therapies must be limited in duration (usually less than 1 week), because chronic administration often leads to immune suppression, wasting of lean tissue, and malnutrition.

REFERENCES

1. Beutler B, Cerami A. Cachectin and tumour necrosis factor as two sides of the same biological coin. Nature 1986; 320:584–8.
2. Fong Y, Moldawer LL, Shires GT, Lowry SF. The biologic characteristics of cytokines and their implication in surgical injury. Surg Gynecol Obstet 1990; 170:363–78.
3. Dinarello CA, Neta R. An overview on interleukin-1 as a therapeutic agent. Biotherapy 1990; 1:245–54.
4. Moldawer LL, Andersson C, Svaninger G, Gelin J, Lundholm K. Regulation of food intake and hepatic protein metabolism by recombinant derived monokines. Am J Physiol 1988; 254:G450–6.
5. Fong Y, Moldawer LL, Marano M, et al. Cachectin/TNF or IL-1α induces cachexia with redistribution of body proteins. Am J Physiol 1989; 256:R659–65.
6. Cady AB, Riveau G, Chedid L, Dinarello CA, Johannsen L, and Krueger JM. Interleukin-1-induced sleep and febrile responses differentially altered by a muramyl dipeptide derivative. Int J Immunopharmacol 1989; 11:887–93.
7. Kluger MJ, Rothenburg BA. Fever and reduced iron: their interaction as a host defense response to bacterial infections. Science 1979; 203:374–6.
8. Sugarman B. Zinc and infection. Rev Infect Dis 1983; 5:137–47.
9. Powanda MC, Beisel WR. Hypothesis: leukocyte endogenous mediator/endogenous pyrogen/lymphocyte activating factor modulates the development of nonspecific and specific immunity and affects nutritional status. Am J Clin Nutr 1982; 35:762–8.
10. Shilo M. Nonspecific resistance to infection. Annu Rev Microbiol 1959; 13:255–79.
11. Kampschmidt RF. Infection, inflammation and interleukin-1. Lymphokine Res 1984; 2:97–110.
12. Dinarello CA, Cannon JG, Wolff SM. New concepts on the pathogenesis of fever. Rev Infect Dis 1988; 10:168–89.
13. Atkins E. Fever: the old and the new. J Infect Dis 1984; 149:229–48.
14. Duff GW, Durum SK. The pyrogenic and mitogen actions of interleukin-1 are related. Nature 1983; 304:449–51.

15. Jampel HD, Duff GW, Gershon RK, Atkins E, Durum SK. Fever and immunoregulation. III. Hyperthermia augments the primary in vitro humoral immune response. J Exp Med 1983; 157:1229–38.
16. Harvey KB, Moldawer LL, Bistrian BR, Blackburn GL. Biological measures for the formulation of a hospital prognostic index. Am J Clin Nutr 1981; 34:2013–22.
17. Buzby GP, Mullen JL, Matthews DC, Hobbs CL, Rosato EF. Prognostic nutritional index in gastrointestinal surgery. Am J Surg 1980; 139:160–7.
18. Murray J, Murray A, Murray N. Anorexia: sentinal of host defense. Perspect Biol Med 1978; 22:134–42.
19. Yamazaki K, Moldawer LL, Maiz A, Bistrian BR, Blackburn GL. Complications associated with overfeeding of infected animals. J Surg Res 1986; 40:152–8.
20. Powanda MC. Changes in body balances of nitrogen and other key nutrients: description and underlying mechanisms. Am J Clin Nutr 1977; 30:1254–68.
21. Koj A. Biological functions of acute phase proteins. *In:* Gordon AH, Koj A, eds. The acute phase response to injury and infection. New York: Elsevier, 1985:146–60.
22. Birkhahn RH, Long CL, Fitkin D, Jeevanadam M, Blakemore WS. Whole body protein metabolism due to trauma in man estimated by L-[^{15}N]alanine. Am J Physiol 1981; 241:E64–71.
23. Moldawer LL, Svaninger G, Gelin J, Lundholm K. Interleukin 1 (alpha or beta) and tumour necrosis factor-alpha do not regulate protein balance in skeletal muscle. Am J Physiol 1987; 253:C766–73.
24. Baracos V, Rodemann HP, Dinarello CA, Goldberg AL. Stimulation of muscle protein degradation and prostaglandin E_2 release by leukocytic pyrogen (interleukin 1). N Engl J Med 1983; 308:553–8.
25. Goldberg AL, Kettlehut IC, Furuno K, Fagan JM, Baracos VM. Activation of protein breakdown and prostaglandin E_2 production in rat skeletal muscle in fever is signalled by a macrophage product distinct from interleukin 1 and other known cytokines. J Clin Invest 1988; 81:1378–81.
26. Flores EA, Bistrian BR, Pomposelli JJ, Blackburn GL, Istfan N. Infusion of tumor necrosis factor/cachectin promotes muscle catabolism in the rat. J Clin Invest 1989; 83:1614–22.
27. Long CL, Birkhahn RH, Geiger JW, Blakemore WS. Urinary excretion of 3-methylhistidine: an assessment of muscle protein catabolism in adult normal subjects and during malnutrition, sepsis and skeletal trauma. Metabolism 1981; 30:765–76.
28. Birkhahn RH, Long CL, Fitkin D, Geiger JW, Blakemore WS. Effects of major skeletal trauma on whole body protein turnover in man measured by L-[1-^{14}C]leucine. Surgery 1983; 88:294–300.
29. Wannemacher RW Jr. Protein metabolism in infections. In: Adibi SA, ed. Total parenteral nutrition. Amsterdam: Elsevier-North Holland, 1976.
30. Rivier C, Vale W, Brown M. In the rat, interleukin-1α and -β stimulate adrenocorticotropin and catecholamine release. Endocrinology 1989; 125:3096–102.
31. George DT, Abeles FB, Mapes CA, Sobocinski PZ, Zenser TV, Powanda MC. Effect of leukocyte endogenous mediators on endocrine pancreas secretory responses. Am J Physiol 1977; 233:E240–5.
32. Roh MS, Moldawer LL, Ekman LG, et al. Stimulatory effect of interleukin 1 upon hepatic metabolism. Metabolism 1986; 35:419–24.
33. Hill MR, Stith RD, McCallum RE. Interleukin 1: a regulatory role in glucocorticoid regulated hepatic metabolism. J Immunol 1986; 137:858–62.
34. Dinarello CA, Cannon JG, Wolff SM, et al. Tumour necrosis factor (cachectin) is an endogenous pyrogen and induces production of interleukin 1. J Exp Med 1986; 163:1433–50.

35. LeMay LG, Vander AJ, Kluger MJ. Role of interleukin 6 in fever in rats. Am J Physiol 1990; 258:R798–803.
36. Dinarello CA, Bernheim HA, Duff GW, et al. Mechanisms of fever induced by recombinant human interferon. J Clin Invest 1984; 74:906–13.
37. Davatelis GA, Wolpe SD, Sherry B, Dayer JM, Chicheportiche R, Cerami A. Macrophage inflammatory protein-I: a prostaglandin independent endogenous pyrogen. Science 1989; 243:1066–8.
38. Brenner DA, Buck M, Feitelberg SP, Chojkier M. Tumor necrosis factor-α inhibits albumin gene expression in a murine model of cachexia. J Clin Invest 1990; 85:248–55.
39. Hooper DC, Steer CJ, Dinarello CA, Peacock AC. Haptoglobin and albumin synthesis in the isolated rat hepatocyte: response to potential mediators of the acute phase reaction. Biochim Biophys Acta 1981; 653:118–29.
40. Ramadori G, Van Damme J, Rieder H, Meyer zum Buschenfelde KH. Interleukin 6, the third mediator of acute-phase reaction, modulates hepatic protein synthesis in human and mouse. Comparison with interleukin 1 beta and tumor necrosis factor-alpha. Eur J Immunol 1988; 18:1259–64.
41. Andus T, Geiger T, Hirano T, Kishimoto T, Heinrich PC. Action of recombinant human interleukin 6, interleukin 1 beta and tumor necrosis factor alpha on the mRNA induction of acute-phase proteins. Eur J Immunol 1988; 18:739–46.
42. Lin BF, Ku NO, Zahedi K, Whitehead AS, Mortensen RF. Induction of hepatocyte synthesis of the mouse acute phase protein serum amyloid P-component (SAP) by IL-1 and IL-6. Ann N Y Acad Sci 1989; 557:534–5.
43. Okusawa S, Gelfand JA, Ikejima T, Connolly RJ, Dinarello CA. Interleukin 1 induces a shock-like state in rabbits. J Clin Invest 1988; 81:1162–72.
44. Waage A, Espevik T. Interleukin-1 potentitates the lethal effect of tumor necrosis factor-α/cachectin in mice. J Exp Med 1988; 167:1987–92.
45. Everaerdt B, Brouchaert P, Shaw A, Fiers W. Four different interleukin-1 species sensitize to the lethal action of tumour necrosis factor. Biochem Biophys Res Commun 1989; 163:378–85.
46. Libert C, Brouckaert P, Shaw A, Fiers W. Induction of interleukin 6 by human and murine recombinant interleukin 1 in mice. Eur J Immunol 1990; 20:691–4.
47. Brouckaert P, Spriggs DR, Demetri G, Kufe DW, Fiers W. Circulating interleukin 6 during a continuous infusion of tumor necrosis factor and interferon gamma. J Exp Med 1989; 169:2257–62.
48. Fong Y, Tracey KJ, Moldawer LL, et al. Antibodies to cachectin/tumor necrosis factor reduce interleukin 1β and interleukin 6 appearance during lethal bacteremia. J Exp Med 1989; 170:1627–33.
49. Gershenwald JE, Fong Y, Fahey TJ III, et al. Interleukin 1 receptor blockade attenuates the host inflammatory response. Proc Natl Acad Sci U S A 1990; 87:4966–70.
50. Ohlsson K, Bjork P, Bergenfeldt M, Hageman R, Thompson RC. An interleukin-1 receptor antagonist reduces mortality in endotoxin shock. Nature 1990; 348:550–552.
51. Wakabayashi G, Gelfand JA, Burke JF, Dinarello CA. A specific receptor antagonist for interleukin-1 prevents *E. coli* induced septic shock in rabbits. FASEB J 1991; 5: 338–343.
52. Starnes Jr. HF, Pearce MK, Tewari A, Yim JH, Zou J-C, Abrams JS. Anti-IL-6 monoclonal antibodies protect against lethal *Escherichia coli* infection and lethal tumor necrosis factor-α challenge in mice. J Immunol 1990; 145:4185–4191.
53. Ikejima T, Okusawa S, Ghezzi P, Van der Meer JWM, Dinarello CA. Interleukin-1 induces tumor necrosis factor (TNF) in human peripheral blood mononuclear cells

in vitro and a circulating TNF-like activity in rabbits. J Infect Dis 1990; 162:215–23.
54. Long NC, Kunkel SL, Vander AJ, Kluger MJ. Antiserum against tumor necrosis factor enhances lipopolysaccharide fever in rats. Am J Physiol 1990; 258:R332–7.
55. Scrimshaw NS, Taylor CE, Gordon JE. Interactions of nutrition and infection. WHO Monog Ser 1968; 57:3–329.
56. Gordon JE, Scrimshaw NS. Infectious disease in the malnourished. Med Clin North Am 1970; 54:1495–508.
57. Hoffman-Goetz L, McFarlane D, Bistrian BR, Blackburn GL. Febrile and plasma iron responses to rabbits injected with endogenous pyrogen from malnourished patients. Am J Clin Nutr 1981; 34:1109–16.
58. Hoffmann-Goetz L, Kluger MJ. Protein deprivation: its effects on fever and plasma iron during bacterial infection in rabbits. J Physiol (Lond) 1979; 295:419–30.
59. Moldawer LL, Hamawy KJ, Bistrian BR, et al. A therapeutic use for interleukin 1 in the protein depleted animal. Br J Rheumatol 1985; 24(suppl):220–4.
60. Drabik M, Schnure FC, Mok KT, et al. Effect of protein depletion and short-term parenteral nutrition on the host response to interleukin 1 administration. J Lab Clin Med 1987: 109:509–16.
61. Keenan RA, Moldawer LL, Yang RD, Kawamura I, Blackburn GL, Bistrian BR. An altered response by peripheral leukocytes to synthesize or release leukocyte endogenous mediator in critically-ill, protein malnourished patients. J Lab Clin Med 1982; 100:844–55.
62. Moldawer LL, Sobrado J, Blackburn GL, Bistrian BR. A rationale for administering leukocyte endogenous mediator (interleukin 1) to protein-malnourished, hospitalized patients. J Theor Biol 1984; 106:119–33.
63. Hamawy KJ, Yamazaki K, Georgieff M, et al. Improvements in host immunity by partially purified interleukin 1 in rats with portocaval anastomosis and splenectomy. J Parent Enter Nutr 1986; 10:146–50.
64. Mochizuki DY, Eisenman JR, Conlon PJ, Larsen AD, Tushinski RJ. Interleukin 1 regulates hematopoietic activity, a role previously ascribed to hematopoietin 1. Proc Natl Acad Sci U S A 1987; 84:5267–71.
65. Zucali JR, Dinarello CA, Oblon DJ, Gross MA, Anderson L, Weiner RS. Interleukin 1 stimulates fibroblasts to produce granulocyte-macrophage colony stimulating factor. J Clin Invest 1986; 77:1857–63.
66. Hangoc G, Williams DE, Falkenburg JHF, Broxmeyer HE. Influence of IL-1α and -1β on the survival of human bone marrow cells responding to hematopoietic colony-stimulating factors. J Immunol 1989; 142:4329–34.
67. Schaafsma MR, Fibbe WE, Van Damme J, et al. Interleukin-6 is not involved in the interleukin-1-induced production of colony-stimulating factors by human bone marrow stromal cells and fibroblasts. Blood 1989; 74:2619–23.
68. Tewari A, Buhles WC, Starnes HF. Preliminary report: effects of interleukin-1 on platelet counts. Lancet 1990; 336:712–714.
69. Campanile F, Binaglia L, Boraschi D, Tagliabue A, Fioretti MC, Puccetti P. Antibacterial resistance induced by recombinant interleukin 1 in myelosuppressed mice: effect of treatment schedule and correlation with colony-stimulating activity in the bloodstream. Cell Immunol 1990; 128:250–60.
70. Van der Meer JWM, Barza M, Wolff SM, Dinarello CA. A low dose of recombinant interleukin 1 protects granulocytopenic mice from lethal gram negative infection. Proc Natl Acad Sci U S A 1988; 85:1620–3.
71. Van der Meer JWM, Helle M, Aarden L. Comparison of the effects of recombinant interleukin 6 and recombinant interleukin 1 on nonspecific resistance to infection. Eur J Immunol 1989; 19:413–6.

72. Vant Wout JW, Van der Meer JW, Barza M, Dinarello CA. Protection of neutropenic mice from lethal *Candida albicans* infection by recombinant interleukin 1. Eur J Immunol 1988; 18:1143–6.
73. Czuprynski CJ, Brown JF. Recombinant murine interleukin 1 alpha enhancement of nonspecific antibacterial resistance. J Immunol 1987; 55:2061–5.
74. Czuprynski CJ, Brown JF, Young KM, Cooley AJ, Kurtz RS. Effects of murine recombinant interleukin 1 alpha on the host response to bacterial infection. J Immunol 1988; 140:962–8.
75. Kurtz RS, Roll JT, Czuprynski CJ. Recombinant human interleukin 1α enhances anti-Listeria resistance in both genetically resistant and susceptible strains of mice. Immunol Lett 1988; 18:289–92.
76. Kurtz RS, Young KM, Czuprynski CJ. Separate and combined effects of recombinant interleukin-1α and gamma interferon on antibacterial resistance. Infect Immun 1989; 57:553–8.
77. McIntyre KW, Unowsky J, DeLorenzo W, Benjamin W. Enhancement of antibacterial resistance of neutropenic, bone marrow-suppressed mice by interleukin-1α. Infect Immun 1989; 57:48–54.
78. Kurlander RJ, Hoffman M, Kratz SS, Gates J. Comparison of the effects of IL-1α and TNF-α on phagocyte accumulation and murine antibacterial immunity. Cell Immunol 1989; 123:9–22.
79. Nakai S, Hirai Y. The therapeutic potential of interleukin-1β in the treatment of chemotherapy and radiation induced myelosuppression and in tumor therapy. Biotherapy 1990; 1:33–354.
80. Bistrian BR, Blackburn GL, Vitale J, Cochran D, Naylor J. Prevalance of malnutrition in general medical patients. JAMA 1976; 235:1567–70.
81. Bistrian BR, Blackburn GL, Hallowell E, Heddle R. Protein status of general surgical patients. JAMA 1974; 230:858–60.
82. Crown J, Gabrilove J, Kemeny C, et al. Phase I-II trial of recombinant human interleukin-1β in patients with metastatic colorectal cancer receiving myelosuppressive doses of 5-fluorouracil. Proc ASCO 1990; 9:708A.
83. Fischen E, Marano MA, Barber A, et al. Interleukin-1α administration can replicate the hemodynamic and metabolic responses to sublethal endotoxemia. (in review)
84. Gasparetto C, Laver J, Abboud M, et al. Effects of interleukin-1 on hematopoietic progenitors: evidence of stimulatory and inhibitory activities in a primate model. Blood 1989; 74:547–50.
85. Johnson CS, Keckler DJ, Topper MI, Braunschweiger PG, Furmanski P. In vivo hematopoietic effects of recombinant interleukin-1α in mice. Blood 1989; 73:678–83.

CHAPTER 14

HEMATOLOGICAL EFFECTS OF CYTOKINES IN VIVO

Thomas R. Ulich

University of California
Irvine, California

INTRODUCTION

Cytokines exert a wide range of hematological effects on white and red blood cells in the bone marrow and in the peripheral circulation. The cytokines whose in vivo hematological effects are reviewed in this chapter can be broadly classified as the classic colony-stimulating factors multi-CSF, granulocyte-macrophage CSF (GM-CSF), G-CSF, M-CSF, and erythropoietin; the interleukins IL-1 to IL-8; the tumor necrosis factors (TNF) α and β; and the interferons (IFN) α, β, and γ. A complete understanding of the hematological effects of cytokines is only possible through the complementary study of both their in vitro and in vivo effects. The in vitro effects of cytokines in colony-forming assays are reviewed by McNiece (Chap. 4). The present chapter focuses on the hematological effects of exogenously administered recombinant cytokines in vivo in healthy nonmyelosuppressed hosts and only briefly alludes to the in vitro and ex vivo effects of cytokines. The interpretation of an exogenously administered cytokine's hematological effects in vivo are unfortunately always clouded by the inability to discern between direct and indirect effects. Most cytokines are well-known to induce the release of other cytokines, so that the indirect hematological effects of exogenously administered cytokines are no doubt of great significance. As monoclonal antisera to the endogenously released cytokines of experimental animals become more readily available, these indirect effects of the "cytokine cascade" will be deciphered. In the meantime, in vitro assays of cytokines on relatively purified bone marrow cell subpopulations provide an important means of dissecting the direct and indirect effects of cytokines on hematopoietic precursors and accessory cells.

Despite the limitations of in vivo experiments, the in vivo study of cytokines provides information that cannot be obtained in vitro. Margination or demargination of peripheral leukocytes, a process that may involve the cytokine-induced expression of leukocyte or endothelial adhesion molecules, can only be studied in vivo. In this regard, one must remember that the number of blood cells as enumerated by phlebotomy represents the circulating number of peripheral blood cells and, because of the existence of a substantial marginated pool, may in some situations (such as paradoxical leukopenias) not be representative of the total number of intravascular cells (1,2). The release of mature marrow cells, such as neutrophils or reticulocytes, from the marrow into the circulation can also not be appreciated in vitro. A cytokine's marrow cell releasing activity and hemoproliferative activity may be functionally reciprocal in that the continued presence of mature cells in the microenvironment of stem cells may initiate negative feedback mechanisms that would disappear in vivo with the release of the mature cells into the circulation. The proliferative effects of cytokines are kinetically different in vivo and in vitro. Proliferative effects in vivo as judged by marrow smears are usually apparent within hours, whereas the results of in vitro colony-forming assays are assessed after days or weeks. The microenvironments of the actual marrow and of bone marrow culture systems are clearly quite different, and thus the in vivo hematological effects of cytokines as determined by the sum total of all a cytokine's direct and indirect effects (permissive, additive, synergistic, or antagonistic) can only be judged by direct examination of the blood and marrow. The catabolism and consequently the half-lives of growth factors in vivo and in vitro must be disparate because of the different mechanisms of clearance in vivo (e.g., renal clearance), with a presumably more prolonged exposure of hematopoietic cells to growth factors in vitro. Finally the spatial limitations imposed on hematopoiesis by the marrow's microanatomy and by the confines of the osseous cortex are not reproduced in vitro, so that the hierarchical expansion of one marrow cell line in preference to another may not be appreciated in vitro. The study of the hematological effects of cytokines in vivo thus provides a complementary perspective to in vitro investigations.

This chapter, as previously mentioned, is largely limited to the description of the hematological effects of the administration of exogenous cytokines to non-myelosuppressed hosts. The therapeutic effects of cytokines in myelosuppressed hosts, which are one of the most promising clinical applications of many cytokines, are a subject of intensive current investigation but are beyond the scope of the present chapter. The in vivo role of hematopoietic negative regulators (3), such as transforming growth factor β, must be mentioned here as a subject that will no doubt grow rapidly in the next decade but as of now is still uncharted. The role of endogenous cytokine release under physiological and pathophysiological conditions is another important facet of the in vivo hematological effects of cytokines that can as of today only be touched upon sketchily. Cytokines no doubt play an important role in normal hematopoiesis as well as during the profound hematological changes noted during endotoxemia and during many other infectious and noninfectious inflammatory diseases. As immunological assays for the measurement of cytokines in serum and in inflammatory effusions become clinically more routinely available, the roles of cytokines in recruiting leukocytes from the marrow into the circulation and inflammatory sites will become more apparent. One of the insights that assays of cytokine levels in the clinic will provide is the knowledge of the pathophysiological (as opposed to the pharmacological) range of cytokine concentrations that are actually achieved in vivo in various diseases. The hematological effects noted after the administration of pharmacological amounts of cytokines may easily be misinterpreted as also being relevant to the effects of endogenously released cytokines during disease states. In this regard one should note that the hematological effects of many cytokines are very dose dependent as well as being dependent upon the route and frequency of administration. Since the kinetics, magnitude, and sources of the endogenous release of many cytokines under both physiological and pathophysiological conditions are still largely unexplored, caution must be exerted in extrapolating the results of pharmacological experiments toward an understanding of physiological and clinical hematological observations.

CLASSIC COLONY-STIMULATING FACTORS AND ERYTHROPOIETIN

Multi–Colony-Stimulating Factor

Multi-CSF, also commonly referred to today as IL-3, is a growth factor acting on proximal hematopoietic stem cells as evidenced by its in vitro direct and indirect effects on cells of erythroid, neutrophil, eosinophil, macrophage, mast cell, and megakaryocytic lineages (4,5).

In vivo, multi-CSF has been reported by several groups of investigators (6–10) to induce a number of hematological effects, although the effects on circulating numbers of peripheral blood cells have been generally much less marked compared to the effects of the other colony-stimulating factors or many other cytokines. In our experience (6,7), human multi-CSF injected intravenously (IV) as a single injection in rats induces a mild neutrophilia and monocytosis peaking at 8 h. The peripheral neutrophilia at 8 h is accompanied by a slight decrease in marrow neutrophils and by a left-shifted myeloid hyperplasia characterized by striking increases in myeloblasts. The marrow also demonstrates a slight increase in pronormoblasts. The peripheral blood and marrow at 24 h after injection are unremarkable. The effects of IL-3 did not demonstrate any significant dose-response relationship over a large range of doses. In vitro culture of rat marrow with human IL-3 did not promote colony formation. On the other hand, culture of rat marrow with human G-CSF also did not result in colony formation, suggesting that the in vitro action of cytokines on marrow cultures is not an absolute predictor of a cytokine's *in vivo* effects since human G-CSF is known to induce a dose-dependent neutrophilia and myeloid hyperplasia in vivo in the rat.

Metcalf et al. (8) studied the effects of homologous multi-CSF in the mouse and reported the occurrence of 2- to 3-fold increases in circulating neutrophils and monocytes and 10-fold increases in peripheral eosinophil numbers after repeated daily injections for up to 6 days. Splenomegaly was observed as a result of increases in the numbers of nucleated erythroid forms, granulocytes, and megakaryocytes and up to 100-fold rises in mast cells. No significant changes were seen in the marrow. Kindler et al. (9) administered multi-CSF via continuous infusion for 3–7 days in a murine model and noted enhancement of the number of myeloid and erythroid precursors in the spleen concomitantly with a decrease in progenitors in the marrow as measured by in vitro assay. The authors postulated that progenitor cells may be stimulated by multi-CSF to leave the marrow and colonize the spleen. Kimoto et al. (10) examined the effect of IL-3 on lymphopoiesis after administration of the cytokine to mice by osmotic minipumps for 1–4 weeks. Although a marked splenomegaly was described due to the accumulation of hematopoietic precursors, no increase in either T or B cells was seen in lymphoid organs. Lord et al. (11) noted that the proliferation rate of colony-forming unit-spleen cells (CFU-S) is rapidly increased after the administration of IL-3 to mice. A similar effect was observed by the same authors after the administration of endotoxin. Since IL-3 was not detectable in the blood of endotoxin-treated mice, the hypothesis was forwarded that lipopolysaccharide (LPS) acts indirectly on blood cell precursors by eliciting the local production of IL-3. In this context, our laboratory group has observed a similarity in the effect of intravenously administered multi-CSF and LPS on the proliferation of myeloblasts in rat marrow smears (6).

Multi-CSF has been reported to synergize with several other growth factors in vitro in colony-forming assays (12–14). In vivo, Donahue et al. (15) showed that multi-CSF and GM-CSF acted synergistically to promote hematopoiesis in primates that had been primed with multi-CSF before receiving GM-CSF. The coinjection of multi-CSF and G-CSF in rats induced only an additive peripheral neutrophilia, an effect that was generally not statistically significant because of the much greater magnitude of the G-CSF- as opposed to the multi-CSF-induced neutrophilia (7). On the other hand, the combination of multi-CSF and G-CSF induced a synergistic myeloid hyperplasia in the marrow after daily injections for 1 week. The combination of multi-CSF and IL-6, in addition to its reported synergistic effects on progenitors in vitro (12), has been reported to induce a synergistic increase in marrow mast cells in vivo (6), a finding that may be of relevance to the observation that IL-3 in the presence of pokeweed mitogen spleen cell-conditioned medium supports the expansion of mast cells in vitro (16).

Granulocyte-Macrophage Colony-Stimulating Factor

GM-CSF in vitro, in addition to supporting the growth of myeloid cells, can cause the growth of erythroid precursors and multipotential cells under appropriate assay conditions (17). GM-CSF in vivo induces peripheral neutrophilia, monocytosis, and eosinophilia in rodents (18,19), nonhuman primates (20,21), and humans (22,24).

Metcalf et al. (18) reported that mice injected intraperitoneally with murine GM-CSF three times daily for 6 days developed a 2-fold increase in blood neutrophils as the only significant change in the peripheral circulation. In the peritoneal cavity, up to a 15-fold increase in macrophages, a 100-fold increase in neutrophils, and a 100-fold increase in eosinophils was noted. The peritoneal macrophages also exhibited increased phagocytic activity for antibody-coated erythrocytes. Increased numbers of neutrophils and monocytes were observed in the liver and lung.

A single IV injection of murine GM-CSF in rats (19) causes a brief initial neutropenia and monocytopenia reaching a nadir at 15 minutes and followed by neutrophilia and monocytosis peaking between 4 and 8 h and subsiding to baseline levels by 12 h. The marrow at 6 h shows a decrease in mature neutrophils and a slight left-shifted myeloid hyperplasia. The marrow differential at 24 h is unremarkable. GM-CSF also causes a mild peripheral lymphopenia. GM-CSF-induced lymphopenia may not reflect a direct effect on lymphocytes but rather may represent GM-CSF-induced gene expression of IL-1 or other cytokines that are known to induce lymphopenia. Daily injection of GM-CSF in rats for 1 week induced a repetitive daily neutrophilia with no evidence of either the development of tolerance or of any cumulative increase in the number of circulating neutrophils.

Donahue et al. (20) reported that continuous infusion of GM-CSF in rhesus macaque monkeys induced an increase in circulating neutrophils, eosinophils, monocytes, and lymphocytes, as well as a modest increase in circulating reticulocytes. GM-CSF in rhesus monkeys was similarly reported by Mayer et al. (21) to steadily increase total circulating leukocyte counts with fivefold increases in granulocytes, two- to fourfold increases in lymphocytes, and three- to fourfold increases in monocytes.

GM-CSF was administered for 3 days by Aglietta et al. (23) to patients who had normal bone marrows. Peripheral neutrophilia, eosinophilia, and monocytosis was noted as well as an increase in morphologically recognizable granulo-monopoietic precursors in posttreatment marrow smears. The left-shifted myeloid hyperplasia in the marrow resulted in a relative decrease in marrow lymphocytes, but no peripheral lymphopenia occurred. As an interesting correlate to the previously mentioned in vitro effect of GM-CSF on erythroid precursors, GM-CSF in vivo caused an increase in the percentage of marrow BFU-E in *S* phase, although no accompanying increase in marrow normoblasts was morphologically recognizable (23).

GM-CSF in vivo also activates circulating neutrophils as evidenced by their enhanced oxidative metabolism and killing of bacteria (21) and by the induction of IgA-mediated phagocytosis (25).

GM-CSF has been observed to act synergistically with other growth factors, such as IL-3, G-CSF, and M-CSF, in vitro (26–28). In vivo, GM-CSF acted synergistically with IL-3 when primates were primed with IL-3 for several days before receiving GM-CSF (15). GM-CSF coinjected with G-CSF in rats as either a single injection or as daily injections for a week induced an approximately additive increase in peripheral neutrophils (19).

Granulocyte Colony-Stimulating Factor

G-CSF supports the proliferation and differentiation of neutrophils in vitro (29) and induces neutrophilia in rodents (30,31), nonhuman primates (32), and humans (24) in vivo. A single injection of G-CSF causes an initial peripheral neutropenia at 15 minutes in rats (31). A similar transient early neutropenia occurs in humans. The mechanism of G-CSF-induced neutropenia is unknown but may conceivably involve G-CSF-induced activation of circulating neutrophils with resultant expression of neutrophil adhesion molecules that would promote systemic margination of neutrophils. Alternatively, neutrophil activation may result in intravascular aggregation and clearance of neutrophils. G-CSF-induced neutropenia is followed by neutrophilia beginning at 30 minutes and peaking at 12 h in rats or hamsters. The number of circulating neutrophils in rats subsides to baseline between 30 and 36 h, but the morphology of the neutrophils at these time points is remarkable for the hypersegmentation of their nuclei. Hypersegmentation of neutrophils has also been reported in humans receiving G-CSF. The marrow of G-CSF-treated rats at 4 and 12 h exhibits an increase in number, mitoses, size, and cytoplasmic granulation of myeloblasts and promyelocytes but a decrease in mature neutrophils, demonstrating that G-CSF acts not only as a mitogen and growth factor for early cells in the myeloid series but also as a releasing factor for mature marrow neutrophils. The bone marrow at 48 h contains slightly increased numbers of myelocytes and metamyelocytes and large numbers of hypersegmented neutrophils. Some of the hypersegmented neutrophils contain nuclear drumsticklike protrusions (31).

Chronic administration of G-CSF to cynomolgus monkeys for 2–4 weeks induces a dose-dependent increase in circulating neutrophils that plateaus after 1 week and is thereafter sustained (32). In rats, single daily IV injections of a constant dose of G-CSF induce an initial large peripheral neutrophilia that is followed on days 2–4 by a decrease in the number of circulating neutrophils and on days 5–7 with an increase in circulating neutrophils (33). The mechanism of the transient trough in neutrophil numbers during daily injection of G-CSF may reasonably be postulated to be due to the marrow-releasing effect of G-CSF and a resultant depleted marrow reserve of neutrophils. The marrow after 3 days of G-CSF injections, however, contains over twice as many mature neutrophils as control or time zero marrows. The trough in peripheral neutrophilia may therefore be postulated to be due to an as yet unidentified inhibitor of neutrophil release, although other mechanisms of tolerance are possible. A similar trough in peripheral neutrophil numbers after daily injections of G-CSF has not been reported in primates or humans. The marrow at 24 h after a week of daily injections of G-CSF shows a striking myeloid hyperplasia at the maturational level of mature neutrophils with little or no increase in numbers of myeloid precursors.

Macrophage Colony-Stimulating Factor

M-CSF in vitro stimulates the proliferation of macrophages and synergizes in regard to this function with multi-CSF, GM-CSF, and TNF (34–36). M-CSF also activates cells of the monocyte-macrophage system as evidenced by the enhancement of macrophage tumoricidal activity (37) and by the induction of monocyte migration (38) in vitro. M-CSF in vivo causes peripheral monocytosis in mice (39–41), rats (42), and primates (43). Human M-CSF is active in vivo in all these species. The increased number of monocytes in the circulation of M-CSF-treated animals may contribute to an increase in reticuloendothelial cells, or M-CSF may cause proliferation of reticuloendothelial cells as evidenced by the increase in Kupffer's cells in M-CSF-treated mice (40).

In mice, Koren et al. (39) reported slight monocytosis, neutrophilia, and lymphopenia after 4 days of M-CSF administration. Also in mice injected with M-CSF for 4 days, Hume et al. (40) reported a 10-fold increase in monocytes, as well as lymphopenia. Broxmeyer et al. (41) also noted an increase in circulating monocytes in M-CSF-treated mice. In rats, a single injection of M-CSF was observed in our laboratory (42) to induce mild peripheral neutrophilia and lymphopenia between 2 and 16 h after injection and monocytosis beginning at 20–24 h, peaking at 28–32 h, and subsiding to baseline levels by 36–48 h. The M-CSF-induced monocytosis was postulated to represent a direct effect of M-CSF on marrow monocyte precursor proliferation, maturation, and release, whereas the neutrophilia and lymphopenia may reflect indirect effects mediated by the known ability of M-CSF to cause the release of other cytokines (44). Unlike neutrophils, which are present in a large reserve pool in the marrow, monocytes are present in the marrow in relatively small numbers (approximately 1–2% of marrow cells) and must therefore first proliferate and mature before they can be released into the circulation in large numbers. Interestingly, the peripheral monocytosis in M-CSF-treated rats was characterized not only by mature monocytes but also by promonocytes with nonlobated nuclei. Garnick et al. (43) noted striking vacuolization and increased Ia antigen expression in the circulating monocytes and macrophage-like cells of M-CSF-treated rats and primates suggesting activation of these cells by M-CSF. In a toxicological study in cynomolgus monkeys by the same authors, a reversible dose-related thrombocytopenia, as well as slight and reversible decreases in the red blood cell count, hemogobin, and hematocrit, was observed.

Erythropoietin

EPO in vitro stimulates erythroid colony formation and also stimulates megakaryocytopoiesis via a direct effect on megakaryocyte progenitors that have receptors for EPO (45).

EPO in vivo given as a single IV injection to rats causes peripheral reticulocytosis beginning within 24 h and reaching a maximum at 3 days (46,47). The reticulocytosis is left-shifted as defined by a relative and absolute increase in immature or so-called type I and II reticulocytes (47). The marrow shows an increase in pronormoblasts and early normoblasts within the first 24 h after the injection of EPO, followed by a right-shifted erythroid hyperplasia on the following days. Daily injection of EPO in rats for 1 week results in a sustained erythroid hyperplasia in the marrow, a striking peripheral reticulocytosis, increases in the hematocrit and hemoglobin, and massive splenomegaly (47). Chronic daily administration of EPO for 12–14 days results in steady-state erythrocyte levels at 20% above control (48). The steady state is associated with a return of reticulocyte levels to control levels despite the continued administration of EPO. EPO administered on the same daily basis also caused an increase in platelets on days 2–8, but not at later time points (48). Interestingly, a transient increase in circulating white blood cells was also reported during the administration of EPO (48).

EPO has been approved by the Food and Drug Administration for the treatment of the anemia associated with chronic renal failure. EPO in anemic renal failure patients raises the hematocrit and hemoglobin and dramatically improves the quality of life (49). EPO is well tolerated by patients, although elevations in blood pressure may be associated with the increased peripheral vascular resistance resulting from the rising hematocrit. Iron supplementation is needed to maintain the therapeutic efficacy of EPO as body iron stores decline as a result of the increase in erythropoiesis. The peripheral blood of EPO-treated patients is reported to contain an increased number not only of blast-forming units-erythroid cells (BFU-E) but also of CFU-GEMM (50). Circulating numbers of CFU-GM were not elevated (50).

INTERLEUKINS

Interleukin-1

IL-1 is a cytokine that no doubt contributed very significantly to the activity of the preparation described by Kampschmidt and his colleagues (51) as leukocyte endogenous mediator (LEM). LEM was shown to induce a neutrophilia at 60–90 minutes after injection into rats. The neutrophilia was accompanied by a decrease in marrow neutrophils, suggesting that the release of marrow neutrophils contributed to the peripheral increase in circulating numbers of neutrophils. Recombinant IL-1α and β at low doses (25 U per rat) were reported by our laboratory (52) to induce a monophasic neutrophilia in rats peaking at 90 minutes after IV injection. IL-1α has been hypothesized to be the membrane form of IL-1α and IL-1β the major cytosolic or secreted form, although the validity of this concept has come into question (53). At the dose studied in our experiments, IL-1β caused a greater peripheral neutrophilia than IL-1α and exhibited more potent neutrophil releasing activity than IL-1α. IL-1β caused the release of 70% of the marrow reserve of mature neutrophils, whereas IL-1α caused the release of approximately 30% of marrow neutrophils. The peripheral neutrophilia was characterized by an increase in circulating band forms as well as by the presence of occasional metamyelocytes, observations that also suggest marrow release of neutrophils. IL-1α and β also both induced a significant absolute lymphopenia accompanying the peripheral neutrophilia. At higher doses, IL-1 induces a rapid and profound granulocytopenia (54). The granulocytopenia is followed at later time points (such as 12 h) by granulocytosis. We also observed that IL-1 induces neutropenia at high doses (unpublished data), although at the high doses studied in our laboratory the rats were clinically hypotensive. IL-1 is known to cause hypotension at high doses (55). Whereas the discrimination between the direct and indirect hematological effects of a cytokine in vivo are problematical in any case, the effects of a cytokine at doses that cause hypotension are even more difficult to interpret since hypotension itself causes neutrophilia (56). At low doses, IL-1 causes neutrophilia in the absence of any changes in blood pressure (52). Since the concentrations of IL-1 measured in septic patients have generally been only three times elevated over background levels (57), the hematological observations made in vivo after the administration of high doses of IL-1 may not be relevant to an understanding of the pathophysiological role of IL-1, although they are certainly of great pharmacological importance. IL-1 at low doses also causes neutrophilia in adrenalectomized rats (52), an observation that is of interest since IL-1 has been reported to possess corticotropin releasing activity (54) and because both adrenocortical and medullary hormones affect circulating numbers of granulocytes and lymphocytes (2).

Daily injection of low doses of IL-1 induces a repetitive daily neutrophilia and a mild myeloid hyperplasia in the marrow at the end of a week (33). The myeloproliferative effect of IL-1 may in part reflect the release of endogenous serum colony-stimulating activity at 3–6 h and the increase in marrow CFU-GM at 48 h after the injection of IL-1 as reported by Stork et al. (58) and similarly by Vogel et al. (59) in mice.

Interleukin-2

IL-2, also known as T cell growth factor, promotes the growth of T cells in vitro. Among the interleukins, the in vivo hematological effects of IL-2 in humans are at present perhaps the best studied because of the use of IL-2 in combination with lymphokine-activated killer (LAK) cells as an experimental therapy for cancer patients by Rosenberg and his colleagues (60).

In rats, daily administration of IL-2 was reported by Anderson et al. (61,62) to cause a dose- and regimen-related lymphocytosis, neutrophilia, eosinophilia, thrombocytopenia, hemolytic anemia, lymphoid hyperplasia, and extramedullary erythropoiesis and eosinopoiesis in the spleen. Large numbers of mononuclear cells accumulated in the hepatic sinusoids. Pleural effusions occurred composed predominantly of large granular lymphocytes (62). In mice receiving repeated injections of IL-2, Ettinghausen et al. (63) observed prominent accumulations of activated lymphocytes in lungs, liver, spleen, kidneys, and mesenteric lymph nodes as confirmed both by an in vivo DNA labeling technique as well as by histological study. In sheep receiving a daily brief infusion of IL-2, Jesmok and Gunther (64) noted a lymphopenia and neutrophilia after the first day's infusion and a more pronounced lymphopenia and neutropenia within 2–4 h after the subsequent days' infusions. Baseline leukocyte levels in the IL-2-treated sheep (i.e., 24 h after the previous day's infusion) increased progressively. As is clear from the foregoing experiments and from the following results in patients, the hematological effects of IL-2 are very dose and regimen dependent as well as dependent upon the time of sampling of the peripheral blood.

A single bolus of IL-2 in humans causes a dramatic decrease in peripheral blood T cells beginning as early as 15 minutes after injection with a progressively greater lymphopenia for the first 4 h followed by a rebound lymphocytosis at 48 h (65). Continuous infusion of IL-2 resulted in an often depressed lymphocyte count during the first week followed by a progressive increase in circulating lymphocytes ranging from 2- to 16-fold over baseline (65). In a review of the hematological effects of IL-2 in combination with LAK cells, Ettinghausen et al. (60) reported that the large majority of patients developed an anemia that could not be explained on the basis of phlebotomy, cytopheresis, or hemodilution and that required red cell transfusions. Anemia was accompanied by reticulocytopenia. IL-2 administration also resulted in an often severe thrombocytopenia, lymphopenia, and eosinophilia. Mild neutropenia and rebound lymphocytosis followed the discontinuation of IL-2 therapy. Colony assays on the peripheral blood of patients showed a decline in circulating erythroid and granulocyte-macrophage progenitors. Furthermore, IL-2 also induced the appearance of circulating interferon-γ, suggesting that IL-2 may also indirectly suppress hematopoiesis.

Interleukin-3

IL-3 is a synonym for multi-CSF, whose hematological effects have already been described.

Interleukin-4

IL-4 in vivo, in addition to its many effects on B cells, downregulates LPS-induced IL-1 and TNF expression by monocytes (66), an action that may potentially implicate IL-4 as a downregulating influence on LPS-induced hematological effects in vivo. Although no published reports of the in vivo effects of IL-4 on peripheral blood and marrow smears are available, Dr. Donna Rennick (DNAX, Palo Alto, CA) has not observed any changes in the total leukocyte count or differential of the peripheral blood after experimental administration of IL-4 (personal communication).

Interleukin-5

IL-5, also known as eosinophil differentiation factor, causes the proliferation of eosinophil colonies in vitro (67). IL-5 also acts as a B cell growth factor in vitro in mice but apparently not in human lymphocyte cultures (67). The concept that the pathogenesis of eosinophilia is regulated in vivo by a lymphokine is suggested by the T cell dependence of parasite-induced eosinophilia in rats (68). Although administration of other cytokines, such as GM-CSF and IL-2, causes peripheral and tissue eosinophilia, IL-5 is especially implicated in the pathogenesis of eosinophilia in vivo because antiserum to IL-5 inhibits the eosinophilia noted during experimental parasitemia in mice (69). Samoszuk and Nansen (70) have found a correlation between the expression of IL-5 mRNA as detected by in situ hybridization in the Reed-Sternberg cells of Hodgkin's disease and tissue eosinophilia in the lymph nodes of these patients. We are unaware of any reports of the hematological effects of recombinant IL-5 after its administration to experimental animals. Our laboratory group injected doses of up to 150 μg of recombinant bacteria-derived human IL-5 to rats without observing any peripheral or marrow eosinophilia within the first 24 h (unpublished data, Ulich, del Castillo, and Yang). However, the cross-species nature of these experiments as well as the nonglycosylated form of the molecule precludes any meaningful conclusions.

Interleukin-6

IL-6 is an extraordinarily multifunctional peptide growth factor that has also been identified under such diverse names as interferon-β_2, B cell stimulating factor, hybridoma growth factor, hepatocyte-stimulating factor, 26 kD protein, and myeloid blood cell differentiation inducing protein (71,72). IL-6 in vitro has been reported to enhance IL-3-dependent proliferation of hematopoietic precursors (12), as well as to enhance colony formation of almost all the hematopoietic lineages when combined with appropriate lineage-restricted growth factors (73). The relative contributions of the direct and indirect effects of IL-6 on the observed in vitro results are still unclear (73). Continuous perfusion of mice with IL-6 for 7 days increases the number of splenic, but not marrow, hematopoietic stem cells (CFU-S) (74).

IL-6 administered as a single IV injection to rats induces a mild peripheral neutrophilia (75). The marrow shows a mild left-shifted hyperplasia but does not show a significant decrease in mature marrow neutrophils, suggesting that IL-6 affects the proliferation of early myeloid precursors but that the source of the increase in peripheral neutrophils may be from the marginated pool rather than from the marrow reserve. The most striking peripheral hematological change after an injection of IL-6 is the reticulocytosis that occurs at 12–24 h. The reticulocytosis is accompanied by an erythroid hyperplasia of late normoblasts in the marrow. The kinetics of the IL-6-induced reticulocytosis and erythroid hyperplasia are different from those of EPO (47). The number of circulating reticulocytes returns to baseline within 48 h after the injection of IL-6, whereas the reticulocyte count is still increasing at 48 h after the injection of EPO and does not reach a maximum until 72 h. Whereas the marrow at 24 h after the injection of IL-6 demonstrates a right-shifted erythroid hyperplasia, the marrow at the same time after injection of EPO shows a more left-shifted erythroid hyperplasia. At 48 h after the injection of IL-6, the marrow differential is unremarkable, whereas at the same time after the injection of EPO a right-shifted erythroid hyperplasia has developed. The foregoing sequence of changes in the marrow is consistent with the hypothesis that EPO acts on an earlier erythroid precursor than IL-6. Furthermore, continued daily injections of IL-6 for 1 week do not result in a continued erythroid hyperplasia, whereas daily injections of EPO causes a progressive reticulocytosis and erythroid marrow hyperplasia (47). With regard to the erythropoietic effect of IL-6 in vivo, one may note that Rennick et al. (76) reported that IL-6 increased the number of erythrocyte colonies supported by IL-4 and EPO, although IL-6 had no erythroid growth-promoting activity of its own. The transient in vivo enhancement of erythropoiesis by IL-6 may thus be an indirect effect or the result of an in vivo interaction with endogenous IL-4, EPO, or another growth factor.

Injections of IL-6 every 12 h for 5 days in mice caused thrombocytosis as well as an increase in the size but not the number of megakaryocytes in the marrow (77). The dual in vivo effect of IL-6 on erythropoiesis and thrombocytopoiesis is qualitatively somewhat reminiscent of the in vivo effect of EPO.

IL-6 has been reported to synergize in vitro with several other growth factors, such as IL-3, IL-4, M-CSF, G-CSF, and erythropoietin (reviewed in Ref. 73). The combination of IL-6 and IL-3 in vivo in rats caused an increase in marrow mast cells not seen after the administration of either factor alone (6). Of potential significance to an understanding of the interactions of the hematological effects of cytokines in vivo is the report of Schindler et al. (78) that IL-6 suppresses TNF and IL-1 production by LPS in human peripheral blood mononuclear cells and the report of Vilcek and his coworkers (79) that IL-6 decreases LPS-induced serum TNF levels in vivo in mice. Our laboratory group recently observed that splenic IL-6 mRNA peaks 1–2 h after the expression of TNF and IL-1 mRNA in LPS-injected rats (unpublished observations), a time sequence that may be consistent with a negative feedback effect of IL-6.

Interleukin-7

IL-7 in vitro supports the growth of early B cells and is a comitogen for T cells (80). IL-7 in vivo has recently been reported to stimulate B-cell and T-cell lymphopoiesis in the lymph nodes and spleen of normal mice (80a).

Interleukin-8

IL-8, also known by such names as monocyte-derived neutrophil chemotactic factor and neutrophil activating factor, is an inflammatory cytokine inducible by IL-1 and TNF and is apparently one of the major neutrophil chemotactic factors in the supernatants of endotoxin-stimulated human peripheral blood mononuclear cells (81). IL-8 has been reported by Rampart et al. (82) to induce an acute neutrophilic inflammatory infiltrate when injected intradermally in combination with the vasodilator prostaglandin E_2 (but not when injected by itself). IL-8 causes an initial peripheral neutropenia followed by neutrophilia.

INTERFERONS

Interferons, originally discovered on the basis of their antiviral effects, also display a wide range of antiproliferative and immunomodulatory effects. In vitro, the IFNs all inhibit myeloid colony formation, with IFN-γ the most potent inhibitor and synergizing in this regard with IFN-α and β (83). The in vitro inhibitory effects of the IFNs can be overcome by the addition of colony-stimulating factor in conditioned medium (83). The occurrence of granulocytopenia is one of the most well known in vivo hematological effects of interferons in humans (84). In mice, all three types of IFNs (α, β, and γ) were reported by Koren et al. (39) to cause a generalized reduction of granulocytes, monocytes, and lymphocytes in the circulation. IFN-γ was 50- to 100-fold more potent in its myelosuppressive activity. IFN-induced peripheral lymphopenia in mice is accompanied by peripheral lymphadenopathy and a decrease in the number of thoracic duct lymphocytes as reported by Gresser et al. (85), who postulated that by inhibiting the egress of lymphocytes from lymphoid tissues IFN may contribute to the lymphadenopathy noted clinically in viral diseases. Interferon has been postulated to be a mediator of the hematopoietic suppression observed in aplastic anemia patients whose sera may contain elevated levels of IFN and whose marrow cells demonstrate an increase in colony formation activity after incubation with antiserum to IFN in vitro (86).

TUMOR NECROSIS FACTOR

TNF-α, also known as cachectin, and TNF-β, also known as lymphotoxin, are proteins that share a moderate amino acid homology and can bind to the same receptor (87). TNF in vitro exerts both stimulatory and inhibitory hematopoietic effects in varying colony-forming assays and the significance of these results to the in vivo effects of the same molecules is sometimes difficult to ascertain (88). TNF-α and β induce similar hematological effects in vivo (52,89) and are therefore discussed together.

TNF in mice was reported by Remick et al. (90) to induce a brief neutropenia followed by a monophasic left-shifted neutrophilia and accompanied by a peripheral lymphopenia characterized by a preferential decrease in B cells. TNF in rats also causes neutropenia at 30 minutes followed at 1–2 h by neutrophilia (52). The neutropenia may be due to transient intravascular margination since epinephrine, a demarginating factor that does not cause the release of marrow neutrophils, reverses TNF-induced neutropenia (2). Further support for the hypothesis that the initial neutropenia is due to intravascular margination is found in the observation that TNF administration causes a reduction in the circulating number of neutrophils during experimental neutrophilia (2), suggesting that TNF actively causes neutrophils to leave the circulation, perhaps by margination resulting from the expression of neutrophil-endothelial adherence molecules. In this regard, Gamble et al. (91) reported that TNF in vitro stimulates the adherence of neutrophils to endothelium by a rapid protein synthesis-independent effect on neutrophils as well as by a slower de novo RNA and protein synthesis-dependent effect on endothelium. TNF in vitro also activates neutrophils, promotes neutrophil aggregation, and is chemotactic for neutrophils and monocytes (92,93). Neutrophil aggregation in vivo after the administration of TNF could hypothetically contribute to neutropenia as a result of microembolization.

At relatively low doses (doses that are not accompanied by hypotension, clinically observable toxicity, or histologically observable tissue injury), the TNF-induced neutrophilia in rats, in contrast to that observed in mice, is biphasic (52). The peripheral neutrophilia is accompanied by a decrease in marrow neutrophils and an increase in circulating band cells, suggesting that the marrow reserve of neutrophils contributes to the increase in circulating neutrophils. The second wave of TNF-induced neutrophilia is of lesser magnitude and is temporally broader (i.e., of longer duration) than the first peak, suggesting that the second wave is due to the release of an endogenous factor. The second wave of neutrophilia is augmented in *Corynebacterium parvum*-primed rats, which exhibit hyperplasia of the reticuloendothelial system (94), and in IFN-γ-primed rats (2). The second wave of neutrophilia has specifically been postulated to be due to the TNF-induced release of endogenous IL-1 (52) on the basis that (1) TNF has been reported to induce the release of IL-1 both in vitro (95) and in vivo (96), (2) indomethacin and dexamethasone, which inhibit IL-1-induced neutrophilia, also abrogate the second peak of TNF-induced neutrophilia (52), and (3) TNF induces a biphasic febrile response in rabbits that has similar kinetics to the biphasic neutrophilia in rats and in which the second wave of fever is accompanied by an increase in serum IL-1 (96). Our laboratory has recently also noted that TNF-injected rats demonstrate an increase in splenic IL-1 mRNA at the time of the second wave of neutrophilia (unpublished observation). TNF in vitro has been shown to induce the synthesis of G-CSF and GM-CSF (97), raising the possibility that these myeloid growth factors contribute to TNF-induced neutrophilia and to the striking myeloid marrow hyperplasia observed in rats treated chronically with high doses of TNF (98). TNF at higher doses in rats induces a more pronounced initial peripheral neutropenia followed by a greater and more sustained monophasic neutrophilia (98). The qualitative and quantitative changes in circulating numbers of neutrophils observed after high doses of TNF are thus indistinguishable from those observed after experimental administration of moderate to high doses of endotoxin (94), a correlation that takes on important pathophysiological significance since endotoxin is known to cause the release of TNF in vivo (99) and because Remick et al. (100) reported that antiserum to TNF inhibits endotoxin-induced neutrophilia in mice. Daily injections of high doses of TNF for 1 week cause a striking myeloid hyperplasia (98), an effect that may in part be postulated to be due to the in vivo release of colony-stimulating factor after administration of TNF (59).

TNF, similarly to endotoxin as well as to a number of other previously mentioned cytokines, causes peripheral lymphopenia. Among the mechanisms that might be postulated to account for the lymphopenia are a cytotoxic effect on lymphocytes, intravascular margination, emigration of lymphocytes into lymphoid or nonlymphoid tissues, or a decrease in recirculation of lymphocytes from the thoracic duct into the circulation (2). The possibility that TNF might induce lympholysis was suggested by Remick et al. (90). However, no in vitro cytotoxicity of TNF for murine peripheral blood mononuclear cells could be demonstrated. A transient decrease in lymphocyte recirculation from the thoracic duct could also explain the observation of peripheral lymphopenia. The importance of thoracic duct recirculation in the maintenance of circulating lymphocyte levels is apparent in the rapid peripheral lymphopenia that occurs in rats from which lymph from the thoracic duct is drained. In rats in which the thoracic duct was cannulated, however, no evidence of a decrease in either lymphocyte recirculation or lymph flow was noted after the administration of TNF (2). The hypothesis that TNF induces lymphopenia via a receptor-mediated interaction between lymphocytes and endothelium is attractive in view of in vitro evidence by Bevilacqua et al. (101) and by Cavender et al. (102) that TNF induces the synthesis of endothelial adhesion molecules that bind lymphocytes and in view of the immunohistochemical finding of Cotran et al. (103) that endothelial adhesion molecules are expressed in vivo within the high endothelium at the site of delayed hypersensitivity reactions. The in vitro binding of lymphocytes to endothelial monolayers reaches a maximum at 4–6 h after TNF treatment (102), kinetics that are quite analagous to our observations on the in vivo kinetics of TNF-induced lymphopenia.

TNF was reported by Michie et al. (104) to be elevated in the serum of healthy men after the experimental intravenous injection of *Escherichia coli* endotoxin. Since endotoxin induces the release of TNF into serum, endotoxin and TNF are likely to be present together in the circulation of patients when endotoxemia occurs during Gram-negative bacterial infections. Coinjection of endotoxin and TNF in rats markedly increases both the magnitude and duration of endotoxin-induced neutropenia, neutrophilia, and lymphopenia (94). TNF also interacts with IL-1 and adrenal hormones in a fashion that suggests that these endogenous factors may all contribute to the changes in circulating numbers of leukocytes noted during Gram-negative infections (2).

In addition to effects on myeloid and lymphoid cells, TNF exerts profound and dose-dependent effects on erythropoiesis in vivo. Cerami and his colleagues (105) noted that rats treated with high doses of TNF developed anemia characterized by a decrease in red blood cell synthesis and a reduced circulating erythrocyte life span. An anemia of similar magnitude was described after the administration of endotoxin, but not after the administration of IL-1, suggesting that TNF may be implicated in the pathogenesis of the anemia of chronic inflammatory diseases. TNF has been reported by Broxmeyer et al. (106) to inhibit erythropoiesis in vitro. Our laboratory (98) noted a peripheral anemia and marrow erythroid hypoplasia in rats treated for a week with high doses of TNF. The erythroid hypoplasia was postulated to in part represent a myelophthisic anemia secondary to a striking myeloid hyperplasia. EPO has been reported to prevent the decrease in hematocrit observed after TNF treatment of mice for 5 days (107).

TABLE 1 Morphologically Recognizable Hematological Effects of Cytokines on the Peripheral Blood and Bone Marrow

Cytokines	Effects
Classic colony stimulating factors	
Multi-CSF	Mild neutrophilia; mild monocytosis; basophilia; moderate eosinophilia; increased marrow blasts; increased splenic megakaryocytes, nucleated erythroid forms, and mast cells
GM-CSF	Initial brief neutropenia followed by neutrophilia; initial monocytopenia followed by monocytosis; eosinophilia; possible basophilia; mild lymphopenia; mild left-shifted myeloid marrow hyperplasia
G-CSF	Initial brief neutropenia followed by marked neutrophilia; marked marrow myeloid hyperplasia; hypersegmented neutrophils; erythroid hypoplasia at high doses
M-CSF	Marked monocytosis; immature, vacuolated, and macrophagelike circulating forms; mild neutrophilia and lymphopenia
EPO	Reticulocytosis; increased peripheral red blood cell indices; thrombocytosis; erythroid marrow hyperplasia; myeloid marrow hypoplasia at high doses
Interleukins	
IL-1	Initial neutropenia at high doses; neutrophilia; lymphopenia; myeloid hyperplasia after repeated administration
IL-2	Initial lymphopenia; lymphocytosis after repeated administration; eosinophilia; anemia
IL-3	Synonym for multi-CSF
IL-4	No effects noted to date (personal communication, Donna Rennick)
IL-5	Eosinophilia is inhibited by antibody to IL-5
IL-6	Mild neutrophilia and lymphopenia; transient reticulocytosis; thrombocytosis; transient late normoblast hyperplasia in marrow; increase in megakaryocyte size in marrow
IL-7	No data
IL-8	Initial brief neutropenia at high doses; neutrophilia
Interferons	Suppression of circulating numbers of neutrophils, monocytes, and lymphocytes
Tumor necrosis factors	Initial neutropenia followed by monophasic or biphasic neutrophilia; lymphopenia; anemia at high doses; erythroid marrow hyperplasia and dysplasia at low doses; myeloid marrow hyperplasia and erythroid hypoplasia at high doses

TNF has also, however, been reported to stimulate erythropoisis in both ex vivo (108) and in vivo experiments (33,98). Johnson et al. (108) found that a single IV injection of a relatively high dose of TNF caused an increase in immature erythroid cells (BFU-E), although inhibiting later stage erythropoiesis as measured by the number of CFU-E in the marrow. Our laboratory group (33,98) observed that low doses of TNF administered to rats as a daily IV dose for 1 week cause an erythroid hyperplasia of late normoblasts. The normoblasts are morphologically dysplastic in their sometimes striking nuclear fragmentation, however, and no increase in circulating red blood cells is observed, suggesting a state of ineffective erythropoiesis (98). Interestingly, TNF has been reported by Clark and Chandri to induce dyserythropoiesis and erythrophagocytosis in experimental malaria (109).

CONCLUSIONS

A summary of the morphologically recognizable hematological effects of the cytokines discussed in this chapter is presented in Table 1. Cytokines are also of course known to affect hematopoietic precursors that are not morphologically recognizable but are readily detectable in ex vivo colony-forming assays of peripheral blood and marrow cells. The short-term and especially the long-term effects of cytokines on these stem cells should not be overlooked. In addition to studying the potential therapeutic uses of pharmacological doses of cytokines, an important puzzle for future investigators is to piece together the way in which the "cytokine cascade" or "cytokine network" functions in vivo to maintain hematopoietic homeostasis during health and to direct the proliferation, trafficking, and activation of blood cells during inflammation and disease.

REFERENCES

1. van Furth R, Sluiter W. Distribution of blood monocytes between a marginating and circulating pool. J Exp Med 1986; 163:474–9.
2. Ulich TR, del Castillo J, Ni RX, Bikhazi N, Calvin L. Mechanisms of TNF-induced lymphopenia, neutropenia, and biphasic neutrophilia. J Leuk Biol 1989; 45:155–67.
3. Axelrad AA. Some hemopoietic negative regulators. Exp Hematol 1990; 18:143–50.
4. Bot F, Dorssers L, Wagemaker G, Lowenberg B. Stimulating spectrum of human recombinant multi-CSF (IL-3) on human marrow precursor: importance of accessory cells. Blood 1988; 71:1609.
5. Prystowsky MB, Otten G, Nanjokas MG, et al. Multiple hemopoietic lineages are found after stimulation of mouse bone marrow precursor cells with interleukin-3. Am J Pathol 1984; 117:171.
6. Ulich TR, del Castillo J, Busser K, Guo K, Yin S. Acute in vivo effects of IL-3 alone and in combination with IL-6 on the blood cells of the circulation and bone marrow. Am J Pathol 1989; 135:663–70.
7. Ulich TR, del Castillo J, McNiece IK, et al. Acute and subacute hematologic effects of multi-CSF in combination with G-CSF in vivo. Blood 1990; 75:48–53.
8. Metcalf D, Bagley CG, Johnson GR, Nicola NA, Lopez AF, Williamson DJ. Effects of purified bacterially synthesized murine multi-CSF (IL-3) on hematopoiesis in normal adult mice. Blood 1986; 68:46–57.

9. Kindler V, Thorens B, de Kossodo S, et al. Stimulation of hematopoiesis in vivo by recombinant bacterial murine IL-3. Proc Natl Acad Sci U S A 1986; 83:1001–5.
10. Kimoto M, Kindler V, Higaki M, Ody C, Izui S, Vassalli P. Recombinant murine IL-3 fails to stimulate T or B lymphopoiesis in vivo, but enhances immune responses to T-cell dependent antigens. J Immunol 1988; 140:1889–94.
11. Lord BI, Molineux G, Testa NG, Kelly M, Spooncer E, Dexter TM. The kinetic response of haematopoietic precursor cells, in vivo to highly purified recombinant IL-3. Lymphokine Res 1986; 5:97–104.
12. Leary AG, Ikebuchi K, Clark SC, Ihle JN, Hirai Y, Ogawa M. Interleukin-6 enhancement of interleukin-3 dependent proliferation of multipotential hematopoietic progenitors. Proc Natl Acad Sci U S A 1987; 84:9035–9.
13. Paquette RL, Zhou JY, Yang YC, Clark SC, Koeffler HP. Recombinant gibbon IL-3 acts synergistically with recombinant human G-CSF and GM-CSF in vitro. Blood 1988; 71:1596–600.
14. Warren DJ, Moore MAS. Synergism among interleukin-1, interleukin-3 and interleukin-5 in the production of eosinophils from primitive hemopoietic stem cells. J Immunol 1988; 140:94.
15. Donahue RE, Seehra J, Metzger M, et al. Human IL-3 and GM-CSF act synergistically in stimulating hematopoiesis in primates. Science 1988; 241:1820.
16. Mori M, Suda T, Suda J, Miura Y, Saito M. The role of IL-3 in the proliferation of murine mast cells in vitro. Acta Haematol Jpn 1987; 50:59–64.
17. Metcalf D, Johnson GR, Burgess AW. Direct stimulation by purified GM-CSF of the proliferation of multipotential and erythroid precursor cells. Blood 1980; 55:138–47.
18. Metcalf D, Begley CG, Williamson DJ, et al. Hemopoietic responses in mice injected with purified recombinant GM-CSF. Exp Hematol 1987; 15:1–9.
19. Ulich TR, del Castillo J, McNiece I, Watson L, Yin S, Andresen J. Hematologic effects of recombinant murine GM-CSF on the peripheral blood and bone marrow. Am J Pathol 1990; 137:369–76.
20. Donahue RE, Wang EA, Stone DK, et al. Stimulation of hematopoiesis in primates by continuous infusion of recombinant human GM-CSF. Nature 1986; 321:872–5.
21. Mayer P, Lam C, Obenans H, Liehl E, Besemer J. Recombinant human GM-CSF induces leukocytosis and activates peripheral blood polymorphonuclear neutrophils in non-human primates. Blood 1987; 70:206–13.
22. Brandt SJ, Peters WP, Atwater SK, et al. Effect of recombinant human granulocyte-macrophage colony stimulating factor on hematopoietic reconstitution after high dose chemotherapy and autologous bone marrow transplantation. N Engl J Med 1988; 318:869–76.
23. Aglietta M, Piacibello W, Sanario F, et al. Kinetics of human hematopoietic cells after *in vivo* administration of granulocyte-macrophage colony stimulating factor. J Clin Invest 1989; 83:551–7.
24. Morstyn G, Lieschke GJ, Sheridan W, Layton J, Cebon J, Fox RM. Clinical experience with recombinant human granulocyte-colony stimulating factor and granulocyte-macrophage colony stimulating factor. Semin Hematol 1989; 26(suppl. 2):9.
25. Weisbart RH, Kacena A, Schuh A, Golde DW: GM-CSF induces human neutrophil IgA-mediated phagocytosis by an IgA Fc receptor activation mechanism. Nature 1988; 332:647–8.
26. McNiece IK, Robinson BE, Quesenberry PJ. Stimulation of murine colony-forming cells with high proliferative potential by the combination of GM-CSF and CSF-1. Blood 1988; 72:191–5.
27. McNiece IK, Stewart MF, Deacon DM, Quesenberry PJ. Synergistic interactions

between hematopoietic growth factors as detected by *in vitro* mouse bone marrow colony formation. Exp Hematol 1988; 16:383–8.

28. McNiece IK, Andrews RG, Stewart MF, Clark S, Boone T, Quesenberry P. Action of interleukin-3, G-CSF and GM-CSF on highly enriched human hematopoietic progenitor cells: synergistic interaction of GM-CSF plus G-CSF. Blood 1989; 74:110.
29. Souza LM, Boone TC, Gabrilove J, et al. Recombinant human granulocyte colony stimulating factor: effects on normal and leukemic myeloid cells. Science 1986; 232:61–5.
30. Cohen AM, Zsebo K, Inoue H, et al. In vivo granulocyte colony stimulating factor. Proc Natl Acad Sci U S A 1987; 84:2484–8.
31. Ulich TR, del Castillo J, Souza L. Kinetics and mechanisms of recombinant human granulocyte colony stimulating factor-induced neutrophilia. Am J Pathol 1988; 133:630–8.
32. Welte K, Bonilla MA, Gillio AAP, et al. Recombinant human granulocyte colony stimulating factor: effects on hematopoiesis in normal and cyclophosphamide-treated primates. J Exp Med 1987; 165:941–8.
33. Ulich TR, del Castillo J, Guo K, Souza L. The hematologic effects of the chronic administration of the monokines tumor necrosis factor, interleukin-1, and granulocyte colony stimulating factor on bone marrow and circulation. Am J Pathol 1989; 134:149–59.
34. Zhan YQ, Stanley RE, Clark SC, et al. Interleukin-3 and interleukin-1a allow early bone marrow progenitors to respond to human colony-stimulating factor-1. Blood 1988; 72:1870.
35. McNiece IK, Stewart FM, Deacon DM, Quesenberry PJ. Synergistic interactions between hematopoietic growth factors as detected by in vitro mouse bone marrow colony formation. Exp Hematol 1988; 16:383.
36. Branch DR, Turner AR, Guilbert LJ. Synergistic stimulation of macrophage proliferation by the monokines tumor necrosis factor-alpha and colony-stimulating factor-1. Blood 1989; 73:307.
37. Ralph P, Nakoinz I. Stimulation of macrophage tumoricidal activity by the growth and differentiation factor CSF-1. Cell Immunol 1987; 105:270.
38. Wang JM, Griffin JD, Rambaldi A, Chen ZG, Mantorani A. Induction of monocyte migration by recombinant macrophage-colony stimulating factor. J Immunol 1988; 141:575.
39. Koren S, Klimpel GR, Fleishman WR. Treatment of mice with macrophage-colony stimulating factor (CSF-1) prevents the in vivo myelosuppression induced by murine alpha, beta and gamma interferons. J Biol Response Mod 1986; 5:481.
40. Hume DA, Parli P, Donahue RE, Fidler IJ. The effect of human recombinant macrophage colony-stimulating factor (CSF-1) on the murine mononuclear phagocyte system in vivo. J Immunol 1988; 141:3405–9.
41. Broxmeyer HE, Geissler K, Cooper S, Williams DE. Influence of purified recombinant human macrophage-colony stimulating factor in mice. Biotech Ther 1988; 1:43–54.
42. Ulich TR, del Castillo J, Watson L, Yin S, Garnick MB. In vivo hematologic effects of recombinant human macrophage-colony stimulating factor. Blood 1990; 75:846–50.
43. Garnick MB, Stoudemire J, Donahue RE, et al. *In vitro* and *in vivo* biological effects of recombinant human macrophage colony stimulatory factor. Proc ASCO 1989; 8:814.
44. Warren MK, Ralph P. Macrophage growth factor CSF-1 stimulates human monocyte production of interferon, tumor necrosis factor and colony stimulating activity. J Immunol 1986; 137:2281.

45. Burstein SA, Ishibashi T. Erythropoietin and megakaryocytopoiesis. Blood Cells 1989; 15:202–4.
46. Eder H, Rosslenbroich B, Failing K. A dose-dependent effect of recombinant erythropoietin in the reticulocyte population of rats. Blut 1989; 59:184–7.
47. Ulich TR, del Castillo J, Yin S, Egrie JC. The erythropoietic effects of IL-6 and erythropoietin in vivo. Exp Hematol 1991; 19:29–34.
48. Berridge M, Fraser JK, Carter JM, Lin FK. Effect of recombinant erythropoietin on megakaryocytes and platelet production in the rat. Blood 1988; 72:970–7.
49. Adamson JW. The promise of recombinant erythropoietin. Semin Hematol 1989; 26:5–8.
50. Ganser A, Bergman M, Volkers B, Gruetzmacher P, Scigalla P, Hoelzer D. In vivo effects of recombinant human erythropoietin on circulating human hemopoietic progenitor cells. Exp Hematol 1989; 17:433–5.
51. Kampschmidt RF, Long RD, Upchurch HF. Neutrophil releasing activity in rats injected with endogenous pyrogen. Proc Soc Exp Biol Med 1972; 139:1224.
52. Ulich TR, del Castillo J, Keys M, Granger GA, Ni RX. Kinetics and mechanisms of recombinant interleukin-1 and tumor necrosis factor alpha-induced changes in circulating numbers of neutrophils and lymphocytes. J Immunol 1987; 139:3406–15.
53. Suttles J, Carruth LM, Mizel SB. Detection of IL-1α and IL-1β in the supernatants of paraformaldehyde-treated human monocytes. J Immunol 1990; 144:170–4.
54. Fibbe WE, Falkenburg JH, Schaafsma MR, Willemze R. The hematopoietic activities of interleukin-1. Biotherapy 1989; 1:263–71.
55. Okusawa S, Gelfand GA, Ikejima T, Connoly RJ, Dinarello C. IL-1 induces a shock-like state in rabbits: synergism with TNF and the effect of cyclooxygenase inhibition. J Clin Invest 1988; 81:1162–72.
56. Ulich TR, Keys M, Ni RX, del Castillo J, Dakay E. The contributions of adrenal hormones, hemodynamic factors, and the endotoxin related stress reaction to stable prostaglandin analog induced peripheral lymphopenia and neutrophilia. J Leuk Biol 1988; 43:5–10.
57. Dinarello CA, Neta R. An overview on interleukin-1 as a therapeutic agent. Biotherapy 1989; 1:245–54.
58. Stork LC, Peterson VM, Rundus CH, Robinson WA. Interleukin-1 enhances murine granulopoiesis in vivo. Exp Hematol 1988; 16:163–7.
59. Vogel SN, Douches SD, Kaufman EN, Neta R. Induction of colony stimulating factor in vivo by recombinant IL-1 and recombinant TNF. J Immunol 1987; 138:2143–8.
60. Ettinghausen SE, Moore JG, White DE, Plataniass L, Young N, Rosenberg S. Hematologic effects of immunotherapy with lymphokine activated killer cells and recombinant interleukin-2 in cancer patients. Blood 1987; 1654–60.
61. Anderson TD, Hayes TJ. Toxicity of human recombinant IL-2 in rats. Pathologic changes are characterized by marked lymphocytic and eosinophilic proliferation and multisystem involvement. Lab Invest 1989; 60:331–46.
62. Anderson TD, Hayes TJ, Gately MK, Bontempo JM, Stern LL, Truitt GA. Toxicity of human recombinant IL-2 in the mouse is mediated by interleukin activated lymphocytes. Lab Invest 1988; 59:598–612.
63. Ettinghausen SE, Lipford E, Mule J, Rosenberg SA. Systemic administration of recombinant IL-2 stimulates in vivo cell proliferation in tissues. J Immunol 1985; 135:1488–97.
64. Jesmok GJ, Gunther R. In vivo biology of recombinant IL-2 infusion in sheep. Inflammation 1989; 3:267–83.

65. Lotze M, Matory Y, Ettinghausen S, et al. In vivo administration of interleukin-2. J Immunol 1985; 135:2865–75.
66. Essner R, Rhoades K, McBride WH, Morton DL, Econom JS. IL-4 downregulates IL-1 and TNF gene expression in human monocytes. J Immunol 1989; 142:3857.
67. Sanderson CJ, Campbell HD, Young IG. Molecular and cellular biology of eosinophil differentiation factor (IL-5) and its effects on human and mouse B cells. Immunol Rev 1988; 102:29–50.
68. Basten A, Beeson PB. Mechanism of eosinophilia. II. Role of the lymphocyte. J Exp Med 1970; 131:1288.
69. Coffman RL, Seymour BP, Hudak S, Jackson J, Rennick D. Antibody to IL-5 inhibits helminth-induced eosinophilia in mice. Science 1989; 308–10.
70. Samoszuk M, Nansen L. Detection of IL-5 mRNA in Reed-Sternberg cells of Hodgkin's disease with eosinophilia. Blood 1990; 75:13–6.
71. Sehgal PB, May LT. Human interferon-beta$_2$. J Interferon Res 1987; 7:521.
72. Shabo Y, Lotem J, Rubenstein M, et al. The myeloid blood cell differentiation-inducing protein MGI-2A is interleukin-6. Blood 1988; 72:2070–3.
73. Le J, Vilcek J. Interleukin-6: a multifunctional cytokine regulating immune reactions and the acute phase protein response. Lab Invest 1989; 61:588–602.
74. Suzuki C, Okano A, Takatsuki F, et al. Continuous perfusion with IL-6 enhances production of hematopoietic stem cells. Biochem Biophy Res Commun 1989; 159:933–8.
75. Ulich TR, del Castillo J, Guo K. In vivo hematologic effects of recombinant IL-6 on hematopoiesis and circulating numbers of RBCs and WBCs. Blood 1989; 73:108–10.
76. Rennick D, Jackson J, Yang G, Wideman J, Lee F, Hudak S. Interleukin-6 interacts with IL-4 and other hematopoietic growth factors to selectively enhance the growth of megakayocytic, erythroid, myeloid, and multipotential progenitor cells. Blood 1989; 73:1828–35.
77. Ishibashi T, Kimura H, Shikama Y, et al. Interleukin-6 is a potent thrombopoietic factor in mice. Blood 1989; 74:1241–4.
78. Schindler R, Mancilla J, Endres S, Ghorbani R, Clark S, Dinarello C. Correlations and interactions in the production of IL-6, IL-1, and TNF in human blood mononuclear cells: IL-6 suppresses IL-1 and TNF. Blood 1990; 75:40–7.
79. Aderka D, Le J, Vilcek J. IL-6 inhibits LPS-induced TNF production in cultured human monocytes, U937 cells, and in mice. J Immunol 1989; 143:3517–23.
80. Armitage RJ, Namen AE, Sassenfeld HM, Grabstein KH. Regulation of human T-cell proliferation by IL-7. J Immunol 1990; 144:938–41.
80a. Morrissey PJ, Conlon P, Charrier K, Braddy S, Alpert A, Williams D, Namen AE, Mochizuki D. J Immunol 1991; 147:561–68.
81. Matsushima K, Oppenheim JJ. Interleukin-8 and MCAF: novel inflammatory cytokines inducible by IL-1 and TNF. Cytokine 1989; 12–3.
82. Rampart M, van Damme J, Zonnekeyn L, Herman AG. Granulocyte chemotactic protein/IL-8 induces plasma leakage and neutrophil accumulation in rabbit skin. Am J Pathol 1989; 135:21–5.
83. Klimpel GR, Fleishmann WR, Klimpel KD. Gamma IFN and IFN alpha/beta suppresses murine myeloid colony formation: magnitude of suppression is dependent upon level of colony stimulating factor. J Immunol 1982; 29:76–80.
84. Kurzrock R, Rosenblum M, Sherwin S, et al. Pharmacokinetics, single dose tolerance, and biological activity of recombinant gamma interferon in cancer patients. Canc Res 1985; 45:2866–72.
85. Gresser I, Guy-Grand D, Maury C, Maunoury MT. Interferon induces peripheral lymphadenopathy in mice. J Immunol 1981; 127:1569–75.

86. Zoumbos NC, Gascon P, Djeu JY, Young N. Interferon is a mediator of the hematopoietic suppression in aplastic anemia in vitro and possibly in vivo. Proc Natl Acad Sci U S A 1985; 82:188–92.
87. Old LJ. Tumour necrosis factor—polypeptide mediator network. Nature 1987; 326:330–1.
88. Le J, Vilcek J. Tumor necrosis factor and interleukin-1: cytokines with multiple overlapping biological activities. Lab Invest 1987; 56:234–48.
89. Ulich TR, del Castillo J, Keys M, Granger GA. Recombinant human alpha lymphotoxin (TNF-b) induces peripheral neutrophilia and lymphopenia in the rat. Am J Pathol 1987; 128:5–12.
90. Remick DG, Kunkel RG, Larrick JW, Kunkel SL. Acute in vivo effects of recombinant TNF. Lab Invest 1987; 56:583–90.
91. Gamble JR, Harlan JM, Klebanoff SJ, Vadas MA. Stimulation of the adherence of neutrophils to umbilical vein endothelium by human recombinant TNF. Proc Natl Acad Sci U S A 1985; 82:8667–71.
92. Larrick JW, Graham D, Toy K, Lin L, Senyk G, Fendly D. Recombinant TNF causes activation of human granulocytes. Blood 1987; 69:640–4.
93. Ming WJ, Bersani L, Mantovani A. TNF is chemotactic for monocytes and polymorphonuclear leukocytes. J Immunol 1987; 138:1469–74.
94. Ulich TR, del Castillo J, Ni RX, Bikhazi N. Hematologic interactions of endotoxin, TNF, IL-1, and adrenal hormones and the hematologic effects of TNF in C. parvum-primed rats. J Leuk Biol 1989; 45:546–57.
95. Bachwich PR, Chensue SW, Larrick JW, Kunkel SL. TNF stimulates IL-1 and PGE_2 production in resting macrophages. Biochem Biophys Res Commun 1986; 136:94.
96. Dinarello CA, Cannon JG, Wolff SM, et al. TNF is an endogenous pyrogen and induces production of IL-1. J Exp Med 1986; 163:1433.
97. Koeffler HP, Gasson J, Ranyard J, Souza L, Shepard M, Munker R. Recombinant human TNF stimulates production of G-CSF. Blood 1987; 70:55–9.
98. Ulich TR, del Castillo J, Yin S. TNF exerts dose-dependent effects on erythropoiesis and myelopoiesis in vivo. Exp Hematol 1990; 18:311–15.
99. Waage A. Production and clearance of TNF in rats exposed to endotoxin and dexamethasone. Clin Immunol Immunopathol 1987; 45:348–55.
100. Remick D, Strieter RM, Eskandari MK, et al. Role of TNF in LPS-induced pathologic alterations. Am J Pathol 1990; 136:49–60.
101. Bevilacqua M, Pober JS, Mendrick DL, Cotran R, Gimbrone MA. Identification of an inducible endothelial-leukocyte adhesion molecule. Proc Natl Acad Sci U S A 1987; 84:9238.
102. Cavender D, Saegusa Y, Ziff M. Stimulation of endothelial cell binding by tumor necrosis factor. J Immunol 1987; 139:1855–60.
103. Munro JM, Pober JS, Cotran RS. TNF and IFN gamma induce distinct patterns of endothelial activation and associated leukocyte accumulation in the skin of *Papio Ánubis.* Am J Pathol 1989; 135:121–33.
104. Michie HR, Manogue KR, Spriggs DR, et al. Detection of circulating TNF after endotoxin administration. Engl J Med 1988; 318:1481–6.
105. Moldawer LL, Marano M, Wei H, et al. Cachectin/TNF-alpha alters red blood cell kinetics and induces anemia in vivo. FASEB J 1989; 3:1637–43.
106. Broxmeyer HE, Williams DE, Lu L, et al. The suppressive influences of tumor necrosis factors on bone marrow hematopoietic progenitor cells from normal donors and patients with leukemia: Synergism of TNF and IFN-gamma. J Immunol 1986; 136:4487.
107. Johnson CS, Cook CA, Furmanski P. In vivo suppression of erythropoiesis by TNF: reversal with exogenous EPO. Exp Hematol 1990; 18:109–13.

108. Johnson CS, Chang MJ, Furmanski P. In vivo hematopoietic effects of TNF in normal and erythroleukemic mice: characterization and therapeutic applications. Blood 1988; 72:1875.
109. Clark IA, Chandri G. TNF may contribute to the anemia of malaria by causing dyserythropoiesis and erythrophagocytosis. Br J Haematol 1988; 70:99.

CHAPTER 15

THE ROLE OF CYTOKINES IN EXPERIMENTAL LUNG INJURY

Jeffrey S. Warren

The University of Michigan Medical School
Ann Arbor, Michigan

INTRODUCTION

Perusal of recent biomedical literature calls attention to the explosive growth of knowledge in cytokine biology. Dozens of lymphokine-cytokine activities were described during the 1960s and 1970s, but it has really been during the last decade that it has been possible to attribute specific biological activities to biochemically defined mediators. Numerous cytokines have been characterized and produced in recombinant form. Cytokines are major mediators of cell-to-cell communication that appear to participate, in at least some manner, in most fundamental pathophysiological processes. For example, tumor necrosis factor and interleukins-1, 6, and 8 are important in acute inflammation (1). Interleukin-2 is a pivotal mediator of T lymphocyte proliferation and such cellular immune processes as delayed-type hypersensitivity (2). Cytokine-associated growth factor activities also appear to be important in chronic inflammation, tissue repair, and neoplasia (3). In view of the pleiotypic nature of cytokine activities, it is not surprising that these mediators participate in systemic as well as local processes, both physiological and pathological (4). Undoubtedly there are locally determined nuances in cytokine function from tissue to tissue. In some cases, local differences in the role of individual cytokines may be a function of anatomy. For example, within the lungs there is a readily accessible reservoir of cytokine-producing alveolar macrophages that orchestrate numerous cytokine-driven responses. The lungs also contain a huge microvascular surface located in close proximity to the airspace. It should be kept in mind that the biologically relevant functions of cytokines are defined not only by their biochemical actions but by the microenvironment.

The focus of this chapter is the role of cytokines in experimental lung injury.

A large number of animal models mimic human pulmonary disease and have thus served as valuable tools for providing insights into understanding basic pathophysiological mechanisms. Attention is directed toward a single well-characterized experimental model of acute lung injury. IgG immune complex-induced alveolitis in the rat serves as a general model of acute inflammation and, more specifically, mimics processes thought to occur in human diseases, such as lupus pneumonitis, rheumatoid pneumonitis, and some types of extrinsic allergic alveolitis. It should be noted that in addition to experimental models of acute lung inflammation, numerous animal models also bear resemblance to more chronic processes. The best characterized models of chronic lung disease include murine *Schistosoma*-induced pulmonary granulomatosis (5), asbestos-induced pulmonary fibrosis (6), and bleomycin-induced pulmonary fibrosis (7). In all these models, there is burgeoning evidence that various cytokines and growth factors are involved.

ACUTE IgG IMMUNE COMPLEX ALVEOLITIS IN THE RAT

Relevance to Human Lung Disease

Deposition of circulating immune complexes and in situ formation of immune complexes in tissue have been invoked as central pathophysiological events leading to injury in many organs, including many human inflammatory and immunological lung diseases (Table 1). In many cases, tissue deposits of immunoglobulin and complement components can be demonstrated by immunofluorescence or electron microscopy (13,14,31,32). In some cases, sensitive tests of systemic complement activation support the premise that immune complex formation leads to complement activation and subsequent tissue injury. For example, pulmonary parenchymal involvement is present to some degree in most patients with systemic lupus erythematosus (14). The severity of pulmonary parenchymal lupus generally correlates with the intensity of systemic disease and ranges from an asymptomatic, clinically unapparent form to an acute fulminating hemorrhagic pneumonitis (33). Deposits containing DNA, IgG anti-DNA, and C3 can be demonstrated in the lungs of patients with acute lupus pneumonitis (31,32,34). Electron-dense immune deposits have also been identified along the alveolar capillary basement membrane in lung biopsies obtained from such patients (35). Despite clinical examples that seem clear-cut, there are many inconsistencies and unknowns. Effector components of complement (e.g., C3a, C3b, C5a, and the membrane attack complex, C5b-9) are thought to be critical mediators of phagocyte activation, inflammatory cell recruitment, and microvascular injury, yet complement components are not always found in lung tissue from patients with lupus pneumonitis (14,33). Immune deposits apparently do not always lead to inflammatory cell recruitment. Inflammatory cells are not always present in lung tissue obtained from patients with lupus pneumonitis (14,33). Histopathological patterns and distributions of inflammation vary considerably among lung diseases considered to be mediated by immune complexes or other immunological mechanisms. It is clear that many factors influence the pathogenesis of immunologically mediated lung disease. Experimental studies of acute immune complex-mediated alveolitis have provided valuable information regarding mechanisms of phago-

Table 1 Human Lung Diseases Associated with Immune Complex Deposition

Disease State (References)	Comments
Idiopathic interstitial pneumontitis[a] (8–12)	Interstitial and alveolar septal deposits of IgG, IgM, and C3 in some patients; elevated levels of circulating immune complexes in some patients
Systemic lupus erythematosus (13,14)	DNA, IgG anti-DNA, and C3 deposits found in most patients, but not all; infiltrating phagocytes are not always present
Rheumatoid pneumonitis (15–17)	Evidence of local complement consumption and immune complex formation
Extrinsic allergic alveolitis (18–20)	Evidence supports immune complex role during acute phase, but biopsies are often negative for immune deposits; thought to be good example of type III hypersensitivity
Goodpasture's syndrome (21)	Prototype type II hypersensitivity; rare patients have circulating immune complexes in addition to anti–basement membrane antibodies
Wegener's granulomatosis (22)	Occasional interstitial pneumonitis and circulating immune complexes
Sjögren's syndrome (23)	Circulating immune complexes
Mixed connective tissue disease (24–26)	Circulating immune complexes
Polymyositis-dermatomyositis (27)	Interstitial lung disease in some patients
Sarcoidosis (28,29)	Circulating immune complexes in some patients; rarely pulmonary immune deposits
Asthma (30)	Unusual patients develop bronchoconstriction later than in classic type I hypersensitivity; some of these patients exhibit stigmata suggestive of type III hypersensitivity reactions

[a] This group includes patients with the following pathological descriptors: usual interstitial pneumonia (UIP), desquamative interstitial pneumonia (DIP), lymphocytic interstitial pneumonia (LIP), and diffuse fibrosis.

cyte-mediated tissue injury, inflammatory cell recruitment, and host defense mechanisms that counterregulate inflammatory tissue damage. In recent years, it has become clear that cytokines play a pivotal role in the pathogenesis of acute immune complex-mediated lung injury.

Rat Model of Immune Complex Alveolitis

The first reported example of experimental immune complex-mediated lung injury was observed by Kniker and Cochrane (36), who identified reversible acute inflammatory reactions in the walls of pulmonary arteries of rabbits with "one-shot" acute serum sickness. It was thought that circulating immune complexes, formed within the vascular space, deposited in the vessel walls. No inflammatory changes were present in the interstitial or alveolar compartments. Brentjens et al. (37) demonstrated irreversible changes in the alveolar interstitium and capillary basement membranes of rabbits with chronic serum sickness. Electron microscopic examination and immunofluorescence studies confirmed the presence of immune complex and complement deposition within the alveolar septa. In 1974, Johnson and Ward (38) characterized an IgG immune complex-mediated acute alveolitis model in rats. The remainder of this section outlines studies that have led to our current understanding of the pathogenesis of this model. The following section focuses on more recent work that addresses the role of cytokines.

In this model, affinity-purified rabbit IgG anti-bovine serum albumin (BSA) is instilled into the alveolar compartment via a tracheal cannula and BSA is infused intravenously. The typical concentrations of anti-BSA (300–600 μg in 0.2–0.4 ml) and BSA (10 mg in 1.0 ml) used to elicit injury have been chosen empirically. Acute alveolitis develops over the ensuing 4–6 h. Lung injury can be quantitated by morphometric analysis by measuring the accumulation of isotope-labeled colloid in the injured lungs or by measuring increases in lung weight. Morphometric analysis allows quantitation of neutrophil influx, alveolar hemorrhage (expressed as red blood cells per alveolus), and endothelial or epithelial injury (expressed as lengths of exposed basement membrane per length of epithelial or endothelial surface). Lung weights and measurements of isotope-labeled colloid reflect pulmonary vascular permeability status and in this model correlate well with morphometric injury measurements (39). The total lung content of [^{125}I] colloid (usually nonspecific rabbit IgG) compared to the amount of [^{125}I] colloid in 1.0 ml whole blood provides a reproducible and quantitative index (permeability index) of lung injury. After development of injury, the heart and lungs are removed en bloc and the lungs perfused via the pulmonary artery to flush out nonparenchymal blood. Comparison of [^{125}I] colloid in the lungs to [^{125}I] colloid in 1.0 ml blood normalizes slight animal-to-animal variations in intravenous injection technique.

Development of lung damage in this model is neutrophil and complement dependent, thus resembling the reversed passive Arthus reaction in skin (40). The physical configuration of immune complexes is an important determinant of the intensity of pulmonary inflammation. There is considerable variation in the capacity for preformed IgG-BSA immune complexes to elicit injury when instilled into the alveolar space. Large, precipitating complexes (formed near antigen-antibody equivalence) are the most potent in terms of inducing lung injury (41). In vitro studies indicate that such complexes generally fix complement more efficiently than small, soluble complexes (42). Precipitating complexes are also potent agonists of phagocyte activation (as measured by respiratory burst or enzyme release) (42). Histological examination of lung tissue obtained from rats with IgG immune complex alveolitis reveals a massive influx of neutrophils (Fig. 1). Electron-dense immune complexes can be seen within neutrophils and alveolar macrophages. The importance of neutrophils in acute immune complex alveolitis has been demonstrated in neutrophil-depleted rats (38). Rats that have been 95% depleted of neutrophils by nitrogen mustard, cyclophosphamide, or antineutrophil antiserum exhibit a 70% reduction in pulmonary vascular permeability compared to positive control animals (38).

There is direct and indirect evidence that complement is required for full development of acute IgG immune complex alveolitis. Indirect immunofluores-

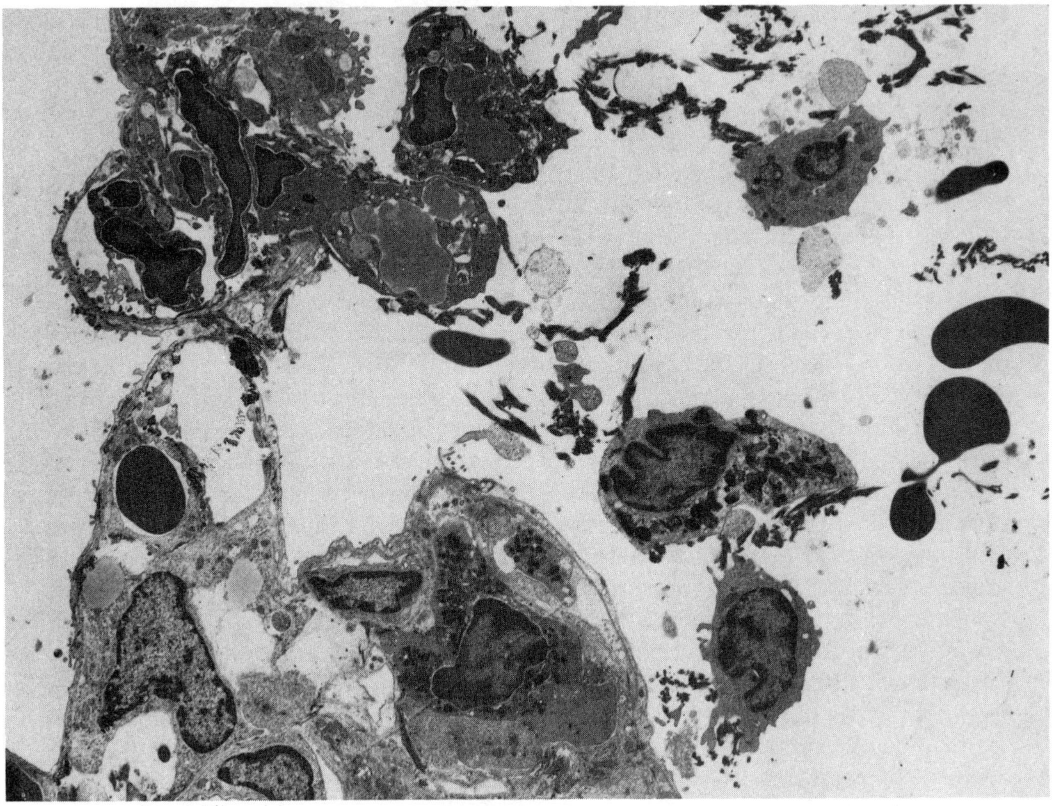

FIGURE 1 Acute IgG immune complex alveolitis in the rat. There is extensive alveolar hemorrhage accompanied by many neutrophils and fibrin strands. Uranyl acetate and lead citrate stain, transmission electron micrograph; ×4200.

cence staining of rat lung sections reveals alveolar septal C3 deposits (38). Numerous in vitro studies implicate complement proteins in acute inflammatory processes, for example, C5a-mediated neutrophil chemotaxis and activation, C5a-mediated phagocyte priming, and C3b opsonization (43,44). Recent studies suggest that the membrane attack complex (MAC; C5b-9) may play a pathogenetic role in some complement-mediated inflammatory lesions (45,46). There is also evidence suggesting that endothelial surface-bound and processed complement components (iC3b) may participate in early neutrophil-endothelial adhesive interactions (47). Several in vivo studies suggest that complement is required for full development of lung injury. Initiation of IgG immune complex alveolitis in rats that have been complement-depleted (through repeated systemic injections of cobra venom factor) results in an attenuated form of lung injury (38). Similarly, deposition of immune complexes in the lungs of mice that are genetically C5 deficient results in negligible lung injury (48).

Pretreatment of rats with superoxide dismutase (SOD), catalase, hydroxyl radical scavengers, or iron chelators suppresses the development of lung injury, supporting the hypothesis that oxygen-derived metabolites play a critical role in neutrophil-mediated tissue injury (39). Suppression of immune complex alveolitis by SOD is time dependent and, early on, is associated with reduced intrapulmonary neutrophil recruitment (49). This observation also supports the hypothesis that oxygen-derived metabolites influence neutrophil recruitment. It is unclear how O_2-influences neutrophil recruitment, but it may be linked to the formation of oxidant-generated chemotactic factors. Several potential oxidant-mediated or oxidant-amplified chemotactic mechanisms have been described. In vitro exposure of plasma to xanthine-xanthine oxidase (a cell-free superoxide anion-generating system) results in the generation of an arachidonate-derived neutrophil chemotactic factor (50,51). Shingu and Nobunaga showed that exposure of purified C5 to an oxygen radical-generating system results in the formation of C5a (52). von Zabern et al. demonstrated that exposure of C5 to H_2O_2 results in conformational changes in C5 and the formation of a membrane attack complex-like aggregate (53). Recently, Lewis et al. showed that exposure of endothelial cell monolayers to H_2O_2 results in platelet-activating factor (PAF) production (54). In vitro studies suggest that endothelium-associated PAF can mediate a rapid neutrophil-endothelial adhesive interaction (55). Platelet-activating factor is also a potent neutrophil activator and chemotactic factor (56). Recent studies suggest that PAF is an important mediator of IgG immune complex alveolitis (see later) (57).

Interactions between oxygen metabolites and lysosomal proteases may also be important in the pathogenesis of immune complex alveolitis. Weiss et al. have shown in vitro that exposure of latent (inactive) gelatinase or collagenase to hypochlorous acid results in enzyme activation (58,59). Hypochlorous acid is derived from myeloperoxidase-H_2O_2 and chloride ions and is produced by activated neutrophils. There is in vivo evidence that proteases and oxygen-derived species may exhibit a synergistic role in immune complex-associated lung injury in rats (60).

It has become clear that the acute inflammatory milieu is exceedingly complex. The capacity for endothelial cells to produce PAF, cytokines, leukocyte adhesion molecules, and even oxidant species bears witness to this premise. For instance, it now appears that conditions of ischemia and some inflammatory mediators can provoke the conversion of endothelial cell xanthine dehydrogenase into xanthine oxidase (61,62). In turn, xanthine oxidase can catalyze the formation of O_2^- (63). The role of such pathways in vivo remains to be determined. Alveolar macrophages, once viewed as passive scavenger cells, clearly orchestrate many acute inflammatory processes. Alveolar macrophages not only produce oxidants, PAF, and complement components, but they are also a major source of cytokines (57). As becomes more clear in the ensuing portions of this chapter, such cytokines play a central role in the pathogenises of both acute and chronic inflammatory processes.

Role of Cytokines in Acute Alveolitis

The best studied cytokine in the context of acute immune complex-induced lung injury is tumor necrosis factor (TNF). Recent studies suggest that formation of IgG-BSA immune complexes within rat alveolar septa results in the elaboration of intrapulmonary TNF, which in turn plays a role in lung injury through a pathway involving neutrophil recruitment (64). Over the 4 h course of evolving lung injury there is a 10-fold increase in TNF activity in retrieved bronchoalveolar lavage fluid compared to that present in fluid from negative controls. Immunohistochemical staining and in vitro studies suggest that resident alveolar macrophages are the chief source of TNF in this model. Coadministration of rabbit polyclonal IgG that specifically neutralizes rat TNF activity results in a marked reduction in lung injury as measured by permeability indices. The reduction in pulmonary microvascular permeability is accompanied by a marked decrease in intrapulmonary neutrophil recruitment. More recent studies suggest that the role of TNF in this alveolitis model is temporally restricted to relatively late in the evolution of injury (3–4 h) (Warren et al., submitted for publication). The mechanisms responsible for TNF-mediated pulmonary neutrophil recruitment are unclear, but several potential mechanisms are likely to contribute. The temporal restriction of TNF-mediated neutrophil recruitment is in agreement with several in vitro studies that indicate that TNF-induced expression of endothelial leukocyte adhesion molecule-1 (ELAM-1) occurs over several hours through a protein synthesis-dependent mechanism (65–68). In turn, ELAM-1 plays a major role in neutrophil-endothelial cell adhesive interactions (69,70). A second TNF-mediated mechanism of neutrophil recruitment involves PAF. Intratracheal administration of anti-TNF antibodies results in a decrease in extractable whole-lung PAF activity in rats with evolving alveolitis (57). Intratracheal administration of specific PAF antagonists (L-652,731 or WEB-2086) results in decreased lung injury and decreased mobilization of neutrophils from the pulmonary vascular and/or interstitial compartment into the alveolar airspace. Exposure of isolated alveolar macrophages to TNF results in dose-dependent PAF secretion. These studies implicate PAF as a TNF-triggered mediator of lung injury. The precise role of PAF is unclear. Platelet-activating factor is a potent chemotactic factor; it can prime neutrophils; it is reported to mediate endothelial-neutrophil adhesive interactions; and it directly increases microvascular permeability (reviewed in Ref. 56). Finally, several investigators here demonstrated that TNF can trigger neutrophil chemotactic factor (NCF; also known as neutrophil activating peptide 1 or interleukin-8) production by several cell types, including endothelial cells (71,72). One can envision a scenario in which local TNF production results in the production of NCF, which in turn is a potent neutrophil chemotactic factor. The biological role of NCF based on in vivo studies has not yet been extensively examined. Additional studies are required to determine the relative importance of these pathways. As emphasized in the introduction, different mediator pathways may be more or less important depending on the anatomic site and the time point examined (Fig. 2).

Less is known regarding the roles of other cytokines in acute immune complex alveolitis. Preliminary studies suggest that interleukin-1 may have a role similar to that of TNF. In vivo neutralization studies in which anti-IL-1β was instilled into rat lungs at the time of induction of alveolitis indicate that IL-1 may also play a role in pulmonary neutrophil recruitment (73). The relative contributions of IL-1α and IL-1β in this model are at present unclear. This issue is clouded by controversy regarding the distribution of IL-1 on cell membranes versus that

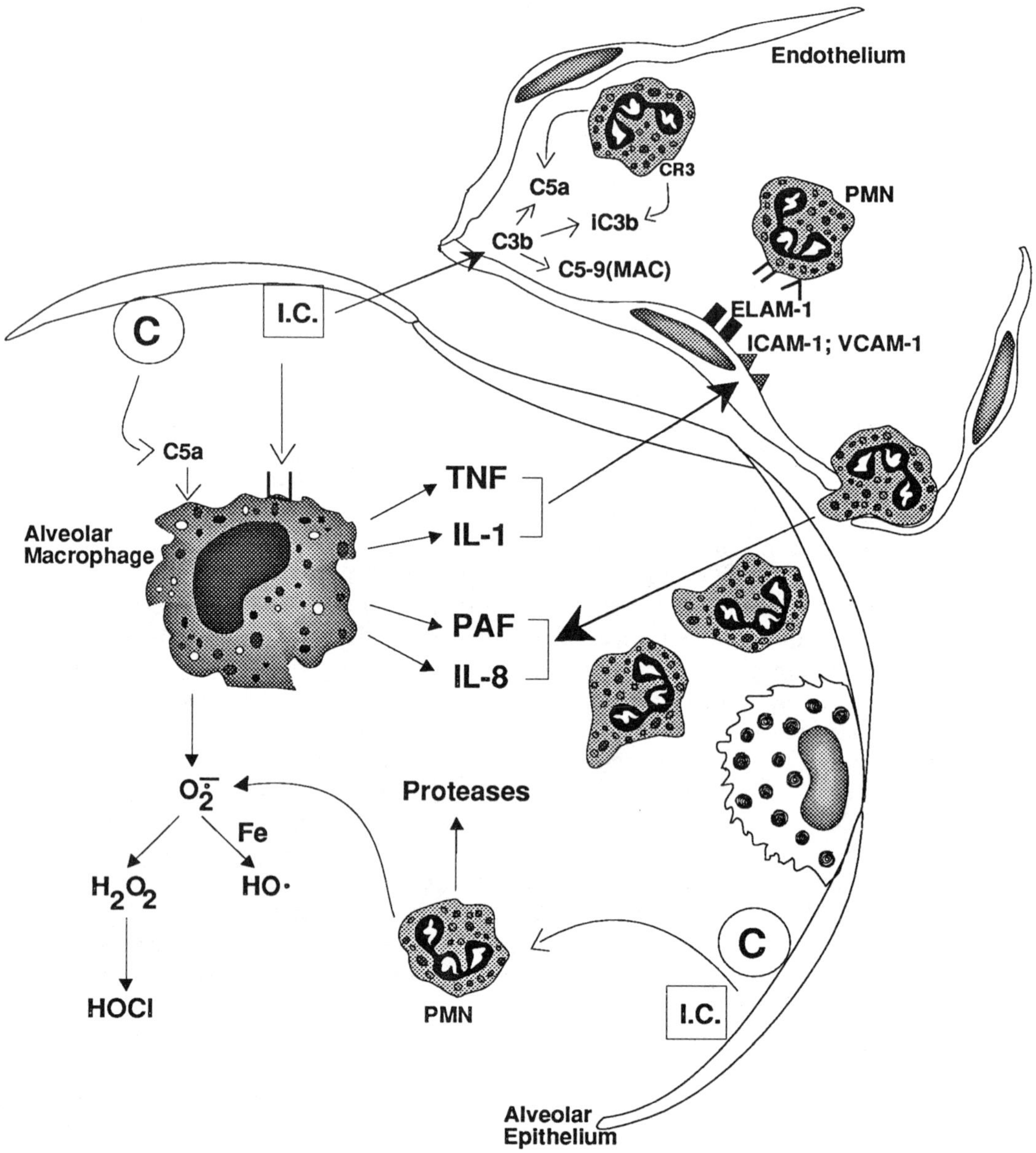

FIGURE 2 Inflammatory mediator pathways in the pathogenesis of acute immune complex alveolitis. Alveolar macrophages play a prominent role in orchestrating the inflammatory response.

secreted in soluble form. There is no direct in vivo evidence that bears on this model, but in vitro studies indicate that IL-1 can, like TNF, induce endothelial ELAM-1 expression and NCF secretion (66,67,69–71). The availability of rat cytokine homologs as well as relevant DNA probes will further our understanding not only of acute immune complex alveolitis but of other lung injuries as well.

Perspectives

The foregoing overview of the role of TNF, and to a lesser extent IL-1, in experimental acute immune complex alveolitis serves to emphasize the complexity of acute inflammatory lung injury. IgG immune complex alveolitis serves not only as a paradigm for acute inflammatory lung disease but acute inflammation in general. For example, Nelson et al. (74) showed that intratracheal administration of endotoxin, a potent secretogog for TNF, into the lungs of rats results in acute alveolitis accompanied by an increase in lung lavage TNF activity and influx of neutrophils. Similar observations have been made in experimental lapine meningitis, in which intracisternal injection of pathogenic bacteria results in acute meningitis that can be blocked with locally instilled anti-TNF antibodies (75,76). Clinical studies suggest that these observations are significant in humans. Mustafa et al. observed a high correlation between spinal fluid TNF activities and suppurative bacterial meningitis (77).

It is particularly exciting to consider the role of cytokines in acute inflammatory processes in the context of the advances that have been made in understanding cell-cell adhesive interactions (e.g., neutrophils and endothelial cells). It appears that cytokine-activated endothelium exhibits a highly regulated set of responses that help dictate the intensity, temporal pattern, and composition of leukocytes that are recruited into an inflammatory site. For instance, TNF or IL-1-activated endothelium expresses ELAM-1 and NCF within hours, a sequence consistent with their putative roles in acute inflammation (65–72). In contrast, ICAM-1 expression occurs more slowly and persists, a time course more compatible with its suspected role in chronic inflammation (78). In vitro and some in vivo studies also suggest that there is redundancy within the system. That is, these are probably several receptor-ligand pairs for each inflammatory cell type. The relative importance of such interactions may be organ, time, and condition dependent. An example of the last is CD18-dependent versus CD18-independent mechanisms of neutrophil to endothelial cell adhesion in which one adhesion interaction is stronger, allowing it to withstand greater shear stress than another (79,80).

The value of recombinant cytokines to the development of models of experimental lung injury is difficult to overestimate. In vitro systems, and to a greater extent in vivo systems, are exceedingly complex. The availability of pure cytokines or derived products (e.g., specific antibodies) have proven invaluable in defining the biological significance of various mediators. This is particularly true in cases in which cytokines exhibit many overlapping activities (e.g., TNF versus IL-1) (81). This chapter has focused on a single model of acute lung injury. It must be kept in mind that numerous other model systems have yielded valuable insights into mechanisms of lung disease.

ACKNOWLEDGMENTS

The author thanks Kimberly Drake and Jennifer Fricke for manuscript preparation and Robin G. Kunkel for artwork and figure preparation. This work was in part supported by the American Heart Association of Michigan and National Institutes of Health Grant HL-40526.

REFERENCES

1. Warren JS. Interleukins and tumor necrosis factor in inflammation. Crit Rev Clin Lab Sci 1990; 28:37–59.
2. Smith K. Interleukin 2: inception, impact, and implication. Science 1988; 240:1169–76.
3. Goustin AS, Leof EB, Shipley GD, Moses HL. Growth factors and cancer. Cancer Res 1986; 46:1015–29.
4. Mizel SB. The interleukins. FASEB J 1989; 3:2379–88.
5. Chensue SW, Remick DG, Higashi GI, Boros DL, Kunkel SL. Modulation of murine Schistosomiasis *mansoni* by exogenously administered prostaglandins. Am J Pathol 1986; 125:28–34.
6. Brody AR, Hill LH, Adkins B, O'Connor RW. Chrysotile asbestos inhalation in rats: deposition pattern and reaction of alveolar epithelium and pulmonary macrophages. Am Rev Respir Dis 1981; 123:640–79.
7. Adamson ITR, Bowden DH. The pathogenesis of bleomycin-induced pulmonary fibrosis in mice. Am J Pathol 1974; 77:185–9.
8. Dreisin RB, Schwarz MI, Theofilopoulos AN, et al. Circulating immune complexes in the idiopathic interstitial pneumonias. N Engl J Med 1978; 298:535–7.
9. Haslam P, Thompson B, Mohammed I, et al. Circulating immune complexes in patients with cryptogenic fibrosing alveolitis. J Immunol 1979; 37:381–90.
10. Schwarz MI, Dreisin RB, Pratt DS, et al. Immunofluorescent patterns in the idiopathic interstitial pneumonias. J Lab Clin Med 1978; 91:929–38.
11. Eisenberg H, Barnett E, Simmons H. Diffuse pulmonary interstitial disease, an immune complex disease. Clin Res 1977; 25:132A.
12. Warwick MT, Haslam P, Weeks J. Antibodies in some chronic fibrosing lung diseases. Clin Allergy 1971; 1:209–19.
13. Silberstein SL, Barland P, Grayzel A, et al. Pulmonary dysfunction in systemic lupus erythematosus. Prevalence, classification, and correlation with other organ involvement. J Rheumatol 1980; 7:187–94.
14. Eagen JW, Memoli VA, Roberts JL, et al. Pulmonary hemorrhage in systemic lupus erythematosus. J Med 1978; 57:545–60.
15. Hunder GG, McDuffie FC, Huston KA, et al. Pleural fluid complement, complement conversions and immune complexes in immunologic and nonimmunologic diseases. J Lab Clin Med 1977; 90:971–9.
16. Wallser WC, Wright V. Pulmonary lesions and rheumatoid arthritis. Medicine (Baltimore) 1968; 47:501–20.
17. DeHoratius RJ, Abruzzo JL, Williams RC. Immunofluorescent and immunologic studies of rheumatoid lung. Arch Intern Med 1972; 129:441–6.
18. Wenzel FJ, Emanual DA, Gray RL. Immunofluorescent studies in patients with farmer's lung. J Allergy Clin Immunol 1971; 48:224–9.
19. Barrowcliff DF, Arblaster PG. Farmer's lung: a study of an early acute fatal case. Thorax 1968; 23:490–500.
20. Geha RS. Circulating immune complexes and activation of the complement sequence in acute allergic bronchopulmonary aspergillosis. J Allergy Clin Immunol 1977; 60:357–9.
21. Poskitt TR. Immunologic and electron microscopic studies in Goodpasture's syndrome. Am J Med 1970; 49:250–7.
22. Shasby DM, Schwarz MI, Forstot JZ, Theofilopoulous AN, Kassan SS. Pulmonary immune complex deposition in Wegener's granulomatosis. Chest 1982; 81:338–40.
23. Lawley TJ, Moutsopoulos HM, Ketz SL, et al. Demonstration of circulating immune complexes in Sjögren's syndrome. J Immunol 1979; 123:1382–7.

24. Parker MD, Marion T. Circulating complement-fixing immune complexes in mixed connective tissue disease. Clin Res 1978; 26:374A.
25. Halla JT, Volanakis JE, Schrohenloher RE. Circulating immune complexes in mixed connective tissue disease. Arthritis Rheum 1979; 22:484–9.
26. Cunningham PH, Andrews BS, Davis JS. Immune complexes in patients with progressive systemic sclerosis and mixed connective tissue disease. Clin Res 1978; 26:374A.
27. Schwarz MI, Matthay RA, Sahn SA, et al. Interstitial lung disease in polymyositis and dermatomyositis: analysis of six cases and review of the literature. Medicine (Baltimore) 1976; 55:89–104.
28. Daniele RP, McMillan LJ, Dauber JH, Rossman MD. Immune complexes in sarcoidosis: a correlation with activity and duration of disease. Chest 1978; 74:261–4.
29. Johnson NM, McNicol MW, Burton-Kee JE, Mowbray JF. Circulating immune complexes in sarcoidosis. Thorax 1980; 35:286–9.
30. Pepys J. Immunopathology of allergic lung disease. Clin Allergy 1972; 3:1.
31. Inoue T, Kanayama Y, Ohe A, et al. Immunopathologic studies of pneumonitis in systemic lupus erythematosus. Ann Intern Med 1979; 91:30–4.
32. Rodriquez-Iturbe B, Garcia R, Rubio L, et al. Immunohistologic findings in the lung in systemic lupus erythematosus. Arch Pathol Lab med 1977; 101:342–4.
33. Eagen JW, Roberts JL, Schwartz MM, et al. The composition of pulmonary immune deposits in systemic lupus erythematosus. Clin Immunol Immunopathol 1979; 12:204–19.
34. Gamsu G, Webb WR. Pulmonary hemorrhage systemic lupus erythematosus. J Can Assoc Radiol 1977; 29:66–8.
35. Kuhn C. Systemic lupus erythematosus in a patient with ultrastructural lesions of the pulmonary capillaries previously reported in the review as due to idiopathic pulmonary hemosiderosis. Am Rev Respir Dis 1972; 106:931–2.
36. Kniker WT, Cochrane CG. Pathogenic factors in vascular lesions of experimental serum sickness. J Exp Med 1965; 122:83–98.
37. Brentjens JR, O'Connell DW, Pawlowski B, Hsu KC, Andres GA. Experimental immune complex disease of the lung. The pathogenesis of a laboratory model resembling certain human interstitial diseases. J Exp Med 1974; 140:105–25.
38. Johnson KJ, Ward PA. Acute immunologic pulmonary alveolitis. J Clin Invest 1974; 54:49–57.
39. Johnson KJ, Ward PA. Role of oxygen metabolities in immune complex injury lung. J Immunol 1981; 126:1365–8.
40. Cochran CG, Janoff A. The Arthus reaction: a model of neutrophil and complement-mediated injury. In: Zweifach B, Grant L, McCluskey R, eds. The inflammatory process, 2nd ed., Vol. 3. New York: Academic Press, 1974, pp 39–51.
41. Scherzer H, Ward PA. Lung injury produced by immune complexes of varying composition. J Immunol 1978; 121:948–52.
42. Ward PA, Duque RE, Sulavik MC, Johnson KJ. In vitro and in vivo stimulation of rat neutrophils and alveolar macrophages by immune complexes: production of O_2^- and H_2O_2. Am J Pathol 1983; 110:297–311.
43. Schreiber RD. The chemistry and biology of complement receptors. Springer Semin Immunopathol 1984; 7:221–34.
44. Ross GD, Medof ME. Membrane complement receptor specific for bound fragments of C3. Adv Immunol 1985; 37:217–29.
45. Kunkel RG, Warren JS, Johnson KJ, Ward PA. Demonstration of the complement membrane attack complex (MAC) in IgA-immune complex induced acute lung injury. Fed Proc 1988; 2:A1176.

46. Muller-Eberhard HJ. The membrane attack complex. Springer Semin Immunopathol 1984; 7:93–118.
47. Marks RM, Todd RJ, Ward PA. Rapid induction of neutrophil-endothelial adhesion by endothelial complement fixation. Nature 1989; 339:314–7.
48. Tvedten HW, Till GO, Ward PA. Mediators of lung injury in mice following systemic activation of complement. Am J Pathol 1985; 119:92–100.
49. Warren JS, Yabroff KR, Mandel DM, Johnson KJ, Ward PA. Role of O_2^- in neutrophil recruitment into sites of dermal and pulmonary vasculitis. Free Radic Biol Med 1990; 8:163–72.
50. Petrone WF, English DK, Wong K, McCord JM. Free radicals and inflammation: the superoxide dependent activation of a neutrophil chemotactic factor in plasma. Proc Natl Acad Sci U S A 1980; 77:1159–63.
51. Perez HD, Weksler BB, Goldstein IM. Generation of a chemotactic lipid from arachidonic acid by exposure to a superoxide-generating system. Inflammation 1980; 4:313–28.
52. Shingu M, Nobunaga M. Chemotactic activity generated in human serum from the fifth component of complement by hydrogen peroxide. Am J Pathol 1984; 117:201–6.
53. von Zabern WV, Hesse D, Nolte R, Haller Y. Generation of an activated form of human C5 (C5b-like C5) by oxygen radicals. Immunol Lett 1987; 14:209–15.
54. Lewis MS, Whatley RE, Cain P, McIntyre TM, Prescott SM, Zimmerman GA. Hydrogen peroxide stimulates the synthesis of platelet-activating factor by endothelium and induces endothelial cell-dependent neutrophil adhesion. J Clin Invest 1988; 82:2045–55.
55. Zimmerman GA, McIntyre TM, Prescott SM. Thrombin stimulates the adherence of neutrophils to human endothelial cells in vitro. J Clin Invest 1985; 76:2235–46.
56. Benveniste J, Arnoux B. Platelet activating factor and structurally related ether-lipids. Amsterdam: Elsevier, 1983.
57. Warren JS, Barton PA, Mandel DM, Matrosic K. Intrapulmonary tumor necrosis factor triggers local platelet-activating factor production in rat immune complex alveolitis. Lab Invest 1990; 63:746–54.
58. Weiss SJ, Peppin G, Ortiz H, Ragsdale CM, Test SI. Oxidative autoactivation of latent collagenase by human neutrophils. Science 1985; 227:747–9.
59. Peppin GJ, Weiss SJ. Activation of the endogenous metalloproteinase, gelatinase, by triggered human neutrophils. Proc Natl Acad Sci U S A 1986; 83:4322–6.
60. Gannon DE, He X, Ward PA, Varani J, Johnson KJ. Time-dependent inhibition of oxygen radical induced lung injury. Inflammation 1990; 14:509–17.
61. Phan SH, Gannon DE, Varani J, Ryan US, Ward PA. Xanthine oxidase activity in rat pulmonary artery endothelial cells and its alteration by activated neutrophils. Am J Pathol 1989; 134:1201–11.
62. Friedl HP, Till GO, Ryan US, Ward PA. Mediator-induced activation of xanthine oxidase in endothelial cells. FASEB J 1989; 3:2512–8.
63. McCord JM, Fridovich I. The reduction of cytochrome c by milk xanthine oxidase. J Biol Chem 1968; 243:5753–60.
64. Warren JS, Yabroff KR, Remick DG, et al. Tumor necrosis factor participates in the pathogenesis of acute immune complex alveolitis in the rat. J Clin Invest 1989; 84:1873–82.
65. Gamble JR, Harlan JM, Klebanoff SJ, Vada MA. Stimulation of the adherence of neutrophil to umbilical vein endothelium by human recombinant tumor necrosis factor. Proc Natl Acad Sci U S A 1985; 82:8667.
66. Pohlman TH, Stanness KA, Beaty PG, Ochs HD, Harlan JM. An endothelial cell surface factor(s) induced in vitro by lipopolysaccharide, interleukin 1 and tumor

necrosis factor-α increases neutrophil adherence by a CDw18-dependent mechanism. J Immunol 1986; 136:4548.

67. Pohlman TH, Harlan JM. Human endothelial cell response to lipopolysaccharide, interleukin-1 and tumor necrosis factor is regulated by protein synthesis. Cell Immunol 1989; 119:41–52.
68. Luscinskas FW, Brock AF, Arnaout MA, Gimbrone MA. Endothelial-leukocyte adhesion molecule-1-dependent and leukocyte (CD11/CD18)-dependent mechanisms contribute to polymorphonuclear leukocyte adhesion to cytokine-activated human vascular endothelium. J Immunol 1989; 142:2257–63.
69. Bevilacqua MP, Pober JS, Mendrick DL, Cotran RS, Gimbrone MA Jr. Identification of an inducible endothelial-leukocyte adhesion molecule. Proc Natl Acad Sci U S A 1987; 84:9238.
70. Bevilacqua MP, Stengelin S, Gimbrone MA Jr, Seed B. Endothelial leukocyte adhesion molecule 1: an inducible receptor for neutrophil related to complement regulatory proteins and lectins. Science 1989; 243:1160.
71. Strieter RM, Kunkel SL, Showell H, et al. Human endothelial cell gene expression of a neutrophil chemotactic factor by TNF-α, LIP, and IL-1β. Science 1989; 243:1468–9.
72. Dixit VM, Green S, Sarma V, et al. Tumor necrosis factor-α induction of novel gene products in human endothelial cells including a macrophage-specific chemotaxin. J Biol Chem 1990; 165:2973–8.
73. Warren JS, Yabroff KR, Remick DG, et al. Intrapulmonary IL-1 and TNF in acute immune complex lung injury in the rat. Fed Proc 1989; 3:A759.
74. Nelson S, Bagby GJ, Bainton BG, Wilson LA, Thompson JJ, Summer WR. Compartmentalization of intraalveolar and systemic lipopolysaccharide-induced tumor necrosis factor and the pulmonary inflammatory response. J Infect Dis 1989; 159:489–94.
75. Leist TP, Frei K, Kam-Hansen S, Zinkernagel RM, Fontana A. Tumor necrosis factor-α in cerebrospinal fluid during bacterial, but not viral meningitis: evaluation in murine model infections and in patients. J Exp Med 1988; 167:1743–8.
76. Mustafa MM, Ramilo O, Olsen KD, et al. Importance of tumor necrosis factor in mediating experimental *Haemophilus influenzae* type b meningitis. J Clin Invest 1989; 84:1253–9.
77. Mustafa MM, Lebel MH, Ramilo O, et al. Correlation of interleukin-1β and cachectin concentrations in cerebrospinal fluid and outcome from bacterial meningitis. J Pediatr 1989; 115:208–13.
78. Pober JS. Cytokine-mediated activation of vascular endothelium. Am J Pathol 1988; 133:426–33.
79. Smith CW, Rothlein R, Hughes BJ, et al. Recognition of an endothelial determinant for CD18-dependent human neutrophil adherence and transendothelial migration. J Clin Invest 1988; 82:1746–56.
80. Smith CW, Marlin SD, Rothlein R, Toman C, Anderson DC. Cooperative interactions of LFA-1 and Mac-1 with ICAM-1 in facilitating adherence and transendothelial migration of human neutrophils. J Clin Invest 1989; 83:2008–17.
81. Le J, Vilcek J. Tumor necrosis factor and interleukin 1: cytokines with multiple overlapping biological activities. Lab Invest 1987; 56:234–48.

CHAPTER 16

FIBROBLASTS AND CYTOKINES

Soverin Karmiol and Sem H. Phan

The University of Michigan Medical School
Ann Arbor, Michigan

INTRODUCTION

The fibroblast, along with the myofibroblast and pericyte, belongs to a group of cells localized primarily in the interstitial space of tissues. These cells arise from mesenchymal tissue and are not always easy to distinguish from each other in culture, despite differences in morphology, contractile protein content and composition, cell surface antigen expression, and extracellular matrix production. Furthermore, fibroblasts from one tissue may show distinguishing features from those in another organ or tissue (1), and even within the same tissue there may be heterogeneity in fibroblast populations (2). However, in many in vitro studies scant attention has been paid to these differences between subpopulations or to differences between fibroblast (and even fibroblastlike) cell lines and primary cell cultures. Since the topic of this chapter is derived primarily from such in vitro studies, it is futile to attempt to differentiate between these cell populations. Consequently, except when clear differences have been unequivocally established, the fibroblast in this chapter refers to any one of these cell populations in a generic manner. To be comprehensive this discussion of fibroblast function covers the results of studies using these various cell types, but all findings may not be strictly applicable to any specific fibroblast population or subpopulation. Hence any cell-specific application of the following discussion and review of fibroblast interaction with cytokines must be considered with this caveat in mind.

The past decade has seen a considerable change in how the fibroblast is viewed in terms of its in vivo role under normal and diseased conditions. Before these recent advances, this cell was viewed primarily as an important structural component of tissues, responsible for the production of interstitial collagens and other extracellular matrix components. Replacement of normal functional organs by fibrotic lesions has long been known to be stereotypically associated with replacement of parenchymal differentiated cells by fibroblasts. By virtue of their inability to express the differentiated and often highly specialized functions of the original parenchymal cells, these fibroblasts have been viewed as passive structural cells devoid of vital functions whose unchecked proliferation is considered inimical to successful repair and regeneration of normal functional parenchyma. Hence early studies focused on fibroblast production of extracellular matrix and enzymes involved in its metabolism, with little attention to its possible active role in paracrine or autocrine regulatory mechanisms. With the realization that these cells are a primary source of the connective tissue found in fibrotic lesions, increasing emphasis is placed on understanding the mechanisms underlying regulation of fibroblast growth, chemotaxis, and extracellular matrix synthesis. These early studies concentrate on the role of exogenous factors or mediators in regulating these cellular functions, primarily treating the fibroblast as a passive target for regulatory signals from other cells. This view gradually begins to change with the discovery that certain fibroblast products, including the extracellular matrix components or their degradation products, have regulatory effects on other cells and the fibroblast itself. Since this cell and cell lines derived from it are readily available as a result of the relative ease of growing and maintaining them in tissue culture, they have been used in many in vitro model systems to study regulation of mediator production in other cells that are more difficult or impossible to culture. These studies serendipitously provide among the first important clues that the fibroblast, not only the cells it is supposed to mimic or be a model for, is in its own right capable of responding to paracrine as well as autocrine signals by the production of mediators of regulatory and pathogenetic consequence on surrounding cells and itself. Hence a wealth of information is now available to convincingly demonstrate that the fibroblast is likely to be an important cell in vivo as a key participant in normal and pathological processes in which these cell-derived mediators or cytokines have been found to be important. Since the fibroblast is ubiquitous, the production of cytokines by this cell is expected to play an important role in most if not all tissues, and considering the myriad activities of the cytokines produced by this cell, it has been postulated as playing a role in an ever expanding repertoire of physiological as well as pathophysiological processes, such as the regulation of tissue differentiation, repair, and fibrosis, hematopoiesis, bone metabolism, inflammation, and immune response.

This chapter is organized into subsections discussing the known classes of cytokines that either are produced by fibroblasts or have an effect on fibroblast function. This organization is certainly not an accurate reflection of the pleiotropic effects of these cytokines, nor does it reflect their diverse multiple cellular sources. As a matter of fact, rigid adherence to this is impossible in view of the well-known and complex interactions between various cytokines. Hence this attempt at providing some structural framework merely represents a starting point by which to review the available literature on fibroblasts and cytokines. In each instance, when sufficient physicochemical and biochemical information on each cytokine, its receptor, and associated signal transduction pathways are available in other chapters, they are not repeated here.

INTERLEUKINS

The interleukin family of cytokines currently consists of some 10 members (3). The nomenclature reflects the original concept that these molecules represent mediators by which leukocytes communicate regulatory signals with each other. Discoveries during the last decade, however, have gradually made this restriction to leukocytes untenable. Although many of these peptides have little in common in terms of their biochemical and functional properties, they have nevertheless been grouped together because of their effects on leukocytes. The discussion that follows is subdivided into interleukins with known effects on fibroblasts or that may be produced by them, namely interleukins-1, 6, and 8. The others either have not been reported to affect, or be produced by, fibroblasts, or their effects on fibroblasts have not been sufficiently well characterized to warrant discussion in separate sections at this time.

Interleukin-1

In accordance with its numbering system, interleukin-1 (IL-1) was the first of this group of mediators to be discovered. Its role in regulating the immune and inflammatory response is well known (4) and is not discussed here. Although there are two distinct forms of IL-1, IL-1α and IL-1β, their functional effects are very similar (5) and mediated by the same receptor (6). Hence the discussion that follows generically refers to IL-1, unless a distinction is necessary to emphasize differences in biological activity.

The effects of IL-1 on fibroblasts are first examined using crude macrophage or monocyte supernatants before it is identified as such (7). These early studies focused on the destructive process in arthritic joints—hence the interest in the synovial fibroblast (8). Studies using purified IL-1 reproduce some of these effects (9). Since arthritis is a destructive process, the discovery of the effects of IL-1 on the inhibition of fibroblast growth and matrix synthesis and stimulation of collagenase production was among the first to be reported (10). The mechanism of inhibition is subsequently found to be at least partly due to the stimulation of prostaglandin E_2 (PGE_2) production by IL-1, which then in autocrine fashion causes downregulation of matrix synthesis and cell proliferation (11). This inhibitory effect is blunted by the addition of cyclooxygenase inhibitors to the target fibroblast during IL-1 treatment (12). Stimulation of prostaglandin production by IL-1 appears to be mediated by upregulation in phospholipase A_2 and cyclooxygenase activities due at least in part to increased synthesis of these enzymes. Additionally, IL-1 amplifies stimulation of PGE_2 production by bradykinin and other agonists by augmenting the bradykinin-induced increase in GTPase activity without a significant alteration in agonist receptor expression (13). IL-1 promotes the increased transcription of the matrix destructive enzymes collagenase (14) and stromelysin (15). With respect to collagenase, the increased transcription does not appear to be mediated by increased PGE_2 production (16). The regulatory mechanisms underlying this stimulation of transcription have not been completely defined. In the case of collagenase, increased transcription is preceded by a rapid but brief burst of c-*jun* transcription, whose gene product is likely to be the component of activator protein 1 (AP-1) which is important for binding to DNA (17). Since binding of AP-1 is enhanced by the formation of a heterodimer between the c-*jun* and c-*fos* gene products and IL-1 also induces c-*fos* expression (18), it has been hypothesized that IL-1 promotes procollagenase gene transcription by increasing AP-1 levels and binding to the responsive element in the 5′ flanking region of the procollagenase gene, which then results in increased collagenase production (19). IL-1 also causes rapid and transient expression of the c-*myc* protooncogene that may be related to its growth factor activity (18). Since the prostromelysin (transin) gene has similar regulatory DNA sequences (20), it is likely that similar mechanisms may be operative in IL-1-induced stimulation of stromelysin production.

The effect of IL-1 on fibroblast collagen gene expression is complicated by the inhibitory effects of PGE_2 on collagen synthesis (21). Thus the conditions of assay are critical in determining whether a stimulatory or inhibitory effect is seen (12). PGE_2 is known to stimulate fibroblast collagenase secretion and elevates intracellular cAMP, which inhibits net collagen production (22). In contrast to this variable inhibitory effect on net collagen synthesis, there is more consistent evidence of IL-1-induced increase in steady-state levels of procollagen mRNA (23). These studies clearly establish the discrepancy between mRNA concentration and net production of collagen, thus suggesting that regulation is occurring at multiple levels of gene expression (12). Complex effects of IL-1 on glycosaminoglycan synthesis have also been reported (24).

Similar unmasking of the growth-promoting properties of IL-1 is also observed when the PGE_2 inhibitory effect is blocked with cyclooxygenase inhibitors or minimized by allowing its metabolism to inactive product before testing for cell proliferation (11). This activity is relatively weak in comparison to other well-defined fibroblast growth-promoting cytokines (25), however, thus making it uncertain that IL-1 can play a significant role in vivo in this regard. In view of these opposing effects, it is also difficult to pinpoint the actual in vivo role of IL-1 vis-à-vis fibroblast function in the pathogenesis of fibrosis. In pulmonary fibrosis there is evidence of an early and relatively brief increase in IL-1 production (26). This in conjunction with the in vitro data suggests that an early IL-1-induced inhibitory effect on fibroblast proliferation and net matrix production, and even the promotion of matrix destruction, may be followed by promotion of fibrogenesis upon metabolism of PGE_2 and removal of its inhibitory effects. On the other hand, a persistent IL-1 effect may result in a sustained destructive process by the continued heightened production of matrix-degrading enzymes and inhibition of matrix production by PGE_2, such as that seen in rheumatoid arthritis (27). The complex regulation of fibroblast proliferation and extracellular matrix production by IL-1 and other cytokines is summarized in Figs. 1 and 2. Alternatively, or in addition to these effects, IL-1 may play a role by regulating the production of other cytokines with similar and additional effects.

In addition to these effects on fibroblasts, IL-1 regulates the production of other cytokines by these cells (Table 1). In addition to stimulating the production of IL-1 itself, it upregulates fibroblast production of IL-6 (28), IL-8, tumor necrosis factor α (TNF-α) (29), monocyte chemotactic protein 1 (MCP-1) (30), and a number of colony-stimulating factors (CSFs) (31) and serum complement components (32). IL-1-dependent regulation of specific cytokines is discussed later in the respective sections. Fibroblasts appear to produce only IL-1β (33), with virtually none of it secreted (34). This lack of secretion may be related to the lack

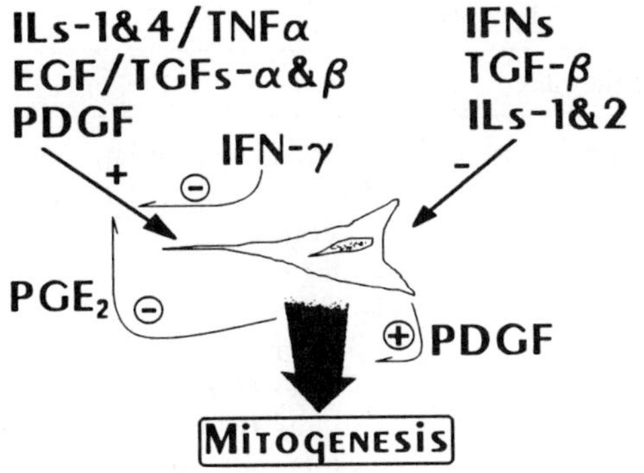

FIGURE 1 Cytokine regulation of fibroblast proliferation. The effects (positive sign indicates stimulation; negative sign indicates inhibition) of cytokines on fibroblast proliferation are shown. The thin lines with half-arrowheads, originating from the fibroblast itself, represent the effects of agents induced by the initial cytokine stimulation and indicate autocrine regulation. The modulatory effect of exogenous IFN-γ is also shown.

of a signal sequence in this molecule (35), and recent data suggest that secretion by monocytes is via a reverse endocytotic process since most of the IL-1β appears to be located inside vesicles. In contrast, U937 cells do not package their IL-1β inside vesicles and do not secrete this cytokine (36). It is possible that the situation in fibroblasts may be similar to that in U937 cells, thus explaining why IL-1β is not secreted even though high levels are encountered intracellularly. In addition to self-regulation, IL-1 production by fibroblasts is upregulated by other cytokines, such as TNF-α (37) and interferon-γ (IFN-γ) (38), and noncytokines, such as phorbol esters, teleocidin, calcium ionophores, ouabain (39), and lipopolysaccharide (LPS) (38), but is downregulated by steroids (40). The diversity of agents

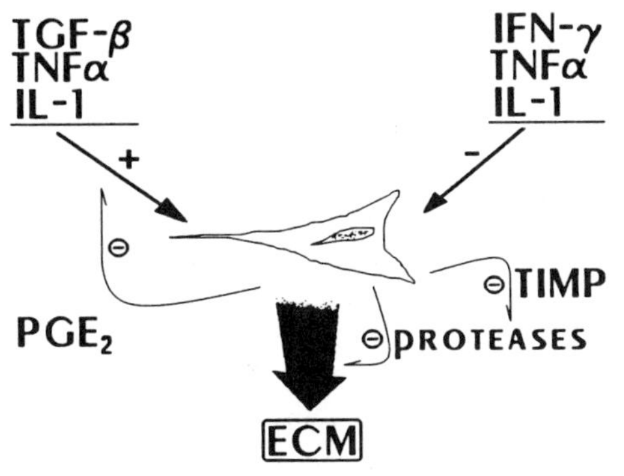

FIGURE 2 Cytokine regulation of extracellular matrix production. The complex effects of cytokines on fibroblast matrix production are shown. The thin and thick arrows have the same significance as in Fig. 1. The figure shows multilevel regulation of net matrix production as exemplified by the paradoxical effects of induction of both matrix-degrading enzymes ("proteases") and their inhibitors (e.g., TIMP). ECM refers to extracellular matrix production.

Table 1 Interleukins and Fibroblasts

IL	Made by fibroblast	Effects on fibroblast
IL-1	Yes: self-induced and induced by TNF-α and IFN-γ	Inhibits or stimulates cell proliferation Inhibits or stimulates extracellular matrix production Induces collagenase and stromelysin Induces IL-1, 6, 8; MCP-1; CSFs; PDGF Stimulates PGE_2 production Induces complement factor B and C3 Inhibits IL-6-induction of antiviral state
IL-6	Yes: self-induced and induced by IL-1 and TNF-α	Induces antiviral state Induces complement factor B and C3 Regulates expression of class I histocompatibility antigens Upregulates TIMP production Inhibits growth-promoting properties of TNF-α
IL-2		Inhibits division
IL-4		Stimulates cell proliferation Inhibits TNF-α-induced factor B production
IL-8	Yes: induced by TNF-α and IL-1	Unknown

suggest multiple regulatory steps, with the evidence suggesting that regulation occurs at both transcriptional and posttranscriptional levels. Although increased intracellular Ca^{2+} and activation of protein kinase C (PKC) appear to upregulate IL-1β production, the exact mechanism remains to be identified. The gene structure for IL-1β is described in detail in a separate chapter, but suffice it to note here that the presence of identifiable regulatory sequences suggests possible sites where these agents could modulate IL-1β gene expression, although definitive data are lacking (41). Increased stability of IL-1β mRNA has been reported in fibroblasts treated by a number of agents, although this may not always be mediated by the AU-rich sequences present in the 3′-untranslated region (42). Inhibition of IL-1 production by steroids may be mediated via the glucocorticoid-responsive element (GRE), which has been described in the IL-1β gene (43). Stimulation of IL-1β production by LPS, unlike that by the other agents, only occurs if the fibroblast has been primed by IFN-γ. The priming stimulus alone is insufficient to induce IL-1β gene expression. This study using synovial fibroblasts also showed significant secretion of IL-1β upon sequential IFN-γ and LPS treatments, which seems to contradict other studies showing no or minimal secretion using other agonists (38). This apparent discrepancy may be due to the cytotoxicity of combined IFN-γ and LPS treatment (44), which has been suggested as a means by which IL-1β is released to the extracellular environment (34). Thus, although it is clear that a number of cytokine and noncytokine agonists are capable of regulating IL-1β production, the lack of significant secretion makes it doubtful that the fibroblast is a significant in vivo source of extracellular IL-1β. However, IL-1β expressed on the cell membrane surface (45) is of consequence since intimate contact with cells in the interstitium may transmit the regulatory signals associated with this cytokine (37).

In addition to regulating the production of other cytokines, IL-1 also stimulates the production of components of the alternative pathway of complement, namely factor B and C3 (Table 1) (46). This effect is enhanced by pretreatment with IFN-γ but is inhibited by dexamethasone and platelet-derived growth factor (PDGF), epidermal growth factor (EGF), and basic fibroblast growth factor (bFGF). Inhibition by the growth factors is specific for factor B only and appears to occur at a pretranslational level (32). Thus IL-1 could also influence complement-dependent pathophysiological events in this manner.

Many of the effects of IL-1 on fibroblasts just described are similar to those induced by TNF-α (47), and synergistic effects have been reported when these two cytokines are used together (28). This occurs despite that they are dissimilar in structure and bind to two different receptors (48). The receptor for IL-1β is described in a separate chapter and is presumed to mediate all the effects described previously.

Interleukin-6

Interleukin-6 (IL-6) represents another example of the multifunctional cytokine with important roles in the acute-phase response, regulation of T cell function, terminal B cell differentiation, and thrombopoiesis (49). Its role in the regulation of fibroblast function is as yet incompletely defined (summarized in Table 1). As with IL-1 and TNF-α, IL-6 is capable of self-induction but does not induce IL-1 or TNF-α in fibroblasts (50). IL-6 is associated with the antiviral state in fibroblasts and was formerly thought to be the endogenous or autocrine mediator for induction of this state by TNF-α, although it inhibits the growth-promoting properties of TNFα (51). More recent data show that IL-1 and PDGF inhibit IL-6 as well as IFN-β_1 induction of the antiviral state (52). IL-6 plays a role in the expression of class I histocompatibility antigens (53) and in the induction of the acute-phase proteins, complement factor B, and C3 (54) in human fibroblasts. A recent report suggests that IL-6 may play a role in fibroblast extracellular matrix metabolism via its ability to enhance the production of tissue inhibitor of metalloproteinase (TIMP) (55). Specific receptors for IL-6 have been reported in a variety of cells (56) and presumably mediate the observed biological functions of this cytokine. Details on this receptor are available in chapter 6.

A great deal more information is available concerning the fibroblast as a source of IL-6 with potential in vivo significance in regulation of the earlier functions mentioned attributed to this cytokine. In the absence of added agonists, IL-6 is produced at very low levels by fibroblasts (57). Upon stimulation by an increasing array of substances, ranging from LPS to cytokines and phorbol esters, increased IL-6 production is detected by increases in cellular IL-6 mRNA content and secretion. Among the cytokines, the effects of IL-1 and TNF-α have been studied extensively (58). Other agonists have also been used as a means of deciphering the stimulus-response coupling mechanisms involved in upregulation of IL-6 production induced by these cytokines. Studies using IL-1 and TNF-α as agonists seem to implicate adenyl cyclase and its attendant effects on intracellular cAMP levels as important in this regard. This conclusion is supported by the observation of the inhibitory effects on IL-6 induction by selective inhibitors of cAMP-dependent protein kinase A (59). PKC appears not to be important in IL-6 induction by IL-1, TNF-α, or TNF-β (49). Other studies, however, show that activators of PKC stimulate IL-6 production (60), suggesting that certain agonists, such as LPS, may work via such a pathway (61). There is also some suggestion of a role for G binding proteins. These increases in IL-6 production are associated with increases in IL-6 mRNA levels, which appear to be due to a combination of increased transcription and stabilization of the mRNA. Addition of cycloheximide causes superinduction (49). Stimulation of transcription appears to be mediated by multiple transcriptional enhancer elements in the 5′ flanking region of the IL-6 gene (62), which could account for the variety of substances capable of regulating IL-6 gene expression. The region from –225 to –111 base pairs of the IL-6 gene appears to be important in induction by a number of stimulants, such as cytokines and viruses (63).

Other Interleukins and Miscellaneous Cytokines

Much less is known about the other interleukins with regard to their effects on and production by fibroblasts (summarized in Figs. 1 and 2 and Table 1). IL-2 has been shown to inhibit proliferation of bone marrow fibroblasts by preventing entry into *S* phase, which is not mediated by IFN-γ (64). The latter is known to have inhibitory effects on fibroblast collagen production and proliferation (65). IFN-α and IFN-β are also known to inhibit fibroblast proliferation (66). Other effects of interferons are discussed in the respective sections on specific cytokines with which they have been shown to have synergistic effects. IL-4 has inhibitory effects on TNF-α-stimulated fibroblast factor B production (67) but appears to stimulate cellular proliferation (68). IL-8 is more completely discussed in the chapter devoted to this cytokine. Of specific note to fibroblasts is their importance as a cellular source for this cytokine in vivo (69). There is no evidence to date that IL-8 has any significant biological effects on the fibroblasts themselves.

More recently, fibroblasts have been also reported to secrete monocyte chemotactic activity in response to TNF-α and IL-1 (30). This activity has now been determined to be similar to that isolated from activated monocyte-conditioned media and endothelial cells (70) and designated variously as monocyte chemotactic and activating factor (MCAF) or monocyte chemotactic protein 1 and has now been identified as the human homolog of the murine *JE* gene product (71). As with IL-8, it has four cysteine residues and has significant sequence homology with a number of proteins belonging to the IL-8 superfamily (70). This chemotactic protein has an apparent molecular weight of approximately 15 kD, and has 76 amino acid residues (72). The chemotactic activity appears to be specific for monocytes and is not active against neutrophils (70). Its effects on fibroblasts have not been evaluated.

TUMOR NECROSIS FACTORS

TNF-α (cachectin) and TNF-β (lymphotoxin) are primarily products of mononuclear phagocytes (73) and lymphoid cells (74), respectively, and share many

TABLE 2 Cytokine Interactions with Fibroblasts

Cytokine	Made by fibroblast?	Fibroblast interactions
IFN-α, β	Yes: β only, induced by IL-6, TNF-α, and IL-1	Inhibits cell proliferation Induces antiviral state
IFN-γ	No	Inhibits cell proliferation Inhibits collagen synthesis Induces IL-1
MCP-1	Yes: induced by TNF-α and IL-1	Unknown
TNF-α	No?	Stimulates cell proliferation Inhibits (stimulates) collagen synthesis Causes class I HLA expression Induces IL-1, 6, 8; MCP-1; factor B Stimulates PGE_2 production
EGF, TGF-α		Stimulates cell proliferation Induces PDGF Stimulates collagen synthesis Is chemotactic (EGF)
TGF-β	Yes: self-induced	Inhibits or stimulates cell proliferation Stimulates extracellular matrix synthesis Stimulates synthesis of protease inhibitors Induces TGF-β and PDGF
PDGF	Yes: self-induced and induced by EGF, TGF-β, and IL-1	Stimulates cell proliferation Is chemotactic

biological activities (75). However, TNF-α has been observed in human peripheral blood lymphocytes carefully depleted of monocytes. The message for the TNF-β gene is also detected in these cells, but the regulation of TNF-β gene expression appears to be independent of the TNF-α gene. Nevertheless, in both the human and mouse, the two genes are closely linked on the same chromosome as their corresponding histocompatibility (HLA) complex (76). It is thus interesting to note that TNF-α activates dermal fibroblasts to express class 1 HLA antigens (77), suggesting an immunoregulatory role for TNF-α that would enhance the participation of cytolytic T lymphocytes in the vascular and interstitial spaces. The proteins are 30% homologous in their primary structure (78), cause necrosis of Meth A sarcoma in vivo, are toxic to selected tumor cells in vitro, and bind to the same receptor on cells (79).

As with other cytokines, the influence of TNF-α on fibroblasts is varied and inseparable from the influences of other cytokines (Figs. 1 and 2 and Table 2). TNF-α inhibits fibroblast collagen synthesis (80), although there is a recent conflicting report showing that it stimulates human lung fibroblasts in the absence of serum to synthesize more types I and III collagens. The basis for this discrepancy is unknown but may be attributable to differences in the conditions of assay.

IFN-γ attenuated the stimulatory effect of TNF-α or IL-1. In the presence of 1% serum, TNF-α has a minor effect on collagen synthesis; however, the combination of IL-1 and TNF-α inhibits collagen production, and IFN-γ inhibits collagen production by itself. Generally these effects correlate with the mRNA levels for these collagens (81).

Human dermal fibroblasts express a membrane-associated IL-1 activity when stimulated with either TNF-α or TNF-β; LPS-stimulated fibroblasts do not. IFN-γ has no effect on the membrane IL-1 expression (82). IFN-γ alone can be cytolytic for normal mouse fibroblasts. The dose required for the cytotoxicity is higher than that required for its antiviral effect or for the activation of macrophages. However, the dose required for cytotoxicity can be reduced 10- to 100-fold by concomitant treatment with TNF-α or IL-1, or both, although neither alone is cytotoxic for these cells. Also, LPS, which alone has no effect on the viability of mouse fibroblasts, induces cytotoxicity in the presence of IFN-γ. Antibodies to TNF-α or IL-1 do not block the cytotoxic effect of LPS and IFN-γ. This toxicity has been shown to be transcription and translation dependent. It is noteworthy that preexposure of fibroblasts to IFN-γ enhances the binding of TNF-α to these cells (83).

Both TNFs have potent mitogenic activity for fibroblasts, which is downregulated by IFN-γ. Stimulation of fibroblasts with TNF-α is accompanied by the phosphorylation of cytosolic proteins of 41 and 43 kD at tyrosine, threonine, and/or serine residues. The mitogenic response correlates well with the increased stimulation of tyrosine phosphorylation (84). TNF-α or IL-1 causes a transient downregulation of EGF binding to quiescent fibroblast monolayers. This results from a reduction in EGF receptor affinity and appears to be mediated by a PKC-independent mechanism, since cytokine-mediated EGF receptor phosphorylation is resistant to staurosporine, a potent inhibitor of PKC (85,86). TNF-α enhances the transcription and translation of IL-6 in human fibroblasts. Human embryonic lung fibroblasts (WI-38) respond to TNF-β and to TNF-α by increasing the accumulation of IL-6 mRNA, with TNF-α about threefold more potent. Stimulation is independent of PKC, does not require new protein synthesis, and is at least in part a result of increased stabilization of the IL-6 mRNA (49). Il-1α or TNF-α, but not LPS, induces the transcription and translation of neutrophil activating peptide (NAP)/IL-8 and MCP-1 in fibroblasts (87).

TNF-α is not chemotactic for fibroblasts, nor does it alter the fibroblast response to other chemoattractants, such as fibronectin. However, whereas fibroblasts do not invade a type I collagen gel, preincubation of the cells with TNF-α markedly increase their invasiveness into the gel. This seems to be associated with specific degradation of type I collagen because TNF-α does not promote the invasion of skin fibroblasts through a reconstituted basement membrane. TNF-α has been observed to induce the synthesis of collagenase in dermal fibroblasts, but at a relatively high dose (88,89).

TNF-α in combination with exogenous arachidonic acid is toxic to confluent fibroblasts in serum-free culture medium. Indomethacin, a cyclooxygenase inhibitor, inhibits this cytotoxic effect. This suggests that TNF-α becomes cytotoxic when arachidonic acid, present in the culture medium, is converted to prostaglandins (90), and it has been shown that TNF-α stimulates the production of PGE_2 in target cells (91).

EPIDERMAL GROWTH FACTOR AND TRANSFORMING GROWTH FACTOR α

There is a family of EGF-like molecules, all of which are encoded by distinct genes. In this section only EGF and transforming growth factor α (TGF-α) are discussed. These molecules are characterized by high-affinity binding to the EGF receptor, inducing mitogenesis in EGF-sensitive cells and the presence of 6 half-cystines within the primary structure of approximately 50–60 residues. These half-cystine residues are essential for EGF biological activity (92). The similarity between EGF and TGF-α is mainly in the cystines, with about 30% identity in the other amino acids (93). Both EGF and TGF-α are processed from larger transmembrane protein precursors. The EGF molecule is synthesized as an active prepro-EGF molecule containing approximately 1200 residues (94,95). TFG-α is synthesized as part of a larger precursor, pro-TGF-α, which is an integral membrane glycoprotein. A 50 amino acid sequence in pro-TGF-α is exposed to the extracellular fluid phase, where it can be cleaved by an appropriate enzyme (93). TGF-α was initially thought to be a fetal form of EGF in that its expression is detected only in fetal or embryonic tissue or ectopically in tumors. However, the expression of TGF-α has been observed in normal adult tissues, such as the pituitary, ovary, keratinocytes, and macrophages. Yet, oncogenic transformation frequently results in enhanced expression of TGF-α, not EGF (96). TGF-α and EGF exert similar biological actions in many systems. There are exceptions, however, and these appear to stem from the ability of various cells to process the EGF receptor differently depending on whether EGF or TGF-α is bound. In NIH-3T3 cells the data suggest that (1) EGF routes the EGF receptor directly to a degradative pathway, whereas TGF-α allows receptor recycling before degradation, and (2) tyrosine phosphorylation could play a role in this differential receptor processing (97).

The EGF receptor is a single 170 kD polypeptide chain of 1186 residues with a substantial amount of N-linked oligosaccharide (98). It is not unlike that of receptors for several other growth factors [PDGF, insulin, Insulinlike Growth Factor-1 (IGF-1), CSF-1, and FGF]. The cytoplasmic tyrosine kinase domain of these receptors is similar to a number of oncogene products (99). With respect to the EGF receptor the tyrosine kinase domain has a high homology to the product of *erb B* (100). Near the carboxyl terminus of the receptor are four sites of EGF-dependent tyrosine autophosphorylation (101), perhaps defining an autoinhibitory region that can be relieved by phosphorylation or truncation (102). Interaction of either TGF-α or EGF with the EGF receptor leads to an increase in the formation of phosphoserine, phosphothreonine, and phosphotyrosine on the EGF receptor. The nontyrosine phosphorylations are attributable to nonreceptor kinases, such as PKC, implicating the activation of these kinases as a consequence of EGF binding (103). The PKC phosphorylation of the EGF receptor inhibits tyrosine phosphorylation and, in some cells, ligand binding (92). Tyrosine kinase-deficient receptors are unable to transduce any biological responses to EGF, although ligand binding is not compromised. Also, it has been demonstrated that agents that interfere with the degradation and processing of the EGF and EGF-receptor complex inhibit the EGF-induced growth response (104). The EGF receptor tyrosine kinase can phosphorylate other proteins, such as phospholipase C-γ1 (PLC-γ1), phosphoinositol 3-kinase, GTPase-activating protein, microtubule-associated protein kinase, and the *raf*-1 gene product (a serine kinase) (99).

The role of phosphatidylinositol turnover in EGF-induced signal transduction has not been fully defined in fibroblasts. Upon addition of EGF to cells, approximately 60% of PLC-γ1 is rapidly phosphorylated on tyrosine residues. PLC-γ1 hydrolyzes phosphoinositol 4,5-bisphosphate, yielding inositol 1,4,5-triphosphate and diacylglycerol. The former acts as a second messenger to liberate stored calcium from the endoplasmic reticulum; the latter is an activator of PKC (105). Most phosphoinositides do not contain a phosphate at the 3 position of the inositol ring, but a small pool phosphorylated at this site has been identified recently in growth factor-stimulated cells (106). All these phosphorylations occur within an hour of EGF binding, but EGF must remain in the extracellular environment for nearly 8 h before the cells become committed to increased DNA synthesis (107). Both EGF and PDGF elicit a mitogenic response. However, during PDGF stimulation, phospholipase C activity remains high, but during EGF stimulation phosphoinositide breakdown is not observed (108). This suggests that polyphosphoinositide hydrolysis is not an exclusive signaling pathway for commitment to DNA replication and cell division. Treatment with α-thrombin following chymotrypsin, EGF, or PDGF pretreatment results in the increase of diacylglycerols primarily through the stimulation of phosphatidylcholine hydrolysis. EGF does not stimulate the hydrolysis of other phospholipids, however, including the phosphoinositides. It thus appears that EGF stimulation is associated with the activation of a PLC specific for phosphatidylcholine, reflecting cytokine-sensitive phosphatidylcholine pools or selective diacylglycerol metabolism (109).

Preexposure of quiescent fibroblasts to PDGF increases the sensitivity to EGF by 10-fold, independent of whether EGF alone is found to be mitogenic (110). IFN-γ inhibits the mitogenic activity of PDGF, EGF, and FGF on fibroblasts. This inhibition is accomplished by blocking the transition of the G_0/G_1 to S phase of the cell cycle (111). Bradykinin, which activates PKC, blocks the IGF-1- and EGF-dependent mitogenic signals without affecting the response to serum or PDGF (112).

The extracellular matrix influences fibroblast responses to cytokines. The addition of EGF to cultures of human skin fibroblasts grown on plastic coated with or without various macromolecules results in repression of collagen synthesis while cell multiplication is slightly stimulated. However, the addition of EGF to fibroblasts grown in a collagen matrix results in stimulation of both noncollagenous protein and collagen synthesis as has been observed in vivo (Fig. 2 and Table 2) (113). Fibroblast chemotaxis is elicited by EGF in vitro, and PDGF and TGF-β can downregulate this activity (Fig. 3) (114).

TRANSFORMING GROWTH FACTOR β

TGF-β belongs to a large superfamily of closely related polypeptides. Currently three distinct forms of TGF-β are identified in mammals: TGF-β_1, TGF-β_2, and TGF-β_3. They are synthesized as larger precursor polypeptides that are processed to yield a C-terminal 112 amino acid monomer of 12.5 kD. The biologically active form is a 25 kD dimer composed of identical disulfide-linked monomers; however,

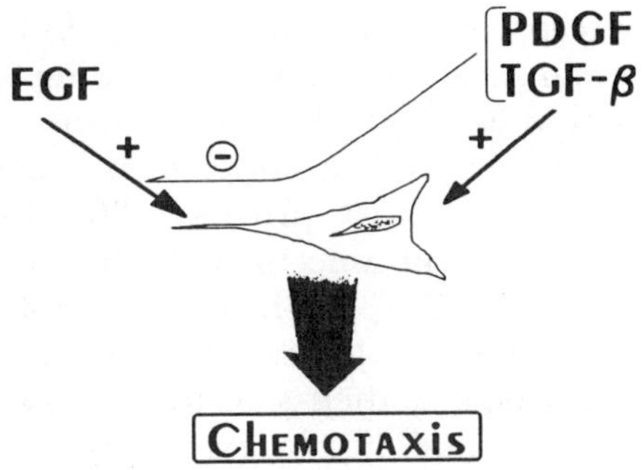

FIGURE 3 Cytokine regulation of fibroblast chemotaxis. All cytokines shown here are chemotactic for fibroblasts. However, as shown by the thin line, PDGF and TGF-β inhibit the chemotactic activity of EGF.

heterodimer molecules also have biological activity (115). Functionally TGF-β_3 exerts activities similar to those of the other two TGF-β species. The distinct differences in the potencies that have been observed between the different TGF-β forms depend on the cell type and assay used. These forms of TGF-β arise from different genes, and the promoter structures and regulatory elements for them are quite different (116). Also there appears to be a very complicated regulatory network by which each of the TFG-βs either upregulates or downregulates each other's expression (117).

The precursor form, which constitutes > 98% of the secreted TGF-β_1, is unable to bind to its cellular receptor without prior activation (118). Normal fibroblasts secrete TGF-β in latent form, whose activation occurs after treatment with acid or proteases, such as plasmin (119). A comparison of the human TGF-B_1, TGF-B_2, and TGF-B_3 precursor cDNAs reveals an amino acid sequence identity of about 75–80% within the mature peptide sequences, but the rest of the precursor sequence is only 25–30% conserved (120,121). Among mammals, the sequence for TGF-B_1 is highly conserved. In human, pig, cow, and monkey the sequence is identical and differs by only one amino acid in the mouse (122).

Three distinct types of TGF-β receptors have been identified on the surface of almost all cell types examined. Two of these receptors, types I and II, are glycoproteins of 53 and 73–95 kD, respectively, and display higher affinity for TGF-B_1 than for TGF-β_2 (123). The third receptor type (type III) is a 300 kD membrane proteoglycan with a core protein of 110 kD that binds TGF-β_1 and TGF-β_2 with similar affinity (124). All three receptors bind all three ligands with high affinity (K_d = 10–200 pM) (125). In human, rodent, and avian fibroblasts, the type III receptor is a larger disulfide-linked multisubunit complex of 565–615 kD (126). These receptors do not seem to autophosphorylate, nor do they possess tyrosine kinase activity. The oligomeric structure of the TGF-β receptor is not induced by receptor occupancy with the ligand (127). An inverse relationship exists between receptor affinity and receptor number per cell such that at low TGF-β concentrations all cells bind a similar number of TGF-β molecules. There is little or no ligand-induced receptor downregulation so that the receptor appears to be essentially unmodulated (128). However, increased cell density and differentiation appear to downregulate TGF-β binding as a result of a decrease in the number of high-affinity receptors, not from a change in receptor affinity (129).

The signal transduction mechanism after TGF binding is not well understood; however, some information is available. The growth stimulatory effect of TGF-B_1 on AKR-2B fibroblastic cells is coupled to a pertussis toxin-sensitive guanine nucleotide regulatory protein (G protein) (130). However, pertussis toxin does not affect TGF-β_1-stimulated fibronectin and collagen mRNA accumulation, nor does it have any effect on TGF-β_1-induced morphological transformation. These observations imply that TGF-β_1-stimulated gene expression is coupled to multiple pathways distinguished by their sensitivity to pertussis toxin (131). In fibroblastic cells that are growth inhibited by TGF-β, FGF- and thrombin-induced alterations in intracellular pH, PKC activity, protein phosphorylation, and phosphoinositide metabolism were not affected by TGF-β (132).

TGF-β is a growth inhibitor for a wide variety of cell types, including selected cell types of mesenchymal origin, although initially it was discovered because of its ability to stimulate anchorage-independent growth of nontransformed fibroblastic cells (133). For cells of mesenchymal origin, however, whether TGF-β stimulates or inhibits proliferation depends on the presence of other growth factors (125). The cell cycle kinetics of TGF-β stimulation of fibroblast proliferation results in an approximate 12 h prolongation of G_1 and appears to be mediated by an indirect mitogenic response. For example, in ARK-2B cells TGF-β induces c-*sis* mRNA associated with an increase in PDGF activity in the conditioned media. Thus, TGF-β indirectly stimulates proliferation by inducing the synthesis of the c-*sis* gene product, PDGF B chain (Fig. 1) (134). TGF-β also stimulates DNA synthesis in human foreskin fibroblasts after a prolonged lag period compared to stimulation by other growth factors, such as PDGF, EGF, or FGF, and appears to be mediated by endogenous production of PDGF A chain gene but not the B chain. This phenomenon may be important in vivo (135). In analogous fashion, mitogenic activity of IL-1 in fibroblasts may be due to autocrine induction of PDGF AA chains (136). In contrast to the mitogenic activity, a recent study shows that selective downregulation of PDGF AA binding is associated with TGF-β-induced inhibition of the mitogenic response to PDGF AA in 3T3 cells (137). The inhibitory effects of TGF-β depend on its concentration and the cell density. At low doses, TGF-β stimulates the proliferation of densely plated human marrow fibroblasts, but it is inhibitory at high concentrations. PDGF-stimulated proliferation of bone marrow cells is inhibited by low concentrations of TGF-β only if plated at low density (138). The high concentrations of TGF-β appear to decrease transcription and expression of PDGF receptor α subunits (139). Transcription of specific genes in response to EGF treatment can also be stably altered by exposure to TGF-β, resulting in a synergistic stimulation of transcription that is not evident using either individually (140).

TGF-β is a potent inducer of extracellular matrix production, stimulating synthesis of collagen types I, III, and V, fibronectin (141) and the fibronectin-receptor complex, and glycosaminoglycans (142). TGF-β inhibits matrix degradation by increased synthesis of inhibitors of proteases involved in matrix degradation, such as metalloproteinase inhibitor and plasminogen activator inhibitor 1 (143) and by inhibiting gene expression and synthesis of the proteases, transin/stromelysin and collagenase (Fig. 2) (144). Regulation of matrix gene expression appears to be at both transcriptional and posttranscriptional levels (145,146).

The effect of TGF-β on matrix production appears to be long lasting, if not irreversible, since an elevated expression of TGF-β, collagen α_2(I), and fibronectin mRNAs persists for at least 96 h after the removal of TGF-β (147). TGF-β stimulates the production of PGE_2 (148), which is paradoxically inhibitory to collagen synthesis (149).

Another key biological activity of TGF-β in fibroblasts and macrophages is chemotaxis (Fig. 3) (150,151). Histological analysis of treated wounds demonstrates an in vivo chemotactic response of macrophages and fibroblasts to both PDGF BB and TGF-β_1, but the response to TGF-B_1 is significantly less than that observed with PDGF BB (152). Intraarticular injection of TGF-β results in a marked synovitis and synovial hyperplasia consistent with its parallel monocyte and fibroblast chemotactic properties and ability to induce macrophage-derived growth factors (153).

Given these properties (summarized in Figs. 1 through 3, and Table 2), TGF-β has been implicated in the pathogenesis of fibrotic lesions. It is spontaneously secreted by synovial and other fibroblastlike cells. For example, human skin fibroblasts from scleroderma patients and normal control donors both produce comparable amounts of TGF-β and possess a comparable number of TGF-β receptors (154). This suggests that an alteration in the activation of latent TGF-β or in postreceptor responsiveness of the scleroderma fibroblasts may be the critical factor in promoting fibrosis. Since TGF-β activity is modulated by other cytokines it is possible that the conditions present in vivo in scleroderma and perhaps other fibrogenic processes may influence the action of TGF-β so that a fibrotic lesion results.

PLATELET-DERIVED GROWTH FACTOR

PDGF is a major mitogen in serum for connective tissue and other cells (Fig. 1). The PDGF from human platelets is a cationic glycoprotein of approximately 30 kD (155). PDGF has been implicated, directly or indirectly, in neoplasia, arthritis, arteriosclerosis, and bone marrow fibrosis. In human platelets, PDGF, which is stored in α granules, is a disulfide-bonded dimer of two similar but not identical polypeptides, denoted A and B. All three combinations of polypeptide chains (PDGF AA, AB, and BB), however, have been identified and purified from platelets or other cells and have been shown to be mitogenic (156). The PDGF isoforms differ in their functional effects on human fibroblasts; whereas PDGF AA induces transmodulation of the receptor for EGF to the same extent as the other isoforms, it is a less potent mitogen and has no stimulatory effect on actin reorganization or chemotaxis (157). PDGF AA is a potent mitogen, however, for Swiss 3T3 cells (158). The functional differences and binding characteristics of the isoforms have led to the identification of two classes of receptors. The PDGF B-type receptor (β-receptor) binds PDGF BB with high affinity and PDGF AB with about 10 times lower affinity but does not bind PDGF AA with any appreciable affinity. The PDGF A-type receptor (α-receptor) binds all three isoforms with high affinity. There is a close structural similarity between the two receptor types; both have extracellular components that can be divided into five immunoglobulinlike domains and cytoplasmic components that possess split protein tyrosine domains (159). The gene product of *raf*-1 is a serine kinase that is a tyrosine phopsphorylation substrate of the PDGF receptor kinase (160).

With human fibroblasts, which contain three to four times more B-type than

A-type PDGF receptors, PDGF AB and PDGF BB were found to be potent mitogens, whereas PDGF AA induced only a limited mitogenic stimulation (161). Whereas both receptors can transduce a mitogenic signal, only the B-type receptor appears to be able to mediate chemotaxis or the formation of circular membrane ruffles in human foreskin fibroblasts. PDGF is a potent chemoattractant for cells that respond to PDGF as a mitogen. The chemotactic response of these cells to PDGF is inversely related to their rate of proliferation, with quiescent cells exhibiting a 25-fold greater chemotactic response than exponentially growing cells. Also, it was suggested that growth factors and transformation and tumor promoters specifically alter the ability of the cell to respond to the PDGF-mediated chemotactic signal and that both transformation and tumor promoters accomplish this by altering PDGF binding to its receptor (162). A transient expression of the gene encoding the PDGF A chain and the synthesis and release of functional A chain homodimers is an early event in the prereplicative phase of normal human foreskin fibroblasts exposed to PDGF or EGF (163). Pretreatment with TGF-β completely abolished binding of radioiodinated PDGF AA and PDGF AB to quiescent 3T3 cells but inhibited the binding of PDGF BB by only 40%. It was suggested that the loss of binding sites may result from direct effects on receptor expression rather than autocrine downregulation by PDGF AA (164).

In addition to its mitogenic effect on fibroblasts, PDGF upregulates IL-1 receptor mRNA levels and expression (165). In the presence of exogenous IL-1, this effect on IL-1 receptor expression may in turn modulate the PDGF mitogenic effect, in view of the regulatory effects of IL-1 on fibroblast growth (11, 12). Cell cycle regulation of human diploid fibroblasts is located in the proximal half of G_1, and to traverse this subphase, cells require certain factors, such as PDGF. Human foreskin fibroblasts exposed to PDGF respond by increasing the mRNA levels of the protooncogenes c-*fos* and c-*myc*. The c-*fos* mRNA level peaked at 30 minutes after exposure; c-*myc* levels peaked after 8 h (166). One strain of Hutchinson-Gilford (progeria) syndrome fibroblasts, AG3513, responded to PDGF by a reduced c-*fos* mRNA induction. The diminished response of AG3513 fibroblasts to PDGF was apparently not due to a reduced PDGF receptor number, affinity, or autophosphorylation (167). PDGF is known to activate the PLC-PKC pathway (168).

The response of fibroblasts to PDGF and/or EGF depends on the type of fibroblasts used. With respect to 3T3 fibroblasts, PDGF and EGF act as a competence and a progression factor, respectively. However, in EL2 rat fibroblasts EGF appears to be able to induce the synthesis of putative intracellular regulatory proteins that govern PDGF-induced competence in 3T3 cells. As a consequence, EGF in EL2 cells may act as both a competence and a progression factor via induction of the mechanisms, regulated in other cell lines by cooperation between different growth factors (169). Exposure to PDGF inhibits high-affinity binding of EGF by several types of fibroblasts. In human fetal lung fibroblasts (WI-38) PDGF-dependent inhibition of EGF binding correlates with PDGF-induced phosphorylation of threonine 654 (a residue phosphorylated when PKC is activated) of the EGF receptor and with inhibition of EGF receptor autophosphorylation on tyrosine residues (170). However, in human foreskin fibroblasts (FS4) PDGF did not stimulate phosphorylation of threonine 654, nor was there an effect on EGF-dependent, tyrosine-specific autophosphorylation of the receptor (171). This variability in cellular responses to a given cytokine underlines the heterogeneity of fibroblast populations as mentioned in the introduction to this chapter and may play an important role in normal and pathological processes.

REFERENCES

1. Conrad GW, Hart GW, Chen Y. Differences in vitro between fibroblast-like cells from cornea, heart, and skin of embryonic chicks. J Cell Sci 1977; 26:119–37.
2. Korn JH, Brinckerhoff CE, Edwards RL. Synthesis of PGE_2, collagenase and tissue factor by fibroblast substrains: substrains are differentially activated for different metabolic products. Collagen 1985; 5:437–47.
3. Hsu D-H, de Waal Malefyt R, Fiorentino DF, et al. Expression of interleukin-10 activity by Epstein-Barr virus protein BCRF1. Science 1990; 250:830–2.
4. Dinarello CA. Interleukin-1. Rev Infect Dis 1984; 6:51–95.
5. Wood DD, Bayne EK, Goldring MB. The four biochemically distinct species of human interleukin-1 all exhibit similar biological activities. J Immunol 1985; 134:895–903.
6. Kilian PL, Kaffha KL, Stern AS. Interleukin-1-alpha and interleukin-1-beta bind to the same receptor on T cells. J Immunol 1986: 136:4509–14.
7. Hamilton JA, Slywka J. Stimulation of human synovial fibroblast plasminogen activator production by mononuclear cell supernatants. J Immunol 1981; 126:851–5.
8. Dayer J-M, Russell RGG, Krane SM. Collagenase production by rheumatoid synovial cells: stimulation by a human lymphocyte factor. Science 1977; 195:181–3.
9. Hamerman D, Wood DD. Interleukin-1 enhances synovial cell hyaluronate synthesis. Proc Soc Exp Biol Med 1984; 177:205–10.
10. Dayer J-M, Bierard J, Chess L, Krane SM. Participation of monocyte/macrophages and lymphocytes in the production of a factor that stimulates collagenase and prostaglandin release by rheumatoid synovial cells. J Clin Invest 1979; 64:1386–92.
11. Elias, JA. Tumor necrosis factor interacts with interleukin-1 and interferons to inhibit fibroblast proliferation via fibroblast prostaglandin-dependent and -independent mechanisms. Am Rev Respir Dis 1988; 138:652–8.
12. Mauviel A. Teyton L, Bhatnagar R, et al. Interleukin-1 α modulates collagen gene expression in cultured synovial cells. Biochem J 1988; 252:247–55.
13. Burch RM, Connor JR, Axelrod J. Interleukin 1 amplifies receptor-mediated activation of phospholipase A_2 in 3T3 fibroblasts. Proc Natl Acad Sci U S A 1988; 85:6306–9.
14. Postlethwaite AE, Lachman LB, Mainardi CL, Kang AH. Interleukin 1 stimulation of collagenase production by cultured fibroblasts. J Exp Med 1983; 157:803–6.
15. Frisch SM, Ruley HE. Transcription from the stromelysin promoter is induced by interleukin-1 and repressed by dexamethasone. J Biol Chem 1987; 262:16300–4.
16. Dayer J-M, de Rochemonteix B, Burrus B, Demczuk S, Dinarello C. Human recombinant interleukin-1 stimulates collagenase and prostaglandin E_2 production by synovial cells. J Clin Invest 1986; 77:645–8.
17. Conca W, Kaplan PB, Krane SM. Increases in levels of procollagenase messenger RNA in cultured fibroblasts induced by human recombinant interleukin-1β or serum follow c-*jun* expression and are dependent on new protein synthesis. J Clin Invest 1989; 83:1753–7.
18. Lin J-X, Vilcek J. Tumor necrosis factor and interleukin-1 cause a rapid and transient stimulation of c-*fos* and c-*myc* mRNA levels in human fibroblasts. J Biol Chem 1987; 262:11908–11.
19. Angel P, Baumann I, Stein B, Delius H, Rahmsdorf HJ, Herrlich P. 12-*O*-tetra-

decanoyl-phorbol-13-acetate induction of the human collagenase gene is mediated by an inducible enhancer element located in the 5′-flanking region. Mol Cell Biol 1987; 7:2256–66.

20. Matrisian LM, Leroy P, Ruhlmann C, Gesnel M-C, Breathnach R. Isolation of the oncogene and epidermal growth factor-induced transin gene: complex control in rat fibroblasts. Mol Cell Biol 1986; 6:1679–86.
21. Bhatnagar R, Penfornis H, Mauviel A, Loyau G, Saklatvala J, Pujol J-P. Interleukin-1 inhibits the synthesis of collagen by fibroblasts. Biochem Int 1986; 13:709–20.
22. Clark JG, Kostal KM, Marino BA. Modulation of collagen production following bleomycin-induced pulmonary fibrosis in hamsters. Presence of a factor in lung that increases fibroblast prostaglandin E_2 and cAMP and suppresses fibroblast proliferation and collagen production. J Biol Chem 1982; 257:8098–105.
23. Postlethwaite AE, Raghow R, Stricklin GP, Poppleton J, Seyer JM, Kang AH. Modulation of fibroblast functions by interleukin 1: increased steady-state accumulation of type I procollagen messenger RNAs and stimulation of other functions but not chemotaxis by human recombinant interleukin 1 α and β. J Cell Biol 1988; 106:311–8.
24. Bronson RE, Argenta JG, Bertolami C. Interleukin-1-induced changes in extracellular glycosaminoglycan composition of cutaneous scar-derived fibroblasts in culture. Collagen 1988; 8:199–208.
25. Raines EW, Dower SK, Ross R. Interleukin-1 mitogenic activity for fibroblasts and smooth muscle cells is due to PDGF-AA. Science 1989; 343:393–6.
26. Jordana M, Richards C, Irving LB, Gauldie J. Spontaneous *in vitro* release of alveolar-macrophage cytokines after the intratracheal instillation of bleomycin in rats. Characterization and kinetic studies. Am Rev Respir Dis 1988; 137:1135–40.
27. Dinarello CA. Biology of interleukin 1. FASEB J 1988; 2:108–15.
28. Elias JA, Freundlich B, Kern JA, Rosenbloom J. Cytokine networks in the regulation of inflammation and fibrosis in the lung. Chest 1990; 97:1439–45.
29. Larsen CG, Anderson AO, Oppenheim JJ, Matsushima K. Production of interleukin 8 by human dermal fibroblasts and keratinocytes in response to interleukin 1 or tumor necrosis factor. Immunology 1989; 68:31–6.
30. Larsen CG, Zachariae CO, Oppenheim JJ, Matsushima K. Production of monocyte chemotactic and activating factor (MCAF) by human dermal fibroblasts in response to interleukin 1 or tumor necrosis factor. Biochem Biophys Res Commun 1989; 160:1403–8.
31. Zucali JR, Dinarello CA, Oblon DJ, Gross MA, Anderson L, Weiner RS. Interleukin 1 stimulates fibroblasts to produce granulocyte-macrophage colony-stimulating activity and prostaglandin E_2. J Clin Invest 1986; 77:1857–63.
32. Circolo A, Pierce GF, Katz Y, Strunk RC. Antiinflammatory effects of polypeptide growth factors. J Biol Chem 1990; 265:5066–71.
33. Mauviel A, Temime N, Charron D, Loyau G, Pujol J-P. Interleukin-1α and β induced gene expression in human dermal fibroblasts. Biochem Biophys Res Commun 1988; 156:1209–14.
34. Young PR, Hazuda DJ, Simon PL. Human interleukin 1β is not secreted from hamster fibroblasts when expressed constitutively from a transfected cDNA. J Cell Biol 1988; 107:447–56.
35. Gray PW, Glaister D, Chen E, Goeddel DV, Pennica D. Two interleukin 1 genes in the mouse: cloning and expression of the cDNA for murine interleukin 1 beta. J Immunol 1986; 137:3644–8.
36. Rubartelli A, Cozzolino F, Talio M, Sitia R. A novel pathway for interleukin-1β, a protein lacking a signal sequence. EMBO J 1990; 9:1503–10.

37. Le J, Weinstein D, Gubler U, Vilcek J. Induction of membrane-associated interleukin 1 by tumor necrosis factor in human fibroblasts. J Immunol 1987; 138:2137–42.
38. Johnson WJ, Breton J, Newman-Tarr T, Connor JR, Meunier PC, Dalton BJ. Interleukin-1 release by rat synovial cells is dependent on the sequential treatment with γ-interferon and lipopolysaccharide. Arthritis Rheum 1990; 33:261–7.
39. Yamato K, El-Hajjaoui Z, Koeffler HP. Regulation of levels of IL-1 mRNA in human fibroblasts. J Cell Physiol 1989; 139:610–6.
40. Larsson E-L. Cyclosporin A and dexamethasone suppress T cell responses by selectively acting at distinct sites of the triggering process. J Immunol 1980; 124:2828–33.
41. Kovacs EJ, Radzioch D, Young HA, Varesio L. Differential inhibition of IL-1 and TNF-α mRNA expression by agents which block second messenger pathways in murine macrophages. J Immunol 1988; 141:3103–5.
42. Caput D, Beutler B, Hartog K, Thayer R, Brown-Shimer S, Cerami A. Identification of a common nucleotide sequence in the 3′-untranslated region of mRNA molecules specifying inflammatory mediators. Proc Natl Acad Sci U S A 1986; 83:1670–4.
43. Lee SW, Tsou A, Chan H, et al. Glucocorticoids selectively inhibit the translation of the interleukin 1β gene and decrease the stability of interleukin 1β mRNA. Proc Natl Acad Sci U S A 1988; 85:1204–8.
44. Dijkmans R, Van Dame J, Cornette F, Heremans H, Billiau A. Bacterial lipopolysaccharide potentiates gamma interferon-induced cytotoxicity for normal mouse and rat fibroblasts. Infect Immun 1990; 58:32–6.
45. Fuhlbrigge RC, Fine SM, Unane ER, Chaplin DD. Expression of membrane interleukin 1 by fibroblasts transfected with murine pro-interleukin 1α cDNA. Proc Natl Acad Sci U S A 1988; 85:5649–53.
46. Katz Y, Strunk RC. IL-1 and tumor necrosis factor: similarities and differences in stimulation of expression of alternative pathway of complement and IFN-β_2/IL-6 genes in human fibroblasts. J Immunol 1989; 142:3862–7.
47. Dinarello CA. Interleukin-1: amino acid sequences, multiple biological activities and comparison with tumor necrosis factor (cachectin). Year Immunol 1986; 2:68–89.
48. Beutler BA, Cerami A. Recombinant interleukin 1 suppressed lipoprotein lipase activity in 3T3-L1 cells. J Immunol 1985; 135:3969–71.
49. Akashi M, Loussararian AH, Adelman DC, Saito M, Koeffler HP. Role of lymphotoxin in expression of interleukin 6 in human fibroblasts: stimulation and regulation. J Clin Invest 1990; 85:121–9.
50. Zhang YH, Lin JX, Yip YK, Vilcek J. Enhancement of cAMP levels of protein kinase activity by tumor necrosis factor and interleukin 1 in human fibroblasts: role in the induction of interleukin 6. Proc Natl Acad Sci U S A 1989; 85:6802–5.
51. Kohase M, Henriksen-DeStefano D, May LT, Vilcek J, Sehgal PB. Induction of β_2-interferon by tumor necrosis factor: a homeostatic mechanism in the control of cell proliferation. Cell 1986; 45:659–66.
52. Kohase M, May LT, Tamm I, Vilcek J, Sehgal PB. A cytokine network in human diploid fibroblasts: interactions of β-interferons, tumor necrosis factor, platelet-derived growth factor, and interleukin-1. Mol Cell Biol 1987; 7:273–80.
53. May LT, Helfgott DC, Sehgal PB. Anti-beta-interferon antibodies inhibit the increased expression of HLA-B7 mRNA in tumor necrosis factor-treated human fibroblasts: structural studies of the beta 2 interferon involved. Proc Natl Acad Sci U S A 1986; 83:8957–61.
54. Katz Y, Revel M, Strunk RC. Interleukin 6 stimulates synthesis of complement proteins factor B and C3 in human fibroblasts. Eur J Immunol 1989; 19:983–8.
55. Sato T, Ito A, Mori Y. Interleukin 6 enhances the production of tissue inhibitor of

metalloproteinases (TIMP) but not that of matrix metalloproteinases of human fibroblasts. Biochem Biophys Res Commun 1990; 170:824–9.
56. Taga T, Kawanishi K, Hardy RR, Hirano T, Kishimoto T. Receptor for B cell stimulatory factor 2 (BSF2): quantitative, specificity, distribution and regulation of the expression. J Exp Med 1987; 166:967–81.
57. Heinrich PC, Castell JV, Andus T. Interleukin-6 and the acute phase response. Biochem J 1990; 265:621–36.
58. Akira S, Hirano T, Taga T, Kishimoto T. Biology of multifunctional cytokines: IL 6 and related molecules (IL 1 and TNF). FASEB J 1990; 4:2860–7.
59. Zhang Y, Lin J-X, Vilcek J. Synthesis of interleukin 6 (interferon-β_2/B-cell stimulatory factor 2) in human fibroblasts is triggered by an increase in intracellular cyclic AMP. J Biol Chem 1988; 263:6177–82.
60. Sehgal PB, Walther Z, Tamm I. Rapid enhancement of β_2-interferon/B cell differentiation factor BSF-2 gene expression in human fibroblasts by diacylglycerols and the calcium ionophore A23187. Proc Natl Acad Sci U S A 1987; 84:3663–7.
61. Dennis GJ, Mond JJ. Corticosteroid-induced suppression of murine B cell immune response antigens. J Immunol 1986; 136:1600–4.
62. Ray A, Tatter SB, May LT, Sehgal PB. Activation of human beta 2-interferon/hepatocyte-stimulating factor/interleukin 6 promoter by cytokines, viruses, and second messenger agonists. Proc Natl Acad Sci U S A 1988; 85:6701–5.
63. Ray A, Sassone-Corsi P, Sehgal PB. A multiple cytokine- and second messenger-responsive element in the enhancer of the human interleukin-6 gene: similarities with *c-fos* gene regulation. Mol Cell Biol 1989; 9:5537–47.
64. MacDonald D, Adams JA, McCarthy D, Barrett AJ. Interleukin-2 inhibits growth of fibroblasts derived from human bone marrow. Acta Haematol (Basel) 1990; 83:26–30.
65. Elias JA, Freundlich B, Kern JA, Rosenbloom J. Cytokine networks in the regulation of inflammation and fibrosis in the lung. Chest 1990; 97:1439–45.
66. Elias JA, Jimenez SA, Freundlich B. Recombinant gamma, alpha, and beta interferon regulation of human lung fibroblast proliferation. Am Rev Respir Dis 1987; 135:62–5.
67. Katz Y, Strunk RC. Enhanced synthesis of factor B induced by tumor necrosis factor in human skin fibroblasts is decreased by IL-4. J Immunol 1990; 144:4675–80.
68. Monroe JG, Haldar H, Prystowsky MB, Lammie P. Lymphokine regulation of inflammatory processes; interleukin-4 stimulates fibroblast proliferation. Clin Immunol Immunopathol 1988; 49:292–8.
69. Strieter RM, Phan SH, Showell HJ, et al. Monokine-induced neutrophil chemotactic factor gene expression in human fibroblasts. J Biol Chem 1989; 264:10621–6.
70. Matsushima K, Oppenheim JJ. Interleukin 8 and MCAF: novel inflammatory cytokines inducible by IL 1 and TNF. Cytokine 1989; 1:2–13.
71. Rollins BJ, Morrison ED, Stiles CD. Cloning and expression of *JE*, a gene inducible by platelet-derived growth factor and whose product has cytokine-like properties. Proc Natl Acad Sci U S A 1988; 85:3738–42.
72. Furutani Y, Nomura H, Notake M, et al. Cloning and sequencing of the cDNA for human monocyte chemotactic and activating factor (MCAF). Biochem Biophys Res Commun 1989; 159:249–55.
73. Carswell EA, Old LJ, Kassel RL, Green S, Fiore N, Williamson B. An endotoxin-induced serum factor that causes necrosis of tumors. Proc Natl Acad Sci U S A 1975; 72:3666–70.
74. Old LJ. Tumor necrosis factor (TNF). Science 1985; 230:630–2.
75. Goeddel DV, Aggarwal BB, Gray PW, et al. Tumor necrosis factors: gene structure and biological activities. Cold Spring Harbor Symp Quant Biol 1986; 51:597–609.

76. Nedospasov SA, Turetskaya RL, Shakhov AN. Cloning and characterization of the rabbit lymphotoxin (TNF-β) gene and its tight linkage to the gene coding for tumor necrosis factor. Nucleic Acids Res 1988; 16:3112.
77. Collins T, Lapierre LA, Fiers W, Strominger JL, Pober JS. Recombinant human tumor necrosis factor increases mRNA levels and surface expression of HLA-A, B antigens in vascular endothelial cells and dermal fibroblasts *in vitro*. Proc Natl Acad Sci U S A 1986; 83:446–50.
78. Rosenblum MG, Donato NJ, Gutterman JU. Characterization of human recombinant tumor necrosis factor-α antiproliferative effects on human cells in culture. Lymphokine Res 1988; 7:107–17.
79. Stauber GB, Aggarwal BB. Characterization and affinity cross-linking of receptors for human recombinant lymphotoxin (tumor necrosis factor-β) on a human histiocytic lymphoma cell line, U-937. J Biol Chem 1989; 264:3573–6.
80. Scharffetter K, Heckman M, Hatamochi A, et al. Synergistic effect of tumor necrosis factor-alpha and interferon-gamma on collagen synthesis of human skin fibroblasts *in vitro*. Exp Cell Res 1989; 181:409–19.
81. Elias JA, Freunlich B, Adams S, Rosenbloom J. Regulation of human lung fibroblast collagen production by recombinant interleukin-1, tumor necrosis factor, and interferon-gamma. Ann N Y Acad Sci 1990; 580:233–44.
82. Kurt-Jones EA, Fiers W, Pober JS. Membrane interleukin-1 induction on human endothelial cells and human dermal fibroblasts. J Immunol 1987; 139:2317–24.
83. Dijkmans R, Van Damme J, Cornette F, Heremans H, Billiau A. Bacterial lipopolysaccharide potentiates gamma interferon-induced cytotoxicity for normal mouse and rat fibroblasts. Infect Immun 1990; 58:32–6.
84. Kohno M, Nishizawa N, Tsujimoto M, Nomoto H. Mitogenic signalling pathway of tumor necrosis factor involves the rapid tyrosine phosphorylation of 41,000 and 43,000-M_r cytosol proteins. Biochem J 1990; 267:91–8.
85. Bird TA, Saklatvala J. Down-modulation of epidermal growth factor affinity in fibroblasts treated with interleukin 1 or tumor necrosis factor is associated with phosphorylation at a site other than threonine 654. J Biol Chem 1990; 265:235–40.
86. Schutze S, Nottrott S, Pfizenmaier K, Kronke M. Tumor necrosis factor signal transduction. Cell-type-specific activation and translocation of protein kinase C. J Immunol 1990; 144:2604–8.
87. Schroder JM, Stichering M, Henneicke HH, Preissner WC, Christophers E. IL-1 alpha or tumor necrosis factor-alpha stimulate release of three NAP-1/IL-8-related neutrophil chemotactic proteins in human dermal fibroblasts. J Immunol 1990; 144:2223–32.
88. Schirren CG, Scharffetter K, Hein R, Braun-Falco O, Krieg T. Tumor necrosis factor alpha induces invasiveness of human skin fibroblasts *in vitro*. J Invest Dermatol 1990; 94:706–10.
89. Lee TH, Lee GW, Ziff EB, Vilcek J. Isolation and characterization of eight tumor necrosis factor-induced gene sequences from human fibroblasts. Mol Cell Biol 1990; 10:1982–8.
90. Hori T, Kashiyama S, Hayakawa M, et al. Tumor necrosis factor is cytotoxic to human fibroblasts in the presence of exogenous arachidonic acid. Exp Cell Res 1989; 185:41–9.
91. Elias JA, Gustilo K, Baeder W, Freundlich B. Synergistic stimulation of fibroblast prostaglandin production by recombinant interleukin-1 and tumor necrosis factor. J Immunol 1987; 138:3812–6.
92. Carpenter G, Wahl MI. Epidermal growth factor. Handbook Exp Pharmacol 1990; 951:69–171.

93. Derynck R. Transforming growth factor-α. Mol Reprod Devel 1990; 27:3–9.
94. Gray A, Dull TJ, Ullrich A. Nucleotide sequence of epidermal growth factor cDNA predicts a 128,000-molecular weight protein precursor. Nature 1983; 303:722–5.
95. Mroczkowski B, Reich M, Chen K, Bell GI, Cohen S. Recombinant human epidermal growth factor precursor is a glycosylated membrane protein with biological activity. Mol Cell Biol 1989; 9:2771–8.
96. Wong DTW, Weller PF, Galli SJ, et al. Human eosinophils express transforming growth factor α. J Exp Med 1990; 172:673–81.
97. Decker SJ. Epidermal growth factor and transforming growth factor-alpha induce differential processing of the epidermal growth factor receptor. Biochem Biophys Res Commun 1990; 166:615–21.
98. Ushiro H, Cohen S. Identification of phosphotyrosine as a product of epidermal growth factor activated protein kinase in A-431 cell membranes. J Biol Chem 1980; 255:8363–5.
99. Carpenter G, Cohen S. Epidermal growth factor. J Biol Chem 1990; 265:7709–12.
100. Ullrich A, Coussens L, Hayflick JS, et al. Human epidermal growth factor receptor cDNA sequence and aberrant expression of the amplified gene in A431 epidermoid carcinoma cells. Nature 1984; 309:418–24.
101. Margolis BL, Lax I, Dombalagian M, et al. All autophosphorylation sites of epidermal growth factor (EGF) receptor and HER2/neu are located in their carboxyl-terminal tails. Identification of a novel site in EGF receptor. J Biol Chem 1989; 264:10667–71.
102. Walton GM, Chen WS, Rosenfeld MG, Gill GN. Analysis of deletions of the epidermal growth factor receptor reveals self-phosphorylation at tyrosine 992 and enhanced *in vivo* tyrosine phosphorylation of cell substrates. J Biol Chem 1990; 265:1750–4.
103. Heisermann GJ, Gill GN. Epidermal growth factor receptor threonine and serine residues phosphorylated *in vivo*. J Biol Chem 1988; 264:13152–8.
104. Chen WS, Lazar CS, Poenie M, Tsien Y, Gill GN, Rosenfeld MG. Requirement of intrinsic protein tyrosine kinase in the immediate and late actions of the EGF receptor. Nature 1987; 328:820–3.
105. Rhee SG, Pann-Ghill S, Sung-Ho R, Lee SY. Studies of inositol phospholipid-specific phospholipase C. Science 1989; 244:546–50.
106. Whitman M, Cantley L. Phosphoinositide metabolism and the control of cell proliferation. Biochim Biophys Acta 1988; 948:327–44.
107. Carpenter G, Cohen S. Human epidermal growth factor and the proliferation of human fibroblasts. J Cell Physiol 1976; 88:227–38.
108. Besterman JM, Watson SP, Cuatrecasas P. Lack, of association of epidermal growth factor-, insulin-, and serum-induced mitogenesis with stimulation of phosphoinositide degradation in BALB/c 3T3 fibroblasts. J Biol Chem 1986; 261:723–7.
109. Pessin MS, Baldassare JJ, Raben DM. Molecular species analysis of mitogen-stimulated 1,2-diglycerides in fibroblasts. Comparison of alpha-thrombin, epidermal growth factor, and platelet-derived growth factor. J Biol Chem 1990; 265:7959–66.
110. Wharton W, Leof E, Olashaw N, O'Keefe EJ, Pledger WJ. Mitogenic response to epidermal growth factor (EGF) modulated by platelet-derived growth factor in cultured fibroblasts. Exp Cell Res 1983; 147:443–8.
111. Oleszak E. Inhibition of mitogenic activity of PDGF, EGF, and FGF by interferon-gamma. Exp Cell Res 1988; 179:575–80.
112. Newman EL, Hyldahl L, Larsson O, Engstrom W, Rees AR. Bradykinin blocks the action of EGF, but not PDGF, on fibroblast division. FEBS Lett 1989; 251:225–9.
113. Colige A, Nusgens B, Lapiere CM. Effect of EGF on the skin fibroblasts is modulated by the extracellular matrix. Arch Dermatol Res 1988; 280(Suppl.: S42–6).

114. Adelmann-Grill BC, Wach F, Cully Z, Hein R, Krieg T. Chemotactic migration of normal dermal fibroblasts toward epidermal growth factor and its modulation by platelet-derived growth factor and transforming growth factor-beta. Eur J Cell Biol 1990; 51:322–6.
115. Derynck R, Jarrett JA, Chen EY, et al. Human transforming growth factor-beta complementary DNA sequence and expression in normal and transformed cells. Nature 1985; 316:701–5.
116. Barton DE, Foellmer BE, Du J, Tamm J, Derynck R, Franke U. Chromosomal mapping of genes for transforming growth factor beta 2 and beta 3 in man and mouse: dispersion of TGF-beta gene family. Oncogene Res 1988; 3:323–31.
117. Bascom CC, Wolfshohl RJ, Coffey J, et al. Complex regulation of transforming growth factor β_1, β_2, and β_3 mRNA expression in mouse fibroblasts and keratinocytes by transforming growth factors β_1 and β_2. Mol Cell Biol 1989; 9:5508–15.
118. Lawrence DA, Pircher R, Krycene-Martinerie C, Jullien P. Normal embryo fibroblasts release transforming growth factors in a latent form. J Cell Physiol 1984; 121:184–8.
119. Sato Y, Rifkin DB. Inhibition of endothelial cell movement by pericytes and smooth muscle cells; activation of a latent transforming growth factor-beta-like molecule by plasmin during co-culture. J Cell Biol 1989; 109:309–15.
120. Derynck R, Lindquist PB, Lee A, et al. A new type of transforming growth factor-beta, TGF-beta 3. EMBO J 1988; 7:3737–43.
121. Madisen L, Lioubin MN, Farrand AL, Brunner AM, Purchio AF. Analysis of proteolytic cleavage of recombinant TGF-β_1: Production of hybrid molecules with increased processing efficiency. Ann N Y Acad Sci 1990; 593:7–25.
122. Roberts AB, Kim S-J, Kondaiah P, et al. Transcriptional control of expression of the TGF-βs. Ann N Y Acad Sci 1990; 593:43–50.
123. Cheifetz S, Weatherbee JA, Tsang ML-S, et al. The transforming growth factor-beta system, a complex pattern of cross-reactive ligands and receptors. Cell 1987; 263:8366–70.
124. Segarini PR, Seyedin SM. The high molecular weight receptor to transforming growth factor-β contains glycosaminoglycan chains. J Biol Chem 1988; 263:8366–70.
125. Barnard JA, Russette ML, Moses HL. The biology of transforming growth factor β. Biochim Biophys Acta 1990; 1032:79–87.
126. Massagué J. Subunit structure of a high-affinity receptor for type β-transforming growth factor: evidence for a disulfide-linked glycosylated receptor complex. J Biol Chem 1985; 260:7059–66.
127. Fanger BO, Wakefield LM, Sporn MB. Structure and properties of the cellular receptor for transforming growth factor type β. Biochem 1986; 25:3983–91.
128. Wakefield LM, Smith DM, Masui T, Harris CC, Sporn MB. Distribution and modulation of the cellular receptor for transforming growth factor-beta. J Cell Biol 1987; 105:965–75.
129. Rizzino A, Kazakoff P, Ruff E, Kuszynski C, Nebelsick J. Regulatory effects of cell density on the binding of transforming growth factor β, epidermal growth factor, platelet-derived growth factor, and fibroblast growth factor. Cancer Res 1988; 48:4266–71.
130. Murthy US, Anzano MA, Stadel JM, Grieg R. Coupling of TGF-beta-induced mitogenesis to G-protein activation in AKR-2B cells. Biochem Biophys Res Commun 1988; 152:1228–35.
131. Howe PH, Cunningham MR, Leof EB. Distinct pathways regulate transforming growth factor beta 1-stimulated proto-oncogene and extracellular matrix gene expression. J Cell Physiol 1990; 142:39–45.

132. Chambard JC, Pouyssegur J. TGF-beta inhibits growth factor-induced DNA synthesis in hamster fibroblasts without affecting the early mitogenic events. J Cell Physiol 1988; 135:101–7.
133. Moses HL, Branum EB, Proper JA, Robinson RA. Transforming growth factor production by chemically transformed cells. Cancer Res 1981; 41:2842–8.
134. Leof EB, Proper JA, Goustin AS, Shipley GD, Dicorleto PE, Moses HL. Induction of *c-sis* mRNA and activity similar to platelet-derived growth factor by transforming growth factor β; a proposed model for indirect mitogenesis involving autocrine activity. Proc Natl Acad Sci U S A 1986; 83:2453–7.
135. Soma Y, Grotendorst GR. TGF-beta stimulates primary human skin fibroblast DNA synthesis via an autocrine production of PDGF-related peptides. J Cell Physiol 1989; 140:246–53.
136. Raines EW, Dower SK, Ross R. Interleukin-1 mitogenic activity for fibroblasts and smooth muscle cells is due to PDGF-AA. Science 1989; 243:393–6.
137. Gronwald RGK, Seifert RA, Bowen-Pope DF. Differential regulation of expression of two platelet-derived growth factor receptor subunits by transforming growth factor β. J Biol Chem 1989; 264:8120–5.
138. Kimura A, Katoh O, Hyodo H, Kuramoto A. Transforming growth factor-beta regulates growth as well as collagen and fibronectin synthesis of human marrow fibroblasts. Br J Haematol 1989; 72:486–91.
139. Battegay EJ, Raines EW, Seifert RA, Bowen-Pope DF, Ross R. TGF-β induces bimodal proliferation of connective tissue cells via complex control of an autocrine PDGF loop. Cell 1990; 63:515–24.
140. Ranganathan G, Getz MJ. Cooperation of specific gene transcription by epidermal growth factor and transforming growth factor type beta 1. J Biol Chem 1990; 265:3001–4.
141. Sporn MB, Roberts AB, Wakefield LM, de Crombrugghe B. Some recent advances in the chemistry and biology of transforming growth factor-beta. J Cell Biol 1987; 105:1039–45.
142. Ignotz RA, Massagué J. Cell adhesion protein receptors as targets for transforming growth factor-beta action. Cell 1987; 51:189–97.
143. Overall CM, Wrana JL, Sodek J. Transforming growth factor-beta regulation of collagenase, 72 kDa-progelatinase, TIMP and PAI-1 expression in rat bone cell populations and human fibroblasts. Connect Tissue Res 1989; 20:289–94.
144. Edwards DR, Murphy G, Reynolds JJ, et al. Transforming growth factor beta modulates the expression of collagenase and metalloproteinase inhibitor. EMBO J 1987; 6:1899–904.
145. Rossi P, Karsenty G, Roberts AB, Roche NS, Sporn MB, deCrombrugghe B. A nuclear factor 1 binding site mediates the transcriptional activation of a type I collagen promoter by transforming growth factor-beta. Cell 1988; 52:405–14.
146. Raghow R, Postlethwaite AE, Keski-Oja J, Moses HL, Kang AH. Transforming growth factor-beta increases steady state levels of type I procollagen and fibronectin messenger RNAs posttranscriptionally in cultured human dermal fibroblasts. J Clin Invest 1987; 79:1285–8.
147. Ishikawa O, Yamakage A, LeRoy EC, Trojanowska M. Persistent effect of TGF-beta 1 on extracellular matrix gene expression in human dermal fibroblasts. Biochem Biophys Res Commun 1990; 169:232–8.
148. Diaz A, Varga J, Jimenez SA. Transforming growth factor-beta stimulation of lung fibroblast prostaglandin E_2 production. J Biol Chem 1989; 264:11554–7.
149. Fine A, Poliks CF, Donahue LP, Smith BD, Goldstein RH. The differential effect of prostaglandin E_2 on transforming growth factor-beta and insulin-induced collagen formation in lung fibroblasts. J Biol Chem 1989; 264:16988–91.

150. Postlethwaite AE, Keski-Oja J, Moses HL, Kang AH. Stimulation of the chemotactic migration of human fibroblasts by transforming growth factor beta. J Exp med 1987; 165:251–6.
151. Wahl SM, Hunt DA, Wakefield LM, et al. Transforming growth factor beta induces monocyte chemotaxis and growth factor production. Proc Natl Acad Sci U S A 1987; 84:5788–92.
152. Pierce GF, Mustoe TA, Lingelbach J, et al. Platelet-derived growth factor and transforming growth factor-beta enhance tissue repair activities by unique mechanisms. J Cell Biol 1989; 109:429–40.
153. Allen JB, Manthey CL, Hand AR, Ohura K, Ellingsworth L, Wahl SM. Rapid onset synovial inflammation and hyperplasia induced by transforming growth factor beta. J Exp Med 1990; 171:231–47.
154. Needleman BW, Choi J, Burrows-Mezu A, Fontana JA. Secretion and binding of transforming growth factor beta by scleroderma and normal dermal fibroblasts. Arthritis Rheum 1990; 33:650–6.
155. Heldin C-H, Wasteson A, Westermark B. Platelet-derived growth factor. Mol Cell Endocrinol 1985; 39:169–87.
156. Ross R, Raines EW, Bowen-Pope DF. The biology of platelet-derived growth factor. Cell 1986; 46:155–69.
157. Nister M, Hammacher A, Mellstrom K, et al. A glioma-derived PDGF A chain homodimer has different functional activities from a PDGF AB heterodimer purified from human platelets. Cell 1988; 52:791–9.
158. Kazlauskas A, Bowen-Pope D, Siefert R, Hart CE, Cooper JE. Different effects of homo- and heterodimers of platelet-derived growth factor A and B chains on human and mouse fibroblasts. EMBO J 1988; 12:3727–35.
159. Hammacher A, Nister M, Heldin C-H. The A-type receptor for platelet-derived growth factor mediates protein tyrosine phosphorylation, receptor transmodulation and mitogenic response. Biochem J 1989; 264:15–20.
160. Morrison DK, Kaplan DR, Escobedo JA, Rapp UR, Roberts TM, Williams LT. Direct activation of the serine/threonine kinase activity of Raf-1 through tyrosine phosphorylation by the PDGF beta-receptor. Cell 1989; 58:649–57.
161. Ostman A, Backstrom G, Fong N, et al. Expression of three recombinant homodimeric isoforms of PDGF in *Saccharomyces cerevisiae*: evidence for difference in receptor binding and functional activities. Growth Factors 1989; 1:271–81.
162. Grotendorst GR. Alteration of the chemotactic response of NIH/3T3 to PDGF by growth factors, transformation, and tumor promoters. Cell 1984; 36:279–85.
163. Paulsson Y, Hammacher A, Heldin C-H, Westermark B. Possible positive autocrine feedback in the prereplicative phase of human fibroblasts. Nature 1987; 328:715–7.
164. Gronwald RG, Seifert RA, Bowen-Pope DF. Differential regulation of expression of two platelet-derived growth factor receptor subunits by transforming growth factor-beta. J Biol Chem 1989; 264:8120–5.
165. Chiou WJ, Bonin PD, Harris PK, Carter DB, Singh JP. Platelet-derived growth factor induces interleukin-1 receptor gene expression in Balb/c 3T3 fibroblasts. J Biol Chem 1989; 264:21442–5.
166. Paulsson Y, Bywater M, Heldin C-H, Westermark B. Effects of epidermal growth factor and platelet-derived growth factor on c-*fos* and c-*myc* mRNA levels in normal human fibroblasts. Exp Cell Res 1987; 171:186–94.
167. Stachniak JB, Sharp ZD, Pool TB, Cameron IL. Impaired proliferation response after PDGF induction in fibroblasts from Hutchinson-Guilford progeria syndrome. Cell Biol Int Rep 1988; 12:621–6.
168. Hesketh TR, Morris JD, Moore JP, Metcalfe JC. Ca^{2+} and pH responses to sequential

additions of mitogens in single 3T3 fibroblasts: correlation with DNA synthesis. J Biol Chem 1988; 263:11879–86.

169. DiFrancesco P, Testa EP, Testa U, Liboi E. Altered growth factor sensitivity in EL2 rat fibroblasts: influence of this biological characteristic on cell growth. Eur J Cell Biol 1989; 49:196–201.

170. Davis RJ, Czech MP. Stimulation of epidermal growth factor receptor threonine 654 phosphorylation by platelet-derived growth factor in protein kinase C-deficient human fibroblasts. J Biol Chem 1987; 262:6832–41.

171. Decker SJ, Harris P. Effects of platelet-derived growth factor on phosphorylation of the epidermal growth factor receptor in human skin fibroblasts. J Biol Chem 1989; 264:9204–9.

CHAPTER 17

FUNCTIONAL RESPONSES ELICITED IN ENDOTHELIAL CELLS BY CYTOKINES

Alberto Mantovani and Elisabetta Dejana

Istituto di Ricerche Farmacologiche Mario Negri
Milan, Italy

INTRODUCTION

Endothelial cells (EC) and leukocytes interact closely in the activation and expression of immunity as well as in inflammatory reactions and hemostasis. Cytokines are an important communication system between leukocytes and EC. A second mode of communication is represented by regulated expression of receptor and counterreceptor pairs on the surface of vessel wall cells and white blood elements that permits the physical interaction of these cell types.

Vascular cells are both a target for and a source of soluble polypeptide mediators. In this chapter we concisely review the responses elicited by cytokines in vascular cells and how vessel wall elements participate in cytokine cascades by producing copious amounts of some polypeptide mediators. Recent reviews of this rapidly expanding area of research provide the background for this chapter (1,2). In the last part of the chapter we discuss pathways of negative regulation of leukocyte-EC interaction.

ACTIVATION OF EC BY CYTOKINES

Cytokines produced by activated lymphoid cells and mononuclear phagocytes elicit complex spectra of responses in vascular cells. Different cytokines activate distinct, largely nonoverlapping sets of functions that can be grouped into programs of activation and differentiation (1). In the discussion of EC activation by cytokines, we highlight the emergence of these distinct activation and differentiation programs (Table 1).

TABLE 1 Functional Responses Elicited in Endothelial Cells by Cytokines

Cytokine	Functions related to	Function
IL-1 and TNF	Inflammation and thrombosis	PGI_2 (vasodilation); tissue factor, PAF; thrombomodulin/protein C; inhibitor of plasminogen activator (thrombosis); adhesion structures for leukocytes and production of cytokines (leukocyte recruitment and inflammation)
IFN-γ	Antigen presentation	Expression of class II MHC and ICAM-1; augmented production of IL-1
FGFs; TGF-β; G- and GM-CSF	Angiogenesis; maintenance of the hematopoietic microenvironment	Proliferation, migration

Interleukin-1 and Tumor Necrosis Factor

The description of the panoply of effects of interleukin-1 (IL-1) and tumor necrosis factor (TNF) on EC occupies a sizable fraction of the literature in this area. All in all, these inflammatory, pleiotropic cytokines orient EC function in a prothrombotic, proinflammatory sense (see Table 2 for summary).

Hemostasis

The antithrombotic properties of EC are profoundly altered by exposure to IL-1 and TNF. Thrombin formation is facilitated on the EC surface by newly synthesized thromboplastin (3) and by a concomitant suppression of thrombomodulin gene transcription (4,5). Moreover, IL-1- and TNF induce "platelet-activating factor" synthesis (6). This phospholipid is a potent platelet and leukocyte activator and is a vasoconstrictor. There are contrasting reports (7,8) on the capacity of IL-1 to induce von Willebrand factor release by EC. If this is the case, this protein can in turn act as a platelet adhesive and aggregating protein. IL-1

TABLE 2 Proinflammatory and Prothrombotic Set of Functions Induced in Endothelial Cells by IL-1 and TNF

EC function	Significance
PGI_2; HO	Vasodilation
Unresponsiveness to norepinephrine	Hypotension
PCA, PAF; TM; PAI	Thrombosis
Adhesion molecules (ICAM-1, ELAM-1, VCAM-1); chemotactic cytokines (IL-8, MCP, CSFs)	Extravasation of circulating cells (leukocytes, tumor cells)

also shifts the fibrinolytic properties of EC by increasing plasminogen activator inhibitor 1 production while leaving unchanged (or decreasing) tissue type plasminogen activator (9–11). Even if the majority of IL-1- and TNF-induced changes facilitate thrombus formation, these cytokines can also stimulate prostacyclin synthesis (see later) and urokinase-type plasminogen activator (12) that can inhibit platelet aggregation and activate the fibrinolitic system, respectively.

Observations made in patients treated with TNF (13) indicate that this cytokine can also induce activation of the coagulation system and plasminogen activator release in vivo in the human.

Vascular Tone

IL-1 and TNF induce the production of prostacyclin (PGI_2) in EC (14). Unlike other agonists active at this level (e.g., thrombin), the effect of IL-1 ensues after ≤2–4 h, is long lasting, and is protein synthesis dependent. Augmented mobilization of arachidonate and enhanced conversion to prostaglandins mediated by induction of expression of the cycloxygenase gene underlie induction of PGI_2 by IL-1 (15–17). PGI_2 is a potent vasodilatory agent. Therefore, cytokine-induced PGI_2 is involved in vasodilation at sites of inflammation and cell-mediated immunity and in the hypotension associated with systemic release (e.g., septic shock) or administration of these mediators. In fact, cyclooxygenase inhibitors prevent hypotension under these conditions (18,19).

Induction of nitric oxide production by IL-1 (20) can also be viewed in the same perspective of vasodilatory responses to these inflammatory cytokines. Exposure of vascular tissue to lipopolysaccharide (LPS) renders it refractory to the contractile activity of adrenergic drugs acting probably via IL-1 and TNF (21). Adrenergic unresponsiveness is also a typical feature of the septic shock syndrome.

IL-1 induces production by EC of endothelin, a potent vasoconstrictor (22). Its significance in the context of alterations of blood flow associated with inflammation remains to be established.

Leukocyte Recruitment

Leukocyte extravasation is a crucial determinant of inflammatory and immunological reactions. IL-1 and TNF injected locally cause leukocyte infiltration in tissues. Both mediators act on EC, but only TNF is directly chemotactic for monocytes and neutrophils (23). As a consequence, protein synthesis inhibitors completely block neutrophil recruitment by IL-1 but do not inhibit the early extravasation caused by TNF (24).

EC participate in leukocyte recruitment caused by inflammatory cytokines by producing chemoattractants that activate and attract leukocytes by expressing in a regulated way adhesion molecules and by altering blood flow.

IL-1 and TNF activation of EC induces the synthesis of adhesive molecules on their surface that mediate leukocyte recruitment (for review see Refs. 2 and 25–27). The endothelial adhesive structures currently known belong to two structural groups: the immunoglobulin (Ig) gene superfamily and the newly discovered selectin family. EC constitutively express at low levels three Ig molecules, intercellular adhesion molecule 1 (ICAM-1), ICAM-2 (27), and INCAM110/VCAM (25,28). IL-1 and TNF treatment strongly increases ICAM-1 (29) and INCAM110/VCAM synthesis (30,31), but ICAM-2 is not modified by these cy-

TABLE 3 Cytokine-Induced Endothelial Adhesive Molecules and Corresponding Leukocyte Receptors

Endothelial molecule		Receptor	
IgG	ICAM-1, ICAM-2	LFA-1, Mac-1	Integrins
	VCAM	VLA-4	
Selectin	ELAM-1	Sugar groups	

tokines (32). ICAM-1 and INCAM110/VCAM expression lasts for several hours (29–31). Ligands of these adhesive receptors are members of the widely distributed integrin family of adhesion molecules: LFA-1 and to a minor extent Mac-1 (belonging to the β_2 or Leu CAM or CD11/18 integrin subfamily) act as receptors for ICAM-1 (27); VLA-4 (β1 or VLA integrin subfamily) is the receptor for INCAM110/VCAM (33) (see Table 3).

The other adhesive protein induced by cytokine treatment of EC is ELAM-1, which is also a member of the selectin family (34). The three components of this group share a similar structure that at the amino-terminal domain resembles the carbohydrate binding sequence of animal lectins, suggesting that they bind to sugars. The ligand for ELAM-1, however, has not been identified yet. Induction of ELAM-1 by IL-1 is short lasting (8–12 h) in comparison to ICAM-1 and INCAM110/VCAM (30).

Monocytes recognize all three IL-1-induced adhesive antigens, but neutrophils can only bind to ICAM-1 and ELAM-1 and lymphocytes in general do not recognize ELAM-1 (25–27). There is evidence, however, that a particular subset of lymphocyte is able to recognize ELAM-1. The reciprocal role of these receptors in promoting adhesion and migration of leukocytes remains to be fully defined. Apparently a concerted action of these adhesive molecules is required for withstanding blood shear stress and for cell migration across the endothelium.

Expression of these EC activation antigens has also been observed in vivo in primates and humans (35–37). ELAM-1 was found essentially in postcapillary venules at sites of delayed-type hypersensitivity reaction and in pathological and inflammatory conditions in the human.

Interestingly, the IL-1- and TNF-induced EC adhesive molecules are not specific for leukocytes but they can also be recognized by solid tumor cells of different origin (30,38). This is likely the mechanism of augmented lung metastasis of human tumor cells injected intravenously into nude mice (39).

As discussed later, EC exposed to inflammatory signals (IL-1 and lipopolysaccaride) produce polypeptide mediators that cause activation and directional locomotion of leukocytes (reviewed in Ref. 1). These include the colony-stimulating factors (CSF) type G (granulocyte), GM (granulocyte and monocyte), and M (monocyte) and members of an emerging superfamily of inflammatory cytokines, in particular IL-8 (also known as neutrophil activating protein-1, NAP-1) and monocyte chemotactic protein (MCP) (40,41).

Chemotactic signals from tissues or produced by vessel wall cells and adhesion molecules are generally considered to determine leukocyte recruitment, but changes in the rheological properties of blood is an important factor contributing to extravasation of white cells. In fact, prostaglandins greatly amplify the activity of locally injected chemoattractants, such as IL-8 (42). Thus, cytokine-induced prostaglandin production (see earlier) acts in concert with expression of adhesion molecules and production of chemotactic cytokines.

EC Proliferation

IL-1, in the absence of other growth factors, is a weak proliferative signal for endothelial cells. When combined with other EC growth factors (e.g., fibroblast growth factor, FGF), IL-1 acts as a growth inhibitory signal (43,44). Moreover, upon in vitro passage EC express increased amounts of IL-1α, and an antisense oligonucleotide extends the in vitro life span of EC (43). These results suggest that IL-1 may represent an endogenous brake for endothelial proliferation and life span.

In vascular smooth muscle cells (SMC; as discussed in a previous review, Ref. 1), IL-1 is a strong inducer of proliferation, provided the production of growth inhibitory prostaglandins is blocked. The effect of IL-1 on SMC is mediated by induction of platelet-derived growth factor (PDGF).

Receptors and Transduction Pathways

Receptors and transduction pathways of IL-1 and TNF on vascular cells have not been extensively studied. We recently characterized the IL-1 receptor on murine endotheliomas and on human umbilical vein endothelial cells (Boraschi et al., in preparation). It was found that EC express high-affinity binding sites for IL-1α. Cross-linking and northern blot analysis showed that EC express the 80 kD fibroblast/T cell-type receptor.

Exposure to IL-1 and TNF induces expression of the immediate early genes c-*fos* and c-*jun*; these encode for proteins that transregulated gene expression. It is therefore likely that c-*fos* and c-*jun* are part of the molecular network that underlies the complex functional reprogramming of vascular cells exposed to monokines (1).

Colony-Stimulating Factors

Until recently, G- and GM-CSF were considered growth and differentiation factors restricted to hematopoietic elements. We found that EC express receptors for G- and GM-CSF and respond to these cytokines with migration and proliferation (45,46).

G-CSF was also found to induce plasminogen activator in EC (47), an enzyme usually associated with cell migration.

In the same vein, it was observed recently that erythropoietin stimulates proliferation of EC (48). Unlike G-CSF and GM-CSF, other molecules that share activity on hematopoietic precursors (M-CSF, IL-3, and IL-6) had no effect on EC proliferation (45,49). Stimulation of EC by G-CSF and GM-CSF was associated with activation of the Na^+ proton antiporter (46).

In an effort to define the pattern of activation of EC induced by CSFs, a series of proliferation-independent functions were examined. Although IL-1 and IFN-γ were used as reference cytokines in these studies; G- and GM-CSF did not affect expression of class II major histocompatibility complex (MHC) antigens or of adhesion structures (ICAM-1 and ELAM-1), nor did they induce thromboplastin and platelet-activating factor. These results are consistent with the hypothesis that G- and GM-CSF do not modulate EC functions related to inflammation and thrombosis or to accessory function.

The in vivo relevance of EC migration and proliferation induced by G- and GM-CSF was examined by evaluating angiogenesis in the rabbit cornea (49). G-CSF was used for these studies since this molecule is not species restricted. It was found that G-CSF is an angiogenic stimulus, although less effective than FGF.

Thus, G- and GM-CSF induce a set of functions in EC related to proliferation and migration and hence to the process of neovascularization. EC are one important component of the hematopoietic microenvironment. The activity of the hematopoietic growth factors G- and GM-CSF on EC may contribute to the maintenance in the bone marrow of microenvironment appropriate for hematopoiesis.

Interferon-γ

IFN-γ was the first molecularly defined immunological cytokine demonstrated to act on EC. IFN-γ induced the expression of class II MHC antigens and of the invariant chain in EC (50). Moreover, it augments the levels of class I MHC. Production of IL-1 by LPS-stimulated EC is augmented by IFN-γ. MHC class expression, as well as IL-1 and IL-6 production, underlies the ability of EC to act as antigen-presenting cells. IFN-γ causes a slow increase in the expression of ICAM-1 and renders EC more adhesive for T lymphocytes. Under conditions of "limiting" class II density, ICAM-1 can be important for antigen presentation (51). Collectively, the available information suggests that IFN-γ has a unique action on EC, distinct from that of other cytokines (for review see Ref. 1). It induces EC to act as accessory cells without inducing proinflammatory-prothrombotic or proliferative-migratory activities.

CYTOKINE PRODUCTION BY EC

In addition to acting as targets for the action of cytokines, EC are important producers of various mediators that regulate the hematopoietic system, the differentiation of T and B cells, and the extravasation of leukocytes at inflammatory sites (Table 4).

IL-1, a cytokine that profoundly affects vascular cells, is also a product of vessel wall elements. Inducers of IL-1 production by vascular cells include LPS, TNF, and IL-1 itself (for review see Ref. 1). EC and SMC also produce large amounts of IL-6 in response to the same stimuli and, at low levels, in the absence of deliberate stimulation (53). IL-1 acts on T cells, at least in part, by inducing production of IL-6, which mediates its action at this level. Since IL-6 does not affect the proinflammatory prothrombotic functions of IL-1 on EC and anti-IL-6 antibodies do not affect the activity of IL-1, it can be concluded that IL-6 is not the ultimate mediator of the effects of IL-1 on EC (52).

EC are an important source of CSFs. Hematopoietic growth factors produced by EC include G-, GM-, and M-CSF. CSF production is induced or augmented

Table 4 Cytokines Produced by Vascular Cells

Cytokine	Relevance
G-, GM-, M-CSF	Leukocyte activation, hematopoiesis, EC activation
PDGF	SMC proliferation
IL-1	Lymphocyte activation; inflammation; acute-phase responses; hematopoiesis
IL-6	Lymphocyte activation, acute-phase protein production; hematopoiesis
IL-8	Regulation of the recruitment of circulating cells[a]
MCP	Recruitment of blood monocytes

[a] EC-produced 77aa IL-8 has been shown to inhibit PMN adhesion to activated EC (58).

by a variety of stimuli, including LPS, IL-1, TNF, and minimally modified low-density lipoproteins (LDL) (53). By producing CSFs, as well as IL-1 and IL-6, which have CSF activity, EC participate in the regulation of hematopoiesis. Since EC respond to certain CSF molecules (G- and GM-CSF and erythropoietin; see earlier), autocrine and paracrine circuits involving EC and CSFs could be important in the generation and maintenance of an appropriate bone marrow milieu.

Vascular cells release cytokines that activate and attract leukocytes. These include CSFs and numbers of an emerging superfamily of chemotactic polypeptides (reviewed in Refs. 54 and 55). Upon exposure to inflammatory signals, EC release IL-8 (also known as neutrophil activating protein-1), GRO, and monocyte chemotactic protein (42,43). IL-8 and GRO are chemoattractants active on neutrophils. In addition to polymorphonuclear leukocytes (PMN), IL-8 affects lymphocytes, basophils (with IL-3), and melanoma cells (56). EC and SMC produce substantial amounts of MCP upon exposure to LPS, IL-1, TNF, and minimally modified LDL (41,57). Similarly, mesangial cells that share properties and possibly ontogenetic origin with SMC produce high levels of MCP (Rambaldi et al., unpublished). Induction of production of MCP and IL-8 by EC is dependent upon activation of gene transcription, as demonstrated by nuclear runoff analysis.

In addition to being relevant for leukocyte extravasation, the production of chemoattractants by vascular elements could be important in the pathogenesis of diseases that affect the vessel wall. Monocyte infiltration is an early event in the natural history of atherosclerosis and a prominent feature of vasculitis. It is likely that local production of MCP, elicited by modified LDL or inflammatory signals, may play a role in these diseases.

NEGATIVE REGULATORY CIRCUITS

The interaction of leukocytes with vascular cells mediated by cytokines is influenced by negative signals that downregulate this ping-pong interplay. Although data in this area are still relatively scanty and fragmentary, information is accumulating rapidly. Activated EC produce inhibitors of leukocyte recruitment.

A cytokine antigenically related to p15E of murine retrovirus produced by IL-1-stimulated EC inhibits chemotaxis of human monocytes (1). Activated EC produce a 77aa version of IL-8 that inhibits binding of PMN to activated EC (58). IL-8 is produced in versions of different length, the most abundant usually being a 73aa molecule (55). The relationship between leukocyte activation and inhibition by IL-8 molecules remains to be fully defined. Transforming growth factor β (TGF-β) inhibits adhesion of PMN to activated EC (59). Finally, IL-4 inhibits a number of proinflammatory functions of activated EC (60). A better understanding of factors and circuits that downregulate the participation of EC to inflammation and immunity may provide tools for the design of novel therapeutic approaches.

OVERVIEW

EC are strategically located at the very interface between circulating blood elements and tissues. It is therefore not surprising that these cells play an important active role in immunity, inflammation, and hemostasis. Cytokine molecules are used as communication signals in the complex bidirectional interaction between leukocytes and EC. EC represent a source of cytokines and, at the same time, a target for the action of various of these polipeptide mediators. Cytokine-induced EC responses follow discrete patterns: a program related to inflammation and thrombosis is activated by IL-1 and TNF, IFN-γ activates accessory cell function, and FGFs and G- and GM-CSF elicit functions related to angiogenesis.

In the complexity of the activation patterns they can express, EC are reminiscent of mononuclear phagocytes: the long-utilized term "reticuloendothelial system," although now largely abandoned, reflected the recognition of this similarity and interrelationship.

ACKNOWLEDGMENTS

This work was supported by the Italian National Research Council (Progetto Finalizzato Biotecnologie e Biostrumentazione, Tecnologie Biomediche e Sanitarie e Oncologia) and by the Association for Cancer Research (AIRC).

REFERENCES

1. Mantovani A, Dejana E. Cytokines as communication signals between leukocytes and endothelial cells. Immunol Today 1989, 10:370–5.
2. Pober J, Cotran RS. Cytokines and endothelial cell biology. Physiol Rev 1990; 70:427–51.
3. Bevilacqua MP, Pober JS, Majeau GR, Cotran RS, Gimbrone MA Jr. Interleukin-1 (IL-1) induces biosynthesis and cell surface expression of procoagulant activity in human vascular endothelial cells. J Exp Med 1984; 160:618–23.
4. Nawroth PP, Stern DM. Modulation of endothelial cell hemostatic properties by tumor necrosis factor. J Exp Med 1986; 163:740–5.
5. Conway EM, Rosemberg RD. Tumor necrosis factor suppresses transcription of the thrombomodulin gene in endothelial cells. Mol Cell Biol 1988; 8:5588–92.
6. Bussolino F, Breviario F, Tetta C, Aglietta M, Mantovani A, Dejana E. Interleukin-

1 stimulates platelet activating factor production in cultured human endothelial cells. J Clin Invest 1986; 77:2027–33.
7. Schorer AE, Moldow CF, Rick ME. Interleukin 1 or endotoxin increases the release of von Willebrand factor from human endothelial cells. Br J Haematol 1987; 67:193–7.
8. de Groot PG, Verweij CL, Nawroth PP. Interleukin-1 inhibits the synthesis of von Willebrand factor in endothelial cells which results in a increased reactivity of their matrix towards platelets. Arteriosclerosis 1987; 7:605–11.
9. Emeis JJ, Kooistra T. Interleukin-1 and lipopolysaccharide induce an inhibitor of tissue type plasminogen activator in vivo and in cultured endothelial cells. J Exp Med 1986; 163:1260–6.
10. Bevilacqua MP, Schleef RR, Gimbrone MA Jr, Loskutoff DJ. Regulation of the fibrinolytic system of cultured human vascular endothelium by interleukin-1. J Clin Invest 1986; 78:587–91.
11. Gramse M, Breviario F, Pintucci G, Millet I, Dejana E, Mussoni L. Enhancement by interleukin-1 (IL-1) of plasminogen activator inhibitor (PA-I) activity in cultured human endothelial cells. Biochem Biophys Res Commun 1986; 139:720–7.
12. van Hinsberg VWM, van der Berg EA, Fiers W, Dooijewaard G. Tumor necrosis factor induces the production of urokinase type plasminogen activator by human endothelial cells. Blood 1990; 10:1991–8.
13. Bauer KA, ten Cate H, Barzegar H, Spriggs DR, Sherman ML, Rosenberg RD. Tumor necrosis factor infusions have a procoagulant effect on the hemostatic mechanism of humans. Blood 1989; 74:165–72.
14. Rossi V, Breviario F, Ghezzi P, Dejana E, Mantovani A. Prostacyclin synthesis induced in vascular cells by interleukin-1. Science 1985; 229:174–6.
15. Raz A, Wyche A, Siegel N, Needleman P. Regulation of fibroblast cyclooxygenase synthesis by interleukin-1. J Biol Chem 1988; 263:3022–28.
16. Breviario F, Proserpio P, Bertocchi F, Lampugnani MG, Mantovani A, Dejana E. Interleukin-1 stimulates prostacyclin production by cultured human endothelial cells by increasing arachidonic acid mobilization and conversion. Arteriosclerosis 1990; 10:129–34.
17. Maier JAM, Hla T, Maciag T. Cyclooxygenase is an immediate-early gene induced by interleukin-1 in human endothelial cells. J Biol Chem 1990; 265:10805–8.
18. Okusawa S, Gelfand JA, Ikeijma T, Connolly RJ, Dinarello CA. Interleukin-1 induces a shock-like state in rabbits. Synergism with tumor necrosis factor and the effect of cycooxygenase inhibition. J Clin Invest 1988; 81:1162–72.
19. Kettelhut IC, Fiers W, Goldberg AL. The toxic effect of tumor necrosis factor in vivo and their prevention by cycooxygenase inhibitors. Proc Natl Acad Sci U S A 1987; 84:4273–7.
20. Fleming I, Gray GA, Julou-Schaeffer MO, Parratt JR, Stoclet JC. Incubation with endotoxin activates the L-arginine pathway in vascular tissue. Biochem Biophys Res Commun 1990; 171:562–8.
21. McKenna T. Prolonged exposure of rat aorta to low levels of endotoxin in vitro results in impaired contractility. Association with cytokine release. J Clin Invest 1990; 86:160–8.
22. Yoshizumi M, Kurihara H, Morita T, et al. Interleukin 1 increases the production of endothelin-1 in cultured endothelial cells. Biochem Biophys Res Commun 1990; 166:324–9.
23. Wang MJ, Walter S, Mantovani A. Reevaluation of the chemotactic activity of tumor necrosis factor for monocytes. Immunology 1990; 71:366–7.
24. Rampart M, De Smet W, Fiers W, Herman AG. Inflammatory properties of recombinant tumor necrosis factor in rabbit skin in vivo. J Exp Med 1989; 169:2227–32.

25. Osborn L. Leukocyte adhesion to endothelium in inflammation. Cell 1990; 62:3–6.
26. Carlos TM, Harlan JM. Membrane proteins involved in phagocyte adherence to endothelium. Immunol Rev 1990; 114:5–28.
27. Springer TA. Adhesion receptors of the immune system. Nature 1990; 346:425–34.
28. Rice EG, Munro JM, Bevilacqua MP. Inducible cell adhesion molecule 110 (INCAM-110) is an endothelial receptor for lymphocytes. J Exp Med 1990; 171:1369–74.
29. Dustin ML, Springer TA. Lymphocyte function-associated antigen-1 (LFA-1) interaction with intracellular adhesion molecule-1 (ICAM-1) is one of at least three mechanisms for lymphocyte adhesion to cultured endothelial cells. J Cell Biol 1988; 107:321–31.
30. Rice GE, Bevilacqua MP. An inducible endothelial cell surface glycoprotein mediates melanoma adhesion. Science 1989; 246:1303–6.
31. Osborn L, Hession C, Tizard R, et al. Direct expression cloning of vascular cell adhesion molecule 1 a cytokine-induced endothelial protein that binds to lymphocytes. Cell 1989; 59:1203–11.
32. Stauton DE, Dustin ML, Springer TA. Functional cloning of ICAM-2 a cell adhesion ligand for LFA-1 homologous to ICAM-1. Nature 1989; 339:61–4.
33. Elices ML, Osborn L, Takada Y, et al. VCAM-1 on activated endothelium interacts with the leukocyte integrin VLA-4 at a site distinct from the VLA-4/fibronectin binding site. Cell 1990; 60:577–84.
34. Bevilacqua MP, Stengelin S, Gimbrone MA Jr, Seed B. Endothelial-leukocyte adhesion molecule 1: an inducible receptor for neutrophils related to complement regulatory proteins and lectins. Science 1989; 243:1160–65.
35. Cotran RS, Gimbrone MA Jr, Bevilacqua MP, Mendrick DL, Pober JS. Induction and detection of a human endothelial activation antigen in vivo. J Exp Med 1986; 164:661–6.
36. Munro JM, Pober JS, Cotran RS. Tumor necrosis factor and interferon gamma induce distinct patterns of endothelial activation and associated leukocyte accumulation in skin of *Papio anubis*. Am J Pathol 1989; 135:121–33.
37. Ruco LP, Pomponi D, Stoppacciaro A, et al. Cytokine production (IL-1 alpha, IL-1 beta and TNF alpha) and endothelial cell activation in reactive lymphadenitis, Hodgkin's disease, and in non-Hodgkin's lymphomas: an immunocytochemical study. Am J Pathol 1990; 137:1163–71.
38. Dejana E, Bertocchi F, Bortolami MC, et al. Interleukin 1 promotes tumor cell adhesion to cultured human endothelial cells. J Clin Invest 1988; 82:1466–70.
39. Giavazzi R, Garofalo A, Bani MR, et al. Interleukin 1 induced augmentation of experimental metastases from human melanoma in nude mice. Cancer Res 1990; 50:4771–5.
40. Strieter RM, Kunkel SL, Showell HJ, et al. Endothelial cell gene expression on a neutrophil chemotactic factor by TNF-α, LPS and IL-1β. Science 1989; 243:1467–9.
41. Sica A, Wang JM, Colotta F, et al. Monocyte chemotactic and activating factor gene expression induced in endothelial cells by IL-1 and TNF. J Immunol 1990; 144:3034–8.
42. Rampart M, Van Damme J, Zonnekeyn L, Herman AG. Granulocyte chemotactic protein/interleukin-8 induces plasma leakage and neutrophil accumulation in rabbit skin. Am J Pathol 1989; 135:21–5.
43. Maier JAM, Vaulalas P, Roeder D, Maciag T. Extension of the life-span of human endothelial cells by an interleukin 1α antisense oligomer. Science 1990; 249:1570–3.
44. Cozzolino F, Torcia M, Aldinucci D, et al. Interleukin-1 is an autocrine regulator of human endothelial cell growth. Proc Natl Acad Sci U S A 1990; 87:6487–91.
45. Bussolino F, Wang JM, Defilippi P, et al. Granulocyte- and granulocyte-macrophage-

colony stimulating factors induce human endothelial cells to migrate and proliferate. Nature 1989; 337:471–3.
46. Bussolino F, Wang JM, Turrini F, et al. Stimulation of the Na^+/H^+ exchanger in human endothelial cells activated by granulocyte and granulocyte macrophage colony stimulating factor. Evidence for a role in proliferation and migration. J Biol Chem 1989; 264:18284–7.
47. Kojima SH, Tadenuma H, Inada Y, Saito Y. Enhancement of plasminogen activator activity in cultured endothelial cells by granulocyte colony-stimulating factor. J Cell Physiol 1989; 138:192–200.
48. Anagnostou A, Lee ES, Kessimian N, Levinson R, Steiner M. Erythropoietin has a mitogenic and positive chemotactic effect on endothelial cells. Proc Natl Acad Sci U S A 1990; 87:5978–82.
49. Bussolino F, Ziche M, Wang JM, et al. In vitro and in vivo activation of endothelial cells by colony-stimulating factors. J Clin Invest in press.
50. Pober JS, Gimbrone MA, Cotran RS, et al. Ia expression by vascular endothelium is inducible by activated T cells and by human γ-interferon. J Exp Med 1983; 157:1339–53.
51. Dransfield I, Buckle AM, Hogg N. Early events of the immune response mediated by leukocyte integrins. Immunol Rev 1990; 114:29–44.
52. Sironi M, Breviario F, Proserpio P, et al. IL-1 stimulates IL-6 production in endothelial cells. J Immunol 1989; 142:549–53.
53. Rajavashisth TB, Andalibi A, Territo MC, et al. Induction of endothelial cell expression of granulocyte and macrophage colony stimulating factors by modified low-density lipoproteins. Nature 1990; 344:254–7.
54. Mantovani A. Tumor-associated macrophages. Curr Opin Immunol 1990; in press.
55. Baggiolini M, Walz A, Kunkel SL. Neutrophil-activating protein-1/interleukin 8 a novel cytokine that activates neutrophils. J Clin Invest 1989; 84:1045–9.
56. Wang, JM, Taraboletti G, Matsushima K, Van Damme J, Mantovani A. Induction of haptotactic migration of melanoma cells by neutrophil activating protein/interleukin 8. Biochem Biophys Res Commun in press.
57. Cushing SD, Berliner JA, Valente AJ, et al. Minimally modified low density lipoprotein induces monocyte chemotactic protein 1 in human endothelial cells and smooth muscle cells. Proc Natl Acad Sci U S A 1990; 87:5134–8.
58. Gimbrone MA, Obin MS, Brock AF, et al. Endothelial interleukin 8: a novel inhibitor of leukocyte-endothelial interactions. Science 1989; 246:1601–3.
59. Gamble JR, Skinner MP, Berndt MC, Vadas MA. Prevention of activated neutrophil adhesion to endothelium by soluble adhesion protein GMP 140. Science 1990; 249:414–7.
60. Thornhill MH, Haskard DO. IL-4 regulates endothelial cell activation by IL-1 tumor necrosis factor or IFN-γ. J Immunol 1990; 145:865–72.

CHAPTER 18

CYTOKINES AND LYMPHOCYTES

Stanley C. Jordan

UCLA School of Medicine and Cedars-Sinai Medical Center
Los Angeles, California

INTRODUCTION

A number of peptide molecules have now been identified that act as intercellular signals during immune activation events. These peptides are termed cytokines and are responsible for the regulation of local and systemic immune inflammatory events. Although the existence of such regulatory peptides that are distinct from antibodies (products of humoral immunity) has been known for more than 40 years, only recently has the full extent of cytokine networks and functions become understood. These progressing revelations are the direct result of advances in cellular and molecular immunology that allows large quantities of purified peptide to be provided for in vitro and in vivo functional studies (1,2). Cytokines are made by a variety of immune and nonimmune cells. Cytokines produced by activated lymphocytes are termed lymphokines. In recent years, substantial progress has been made in elucidating the mechanism by which cytokines modulate the immune response of lymphocytes. Use of advanced molecular biology and immunological techniques has provided success in defining the diverse functional properties of cytokines. Knowledge of cytokine structure and function holds great potential benefit since modification or abrogation of cytokine effects should be of great potential value in controlling inflammatory diseases and aberrant or dysfunctional immune cell activation, such as that occurring in autoimmune diseases and allograft rejection. The goals of this chapter are to define how the panoply of cytokines interacts with and regulates lymphocyte functions and how this may be modified to achieve immunoregulation.

HISTORICAL PERSPECTIVE

Among the first demonstrations of soluble mediators distinct from antibodies were the studies by David et al. (3) and Bloom and Bennett (4). These investigators described the existence of a soluble mediator present in the culture supernatants of activated lymphocytes that was inhibitory to migration of normal macrophages. This factor was designated macrophage inhibitory factor (MIF). The mechanisms of action of MIF were unclear, but these papers fundamentally established that lymphocyte responses to antigen are not exclusively limited to the production of antibody.

The discovery of MIF resulted in an intense search for other mediators. Among the early cytokines discovered were lymphotoxin, macrophage activating factor (MAF), and interferon (5–7). Subsequently, these factors derived from activated lymphocyte cultures were termed lymphokines by Dumonde et al. (8). The discovery of lymphokines and their regulation of cell functions brought new meaning to the traditional concept of cell-mediated immunity and lymphocyte functions (2). No longer were lymphocytes believed to be mere appendages of circulating red blood cells, and the discovery of lymphokines heralded the new dawn of modern immunology.

The lymphokine concept provided an explanation of immunologically mediated inflammatory events, including autoimmune diseases and allograft rejection. In addition, acquired resistance to intracellular infections and delayed-type hypersensitivity could also be explained (2). Since lymphokines appeared to be of pivotal importance in mediating immune effector functions, investigators then turned their attention to factors that could regulate T and B lymphocyte functions. Gery and Waksman (9) observed that adherent nonlymphoid cells released a soluble mediator that augmented the growth of lymphocytes. This factor was called lymphocyte activating factor (LAF) and is now known to be interleukin-1 (IL-1) (2).

In 1974, Cohen et al. (10) proposed the term "cytokine," which comprises a broader array of soluble factors produced by lymphoid and nonlymphoid cells having the capacity to interact with immune and nonimmune cells. The dawn of modern molecular biology enabled immunologists to make spectacular advances in the understanding of cytokines and their functions. Gene cloning provided the key technical tool for isolating cytokine genes and producing recombinant proteins. The data obtained from experiments confirmed the pleiotropism and redundancy of activity of specific cytokine proteins. The role of cytokines in the regulation of lymphocyte functions is the focus of the remainder of this chapter.

CYTOKINES AND T CELLS

T Cell Activation and Cytokine Production

T cells recognize and respond to antigen in the context of HLA-DR (class II) or HLA-A, B, and C (class I) antigens. These HLA molecules "restrict" which subset of T cell ($CD4^+$ T cell or $CD8^+$ T cell) the antigen-presenting cell (APC) interacts with (Fig. 1). The classic concept of $CD4^+$ T cell activation involves antigen presentation via HLA-DR molecules on an APC. This presentation to the T cell

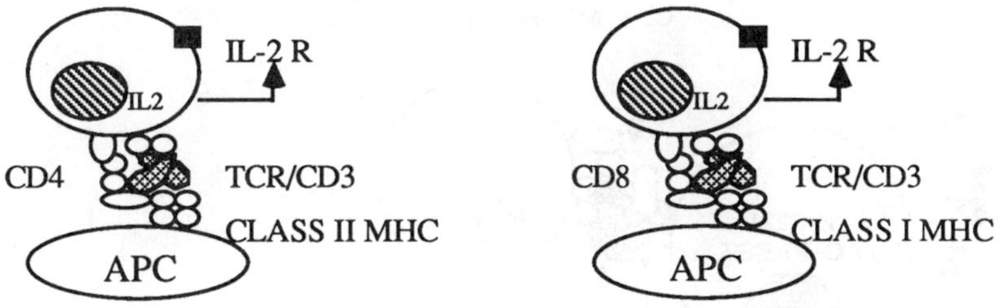

FIGURE 1 MHC restrictions of CD4 and CD8 cell activation. $CD4^+$ T cells can only be activated by HLA class II antigen-presting cells (APC). $CD8^+$ T cells are activated only by class I-positive APCs. The CD4 and CD8 molecules in both circumstances help to stabilize this interaction.

receptor complex then activates the T cell through calcium-dependent pathways and induces the expression of interleukin-2 receptors (IL-2R) on the cell surface. The T cells subsequently produce IL-2, which is consumed in an autocrine and paracrine fashion. Macrophages were initially thought to be the only cells capable of presenting antigen to T cells, but any HLA-DR-expressing cell can serve the same function. These include dendritic cells, endothelial cells, and B cells (11). Indeed, B cell presentation of antigen recognized by surface immunoglobulin molecules and presented by HLA-DR to $CD4^+$ T cells is a potent activator of T cells and production of cytokines that rapidly results in the activation, proliferation, and differentiation of B cells into antigen-specific antibody-producing plasma cells (Fig. 2).

After antigen presentation to T cells, a number of cytokines are produced that regulate subsequent T cell activation and differentiation. A limited discussion of the cytokines produced by activated T cells is presented here because more exhaustive reviews appear in other chapters.

Interleukin-2

IL-2 is a lymphokine produced by activated T cells. This lymphokine has a broad range of biological activities in vitro that results primarily from its ability to expand and differentiate different subpopulations of T cells and B cells (12). Induction of proliferation in antigen- and mitogen-activated T cells appears to be mediated through binding of IL-2 to its high-affinity receptors (75 and 55 kD) that appear on the cell surface of activated T cells. IL-2-IL-2R interaction appears to activate T cells through a translocation of protein kinase C (PKC) from cytosol to plasma membrane. Hydrolysis of phosphatidylinositol to form inositl triphosphate (IP_3) and diacylglycerol (DAG) subsequently results in an intracellular rise of Ca^{2+} with subsequent increase in PKC activation. Thus, the interaction of IL-2 with IL-2R results in the activation of intracellular signaling mechanisms that transmit the signal to the nucleus for cell proliferation and differentiation (13). This ligand-receptor activation sequence is probably common to other cytokine-receptor couplets as well. In addition to its ability to activate T cells, IL-2 can also induce the release of other lymphokines from activated T cells. These include interferon-γ (IFN-γ), IL-4, IL-5, and tumor necrosis factor β (TNF-β) (14–18).

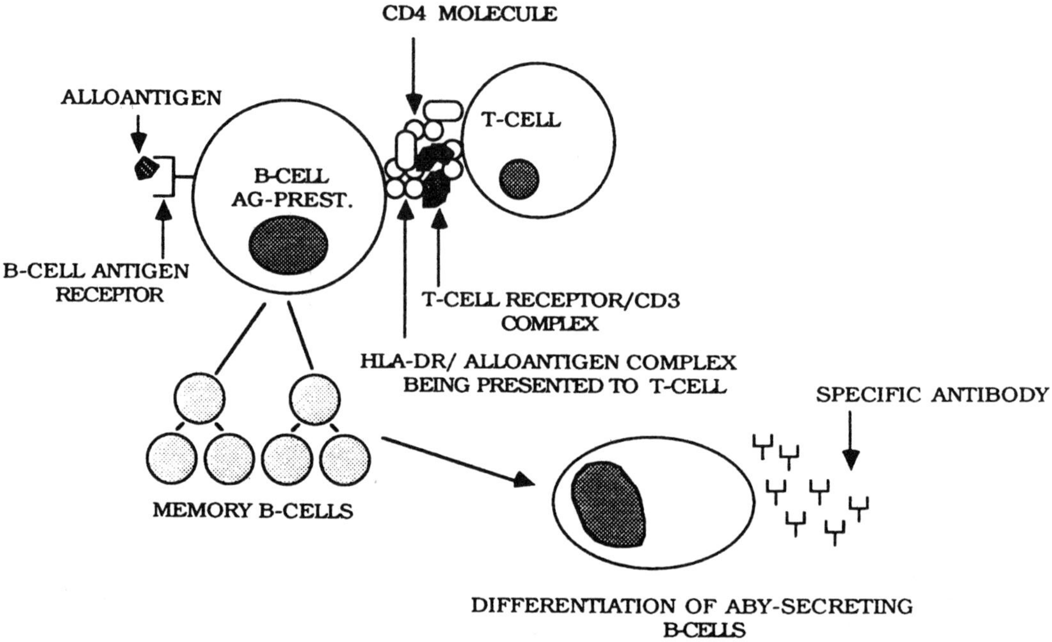

FIGURE 2 Antigen presentation by B cells. HLA-DR$^+$ B cells bind antigen (alloantigen shown here) via surface Ig receptors. This antigen is processed and presented to T cells through class II–TCR-CD3 interactions. Subsequent activation of the T cells results in the production of B cell stimulating (IL-2, IL-4, and IL-5) and proliferating cytokines (IL-6). This results in the rapid differentiation of B cells into antibody-secreting plasma cells.

Interferon-γ

IFN-γ was first described by Wheelock (19) as an IFN-like molecule produced in supernatants of lymphocytes stimulated with phytohemagglutinin (PHA). Human IFN-γ has been cloned (20). The gene is located on human chromosome 12 (21). The important biological functions of IFN-γ include activation of class I and class II antigen (22,23) (induction of targets for T cell-mediated cytotoxity), induction of Fc receptors on macrophages (24,25), activation of natural killer (NK) cells (26,27), and activation of cytotoxic T cells (28). IFN-γ is also a potent activator of macrophage killing (29), a function of prime importance in tumor immunity, allograft rejection, and antimicrobial activity (30).

Lymphotoxin

TNF-β is a cytolytic cytokine produced by activated T cells. Human TNF-β appears to be coded for by a single gene (30,31). TNF-β is implicated as having many roles in human immune function that are exclusive of its role as a cytolytic lymphokine. TNF-β has been implicated in the mediation of cytolytic T lymphocyte-mediated cytotoxicity (32), antibody-dependent cell-mediated cytotoxicity (ADCC) (33), and NK cell cytotoxic reactions (34). In addition, it has been shown that TNF-β can synergize with other cytokines (i.e., IFN-γ) to increase growth inhibitory effects (35). We recently showed that polyclonal antibodies specific for TNF-β can significantly inhibit the cell-mediated tissue injury seen in a rat model of lung allograft rejection. TNF-β therefore appears to be a potent cytolytic and immunoregulatory cytokine produced after T cell activation and may be an important effector cytokine in autoimmune disease and allograft rejection.

Interleukin-3

IL-3 is also known as multi-CSF (colony-stimulating factor). IL-3 is produced by activated helper T cells. Among its actions are included various growth and differentiation effects on hematopoietic precursor cells. IL-3 stimulates the growth of multilineage colonies from bone marrow stem cells, which include erythroid, granulocyte-macrophage, and megakaryocyte precursors. IL-3 also has potent growth-promoting properties for most cells (2,36).

Granulocyte-Macrophage Colony-Stimulating Factor (GM-CSF)

GM-CSF is another T cell cytokine with the ability to stimulate the growth and differentiation of hematopoietic stem cells along the granulocyte and monocyte pathways. GM-CSF also has the ability to activate macrophages to kill tumor cells. GM-CSF is produced by T cells and by macrophages and endothelial cells. Recombinant GM-CSF is currently being evaluated in clinical trials for treatment of severe neutropenias, but initial data suggest that recombinant G-CSF is equally effective without the severe side effects (including eosinophilia and vascular leak syndrome) noted with administration of GM-CSF (2,37,38).

Interleukin-4

IL-4 was also referred to as B-cell stimulating factor-1 (BSF-1) and IgG_{-1} inducing factor. Like IL-2, it is produced primarily by activated T helper cells. This cytokine acts primarily on B cells to induce class II antigen expression and by priming the cells for activation. IL-4 can also activate macrophages and is important in promoting isotype switch to IgE production in B cells. In this regard, dysfunctional activation and production of IL-4 may be responsible for many hypersensitivity disorders observed in the human (2,39).

Interleukin-5

IL-5 is a T cell cytokine with pleiotropic effects on both T and B cell populations. IL-5, also known as T-cell replacing factor (TRF) and B-cell growth factor-II (BCGF-II), has both early and late activating effects on B cells. In early B cell activation, IL-5 costimulates B cells activated with mitogen. Late effects on B cell function include stimulation of IgM production by activated B cells and promotion of isotype switch to IgA production. Dys-regulation of IL-5 production by T cells could play a role in such diseases as IgA nephropathy and Henoch-Schönlein purpura where excessive IgA responses result in IgA immune complex injury. IL-5 affects T cells by promoting T cell proliferation and differentiation to cytotoxic T cells (2,40).

Interleukin-6

IL-6 is a pleiotropic cytokine that was previously described as IFN-β_2, BSF-2, and hepatocyte-stimulating factor. Although IL-6 is produced primarily by macrophages and has a potent costimulatory activity on T cells, it is also produced by T cells primarily as a late-acting factor responsible for B cell Ig production. IL-6 has endogenous pyrogenic and acute-phase reactant promoting properties and has recently been identified as a growth factor for mesangial cells. In this regard IL-6 appears to have an important pathogenic role in the mediation of mesangial proliferative glomerulonephritis (2,41–43).

Transforming Growth Factor β (TGF-β)

TGF-β is a multifunctional peptide with pleiotropic effects on a number of cell types. Receptors for TGF-β are present on a number of cells, and T cells are known to be a good source for TGF-β. TGF-β appears to block the stimulatory effects of other T cell growth factors (i.e., IL-2) and therefore may serve to downregulate T cell immune responses (2,44).

Cytokine Regulation of T Cell Functions

T cells not only produce a wide array of cytokines but their functions are also controlled by endogenous cytokines (autocrine effect) or exogenous cytokines (paracrine effect) produced by a number of cell types in the vicinity of an immune activation event. The purpose of this section is to summarize the cytokines that are most important in regulation of T cell activation. Some of this information was mentioned in the previous section on cytokines produced by T cells. An in-depth review of each cytokine is not presented because this is covered in other chapters.

Interleukin-1

IL-1 is a term applied to two polypeptides (IL-1α and β) that possess a number of immunological and nonimmunological activities. Both forms of IL-1 are distinct gene products, but they share the same IL-1 receptor and have indistinguishable biological activities. For the purpose of this review, we concentrate on the role of IL-1 in regulating T cell activation and function.

IL-1 and T Cell Activation. There can now be little doubt that IL-1 is an important coactivator of T cells during antigen stimulation events. This was confirmed in experiments using recombinant IL-1, which was shown conclusively to augment T cell responses to antigen, increase T cell IL-2 production, increase IL-2R expression, synergize with recombinant IL-4 in T cell activation, and induce and synergize with IL-6 in T cell activation. In addition, some T cells synthesize IL-1, suggesting an important role for IL-1 in T and B cell activation (45–48). Rat thymocytes do not proliferate in response to concanavalin A (ConA) when depleted of macrophages. This response can be restored by the addition of IL-1 to the cultures, indicating that IL-1 is an important stimulator of IL-2 and IL-2R in rat thymocytes (45). In human peripheral blood T cell populations, IL-1 serves as an important cofactor for activation in the absence of macrophages. In these experiments, IL-1 partially restores the role of the macrophage by inducing IL-2 production and IL-2R expression (45). Recently, the identification of a unique cytokine, IL-1 receptor antagonist, which functions by competitive inhibition of both IL-1α and IL-1β, was described (49). The ability of this IL-1 receptor antagonist to inhibit T cell activation has been shown, suggesting an important role for IL-1 in coactivation of T cells.

Interleukin-2, a Regulator of T Cell Growth and Differentiation

IL-2 is probably the most important regulatory cytokine for T cell growth and differentiation. IL-2 is important in the amplification of antigen-primed T cells, it may also regulate B cell growth and differentiation, and it probably has a role in the regulation of monocytes, NK cells, and other cells that participate in the immune responses (50). The physiology of IL-2-IL-2R interaction is not reviewed here. IL-2 is produced by T cells upon stimulation with antigen. Although $CD4^+$ T cells are thought to be the primary producers of IL-2, it is well known that both $CD4^+$ T cells and $CD8^+$ T cells are capable of producing IL-2 (51,52). The interaction of MHC protein (+) antigen with the T cell receptor complex on T cells results in the expression of IL-2R and production of IL-2. IL-2 interactive with the IL-2R results in a series of signal transduction events that ultimately leads to T cell activation and differentiation into terminal effector cells. For IL-2 to exert these effects on target cells (autocrine or paracrine), it is essential that the generation of a series of intracellular signals occurs, which are triggered via the interaction of IL-2 with IL-2R. The intracellular signals result in the expression of new genes that play important roles in regulating T cell growth and differentiation (50). A full discussion of these intracellular signaling mechanisms is beyond the scope of this chapter, but activation of protein kinase C and increases in intracellular Ca^{2+} probably play critical roles in T cell activation initiated by IL-2-IL-2R interactions.

In addition to its direct effect on T cell activation, IL-2 also amplifies its effect on immune responses by stimulating the production of other cytokines. IL-2 is known to stimulate the secretion of IFN-γ (53,54). In addition, IL-2 has been shown to stimulate IL-4 production (55). Other investigations have shown that IL-2 increases the secretion of IL-3 (56) and GM-CSF (57). In addition to a direct effect on stimulating T cell secretion of lymphokines, IL-2 may also act as a costimulus for the release of other cytokines (58).

Tumor Necrosis Factor and T Cell Function

TNF-α is a cytokine produced primarily by lipopolysaccharide (LPS)-stimulated macrophages that mediates necrosis of transplanted tumors in vivo (59). Despite its role as an inflammatory cytokine, TNF-α has recently been shown to have potent immunoregulatory functions in human and animal experimental systems (59). Bonavida et al. (59) showed that the addition of recombinant human TNF (1–10 μ g/ml) results in a dose-dependent inhibition of pokeweed mitogen (PWM)-induced antibody production by human peripheral blood cells in vitro.

Further experiments by this group showed that TNF suppresses PWM-induced B cell differentiation without affecting B cell proliferation. These notions were given further credence by the observations of Satoh et al. (60), who showed that recombinant TNF is a potent inhibitor of the development of autoimmune diabetes mellitus in the nonobese diabetic mice (NOD strain). These investigators tested a number of recombinant cytokines in these experiments, including recombinant IL-1α, INF-γ, IL-2, and GM-CSF. Only TNF showed this remarkable ability to inhibit T cell-mediated destruction of NOD mice β cells. These investigators thought that the ability to produce TNF in various mouse strains correlated with their propensity to develop autoimmune disease. NOD mice were poor producers of TNF; it was therefore postulated that the lack of TNF production allowed autoimmune events to proceed. Exogenous administration of TNF inhibited the dysfunctional T cell activation and prevented autoimmune disease by induction of suppressor T cells (61). Other investigators have shown that TNF administration to (NZB × NZW)F hybrid mice suppresses the progression of murine systemic lupus erythematosus (SLE). This is, again, presumably through induction of suppressor T cell networks by TNF (62).

Interleukin-6 and T Cell Function

The effect of IL-6 on lymphocytes and bone marrow stem cells is broadly based. IL-6 exhibits typical comitogenic activity on murine T cells. IL-6 has been shown to increase the production of IL-2 and expression of IL-2R on these cells (45). Other authors have suggested that the IL-1-mediated comitogenic signal for T cells is actually mediated by IL-6 since IL-1 rapidly stimulates IL-6 production (63). IL-6 is a weak inflammatory peptide but appears to have potency similar to that of IL-1 in coactivation of human T cells (45). IL-6 appears to have a much more profound effect on human B cell proliferation and immunoglobulin production. This is discussed in the next section.

CYTOKINES AND B CELLS

Cytokine Regulation of B Cell Functions

There is currently no clear consensus regarding the mechanisms responsible for B cell activation with subsequent differentiation to antibody-producing plasma cells. The problems are many and include the individual regulation of specific immunoglobulin isotype production by specific cytokines and the entry of new cytokines into the B cell regulation derby on a daily basis (64). Another problem complicating an analysis of cytokine effects on B cell function is the multiplicity and redundancy of cytokine effects on a mixed cell population. The advent of recombinant cytokines and monoclonal antibodies inhibitory to specific cytokine functions has helped to define the role of specific cytokines in regulating B cell functions. Despite these advances, much effort is still needed to define how the numerous cytokines known to affect B cell functions interact to stimulate a specific isotype response to a particular antigen. In addition, a better understanding of cytokine regulation of B cell function will aid in understanding inflammatory processes in which hyperactive B cell responses are seen, as in autoimmune diseases, allergic disorders, and allograft rejection. In this section we review the cytokines that have the most relevance to regulation of B cell functions.

Interleukin-2 and B Cell Function

IL-2 is known to be a potent stimulator of B cell activity (65–69). A great deal of skepticism arose surrounding these early studies since the prevailing knowledge suggested that IL-2R were present only on activated T cells and that the growth effects of IL-2 on B cell populations were probably due to IL-2-induced activation signals in contaminating T cells present in B cell cultures (64). Further proof that B cells could respond directly to IL-2 was shown by Malek et al. (70) and Ortega et al. (71), who demonstrated that the p55 Tac antigen (IL-2R) was present on B cells. Data from our laboratory also support a direct role for IL-2 action on human B cells (72). In our experiments, we demonstrated that the lymphocytes isolated from active SLE patients expressed high levels of IL-2R. Cell-sorting experiments established that the majority of cells expressing IL-2R were B cells and that addition of IL-2 to active SLE lymphocyte cultures significantly increased the level of immunoglobulin production from these cells (72). Zubler et al. (73) suggest that IL-2 functions to clonally expand activated B cells. In addition, IL-2 increases IgM production and has been shown to significantly increase mRNA for J chain and μ chain in normal B cells (64,74,75). Other investigators (76) have also shown that IL-2 is a potent regulator of J chain mRNA levels in B cells.

These data present a strong case for a role of IL-2 in B cell activation and IgM production. An additional piece of evidence is also useful in this regard. Tigges et al. (77) showed that recombinant IL-4 added to BCL-1 cells inhibited the J chain mRNA accumulation stimulated by IL-2. This information suggests a possible mechanism for isotype switch mediated by IL-4, since other investigators have shown that IL-4 downregulates IgM production and increases IgG_1 production in B cell lines (64,78).

Interleukin-4 and B Cell Function

The existence of IL-4 was first demonstrated by its ability to induce the production of IgG antibody in LPS-stimulated B cells and to act synergestically with anti-IgM antibody to induce proliferation of B cells (64,79,80). IL-4 also has the ability to enhance MHC class II antigen expression, which enhances the ability of the B cell to act as an antigen-presenting cells (Fig. 2) (81). IL-4 also stimulates the synthesis and expression of low-affinity Fc receptors for IgE (FcE RII) (82). IL-4 appears to have two important functions in human B cell responses. These are the enhancement of IgG_1 synthesis by activated B cells and the enhanced production of IgE by LPS-activated B cells. In addition to these findings, there is a concomitant suppression of IgG_3 and IgG_{2b} subclasses in these cultures (64,83,84). In murine B cells, IFN-γ is a potent inhibitor of most of the actions of IL-4 (85). This effect is less clear in human B cell populations (86).

Interferon-γ and B Cell Function

IFN-γ is known to have a profound effect on B cell function. IFN-γ is primarily a late-acting factor in B cell proliferation, and studies with recombinant IFN-γ and monoclonal or polyclonal antibodies specific for IFN-γ have established its importance as a regulator of B cell activity (64,87). IFN-γ appears to be very important in the enhancement of IgG_{2a} production (88). In addition, IFN-γ suppressed the production of IgG_3 and IgG_{2b} (64,88). Since IL-4 is thought to act by selectively propogating IgG_1- and IgE-producing clones, IFN-γ is believed to act in a similar way by enhancing the proliferation of IgG_{2a}-producing clones while suppressing the development of other B cell isotype-bearing cells. As previously mentioned, the effect of IFN-γ on IL-4-driven B cell responses is particularly striking. IFN-γ tends to inhibit these responses profoundly (85,86).

These observations are of interest since evidence exists for restriction of cytokine production to selective subsets of T helper (TH) cells. TH-1 cells are thought to produce primarily IL-2 and IFN-γ; TH-2 cells produce IL-4 and IL-5. Other cytokines may also segregate to a particular subset of TH cells (89). Since effector functions are mediated by different immunoglobulin classes (i.e., IgE mediates hypersensitivity reactions and IgG_{2a} mediates complement-dependent cytotoxicity), one can postulate that T cells have developed the unique capacity to modify their immune responses to fit the characteristics of the invading pathogen (64,89).

Interleukin-5 and B Cell Function

IL-5 exists as a 13 kD polypeptide and as a natural oligomeric glycoprotein of 30–60 kD (86,90). IL-5 is known to have differentiating effects on murine B cells and to induce the CD25 component of the IL-2R (86,91). IL-5 is also known to enhance the growth and differentiation of eosinophils (92). In addition, IL-5 enhances the production of IgA by LPS-stimulated murine B cells. These observations have not been confined in human B cells. In conclusion, IL-5 appears to be an important B cell growth and differentiating factor for murine B cells but has no direct action on human B cells in vitro (86).

Interleukin-6 and B Cell Function

IL-6 is a 26 kD cytokine produced by a variety of cell types, including T cells, monocytes, and fibroblasts. It is a weak pyrogen but has potent effects on B cell differentiation. Resting B cells do not express IL-6 receptors; therefore one does not expect IL-6 alone to have the capacity to induce B cell responses (42,86).

The main function of IL-6 appears to be the promotion of B cell differentiation into antibody-producing plasma cells. The role of IL-6 in enhancing Ig production in Epstein-Barr virus (EBV)-transformed cells and human peripheral blood lymphocytes stimulated with PWM is substantial (93). Muraguchi et al. (93) showed that Ig production in human lymphocyte cultures stimulated with PWM was substantially inhibited when antibody to IL-6 was added to cultures. IL-6 appears to augment Ig secretion from B cells independent of an action on B cell proliferation. This is consistent with the role of IL-6 on a late-acting factor in B cell differentiation (86).

In summary, IL-6 promotes B cell activation, and enhances Ig production without a subsequent effect on B cell proliferation. These actions are dependent upon IL-2 in cultures (86).

Interleukin-1 and B Cell Function

IL-1 is known to activate the proliferation of murine B cells stimulated with anti-IgM antibody (86,94). In other studies, IL-1 was found to be an important coactivator of suboptimally activated B cells, suggesting that IL-1 is an important early activating factor in B cell proliferation (95). IL-1 also enhances Ig secretion by preactivated B cells in response to IL-2, demonstrating that a specific effect of IL-1 is to enhance IL-2 directed B cell differentiation (86). The mechanism by which IL-1 induces B cells to proliferate is not known but probably does not relate to increased intracellular cAMP levels since increased cAMP tends to suppress B cell activation (96).

Transforming Growth Factor β and B Cell Function

TGF-β is produced by a wide variety of normal and transformed cells, including B cells (86,97). TGF-β inhibits the growth of many cell types, including B cells. TGF-β has been reported to promote IgA synthesis in murine B cells stimulated with LPS. This appears to be mediated by a promotion of class switch (98). There are currently no reports on the regulation of IgA synthesis in human B cells (86).

SELECTIVE INHIBITION OF CYTOKINE-LYMPHOCYTE INTERACTIONS IN THE TREATMENT OF HUMAN DISEASE

Vigorous immune responses are desirable to maintain the integrity of the individual's health. However, undesirable immune responses can often occur and result in such diseases as systemic autoimmunity, uncontrolled allergic responses, allograft rejection, and nephritogenic immune responses (99).

Concomitant with advances in our understanding of the immune system were the development and application of the potent T cell inhibitory drug cyclosporine-A (CsA). The potent T cell regulatory effects of CsA can be attributed to its inhibition of cytokine mRNA expression in T cells (100). Among its most important targets is the IL-2 gene, in which a potent and dose-dependent inhibition of mRNA accumulation occurs (101). The ability of CsA to specifically inhibit cytokine mRNA accumulation and subsequent translation has opened new doors of therapeutic opportunities in our quest to control undesirable immune responses. CsA celebrated a decade of service to transplantation in 1990. During the past 11 years, remarkable advances were made in every field of transplantation. A major step forward was made in our ability to control the allograft rejection response through inhibition of cytokine production. CsA is also a potent inhibitor of IFN-γ production (100,101). IFN-γ plays a significant role in allograft rejection through activation of cytodestructive mechanisms in macrophages and through activation of HLA class I and II molecules on target tissues. Controlling these responses is critical to preservation of the functional integrity of transplanted organs.

CsA will also play an important role in regulating nephritogenic and autoimmune disorders through its ability to inhibit T cell-mediated inflammatory events. We have recent experience in treating patients with idiopathic nephrotic syndrome (NS) with CsA (102). Our experience suggests that many patients with NS present with high levels of circulating IL-2 in their plasma. Both IL-2 levels and NS symptoms respond rapidly to institution of CsA therapy, suggesting a T cell-mediated pathogenesis for this disorder. CsA is also being investigated as a potential therapeutic agent in a number of other autoimmune disorders (100).

Monoclonal antibodies have played an important role in defining functional characteristics of specific T cell molecules. In addition, these molecules have often become targets for immunosuppressive regimens. The T cell receptor complex (TRC/CD3) serves a critical role in transmitting signals initiated by antigen-presenting cell-T cell interactions. The CD3 component plays a critical role in transducing this signal to the interior of the T cell (99,103). The monoclonal antibody OKT3, which recognizes the CD3 complex on T cells, is a potent immunosuppressive agent. This immunosuppression appears to be mediated through effacement of the TCR/CD3 complex from all T cells, thus rendering them incapable of recognizing alloantigen presented in the context of a major histocompatibility complex (MHC)-restricted fashion. A unique side effect of anti-CD3 therapy is an almost instantaneous syndrome of fever, chills, myalgias, and capillary leak. This syndrome appears to be mediated by the ability of OKT3 to perturb the CD3 molecules on T cells, thus sending an activation signal to virtually every T cell in the body. These symptoms result from a massive release of proinflammatory cytokines, including TNF, IL-2, and IFN-γ (99). To date, OKT3 has proven to be an extremely potent and effective immunosuppressive agent, but the cytokine release syndrome and its predisposition of patients to infections and neoplastic complications may limit its use.

A more ideal immunosuppressive agent would be one that targets a selective population of cytokine-producing T cells involved in a specific immunological event (i.e., mediation of allograft rejection or autoimmunity). One such target is the p55 kD IL-2R. Experimental data from animal transplants suggest that anti-IL-2R is a potent immunosuppressive agent (99,104). In addition, recent studies in human renal transplantation have shown that anti-IL-2R monoclonal antibody therapy is a useful prophylactic agent for the prevention of allograft rejection compared with standard antithymocyte globulin (105). Numerous other studies have also shown that anti-T cell, anti-IL-2, and anti-CD4 monoclonal antibodies are effective in blocking autoimmune diseases (99,106–108).

More recently, an IL-2 toxin was shown to be an extremely potent and selective immunotherapeutic agent (109). IL-2 toxin suppresses the delayed-type hypersensitivity reaction more potently than that seen with IL-2R monoclonal antibody (99). It also has potent anti-rejection properties (110). In animal models of cardiac transplantation, use of the IL-2 toxin results in permanent engraftment of transplanted hearts (99).

Thus, IL-2 toxin may prove an extremely potent method of targeting IL-2R$^+$ cells and eliminating them from the immune response scenario (99). Other cytokine-toxin hybrids will prove useful in aiding our understanding of T cell activation events and their role in the mediation of undesirable inflammatory events. This should also lead to more novel and selective approaches to immunosuppression in the future.

REFERENCES

1. Menkin V. Chemical basis of injury in inflammation. Arch Pathol 1943; 36:269.
2. Neta R, Oppenheim JJ, Durum S. The cytokine concept: historical perspectives and current status of cloned cytokines. In: Cohen S, ed. Lymphokines and the immune response. Boca Raton, FL: CRC Press, 1990; 30–40.
3. David JR, Al-Askari S, Lawrence HS, Thomas L. Delayed hypersensitivity in vitro. I. The specificity of inhibition of cell migration by antigens. J Immunol 1964; 93:264.
4. Bloom BR, Bennett B. Mechanism of a reaction in vitro associated with delayed type hypersensitivity. Science 1966; 153:80.
5. Ruddle NH, Waksman BH. Cytotoxicity mediated by soluble antigen and lymphocytes in delayed hypersensitivity. III. Analysis of mechanisms. J Exp Med 1968; 128:1267.
6. Kolb WP, Granger GA. Lymphocyte in vitro cytotoxicity: characterization of human lymphotoxin. Proc Natl Acad Sci U S A 1968; 61:1250.
7. Green JA, Cooperband SR, Kibnick S. Immune specific induction of interferon production in cultures of human blood lymphocytes. Science 1969; 164:1415.
8. Dumonde DC, Wolstencroft RA, Panayi G, Matthew M, Morley J, Howson WT. "Lymphokines": non-antibody mediators of cellular immunity generated by lymphocyte activation. Nature 1969; 224:38.
9. Gery I, Waksman BH. Potentiation of the T-lymphocyte response to mitogens. II The cellular source of the potentiating mediators. J Exp Med 1972; 136:143.
10. Cohen S, Bigazzi PE, Yoshida T. Similarities of T-cell function in cell-mediated immunity and antibody production. Cell Immunol 1974; 12:150.

11. Inaba K, Steinman RM. Resting and sensitized T-lymphocytes exhibit distinct stimulatory (antigen-presenting cell) requirements for growth and lymphokine release. J Exp Med 1984; 160:1717.
12. Morgan DA, Ruscett F, Gallo R. Selective in vitro growth of T-lymphocytes from normal human bone marrows. Science 1976; 193:1007.
13. Fresa K, Hameed M, Cohen S. Intracellular and extracellular factors promoting lymphocyte activation and proliferation. In: Cohen S, ed. Lymphokines and the immune response. Boca Raton, FL: CRC Press, 1990:70–84.
14. Strotter H, Rude E, Wagner H. T-cell factor (interleukin-2) allows in vivo induction of T help cells against heterologous erythrocytes in athymic (nu/nu) mice. Eur J Immunol 1980; 10:719.
15. Wagner H, Hardt C, Heeg K, Rollinghoff M, Pfizenmaier K. T-cell derived helper fact allows in vivo induction of cytotoxic T cells in nu/nu mice. Nature 1980; 284:278.
16. Gillis S, Smith K. Long-term culture of tumor-specific cytotoxic T-cells. Nature 1977; 268:154.
17. Yamamoto JK, Farrar WL, Johnson HM. Interleukin 2 regulation of mitogen induction of immune interferon (IFN) in spleen cells and thymocytes. Cell Immunol 1982; 66:333.
18. Howard M, Matis L, Malek TR, et al. Interleukin-2 induces antigen-reactive T cell lines to secrete BCGF-1. J Exp Med 1983; 158:202.
19. Wheelock EF. Interferon-like virus-inhibitor induced in human leukocytes by phytohemagglutinin. Science 1965; 149:310.
20. Vilcek J, Gray PW, Rinderknecht E, Sevastopoulos CG. Interferon: a lymphokine for all seasons. In: Pick E, ed. Lymphokines, Vol. 11. Orlando, FL: Academic Press, 1985:1.
21. Naylor SL, Sakaguchi AY, Shows TB, Law ML, Goeddel DV, Gray PW. Human immune interferon gene located on chromosome T2. J Exp Med 1983; 157:1020.
22. Steeg PG, Moore RN, Johnson HM, Oppenheim JJ. Regulation of murine macrophage Ia antigen activity. J Exp Med 1982; 156:1780.
23. King DP, Jones PP. Induction of Ia and H-2 antigens on a macrophage cell line by immune interferon. J Immunol 1983; 131:315.
24. Guyre PM, Morganelli PM, Miller R. Recombinant immune interferon increases immunoglobulin G Fc receptors on cultured human mononuclear phagocytes. J Clin Invest 1983; 72:393.
25. Perussia B, Dayton ET, Lazarus R, Fanning V, Trinchieri G. Immune interferon induces the receptor for monomeric IgG_1 on human monocytic and myeloid cells. J Exp Med 1983; 158:1092.
26. Weigent DA, Langford MP, Fleishmann WR Jr, Stanton GJ. Potentiation of lymphocyte natural killing by mixtures of alpha or beta interferon with recombinant gamma interferon. Infect Immun 1983; 40:35.
27. Svedersky LP, Shepard HM, Spencer SA, Shalaby MR, Palladino MA. Augmentation of human natural cell-mediated cytotoxicity by recombinant human interleukin 2. J Immunol 1984; 133:714.
28. Farrar WL, Johnson HM, Farrar JJ. Regulation of the production of immune interferon and cytotoxic T lymphocytes by interleukin 2. J Immunol 1981; 126:1120.
29. Pace JL, Russell SW, Torres BA, Johnson HM, Gray PW. Recombinant mouse g-interferon induces the priming step in macrophage activation for tumor cell killing. J Immunol 1983; 130:2011.
30. Cohen MC. Lyphokines and tumor immunity. In: Cohen S, ed. Lymphokines and the immune response. Boca-Raton, FL: CRC Press, 1990:238–247.
31. Gray PA, Aggarwal BB, Benton CV, et al. Cloning and expression of cDNA for

human lymphotoxin, a lymphokine with tumor necrosis activity. Nature 1984; 312:721.

32. Ware CF, and Granger GA. Mechanisms of lymphocyte-mediated cytotoxicity. The effect of anti-human lymphotoxin antisera on the cytolysis of allogenic B cell lines by MLC-sensitized human lymphocytes in vitro. J Immunol 1981; 126:1131.
33. Kondo LL, Rosenua W, Wara DW. Role of lymphtoxin in antibody-dependent cell-mediated cytotoxicity (ADCC). J Immunol 1981; 126:1131.
34. Wright SC, Bonavida B. Selective lysis of NK-sensitive target cells by a soluble mediator released from murine spleen cells and human peripheral blood lymphocyte. J Immunol 1981; 125:1516.
35. Williams TW, Bellanti JA. In vitro synergism between interferons and human lymphotoxin: enhancement of lymphotoxin-induced target cell killing. J Immunol 1983; 130:518.
36. Fung M, Hapel A, Ymer S, et al. Molecular cloning of cDNA for murine IL-3. Nature 1984; 307:233.
37. Gough N, Gough H, Metcalf D, et al. Molecular cloning of cDNA encoding a murine hematopoietic growth regulation: granulocyte-macrophage colony stimulating factor. Nature 1984; 309:763.
38. Boxer L. Clinical efficacy of recombinant human granulocyte colony stimulating factor in patients with severe chronic neutropenia (abstract). Future directions in cytokine and immunoglobulin therapy. Tucson, AZ. January 11–12, 1991.
39. Noma Y, Sideras P, Naito T, et al. Cloning of cDNA encoding the murine IgG_1 inducting factor by a novel strategy using SPG promoter. Nature 1986; 319:640.
40. Kinashi T, Harada N, Severinson E, et al. Cloning of complementary DNA encoding T-cell replacing factor and identity with B-cell growth factor II. Nature 1986; 324:70.
41. Hirano T, Yasukawa K, Harada H, et al. Complementary DNA for a novel human interleukin (BSF-2) that induces B-cells to produce immunoglobulin. Nature 1986; 324:73.
42. Kishimoto T. The biology of IL-6. Blood 1989; 74:1–10.
43. Yashiro H, Atsush M, Masaynki I, et al. Involvement of IL-6 in mesangial proliferative glomerulonephritis. J Immunol 1989; 143:3949.
44. Derynck R, Jarrett J, Chen E, et al. Human transforming growth factor-B complementary DNA sequence and expression in normal and transformed cells. Nature 1985; 316:701.
45. Dinarello CA. Interleukin-1 and biologically related cytokines. In: Cohen S, ed. Lymphokines and the immune response. Boca Raton, FL: CRC Press, 1990:146–172.
46. Acres RB, Larsen A, Conlon PJ. IL-1 expression in a clone of human T-cells. J Immunol 1987; 138:2132.
47. Ho S, Abraham RT, Nilson A, Handwerger B, McKean D. Interleukin 1-mediated activation of interleukin-4 (IL-4) producing T. lymphocytes proliferation by IL-4 dependent and IL-4 independent mechanisms. J Immunol 1987; 139:1532.
48. Tartakovsky B, Kovacs E, Takacs L, Durum SK. T-cell clone producing an IL-1-like activity after stimulation by antigen-presenting B-cells. J Immunol 1986; 137:160.
49. Hannum CH, Wilcox CJ, Arend WP, et al. Interleukin-1 receptor antagonist activity of a human interleukin-1 inhibitor. Nature 1990; 343:336–40.
50. Sabath D, Prystoiwsky M., The molecular basis of interleukin-2 action. In: Cohen S, ed. Lymphokines and the immune response. Boca Raton, FL: CRC Press, 1990: 182–91.
51. Jordan SC, Toyoda M, Prehn J, Lemire J, Sakai R, Adams J. 1,25-Dihydroxyvitamin-

D_3 regulation of interleukin-2 and interleukin-2 receptor levels and gene expression in human T-cells. Mol Immunol 1989; 26:979–84.

52. Meuer SC, Hussey R, Penta A, et al. Cellular origins of IL-2 production by T-4+ and T-8+ lymphocytes. J Immunol 1982; 129:1076–9.
53. Benjamin WR, Steeg PS, Farrar JJ. Production of immune interferon by an interleukin 2-dependent murine T cell line. Proc Natl Acad Sci U S A 1982; 79:5379.
54. Vilcek J, Jenriksen-Destefano D, Siegel D, Klion A, Robb R, Le J. Regulation of IFN-γ production in human peripheral blood cells by exogenous and endogenously produced interleukin 2. J Immunol 1985; 135:1851.
55. Lee F, Yokota T, Otsuka T, et al. Isolation and characterization of a mouse interleukin cDNA clone that expresses B-cell stimulatory factor 1 activities and T-cell and mast-cell stimulating activities. Proc Natl Acad Sci U S A 1986; 83:2061.
56. Kelso A, Metcalf D, Gough NM. Independent regulation of granulocyte-macrophage colony-stimulating factor and multilineage colony-stimulating factor production in T lymphocyte clones. J Immunol 1986; 136:1718.
57. Kelso A, Gough N. Expression of hemopoietic growth factor genes in murine T lymphocytes. Lymphokines 1987; 13:209.
58. Otten G, Fitch F. T-cell clones as a source of lymphokines. In: Cohen S, ed. Lymphokines and the immune response. Boca Raton, FL: CRC Press, 1990:44–52.
59. Bonavida B, Wright S, Kashiwa H, et al. Immunoregulation and cytotoxicity by tumor necrosis factor. In: eds: B Bonavida, GE Gifford, H Kirchner, LJ Old. Tumor necrosis factor/cachectin and related cytokines. Basel: Karger, 1988:53–8.
60. Satoh J, Seino H, Abo T, et al. Recombinant human tumor necrosis factor-alpha suppresses autoimmune diabetes in nonobese diabetic mice. J Clin Invest 1989; 84:1345–8.
61. Serreze DV, Leiter E. Defective activation of T-suppressor function in nonobese diabetic mice. Potential relation to cytokine deficiencies. J Immunol 1988; 140:3801–7.
62. Jacob CO, McDevitt HO. Tumor necrosis factor alpha in murine autoimmune "lupus" nephritis. Nature 1988; 331:356–8.
63. Garman RO, Jacobs KA, Clark SC, Raulet DH. Proc Natl Acad Sci U S A 1987; 84:7251.
64. Roehm N. Lymphokine regulation of B-cell function. In: Cambier J, ed. Ligands, receptors and signal transduction in regulation of lymphocyte function. Washington, DC: American Society for Microbiology, 1990:97–116.
65. Leibson HJ, Marrack P, Kapple J. B cell helper factors. II. Synergy among three helper factors in the response of T cells and macrophage depleted B cells. J Immunol 1982; 129:1398–402.
66. Nakanishi K, Malek TR, Smith KA, Hamaoka T, Shevach EM, Paul WE. Both interleukin 2 and a second T cell derived factor in EL4 supernatant have activity as differentiation factors in IgM synthesis. J Exp Med 1984; 160:1605–21.
67. Roehm NW, Marrack P, Kappler JW. Helper signals in the plaque forming cell response to protein haptens. J Exp Med 1983; 158:317–33.
68. Parker D. Separable helper factors support B-cell proliferation and maturation to Ig secretion. J Immunol 1982; 129:469–74.
69. Pike BL, Nossal GJV. Interleukin 1 can act as a B-cell growth and differentiation factor. Proc Natl Acad Sci U S A 1985; 82:8153–7.
70. Malek TR, Robb RJ, Shevach EM. Identification and initial characterization of a rat monoclonal antibody reactive with the murine interleukin 2 receptor-ligand complex. Proc Natl Acad Sci U S A 1983; 80:5694–8.
71. Ortega GR, Robb RJ, Shevach E, Malek TR. The murine IL2 receptor. 1. Monoclonal

antibodies that define distinct functional epitopes on activated T-cells and react with activated B-cells. J Immunol 1984; 133:1970–5.
72. Wigfall DR, Sakai R, Wallace DJ, Jordan SC. IL-2 receptor expression in peripheral blood lymphocytes from SLE patients: Relationship to clinical activity. Clin Immunol Immunopathol 1988; 354–62.
73. Zubler RH, Lowenthal JW, Erard F, Hashimoto N, Devos R, MacDonald HR. Activated B cells express receptors for and proliferate in response to pure interleukin 2. J Exp Med 1984; 160:1170–83.
74. Berton MT, Uhr JW, Vitetta ES. Synthesis of germ line γ1 immunoglobulin heavy chain transcripts in resting B cells: induction by interleukin 4 and inhibition by interferon-γ. Proc Natl Acad Sci U S A 1989; 86:2829–33.
75. Nakanisi K, Cohen DI, Blackman E, et al. Ig RNA expression in normal B cells stimulated with anti-IgM antibody and T cell derived growth, and differentiation factors. J Exp Med 1984; 160:1736–51.
76. Blackman MA, Tigges MA, Minie ME, Koshland ME. A model system for peptide hormone action in differentiation: interleukin 2 induces a B lymphoma to transcribe the J chain gene. Cell 1986; 47:609–17.
77. Tigges MA, Casey LS, Koshland ME. Mechanism of interleukin 2 signaling: mediation of different outcomes by a single receptor and transduction pathway. Science 1989; 243:781–6.
78. Snapper CM, Finkelman FD, Paul WE. Differential regulation of IgG1 and IgE synthesis by interleukin-4. J Exp Med 1988; 167:183–97.
79. Isakson PC, Pure E, Vitetta ES, Krammer PH. T cell derived B cell differentiation factor(s). Effect on the isotype switch of murine B cells. J Exp Med 1982; 155:734–48.
80. Howard MJ, Farrar J, Hilfiker M, et al. Identification of a T cell derived B cell growth factor distinct from interleukin 2. J Exp Med 1982; 155:914–23.
81. Noelle RJ, Kuziel WA, Maliszewski CR, McAdams E, Vitetta ES, Tucker PW. Regulation of expression of multiple class II genes in murine B cells by B cells stimulatory factor-1 (BSF-1). J Immunol 1986; 137:1718–23.
82. Conrad DH, Waldschmidt TJ, Lee WT, et al. Effect of B cell stimulatory factor-1 (interleukin 4) on Fcε and Fcγ receptor expression on murine B lymphocytes and B cell line. J Immunol 1987; 139:2290–6.
83. Sideras PS, Bergstedt-Lindqvist HR, MacDonald HR, Severinson E. Secretion of IgG_1 induction factor by T cell clones and hybridomas. Eur J Immunol 1985; 15:586–93.
84. Coffman RL, Ohara J, Bond MW, Carty J, Zlotnik A, Paul WE. B cell stimulatory factor-1 enhances the IgE response of lipopolysaccharide activated B cells. J Immunol 1986; 136:4538–41.
85. Snapper C, Paul W. Interferon-gamma and B cell stimulatory factor-1 reciprocally regulate Ig isotype production. Science 1987; 236:944–7.
86. Splanski J, Lipsky P. Human B-cell regulation by growth and differentiation factors. In: Cambier J, ed. Ligands, receptors, and signal transduction in regulation of lympyhocyte function. Washington DC: American Society for Microbiology, 1990: 149–195.
87. Brunswick M, Lake P. Obligatory role of gamma interferon in T cell replacing factor dependent antigen specific murine B cell responses. J Exp Med 1985; 161:953–71.
88. Snapper CM, Paul WE. Interferon-γ and B cell stimulatory factor 1 reciprocally regulate Ig isotype production. Science 1987; 236:944–7.
89. Mossman TR, Coffman RL. Th1 and Th2 cells: different patterns of lymphokine secretion lead to different functional properties. Annu Rev Immunol 1989; 7:145–74.
90. Yokota TR, Coffman R, Hagiward D, et al. Isolation and characterization of lym-

phokine cDNA clones encoding mouse and human IgA enhancing factor and eosinophil colony-stimulating factor activities: relationship to interleukin 5. Proc Natl Acad Sci U S A 1987; 84:7388–92.
91. Kishimoto R. B-cell stimulatory factors (BSFs): molecular structure, biological function, and regulation of expression. J Immunol 1987; 7:343–55.
92. O'Garra A, Umland S. Defrance T, Christiansen J. B-cell factors are pleiotropic. Immunol Today 1988; 9:45–54.
93. Muraguchi A, Hirano T, Tang B, et al. The essential role of B cell stimulatory factor 2 (BSF-2/IL-6) for the terminal differentiation of B cells. J Exp Med 1988; 167:332–44.
94. Chiplunkar S, Langhorne J, Kaufmann S. Stimulation of B cell growth and differentiation by murine recombinant interleukin 1. J Immunol 137:3748–52.
95. Lipsky P, Thompson P, Rosenwasser L, Dinarello C. The role of interleukin 1 in human B cell activation: inhibition of B cell proliferation and the generation of immunoglobulin-secreting cells by an antibody against human leukocyte pyrogen. J Immunol 1983; 130:2708–14.
96. Simkin N, Jelinek D, Lipsky P. Inhibition of human B cell responsiveness by prostaglandin E_2. J Immunol 1987; 138:1074–81.
97. Sporn M, Roberts L, Wakefield L, Assoian R. Transforming growth factor B: biological function and chemical structure. Science 1986; 233:532–4.
98. Coffman RL, Lebman DA, Schrader B. Transforming growth factor B specifically enhances IgA production by lipopolysaccharide-stimulated murine B lymphocytes. J Exp Med 1989; 170:1039–44.
99. Strom TB, Kelley V. Toward more selective therapies to block undesired immune responses. Kidney Int 1989; 31:1026–33.
100. Lafferty K, Paris L. Cyclosporin A and the regulation of autoimmune disease. J Autoimmun 1988; 1:519–32.
101. Hess AD, Colomnani PM. Mechanism of action of CSA: unifying hypothesis. Adv Exp Med Biol 1987; 213:309.
102. Jordan SC, Querfeld V, Toyoda M, Prehn J. Serum IL-2 levels in a patient with focal segmental glomerulosclerosis: relationship to clinical course and CSA therapy. Pediatr Nephrol 1990; 4:166–8.
103. Weiss A, Imboden J, Hardy K, et al. The role of T_3 antigen receptor complex in T-cell activation. Ann Rev Immunol 1986; 4:593–619.
104. Shapiro ME, Kirkman RL, Reed MH, et al. Monoclonal anti-IL-2R antibody in primate renal transplantation. Transplant Proc 1987; 19:594–8.
105. Soulillous JP, Cantarovich D, LeMauff B, et al. Randomized controlled trial of a monoclonal antibody against the interleukin-2 receptor (33B3.1) as compared with rabbit antithymocyte globulin for prophylaxis against rejection of renal allografts. N Engl J Med 1990; 322:1175–82.
106. Wofsy D, Ledbetter JA, Hendler PL, Seaman WE. Treatment of murine lupus with monoclonal anti-T cell antibody. J Immunol 1985; 134:852–7.
107. Wofsy D, Seaman WE. Successful treatment of autoimmunity in NZB × NZWF1 mice with monoclonal antibody to L3T4. J Exp Med 1986; 161:378–91.
108. Wofsy D, Seaman WE. Reversals of advanced murine lupus in NZB × NZWF1 mice by treatment with monoclonal antibody to L3T4. J Immunol 1987; 138:3247–53.
109. Kelley VE, Bacha P, Panekewycz O, Nicholas JC, Murphy JR, Strom TB. Interleukin 2-diphtheria toxin fusion protein can abolish cell mediated immunity in vivo. Proc Natl Acad Sci U S A 1988; 85:3980–4.
110. Pankewycz O, Mackie J, Hassarjian R, et al. Interleukin 2-diphtheria toxin fusion protein prolongs murine islet cell engraftment. Transplantation 1989; 47:318–22.

CHAPTER 19

CYTOKINES AND MACROPHAGES

Mark D. Wewers

The Ohio State University
Columbus, Ohio

INTRODUCTION

In the day-to-day surveillance and regulation of the body's interactions with foreign substances, it is difficult to find a more central player than the mononuclear phagocyte. Composed of monocytes and macrophages stationed at sentinel posts throughout the body, these cells function as critical regulators of immune response to foreign invasion. This chapter focuses on the role of cytokines in providing the communication network that places this array of macrophage defenders in direct contact with each other and with the vascular, mesenchymal, and inflammatory cells important in the defense of self.

Macrophage Life Cycle

The capacity to *produce* cytokines is the forte of the macrophage and is the focus of this chapter. However, afferent cytokines also have a direct effect on mononuclear phagocytes, such as controlling the numbers of macrophages, their state of differentiation, and their state of activation. It is now recognized that macrophages are derived from bone marrow precursors induced by colony-stimulating factors to differentiate from a myelocytic precursor to the monocyte lineage (1–3). These bone marrow progenitors develop into monocytes within a week and are released as blood monocytes that circulate in the blood from 1 to 3 days. Apparently at random, these mononuclear phagocytes then migrate into the tissues of the body to differentiate into tissue macrophages (3). Proof that alveolar macrophages are of bone marrow origin comes from observing the phenotypic and genotypic changes that occur within the lung population several months after either bone marrow transplantation or lung transplantation (4,5). In both instances, the lung becomes populated by macrophages autologous with the cell type of the functioning bone marrow.

The movement of macrophages from the blood to the tissues represents an important crossroads in the functional role of the macrophage. Macrophages that have differentiated perform very different functions. In this context cytokine differences occur in accordance with differentiation. Monocytes are characterized by peroxidase-positive granules that are rich in leukocyte elastase and cathepsin G (6), which are lost with maturation into macrophages. Conversely, monocytes are potent releasers of interleukin-1 (IL-1) in response to endotoxin; however, this potency wanes with maturation in vitro and in vivo (7,8). In contrast, tumor necrosis factor (TNF) and platelet-derived growth factor release by mononuclear phagocytes is enhanced with maturation into macrophages (9–12). These differentiation-induced cytokine regulatory changes broaden our understanding of macrophage activation. They suggest that some of the activities previously attributed to macrophage activation may also be a reflection of relative stages of differentiation in the macrophage life cycle.

Macrophage Functions

After setting up tissue residence, macrophages have at least three classic functions (2). First, they operate as housekeepers by removing dead cells and both endogenous and exogenous debris. In the process of this "garbage collection," macrophages scrutinize the environment for microorganisms. Their second function is the body's primary defense against microorganisms, that is, the phagocytosis and killing of these invaders. The destruction of microorganisms first requires recognition of the invaders, which is aided by cell surface receptors for opsonins, such as immunoglobulins (Fc receptors) and components of C3. Interaction with these receptors not only enhances phagocytosis but also "activates" the macrophages to heightened oxidant production and, as discussed later, cytokine production. The third function, related to phagocytic digestion of foreign material, involves processing and presenting foreign antigen to lymphocytes, inducing the proliferation of specific T lymphocytes as well as triggering the effector cells of the humoral system. It is now recognized that cytokine production by macrophages is intimately a part of these classic functions and that in addition to these "classic" functions macrophages may have long-range effects on virtually any cell type by the hormonal modulation of macrophage-derived cytokines.

HISTORY OF MACROPHAGE LINK TO CYTOKINES

Macrophages have been linked to cell-derived messenger proteins since the first descriptions of cytokines in the early 1960s. The first well-characterized cytokine was a lymphokine (lymphocyte product) that inhibited the in vitro migration of macrophages. Termed macrophage migration inhibitory factor (MIF), this cytokine, produced in response to a sensitized antigen, demonstrated that soluble nonimmunoglobulin cell proteins could have significant effects upon cell function (13,14). (MIF activity has subsequently been further characterized; it is now known to represent one of the functions of interferon-γ.)

Later it was recognized that these "kines" had effects on other functions besides kinetic (cell movement) phenomena. From the perspective of macrophage-produced cytokines, the discovery of interleukin 1 represents a typical history of the recognition and then refinement of understanding of particular cytokines. IL-1 was first recognized as a soluble factor in rabbit peritoneal exudates that could cause fever when injected into other animals (15). It was called endogenous pyrogen (EP) to distinguish it from exogenous pyrogens, such as endotoxin. EP was determined to be a macrophage product, and an independent body of literature was generated in the EP field for the next 30 years. It was not until the late 1970s that it was appreciated that EP and IL-1 represented the same molecule.

The other alias for IL-1 was lymphocyte activating factor (LAF). As such it was first identified in the early 1970s as the soluble macrophage protein (LAF) that substituted for the macrophage requirement in lymphocyte proliferation (16,17). LAF became the first interleukin in 1979 at the Second International Lymphokine Workshop (18). This term suggested its function as a messenger between leukocytes, in this specific case as an activated macrophage signaling a lymphocyte to produce IL-2, the growth factor for T lymphocytes. This nomenclature unintentionally ignored the multifunctional components of IL-1, particularly its effects upon nonleukocyte cells (such as its function as an endogenous pyrogen) but set the precedent for the current practice of giving new cytokines an interleukin nomenclature once the amino acid sequence has been determined.

MACROPHAGE INTERACTIONS IMPORTANT IN CYTOKINE PRODUCTION

Cytokine production by macrophages generally requires stimulation or activation, as resident "resting" macrophages are typically not constitutive cytokine producers. Stimulation can come from various particulate and cell interactions with macrophages. Endotoxin (one of the most potent "activators" of macrophages), interferon-γ (a lymphocyte-derived macrophage activating cytokine responsible at least in part for MIF activity), and interactions with macrophage Fc receptors and complement receptors (processes linked to their classic phagocytic function) have all been extensively studied as macrophage stimulators.

Macrophage-Endotoxin Interactions

Endotoxin represents the classic in vitro stimulator of macrophages. It is likely an important in vivo stimulator as well, since it is the single moiety that represents the bacterial cell component responsible for activating the immune response. Current concepts are that macrophages are key regulators of host response to bacterial lipopolysaccharides, particularly important to the linkage of macrophage-generated cytokines and sepsis (19). In this context, the predominant cell responsible for endotoxin handling is the macrophage. When radiolabeled endotoxin is injected into animals, it is cleared almost exclusively by tissue macrophages (20). When measured per gram of tissue, the highest concentrations occur in the liver, spleen, and lung (20). Thus the mononuclear phagocyte defense system (formerly known as the reticuloendothelial system) represents the first-line defense against bacteria.

Understanding the macrophage's role in defense against Gram-negative infection has been expanded greatly by the model provided by the endotoxin-nonresponsive mouse strain. C3H/HeJ mice are resistant to endotoxin shock at LPS concentrations that are lethal to endotoxin-responsive strains (C3H/HeN) (21). At least part of this resistance can be attributed to the inability of the macrophage from the C3H/HeJ strain to release TNF in response to endotoxin (22). Of note, however, is that the endotoxin nonresponder strain is more susceptible to infection with *Salmonella* (23). These observations suggest that the ability to produce cytokines like TNF may be beneficial in fighting infection but that an overwhelming release of TNF may, on the other hand, be lethal.

Endotoxin Receptors

The exact mechanism of how lipopolysaccharide interacts with macrophages is under active investigation. Studies are complicated by the heterogeneity and complexity of endotoxin molecules. Although lipophilic endotoxin may interact with cells directly via the plasma membrane, several candidate receptors have been identified. For example, the adhesion-promoting integrins of the CD11/CD18 family interact with endotoxin (24), and using radiolabeled endotoxin, specific macrophage binding to a surface receptor has been reported (25). Recently, CD14, a surface marker specific for mononuclear phagocytes, has been demonstrated to complex with endotoxin. This endotoxin complex, however, requires a second protein, lipopolysaccharide binding protein (LBP). CD14 will complex with LBP, which is an acute-phase protein, but it does so only after LBP has first bound endotoxin (lipopolysaccharide; Fig. 1) (24,26,27). Endotoxin incorporated into red blood cell membranes will rosette macrophages only if the red cell-endotoxin complex has been preincubated with LBP (28). CD14 antibodies can block this interaction, and LBP is required for endotoxin to be recognized by CD14. This interaction is of interest, first, because it demonstrates the complexity of the in vivo response to endotoxin. Second, this model is intriguing because it completes a cycle by linking endotoxin-induced cytokines, which have potent effects on acute-phase proteins (e.g., IL-6, IL-1, and TNF), to the ability of the macrophage to interact with endotoxin.

Endotoxin Sensitivity

Endotoxin stimulation produces a burst of proinflammatory cytokines from macrophages, including IL-1, TNF, and IL-6 (29–31). Its interaction with the circulating mononuclear phagocyte, the blood monocyte, is astonishingly potent. The monocyte's sensitivity to endotoxin is in the pg/ml range for IL-1 production, rivaling the *Limulus* amebocyte lysate for sensitivity in this regard (32–34). The reason for the marked endotoxin sensitivity can partly be explained by new information from lipopolysaccharide receptor studies, but this work continues.

Since host response to sepsis is to a large part linked to the ability of the macrophage to interact with endotoxin, it is also notable that macrophages downregulate their responsiveness to endotoxin in response to corticosteroids and to endotoxin itself (22,35,36). Interestingly, most of the endotoxin-induced cytokines share a 3′-untranslated repetitive TTATTTAT consensus sequence (37). Recent data argue that this region of the genetic message may be responsible for post-transcriptional control of cytokine expression; this has been demonstrated convincingly for TNF biosynthesis using a CAT gene construct (38).

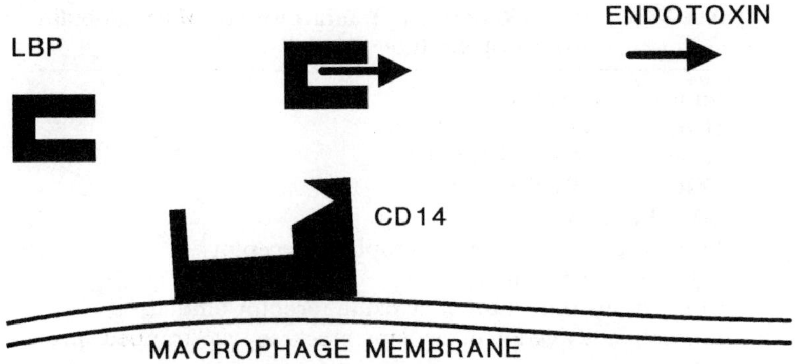

FIGURE 1 Interaction required between lipopolysaccharide binding protein (LBP) and lipopolysaccharide (endotoxin) to permit binding to the CD14 receptor.

Inflammatory cells recruited by macrophages may also affect the sensitivity of macrophages for endotoxin. For example, tissue toxicity caused by lipopolysaccharides can be dramatically reduced by an enzymatic activity (acyloxyacyl hydrolase) from human neutrophils that removes acyl groups (39,40). Deacylated endotoxin has markedly depressed activity. Thus, endotoxin-induced release of neutrophil chemoattractants, such as IL-8, may provide a means to detoxify endotoxin by the recruitment of neutrophil acyloxyacyl hydrolase. Ongoing investigations into the regulation of endotoxin receptor density and into the regulation of cytokine and endotoxin stability will provide new insights for therapeutic strategies in management of diseases characterized by endotoxin-induced cytokine excess.

α_2-Macroglobulin and Macrophage Cytokines

Macrophages interact with cytokines via specific cytokine receptors but likely also interact in various indirect ways, such as with α_2-macroglobulin (α_2-MG). Interaction with the serum antiprotease α_2-MG represents a mechanism that has been evolutionarily preserved for more than 550 million years, phylogenetically dating back to arthropodia (41). Macrophages express a 420 kD cell surface glycoprotein that binds the activated conformation of α_2-MG (42). The activated conformation ("fast" α_2-MG) is the protease-complexed form of α_2-MG that is rapidly cleared from the circulation ($T_{1/2}$ of 6 min.) (43). A number of investigations now suggest that this "fast" α_2-MG may also noncovalently complex various cytokines, such as IL-1 (44), transforming growth factor β (TGF-β) (45), platelet-derived growth factor (PDGF) (46), IL-6 (47), and others, such as macrophage activating factor (MAF), nerve growth factor (NGF), and fibroblast growth factor (FGF) (Table 1) (48). The significance of this interaction is not known at present but suggests that not only may macrophage receptors for α_2-MG rapidly clear cytokines in preference of their natural receptors, but they may also regulate cytokine-receptor interactions and macrophage function. It is clear that in vitro systems that use sera must take into account the possible interference of α_2-MG in functional measurements (45). Furthermore, since macrophages are capable of α_2-MG synthesis, autocrine effects on macrophage cytokine release must be considered as well.

TABLE 1 Cytokines Reported to Interact with α_2-Macroglobulin and Potential Effects of the Interaction

Interacting cytokines		
IL-1β	TNF	IL-2
IL-6	FGF	MAF
TGF-β	PDGF	NGF
Potential effects		
Enhanced clearance via macrophage receptor		
Inhibition of function		
Competitive inhibition of cytokine receptor binding		
Proteolytic activation of cytokine precursor via "trapped" protease		

Source: Adapted from James (48).

Macrophage Fc Receptors and Cytokines

The interaction of antigen-antibody complexes with macrophages is a key activation signal for macrophages. Bacteria coated with antibody are opsonized or more readily phagocytosed by macrophages. This event is mediated by the expression of receptors for the Fc component of immunoglobulin. It is now recognized that macrophages express three distinct types of Fc receptors (FcRI, FcRII, and FcRIII) (49) and that these receptors have important links to cytokines. Certain cytokines effect the expression of the Fc receptors, and conversely, Fc receptor triggering may regulate the expression of cytokines.

Fc Receptor Expression

In vitro, recombinant interferon-γ induces monocytes to increase their Fc receptor density by 5 to 10-fold, thus sensitizing the macrophage to opsonized particles and immune complexes (50). This may be one of the mechanisms by which interferon-γ acts as macrophage activating factor (MAF or MIF). Interestingly, other cytokines have potentially relevant functions in regard to Fc receptor expression. For example, IL-4, which itself may be induced by Fc receptor cross-linking of non-B, non-T cells from spleen and certain mast cell lines (51), can inhibit the interferon-γ-induced upregulation of Fc receptor expression (52). Endotoxin, IL-1, and to a lesser extent TNF have also been shown to counteract interferon-γ effects on Fc receptor density (53). Thus cytokines may regulate the density of Fc receptors on macrophages.

Fc Receptor Triggering of Cytokines

From the perspective of function, Fc receptors may direct the production and release of various cytokines. The best studied examples are with TNF. Cross-linking of FcRI on monocytes induces TNF-α release within 2 h (54,55). Of note, monocyte subsets that are Fc receptor positive are much better producers of TNF than Fc receptor-negative subsets (56). IL-6 is induced by aggregated IgG and the Fc fragment of IgG in monocytes (57). The story with IL-1 is more involved. Although several studies have implicated Fc receptor cross-linking with IL-1 release by monocytes (58–61), this finding is not universal and is complicated by concerns of endotoxin contamination with antibody preparations (62).

The role of Fc receptors and IL-1 has become even further complicated with the recent cloning of a specific IL-1 inhibitory protein, the IL-1 receptor antagonist (IL-1ra) (63). IL-1ra is produced most efficiently by the cross-linking of Fc receptors on immunoglobulin-coated plates (see later discussion).

Antigen Presentation: Cytokines and Macrophages

Classic Concept

The macrophage has long been linked to lymphocyte proliferation as the cell responsible for antigen presentation. As mentioned earlier, monocytes were demonstrated to be critical for lymphocyte proliferation (16,17) and a monocyte-derived cytokine, LAF, was thought to be a required signal in inducing this proliferation (17,64). Indeed, it was this function that was largely responsible for the consensus that LAF be termed IL-1 and that T cell growth factor (TCGF) be termed IL-2 (18,65,66). This intimate interaction of the macrophage and lymphocyte is called antigen presentation. Having phagocytosed, processed, and displayed the foreign antigen on its surface in association with a histocompatibility antigen (HLA-DR, HLA-DP, or HLA-DQ), macrophages bind to T lymphocytes bearing the specific antigen receptor. This complex interaction is responsible for T lymphocyte production of IL-2 (67) and the expression of IL-2 receptors that drive the T lymphocyte proliferation. IL-1 production by the presenting cell (either as a soluble mediator or as a membrane-bound form of IL-1) was believed to provide T lymphocyte competency via induction of IL-2 receptor expression on the lymphocyte (68–71).

Revised Concept

However, this classic concept about the macrophage as *the* antigen-presenting cell has been dramatically revised in the recent past. First, other HLA-DR-bearing cell types are also clearly capable of presenting antigen. Endothelial cells can function in this regard, and importantly, the recently characterized dendritic cell (72,73) is an extremely potent antigen presenter. In this context, the dendritic cell does not produce IL-1 (74,75). Furthermore, the requirement for IL-1 in macrophage-induced antigen presentation has been challenged (74,76,77). Likewise, studies using formaldehyde-fixed macrophages that suggest that IL-1α is a "membrane" form of IL-1 (70) responsible in large part for lymphocyte activation in antigen presentation have also been disputed. Ultrastructural studies have been unable to demonstrate a cell membrane component of IL-1 (78). Better understanding of the nature of intracellular IL-1α and β precursors (especially that the IL-1α precursor is functional and the IL-1β precursor is not) and the reasonable possibility that the "membrane" activity can readily be explained by the leakage of IL-1α precursor from fixed cells combine to produce doubt that membrane IL-1 is a physiological IL-1 that has a role in antigen presentation (79,80). A conservative concept regarding macrophage-derived IL-1 is that it may function to augment lymphocyte proliferation in the process of antigen presentation but it is not required. Furthermore, newer macrophage cytokines, such as IL-6, are likely to be equally important in the accessory cell function of macrophages (81–83).

Macrophage Interactions with Fibrogenic Dust

It has long been held that certain types of dusts are fibrogenic in humans and other animals and that the fibrogenicity is related to the interaction of the dust particles with macrophages. Of the fibrogenic dusts, silica and asbestos are the prime examples. These particles have long been known to have a profound effect upon macrophages. The induction of cytokine production by fibrogenic dusts is recently an area of active investigation.

Silica represents a powerful membrane perturbation to macrophages and produces a selective toxicity to macrophages. Silicosis has been linked to diseases of macrophage dysfunction, such as alveolar proteinosis (inability to clear surfactant) and tuberculosis (impaired killing of the tubercle bacillus) (84). Therefore, it is reasonable to hypothesize that silica-induced cytokine production by macrophages may also be involved in disease states. Silica is a potent inducer of IL-1 from monocytes and macrophages (85). It appears to have a greater effect upon inducing the release of IL-1 precursor stores than endotoxin, an effect that is possibly related to its cytotoxicity (85–88). Furthermore, silica sensitizes macrophages to endotoxin with respect to IL-1 release (89).

Silicotic lung disease is primarily a granulomatous and fibrotic disease, which suggests the release of fibroblast growth factors. IL-1 may have growth-promoting activity (90). In vitro, silica induces fibroblast growth factor activity but without the concomitant prostglandin E2 (PGE2) release that blocks this activity in endotoxin-induced macrophages (91). Silica also releases TNF in both in vitro and in vivo models (92,93). An exciting recent study linked the lung fibrosis of silica to TNF (94). Rats given intratracheal silica developed pulmonary fibrosis associated with the continued expression of TNF mRNA for over 70 days without a demonstrable increase in IL-1 or TGF-β. Furthermore, an antibody to TNF prevented the increased collagen deposition in this model.

Asbestos is also linked to fibrotic changes in the lung, and like silica, asbestos is cytotoxic for macrophages. Although less is known about the ability of asbestos to induce cytokines, it has been linked to TNF release (93) and to alveolar macrophage-derived growth factor (95). Of note, the mononuclear phagocytes harvested by bronchoalveolar lavage of asbestos workers demonstrate an increase in the population of younger macrophages (96). This change in the population has implications regarding the sensitivity of this lung population to cytokine release, since monocyte and macrophages differ with respect to IL-1 and TNF release (10,11,97,98).

Miscellaneous Macrophage Stimuli and Cytokines

As information about cytokines expands, the types of macrophage interactions that may play a physiological role in macrophage cytokine production is growing exponentially. The largest body of new data centers around deciphering the messages that cytokines produce when they are presented in concert. However, changes induced by viruses, diet, and bacterial exotoxins have been recognized

TABLE 2 Examples of Macrophage Cytokine Inducers[a]

Inducer	Cytokine
Infectious material	
Endotoxin	IL-1 (10), TNF-α (10), IL-6 (182), IL-8 (183)
Virus	
RSV	IL-1 (104)
influenza	IL-1 (104); TNF (184)
S. aureus (toxic shock toxin)	IL-1 (103)
Immune complexes: Fc receptor triggering	TNF (55), IL-1 (59), IL-1ra (62,63,185), PDGF (160)
Fibrogenic material	
Silica	IL-1 (85,89,93), TNF (93,94)
Asbestos	TNF (92,93)
Complement C5a	IL-1 (111)
Cytokines	
IL-1	PDGF (161), IL-8 (157)
TNF	IL-8 (157), IL-1 (179)
GM-CSF + IFN	TNF (171)
Neuropeptides: substance P	IL-1 (186)

[a] Cytokines released by macrophages directly in response to the interacting agent. References documenting these effects are in parentheses after each cytokine.

as important macrophage modulators as well. (Table 2 provides a quick reference to the types of cytokines that various agents induce.)

Diet

A fish oil diet (high in N-3 polyunsaturated fatty acids) has surprisingly potent effects upon macrophage cytokine release (99). Within 6 weeks of supplementation inducible levels of IL-1α, IL-1β, and TNF-α were decreased in normal individuals. These changes were accompanied by changes in PGE_2 inducibility and in a decrease in the arachidonic acid to eicosapentaenoic acid ratio in mononuclear cell membranes. The mechanism of this effect on cytokines is not known but may be at least partly explained by previous in vitro observations with prostanoids (100–102).

Infectious Agents

As mentioned, bacterial endotoxins are the classic inducers of macrophage cytokines, but other infectious agents have striking effects also. The toxin produced by the strain of *Staphylococcus aureus* responsible for toxic shock syndrome is an inducer of IL-1 from monocytes (103). Viral particles from influenza and respiratory syncytial virus (RSV) both can induce IL-1, although RSV induces a high-molecular-weight IL-1 inhibitor concomitantly (104). Human immunodeficiency virus type 1 HIV-1 has been examined extensively with conflicting results regarding cytokines. As with RSV, part of the conflict has to do with the concomitant production of inhibitors that has been demonstrated for IL-1 (105,106). In addition, the stage of infection with HIV has an effect. For example, endotoxin-induced TNF release may be high with asymptomatic HIV infection but drops progressively with advancement through acquired immunodeficiency virus (AIDS)-related complex and full-blown AIDS (107). Of note, however, is that normal macrophages are not induced to produce IL-1, IL-6, or TNF with HIV or with purified envelope protein (108,109). Furthermore, when hyperplastic lymph nodes of HIV-infected individuals have been studied, although IL-1 and IL-6 can be detected in sinus cells they do not differ from non–HIV-infected lymph nodes in this regard (110). In contrast, there is a marked enhancement of interferon-γ expression in the HIV lymph node cells that are in direct contact with HIV-infected cells, suggesting an ongoing anti-HIV T cell immune response (110).

Complement

Complement effects on macrophages have been linked to cytokine release. C5a may act upon macrophages to induce cytokines. It has been shown that C5a can induce IL-1 release. It also synergizes with endotoxin or with interferon-γ (111) and is believed to work by acting upon macrophage receptors for C5a (112). As another example, monocytes that are enriched for CR3 are better IL-1 producers than $CR3^-$ monocytes, implying a complement connection (113).

MACROPHAGE CYTOKINES

The macrophage-produced cytokines fall largely into the group of cytokines termed proinflammatory. These cytokines are the first messengers that macrophages release in response to perturbations in their environment and represent one of the more potent ways that macrophages serve to coordinate and direct immune reactions. These proinflammatory cytokines are briefly reviewed here and in more detail in specific chapters.

Interleukin-1

Formerly known as endogenous pyrogen and lymphocyte activating factor, IL-1 is really two distinct proteins of 17,000 molecular weight encoded on chromosome 2 (114). Termed IL-1α and IL-1β, these proteins are both produced as 35,000 D precursor proteins produced in large quantities by macrophages in response to many stimuli, most notably endotoxin. IL-1β may represent as much as 1–2% of the mRNA produced after endotoxin challenge (79). IL-1α is the pI 5 molecule that is functional in the propeptide state; IL-1β is the pI 7 protein that requires processing to the 17,000 D protein for functional activation. These molecules share 50% homology at the gene level and 26% homology at the protein level, react with the same receptor molecules, and have almost if not complete overlap in functional characteristics (79,115). When stimulated, monocytes produce about 10 times more IL-1β than IL-1α (79). Since IL-1α is functional in the precursor state, it may represent the molecule important in reactions within the localized milieu of the macrophage, whereas IL-1β may represent the more hormonal of the two.

Function

IL-1 acts upon many cell types, including lymphocytes, hepatocytes, endothelial cells, fibroblasts, chrondrocytes, and neutrophils (116). With lymphocytes the effects include augmentation of T cell proliferation and B cell activation in response to antigen challenge (77,116,117). With hepatocytes, IL-1 is an inducer of the acute-phase response (118). Endothelial cells present new neutrophil adherence molecules, such as ELAMs, and may change permeability characteristics (119,120). IL-1 enhances fibroblast proliferation and induces fibroblast collagenase and PGE_2 release (90,121). Neutrophils experience heightened oxidant production and smooth muscle cells are induced to relaxation in response to IL-1 (97,122). From this perspective IL-1 synergizes with other cytokines for much of its activity, the best studied examples being with TNF (8,123,124).

Regulation

IL-1 release decreases with maturation of monocytes into macrophages (7,10); its production is inhibited by corticosteroids (36) and is greatly upregulated after interferon-γ (125). Its production can be superinduced with cycloheximide, suggesting that there is a repressor protein, and its processing requires the coexpression of a convertase activity (126–130). Its half-life in the circulation is short (minutes), and its function is counteracted by a number of inhibitors, such as uromodulin (131,132) and the exciting, recently discovered, IL-1 receptor antagonist (133).

Interleukin-1 Receptor Antagonist

IL-1ra represents a new and unique cytokine that functions by acting as a competitive inhibitor for both IL-1α and IL-1β (133). It was first purified and subsequently characterized from the inhibitory supernatant molecules produced by monocytes grown on adherent immune complexes or IgG (133). IL-1ra is similar in structure to IL-1β and IL-1α (26 and 19% homology at the gene level, respectively) (63) and functions by competing with IL-1 for its receptor. The significance of this molecule has yet to be elucidated, but its unique function as a pure receptor antagonist to IL-1α and IL-1β introduces an exciting new perspective to cytokine interactions.

Tumor Necrosis Factor

A cytokine that is completely distinct in structure from IL-1 but that has enormous functional overlap is TNF-α. TNF-α is a 17,000 D protein that circulates as a dimer of 35,000 D. Like IL-1, it is largely a macrophage product that is produced in large quantities within 90 minutes of endotoxin challenge (134). It exists on chromosome 6 in tandem with TNF-β within the major histocompatibility complex (64,135). (TNF-β, also known as lymphotoxin, is the lymphocyte product and TNF-α, also known as cachectin, the macrophage product. Like IL-1α and β, these TNF proteins have significant homology at both the gene and protein levels, interact with the same TNF receptor, and have almost identical functional characteristics.)

Functions

The classic functions of tumor necrosis factor are its ability to cause necrosis of tumors transplanted into mice and its ability to cause cachexia (136). The phys-

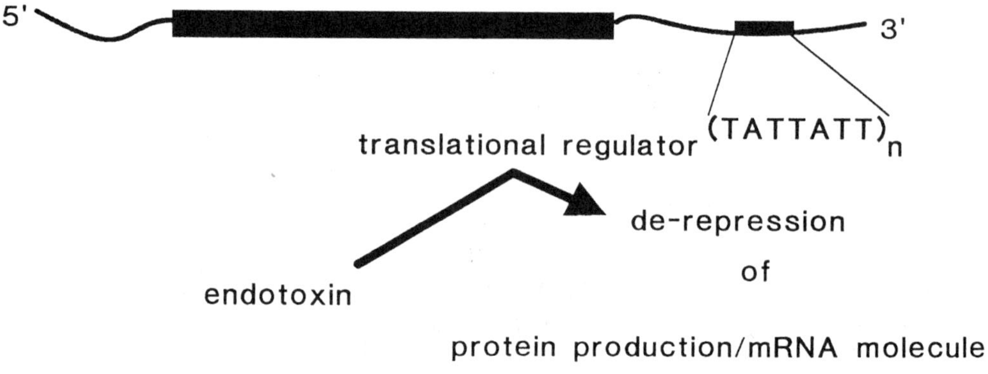

FIGURE 2 How the 3′-untranslated mRNA consensus sequence present on a number of inflammatory mediators may represent a regulator of protein translation.

iological revelance of these classic functions have been questioned, but TNF also has important effects on many cells that overlap almost completely with those of IL-1, including lymphocyte proliferation (137), fibroblast PGE_2 and collagenase release (138), fever (139), endothelial expression of ELAM (140), induction of acute-phase proteins (83), and activation of neutrophils (141,142). TNF has been singled out as a critical if not central player in the cascade of events that occurs with the syndrome of septic shock (143–145).

Regulation

In contrast to IL-1, TNF release is enhanced in macrophages compared to monocytes, but like IL-1 its production is also enhanced by interferon-γ (125,146) and inhibited by corticosteroids (147). As mentioned earlier, TNF (and most proinflammatory peptides) contains a 3′-untranslated repeating sequence, TTATTTAT, that for TNF has been shown to be important in regulating translation (Fig. 2) (37,38). TNF is produced within 90 minutes of endotoxin challenge in humans (134) (Fig. 3), but its production in response to repeated endotoxin stimulation is downregulated (148). Endotoxin undoubtedly institutes the expression and repression of a variety of modulatory factors.

Interleukin-6

IL-6 is a macrophage-derived cytokine (also produced by many other cell types) that is 21,000 D in size and that has multiple functions, many of which overlap with those of IL-1 and TNF (149,150). IL-6 classically is a B cell growth factor but has important effects as the major hepatic acute-phase protein inducer, as a T cell activator, and as a thrombopoietin (83). As mentioned earlier, IL-1 and TNF are potent inducers of IL-6 production, and many of the functions previously attributed to IL-1 or TNF may be IL-6 effects (e.g., acute-phase protein production, thymocyte proliferation, and T cell activation). IL-6 does not induce IL-1 or TNF but feeds back to inhibit endotoxin-induced TNF and IL-1 production.

The control of IL-6 production is intimately linked to that of IL-1 and TNF. IL-1 and TNF rapidly induce IL-6 release. The mechanism of this effect is rapidly

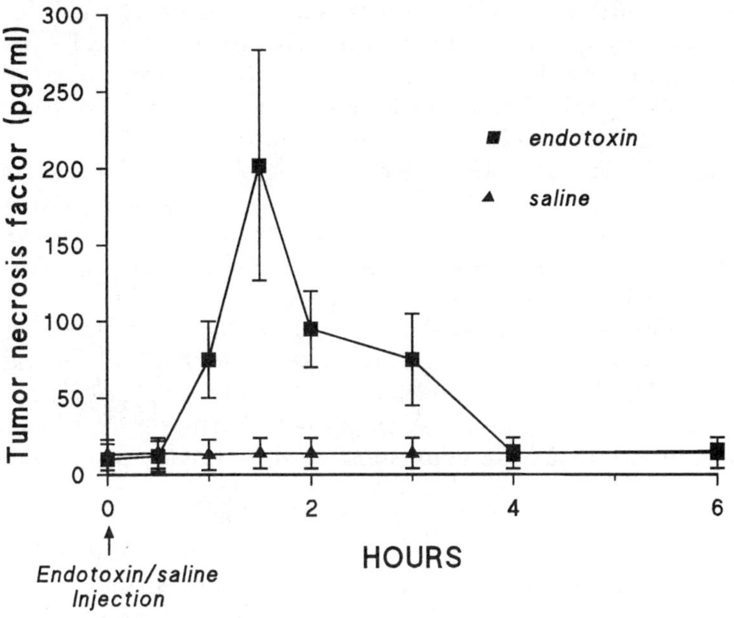

FIGURE 3 Effect of a single injection of endotoxin in normal humans on the levels of circulating TNF. (Adapted from Ref. 134.)

being dissected. For example, some of the function of IL-1 on cells has been linked to the induction of NF-κB (151,152). NF-κB is a gene regulatory protein that was first recognized to interact with the immunoglobulin κ regulatory gene (153). An NF-κB-like factor, produced in response to IL-1 or TNF, interacts with an NF-κB site on the IL-6 promoter (83). Other regulatory sequences in the IL-6 promoter are also responsive to IL-1 and TNF (83). Cycloheximide superinduces IL-6 in addition to IL-1 and TNF. Interestingly, IL-6 does not appear to contain the TATTTATT sequence in the 3′-untranslated region, which is standard for most of the proinflammatory cytokines (37).

Interleukin-8

IL-8 (formerly monocyte-derived chemotactic factor or neutrophil activating peptide 1) is an 8000 D peptide produced by mononuclear phagocytes (and other cell types) that is a potent neutrophil attractant and stimulant (154–156). As with IL-6, IL-8 can be induced by endotoxin, IL-1, and TNF (157,158). Also like IL-1, TNF, and IL-6, it is superinducible by cycloheximide (154). IL-8 is likely responsible for many of the neutrophil chemotactic properties that have been previously attributed to IL-1 and TNF in animal experiments in vivo (159).

Growth Factors

Platelet-derived Growth Factor

Platelet-derived growth factor is a 31,000 D glycoprotein product of platelets and macrophages that functions as a potent mesenchymal cell chemoattractant and as a fibroblast growth factor (160). It acts as a "competence" factor for fibroblast growth by inducing entrance into the early G_1 phase of the cell cycle, allowing the cell to respond to subsequent "progression" factors for proliferation. PDGF is released in exaggerated amounts in idiopathic pulmonary fibrosis (160) and may play a pathogenetic role in the fibrotic reaction.

Of note, PDGF does complex with α_2-macroglobulin, and in this regard when studied in vitro, its function often requires a pretreatment step to allow its expression (46,48). For example, supernatants from macrophages are dialyzed against 1 M acetic acid to allow full expression of chemotactic activity (160); it is conceivable that this step removes the α_2-macroglobulin. However, a role for α_2-macroglobulin in the in vivo regulation of PDGF has not been demonstrated.

In the context of cytokine interactions, it is of note that IL-1 can induce PDGF from fibroblasts and smooth muscle cells, which may explain in part the ability of IL-1 to induce fibroblast proliferation (90,161). Furthermore, it has been shown that PDGF can induce TGF-β expression in wound macrophages (162).

Insulinlike Growth Factors

Insulinlike growth factors are 7500 D peptides that have considerable homology with each other and with proinsulin, which function as stimulators of cellular proliferation and differentiation (163). Virtually all cells have IGF receptors, with IGF-2 primarily important in prenatal growth and development and IGF-1 the postnatal growth factor (163). IGF-1 is known to be produced by alveolar macrophages, and it may represent most if not all of the activity formerly known as alveolar macrophage-derived growth factor (AMDGF) (164). Like AMDGF, IGF-1 acts as a progression factor; that is, it can take a cell made "competent" by PDGF or fibronectin and push it through the G_1 phase of the cell cycle (164). It has been speculated that IGF-1 may be a key cytokine in the induction and maintenance of the fibrosis of certain interstitial lung disorders (164).

Transforming Growth Factor β

Transforming growth factor β (TGF-β) is a 25,000 D dimer that is a multifunctional regulator of cell growth and differentiation produced and stored by platelets (165) but also by macrophages (166). Its function overlaps with that of epidermal growth factor and PDGF in their effects upon fibroblasts. TGF-β is chemotactic for fibroblasts (167). Of note, TGF-β mRNA appears to be constitutively expressed in monocytes and macrophages, but translation and protein release require mononuclear phagocyte activation (166).

The bleomycin model of lung fibrosis has been demonstrated to be linked to TGF-β production by macrophages (168). TGF-β, like IL-6, induces the production of acute-phase proteins, an effect that is both direct and due to modulation of the IL-6 effect (169). It may be linked to PDGF in that PDGF can induce its expression in experimental wounds (162). In this context TGF-β belongs with other macrophage cytokines, like PDGF and IGF-1, that may be critical regulators of fibrotic disorders of the lung (168). Distinct functions have been noted as well. For example, an interesting new twist to the repertoire of cytokine functions is provided by the recent observation that TGF-β may also have antiinflammatory functions. TGF-β can produce burst suppression for H_2O_2 production by macrophages (170).

CYTOKINE NETWORKS

Cytokine networks have been likened to a language. Just as the letters of the alphabet are to a message, the context of a particular cytokine to coexistent cytokines determines its meaning. The deciphering of this language has only begun. The effect of granulocyte-macrophage colony-stimulating factor (GM-CSF) upon monocytes provides an example. GM-CSF alone has no effect upon the production of IL-1, TNF, or PGE_2 production but when added in the context of interferon-γ it specifically enhances TNF release but not IL-1 release (171). On the other hand, interferon-γ synergizes with endotoxin for the induction of both TNF and IL-1 (172–176). Another example, is the effects of IL-3 on macrophages. IL-3 (a multipotent CSF) synergizes with interferon-γ for the induction of Ia determinants on macrophages (177) but not for IL-1 release (178). However, it synergizes with endotoxin for IL-1 release (178).

An experimental problem that this scenario produces is that it is often difficult to determine if the effects of a particular cytokine are direct or produced by secondary cytokine cascades. TNF, for example, overlaps significantly with IL-1 in many proinflammatory functions. Interestingly, TNF may work in part via the induction of IL-1 (179,180). IL-1 acts in the thymocyte assay to induce thymocyte proliferation (181), yet IL-6 can be induced by IL-1 acting upon fibroblasts (81) and or thymocytes (82). IL-6 may represent the final pathway for many of the effects of IL-1 (150). These examples refer only to incidences of single cytokines inducing secondary single cytokines, however. The more complex language of cytokines will undoubtedly be more difficult to decipher.

SUMMARY

Macrophages are key regulators of the immune response. They function at multiple levels of sophistication. Although they often work as day laborers performing normal cleanup and maintenance procedures, they may also function as "quality control advisors" and as "administrators," recognizing problems and communicating the appropriate response. These more sophisticated functions require a sophisticated communication network. Cytokines represent one means by which the information can be transferred to appropriate members of the defense system to maintain a coordinated response. This coordination is important in the functioning of the immune system and its interaction with the body's processes of growth, repair, and differentiation.

REFERENCES

1. van Furth R, Cohn ZA. The origin and kinetics of mononuclear phagocytes. J Exp Med 1968; 128:415–33.
2. Cline MJ, Lehrer RI, Territo C, Golde DW. Monocytes and macrophages: functions and diseases. Ann Intern Med 1978; 88:78–88.
3. Johnston RB Jr. Monocytes and macrophages. N Engl J Med 1988; 318:747–52.
4. Thomas ED, Ramberg RE, Sale GE, Sparkes RS, Golde DW. Direct evidence for a bone marrow origin of the alveolar macrophage in man. Science 1976; 192:1016–8.
5. Fung JJ, Zeevi A, Kaufman C, et al. Interactions between bronchoalveolar lym-

phocytes and macrophages in heart-lung transplant recipients. Hum Immunol 1985; 14:287–94.

6. Kargi HA, Campbell EJ, Kuhn C III. Elastase and cathepsin G of human monocytes: heterogeneity and subcellular localization to peroxidase-positive granules. J Histochem Cytochem 1990; 38:1179–86.
7. Wewers MD, Saltini C, Sellers S, et al. Evaluation of alveolar macrophages in normals and individuals with active pulmonary sarcoidosis for the spontaneous expression of the interleukin-1 beta gene. Cell Immunol 1987; 107:479–88.
8. Elias JA, Gustilo K, Freundlich B. Human alveolar macrophage and blood monocyte inhibition of fibroblast proliferation: evidence for synergy between interleukin-1 and tumor necrosis factor. Am Rev Respir Dis 1988; 138:1595–603.
9. Martinet Y, Yamauchi K, Crystal RG. Differential expression of the tumor necrosis factor/cachectin gene by blood and lung mononuclear phagocytes. Am Rev Resp Dis 1988; 138:659–65.
10. Wewers MD, Herzyk DJ. Alveolar macrophages differ from blood monocytes in human interleukin 1 beta release: quantitation by enzyme linked immunoassay. J Immunol 1989; 143:1635–41.
11. Rich EA, Panuska JR, Wallis RS, et al. Dyscoordinate expression of tumor necrosis factor-alpha by human blood monocytes and alveolar macrophages. Am Rev Respir Dis 1989; 139:1010–6.
12. Mornex JF, Martinet Y, Yamauchi K, et al. Spontaneous expression of the *c-sis* gene and release of a platelet-derived growth factor like molecule by human alveolar macrophages. J Clin Invest 1986; 78:61–6.
13. Bloom BR, Bennett B. Mechanism of a reaction in vitro associated with delayed-type hypersensitivity. Science 1966; 153:180–2.
14. David JR. Delayed hypersensitivity in vitro: its mediation by cell-free substances formed by lymphoid-cell-antigen interactions. Proc Natl Acad Sci U S A 1966; 56:73–7.
15. Beeson PB. Temperature-elevating effect of a substance obtained from polymorphonuclear leukocytes. J Clin Invest 1948; 27:524.
16. Bach FH, Alter BJ, Solliday S, Zoschke DC, Janis M. Lymphocyte reactivity in vitro. II. Soluble reconstituting factor permitting response of purified lymphocytes. Cell Immunol 1970; 1:219–27.
17. Gery I, Waksman BH. Potentiation of the T-lymphocyte response to mitogens II. The cellular source of potentiating mediator(s). J Exp Med 1972; 136:143–55.
18. Aarden LA, Burnner TK, Cerottini JD, et al. Letter to the editor. Revised nomenclature for antigen-nonspecific T cell proliferation and helper factors. J Immunol 1979; 123:2928.
19. Ulevitch RJ, Wolfson N, Virca GD, Kim S, Kline L, Mathison JC. Macrophages regulate the host response to bacterial lipopolysaccharides. In: Perspectives in shock research: metabolism, immunology, mediators, and models. New York: Alan R. Liss, 1989:193.
20. Mathison JC, Ulevitch RJ. The clearance, tissue distribution, and cellular localization of intravenously injected lipopolysaccharide in rabbits. J Immunol 1979; 123:2133–43.
21. Michalek SM, Moore RN, McGhee JR, Rosenstreich DL, Mergenhagen SE. The primary role of lymphoreticular cells in the mediation of host responses to bacterial endotoxin. J Infect Dis 1980; 141:55–63.
22. Beutler B, Krochin N, Milsark IW, Leudke C, Cerami A. Control of cachectin (tumor necrosis factor) synthesis: mechanisms of endotoxin resistance. Science 1986; 232:977–80.

23. von Jeney N, Gunther E, Jann K. Mitogenic stimulation of murine spleen cells: relation to susceptibility to *Salmonella* infection. Infect Immun 1977; 15:26–33.
24. Wright SD, Jong MTC. Adhesion-promoting receptors on human macrophages recognize *E. coli* by binding to lipopolysaccharide. J Exp Med 1986; 164:1876–88.
25. Haeffner-Cavaillon N, Chaby R, Cavaillon J-M, Szabo L. Lipopolysaccharide receptor on rabbit peritoneal macrophages: binding characteristics. J Immunol 1982; 128:1950–4.
26. Tobias PS, Mathison JC, Ulevitch RJ. A family of lipopolysaccharide binding proteins involved in responses to Gram-negative sepsis. J Biol Chem 1988; 263:13479–81.
27. Ferrero E, Hsieh C-L, Francke U, Goyert SM. CD14 is a member of the family of leucine-rich proteins and is encoded by a gene syntenic with multiple receptor genes. J Immunol 1990; 145:331–6.
28. Wright SD, Tobias PS, Ulevitch RJ, Ramos RA. Lipopolysaccharide (LPS) binding protein opsonizes LPS-bearing particles for recognition by a novel receptor on macrophages. J Exp Med 1989; 170:1231–41.
29. Durum SK, Schmidt JA, Oppenheim JJ. Interleukin 1: an immunological perspective. Ann Rev Immunol 1985; 3:263–87.
30. Dinarello CA, Human pyrogen: a monocyte product mediating host defenses. In: Gallin JI, Fauci AS, eds. Advances in host defense mechanisms. Raven Press, New York: 1982:57.
31. May LT, Ghrayeb J, Santhanam U, et al. Synthesis and secretion of multiple forms of beta 2-interferon/B-cell differentiation factor 2/hepatocyte-stimulating factor by human fibroblasts and monocytes. J Biol Chem 1988; 263:7760–6.
32. Duff GW, Atkins E. The detection of endotoxin by in vitro production of endogenous pyrogen: comparison with *Limulus* amebocyte lysate gelation. J Immunol Methods 1982; 52:323–31.
33. Wood DD, Cameron PM. The relationship between bacterial endotoxin and human B cell-activiting factor. J Immunol 1978; 121:53–60.
34. Northoff H, Gluck D, Wolpl A, Kubanek B, Galanos C. Lipopolysaccharide-induced elaboration of interleukin 1 by human monocytes: use for detection of lipopolysaccharide in serum and the influence of serum-lipopolysaccharide interactions. Rev Infect Dis 1987; 9:S599–601.
35. Virca GD, Kim SY, Glaser KB, Ulevitch RJ. Lipopolysaccharide induces hyporesponsiveness to its own action in RAW 264.7 cells. J Biol Chem 1990; 264: 21951–6.
36. Kern JA, Lamb RJ, Reed JC, Daniele RP, Nowell PC. Dexamethasone inhibition of interleukin 1 beta production by human monocytes: posttranscriptional mechanisms. J Clin Invest 1988; 81:237–44.
37. Caput D, Beutler B, Hartog K, Thayer R, Brown-Shimer S, Cerami A. Identification of a common nucleotide sequence in the 3′-untranslated region of mRNA molecules specifying inflammatory mediators. Proc Natl Acad Sci U S A 1986; 83:1670–4.
38. Han J, Brown T, Beutler B. Endotoxin-responsive sequences control cachectin/ tumor necrosis factors biosynthesis at the translational level. J Exp Med 1990; 171:465–75.
39. Munford RS, Hall CL. Detoxification of bacterial lipopolysaccharides (endotoxins) by a human neutrophil enzyme. Science 1986; 234:203–5.
40. Kovach NL, Yee E, Munford RS, Raetz CRH, Harlan JM. Lipid IVa inhibits synthesis and release of tumor necrosis factor induced by lipopolysaccharide in human whole blood ex vivo. J Exp Med 1990; 172:77–84.
41. Sottrup-Jensen L, Borth W, Hall M, Quigley JP, Armstrong PB. Sequence similarity between α_2-macroglobulin from the horseshoe crab, *Limulus polyphemus*, and proteins

of the α_2-macroglobulin family from mammals. Comp Biochem Physiol [B] 1990; 96B:621–5.

42. Ashcom JD, Tiller SE, Dickerson K, Cravens JL, Argraves WS, Strickland DK. The human α_2-macroglobulin receptor: identification of a 420-kD cell surface glycoprotein specific for the activated conformation of α_2-macroglobulin. J Cell Biol 1990; 110:1041–8.
43. Starkey PM, Barrett AJ. Alpha 2-macroglobulin, a physiological regulator of proteinase activity. In: Barrett AJ., ed. Proteinases in mammalian cells and tissues. Amsterdam: Elsevier/North-Holland Biomedical Press, 1977:663.
44. Borth W, Urbanski A, Prohaska R, Susani M, Luger TA. Binding of recombinant interleukin-1β to the third complement component and α_2-macroglobulin after activation of serum by immune complexes. Blood 1990; 75:2388–95.
45. Danielpour D, Sporn MB. Differential inhibition of transforming growth factor β1 and β2 activity by α_2-macroglobulin. J Biol Chem 1990; 265:6973–7.
46. Bonner JC, Hoffman M, Brody, AR. Alpha-macroglobulin secreted by alveolar macrophages serves as a binding protein for a macrophage-derived homologue of platelet-derived growth factor. Am J Resp Cell Mol Biol 1989; 1:171–9.
47. Matsuda T, Hirano T, Nagasawa S, Kishimoto T. Identification of alpha-2-macroglobulin as a carrier protein for IL-6. J Immunol 1989; 142:148–52.
48. James K. Interactions between cytokines and α_2-macroglobulin. Immunol Today 1990; 11:163–6.
49. Anderson CL, Shen L, Eicher DM, Wewers MD, Gill JK. Phagocytosis mediated by three distinct Fc gamma receptor classes on human leukocytes. J Exp Med 1990; 171:1333–45.
50. Guyre PM, Morganelli PM, Miller R. Recombinant immune interferon increases immunoglobulin G Fc receptors on cultured human mononuclear phagocytes. J Clin Invest 1983; 72:393–7.
51. Conrad DH, Ben-Sasson SZ, Le Gros G, Finkelman FD, Paul WE. Infection with *Nippostrongylus bransiliensis* or injection of anti-IgD antibodies markedly enhances Fc-receptor-mediated interleukin 4 production by non-B, non-T cells. J Exp Med 1990; 171:1497–508.
52. Te Velde AA, Huijbens RJF, De Vries J, Figdor CG. IL-4 decreases FcgammaR membrane expression and FcgammaR-mediated cytotoxic activity of human monocytes. J Immunol 1990; 144:3046–51.
53. Arend WP, Ammons JT, Kotzin BL. Lipopolysaccharide and interleukin 1 inhibit interferon-gamma induced Fc receptor expression on human monocytes. J Immunol 1987; 139:1873–9.
54. Debets JMH, Van der Linden CJ, Dieteren IEM, Seeuwenberg JFM, Buurman WA. Fc-receptor cross-linking induces rapid secretion of tumor necrosis factor (cachectin) by human peripheral blood monocytes. J Immunol 1988; 141:1197–201.
55. Debets JMH, Van de Winkel JGJ, Ceuppens JL, Dieteren IEM, Buurman WA. Cross-linking of both Fc gamma RI and Fc gamma RII induces secretion of tumor necrosis factor by human monocytes, requiring high affinity Fc-Fc gamm R interactions: functional activation of Fc gamma RII by treatment with proteases or neuraminidase. J Immunol 1990; 144:1304–10.
56. Szabo G, Miller-Graziano CL, Wu J-Y, Takayama T, Kodys K. Differential tumor necrosis factor production by human monocyte subsets. J Leukoc Biol 1990; 47:206–16.
57. Ling Z-D, Ziltener HJ, Webb BT, Matheson DS. Aggregated immunglobulin and Fc fragment of IgG induce IL-6 release from human monocytes. Cell Immunol 1990; 129:95–103.

58. Blyden G, Handschumacher RE. Purification and properties of human lymphocyte activating factor (LAF). J Immunol 1977; 118:1631–8.
59. Morgan EL, Hobbs MV, Noonan DJ, Weigle WO. Induction of IL-1 secretion from human monocytes by Fc region subfragments of human IgG_1. J Immunol 1988; 140:3014–20.
60. Chou YK, Sherwood T, Virella G. Erythrocyte-bound immune complexes trigger the release of interleukin-1 from human monocytes. Cell Immunol 1985; 91:308–14.
61. Dayer JM, Passwell JH, Schneeberger EE, Krane SM. Interactions among rheumatoid synovial cells and monocyte-macrophages: production of collagenase-stimulatory factor by human monocytes exposed to concanavalin A or immunoglobulin Fc fragments. J Immunol 1980; 124:1712–20.
62. Arend WP, Joslin FG, Massoni RJ. Effects of immune complexes on production by human monocytes of interleukin 1 or an interleukin 1 inhibitor. J Immunol 1985; 134:3868–75.
63. Eisenberg SP, Evans RJ, Arend WP, et al. Primary structure and functional expression from complementary DNA of a human interleukin-1 receptor antagonist. Nature 1990; 343:341–6.
64. Carroll MC, Katzman P, Alicott EM, et al. Linkage map of the human major histocompatibility complex including the tumor necrosis factor genes. Proc Natl Acad Sci U S A 1987; 84:8535–9.
65. Maizel AL, Mehta SR, Hauft S, Franzini D, Lachman LB, Ford RJ. Human T lymphocyte/monocyte interaction in response to lectin: kinetics of entry into the S-phase. J Immunol 1981; 127:1058–64.
66. Smith KA, Lachman LB, Oppenheim JJ, Favata MF. The functional relationship of the interleukins. J Exp Med 1980; 151:1551–6.
67. Smith KA, Gilbride KJ, Favata MF. Lymphocyte activating factor promotes T-cell growth factor production by cloned murine lymphoma cells. Nature 1980; 287:853–5.
68. Teshigawara K, Wang HM, Kato K, Smith KA. Interleukin 2 high-affinity receptor expression requires two distinct binding proteins. J Exp Med 1987; 165:223–8.
69. Cantrell DA, Smith KA. The interleukin-2 T-cell system: a new cell growth model. Science 1984; 224:1312–6.
70. Kurt-Jones EA, Beller DL, Mizel SB, Unanue ER. Identification of a membrane-associated interleukin in macrophages. Proc Natl Acad Sci U S A 1985; 82:1204–8.
71. Beuscher HU, Colten HR. Structure and function of membrane IL-1. Mol Immunol 1988; 25:1189–99.
72. Inaba K, Steinman RM, Voorhis WC, Muramatsu S. Dendritic cells are critical accessory cells for thymus-dependent antibody responses in mouse and in man. Proc Natl Acad Sci U S A 1983; 80:6041–5.
73. Inaba K, Steinman RM. Resting and sensitized T lymphocytes exhibit distinct stimulatory (antigen-presenting cell) requirements for growth and lymphokine release. J Exp Med 1984; 160:1717–35.
74. Koide S, Steinman RM. Induction of murine interleukin 1: stimuli and responsive primary cells. Proc Natl Acad Sci U S A 1987; 84:3802–6.
75. Nicod LP, Galve-de Rochemonteix B, Dayer J-M. Dissociation between allogeneic T cell stimulation and interleukin-1 or tumor necrosis factor production by human lung dendritic cells. Am J Resp Cell Mol Biol 1990; 2:515–22.
76. Tsakalos ND, Lachman LB, Newhouse YG, Whisler RL. Lipopolysaccharide (LPS) modulation of human monocyte accessory cell function in promoting T-cell colonies:

inability of LPS and IL-1 to abrograte the need for monocytes with high HLA-DR expression. Cell Immunol 1984; 83:229–41.
77. Bhardwaj N, Lau LL, Friedman SM, Crow MK, Steinman RM. Interleukin 1 production during accessory cell-dependent mitognesis of T lymphocytes. J Exp Med 1989; 169:1121–36.
78. Singer II, Scott S, Hall GL, Limjuco G, Chin J, Schmidt JA. Interleukin 1 beta is localized in the cytoplasmic ground substance but is largely absent from the Golgi apparatus and plasma membranes of stimulated human monocytes. J Exp Med 1988; 167:389–407.
79. March CJ, Mosely B, Larsen A, et al. Cloning, sequence and expression of two distinct human interleukin-1 complementary DNAs. Nature 1985; 315:641–7.
80. Minnich-Carruth LL, Suttles J, Mizel SB. Evidence against the existence of a membrane form of murine IL-1 alpha. J Immunol 1989; 142:526–30.
81. Elias JA, Trinchieri G, Beck JM, et al. A synergistic interaction of IL-6 and IL-1 mediates the thymocyte-stimulating activity produced by recombinant IL-1-stimulated fibroblasts. J Immunol 1989; 142:509–14.
82. Helle M, Boeije L, Aarden LA. IL-6 is an intermediate in IL-1-induced thymocyte proliferation. J Immunol 1989; 142:4335–8.
83. Akira S, Hirano T, Taga T, Kishimoto T. Biology of multifunctional cytokines: IL 6 and related molecules (IL 1 and TNF). FASEB J 1990; 4:2860–7.
84. Ziskind M, Jones RN, Weill H. Silicosis. Am Rev Respir Dis 1976; 113:643–65.
85. Schmidt JA, Oliver CN, Lepe-Zuniga JL, Green I, Gery I. Silica-stimulated monocytes release fibroblast proliferation factors identical to interleukin 1: a potential role for interleukin 1 in the pathogenesis of silicosis. J Clin Invest 1984; 73:1462–72.
86. Gery I, Davies, P, Derr J, Krett N, Barranger JA. Relationship between production and release of lymphocyte-activating factor (interleukin 1) by murine macrophages: effects of various agents. Cell Immunol 1981; 64:293–303.
87. Apte RN, Durum SK, Oppenheim JJ. Opioids modulate interleukin-1 production and secretion by bone-marrow macrophages. Immunol Lett 1990; 24:141–8.
88. Lepe-Zuniga JL, Gery I. Production of intra- and extracellular interleukin-1 (IL-1) by human monocytes. Clin Immunol Immunopath 1984; 31:222–30.
89. Vogel SN, English KE, O'Brien AD. Silica enhancement of murine endotoxin sensitivity. Infect Immun 1982; 38:681–5.
90. Schmidt JA, Mizel SB, Cohen D, Green I. Interleukin 1, a potential regulator of fibroblast proliferation. J Immunol 1982; 128:2177–21.
91. Brown GP, Monick M, Hunninghake GW. Fibroblast proliferation induced by silica-exposed human alveolar macrophages. Am Rev Respir Dis 1988; 138:85–9.
92. Dubois CM, Bissonnete E, Rola-Pleszczynski M. Asbestos fibers and silica particles stimulate rat alveolar macrophages to release tumor necrosis factor: autoregulatory role of leukotriene B_4. Am Rev Respir Dis 1989; 139:1257–64.
93. Driscoll KE, Sindenschmidt RC, Maurer JK, Higgins JM, Ridder G. Pulmonary response to silica or titanium dioxide: inflammatory cells, alveolar macrophage-derived cytokines, and histopathology. Am J Respir Cell Mol Biol 1990; 2:381–90.
94. Piguet PF, Collart MA, Grau GE, Sappino A-P, Vassalli P. Requirement of tumour necrosis factor for development of silica-induced pulmonary fibrosis. Nature 1990; 344:245–7.
95. Rom WN, Bitterman PB, Rennard SI, Cantin A, Crystal RG. Characterization of the lower respiratory tract inflammation of nonsmoking individuals with interstitial lung disease associated with chronic inhalation of inorganic dusts. Am Rev Respir Dis 1987; 136:1429–34.
96. Spurzem JR, Saltini C, Rom W, Winchester RJ, Crystal RG. Mechanisms of mac-

rophage accumulation in the lungs of asbestos-exposed subjects. Am Rev Respir Dis 1987; 136:276–280.

97. Wewers MD, Rennard SI, Hance AJ, Bitterman PB, Crystal RG. Normal human alveolar macrophages obtained by bronchoalveolar lavage have a limited capacity to release interleukin-1. J Clin Invest 1984; 74:2208–18.
98. Elias JA, Schreiber AD, Gustilo K, et al. Differential interleukin 1 elaboration by unfractionated and density fractionated human alveolar macrophages and blood monocytes: relationship to cell maturity. J Immunol 1985; 135:3198–204.
99. Endres S, Ghorbani R, Kelley VE, et al. The effect of dietary supplementation with N-3 polyunsaturated fatty acids on the synthesis of interleukin-1 and tumor necrosis factor by mononuclear cells. N Engl J Med 1989; 320:265–71.
100. Kunkel SL, Spengler M, May MA, Spengler R, Larrick J, Remick D. Prostaglandin E_2 regulates macrophage-derived tumor necrosis factor gene expression. J Biol Chem 1988; 263:5358–84.
101. Rola-Pleszczynski M, Lemaire I. Leukotrienes augment interleukin 1 production by human monocytes. J Immunol 1985; 135:3058–61.
102. Kunkel SL, Chensue SW, Phan SH. Prostaglandins as endogenous mediators of interleukin 1 production. J Immunol 1986; 136:186–92.
103. Ikejima T, Dinarello CA, Gill DM, Wolff SM. Induction of human interleukin-1 by a product of *Staphylococcus aureus* associated with toxic shock syndrome. J Clin Invest 1984; 73:1312–20.
104. Roberts NJ, Prill AH, Mann TN. Interleukin 1 and interleukin 1 inhibitor production by human mcrophages exposed to influenza virus or respiratory synctial virus. J Exp Med 1986; 163:511–9.
105. Berman MA, Sandborg CI, Calabia BS, Andrews BS, Friou GJ. Interleukin 1 inhibitor masks high interleukin 1 production in acquired immunodeficiency syndrome (AIDS). Clin Immunol Immunopathol 1987; 42:133–40.
106. Pennica D, Kohr W, Kuang W-J, et al. Identification of human uromodulin as the Tamm-Horsfall urinary glycoprotein. Science 1987; 236:83–8.
107. Cox RA, Anders GT, Cappell PJ, et al. Production of tumor necrosis factor-alpha and interleukin-1 by alveolar macrophages from HIV-1-infected persons. AIDS Res Hum Retroviruses 1990; 6:431–41.
108. Molina J-M, Scadden DT, Amirault C, et al. Human immunodeficiency virus does not induce interleukin-1, interleukin-6, or tumor necrosis factor in mononuclear cells. J Virol 1990; 64:2901–6.
109. Molina J-M, Schindler R, Ferriani R, et al. Production of cytokines by peripheral blood monocytes/macrophages infected with human immunodeficiency virus type I (HIV-1). J Infect Dis 1990; 161:888–93.
110. Emilie D, Peuchmaur M, Maillot MC, et al. Production of interleukins in human immunodeficiency virus-1-replicating lymph nodes. J Clin Invest 1990; 86:148–59.
111. Okusawa S, Dinarello CA, Yancey KB, et al. C5a induction of human interleukin 1: synergistic effect with endotoxin or interferon gamma. J Immunol 1987; 139:2635–40.
112. Goodman MG, Chenoweth DE, Weigle WO. Induction of interleukin 1 secretion and enhancement of humoral immunity by binding of human C5a to macrophage surface C5a receptors. J Exp Med 1982; 1156:912–7.
113. Whisler RL, Newhouse YG, Lachman LB. Heterogeneity of human monocyte subsets in the promotion of B cell colonies and the role of interleukin 1. J Immunol 1982; 129:455–60.
114. D'Eustachio P, Jadidi S, Fuhlbrigge RC, Gray PW, Chaplin DD. Interleukin-1 alpha and beta genes: linkage on chromosome 2 in the mouse. Immunogenetics 1987; 26:339–43.

115. Rupp EA, Cameron PM, Ranawat CS, Schmidt JA, Bayne EK. Specific bioactivities of monocyte-derived interleukin 1 alpha and interleukin 1 beta are similar to each other on cultured murine thymocytes and on cultured human connective tissue cells. J Clin Invest 1986; 78:836–9.
116. Dinarello CA, Cannon JG, Mier JW, et al. Multiple biological activities of human recombinant interleukin 1. J Clin Invest 1986; 77:1734–9.
117. Durum SK, Gershon RK. Interleukin 1 can replace the requirement for I-A-positive cells in the proliferation of antigen-primed T cells. Proc Natl Acad Sci U S A 1982; 79:4747–50.
118. Dinarello CA. Interleukin-1 and the pathogenesis of the acute-phase response. N Engl J Med 1984; 311:1413–8.
119. Pober JS, Bevilacqua MP, Mendrick DL, Lapierre LA, Fiers W Jr, Gimbrone MA. Two distinct monokines, interleukin 1 and tumor necrosis factor, each independently induce biosynthesis and transient expression of the same antigen on the surface of cultured human vascular endthelial cells. J Immunol 1986; 135:1680–7.
120. Goldblum SE, Yoneda K, Cohen DA, McClain CJ. Provocation of pulmonary vascular endothelial injury in rabbits by human recombinant interleukin-1 beta. Infect Immun 1988; 56:2255–63.
121. Dayer J-M, de Rochemonteix B, Burrus B, Demczuk S, Dinarello CA. Human recombinant interleukin 1 stimulates collagenase and prostaglandin E_2 production by human synovial cells. J Clin Invest 1986; 77:645–8.
122. Beasley D, Cohen RA, Levinsky NG. Interleukin 1 inhibits contraction of vascular smooth muscle. J Clin Invest. 1989; 83:331–5.
123. Elias JA, Lentz V. IL-1 and tumor necrosis factor synergistically stimulate fibroblast IL-6 production and stabilize IL-6 messenger RNA. J Immunol 1990; 145:161–6.
124. Oksusawa S, Gelfand JA, Ikejima T, Connolly RJ, Dinarello CA. Interleukin 1 induces a shock-like state in rabbits: synergism with tumor necrosis factor and the effect of cyclooxygenase inhibition. J Clin Invest 1988; 81:1162–72.
125. Burchett SK, Weaver WM, Westall JA, Larsen A, Kronheim S, Wilson CB. Regulation of tumor necrosis factor/cachectin and IL-1 secretion in human mononuclear phagocytes. J Immunol 1988; 140:3473–81.
126. Dalboge H, Bayne S, Christensen T, Hejnaes KR. Cloning and expression of an interleukin-1 beta precursor and its conversion to interleukin-1 beta. FEBS Lett 1989; 246:89–93.
127. Kostura MJ, Tocci MJ, Limjuco G, et al. Identification of a monocyte specific pre-interleukin 1 beta convertase activity. Proc Natl Acad Sci U S A 1989; 86:5227–31.
128. Black RA, Kronheim SR, Sleath PR. Activation of interleukin-1 beta by a co-induced protease. FEBS Lett 1989; 247:386–90.
129. Black RA, Kronheim SR, Merriam JE, March CJ, Hopp TP. A pre-aspartate-specific protease from human leukocytes that cleaves pro-interleukin-1 beta. J Biol Chem 1989; 264:5323–6.
130. Kobayashi Y, Yamamoto K, Saido T, Kawasaki H, Oppenheim JJ, Matsushima K. Identification of calcium-activated neutral protease as a processing enzyme of human interleukin 1α. Proc Natl Acad Sci U S A 1990; 87:5548–52.
131. Brown KM, Muchmore AV, Rosenstreich DL. Uromodulin, an immunosuppressive protein derived from pregnancy urine, is an inhibitor of interleukin 1. Proc Natl Acad Sci U S A 1986; 83:9119–23.
132. Larrick JW. Native interleukin 1 inhibitors. Immunol Today 1989; 10:61–6.
133. Hannum CH, Wilcox CJ, Arend WP, et al. Interleukin-1 receptor antagonist activity of a human interleukin-1 inhibitor. Nature 1990; 343:336–40.
134. Michie HR, Manogue KR, Spriggs DR, et al. Detection of circulating tumor necrosis factor after endotoxin administration. N Engl J Med 1988; 318:1481–6.

135. Spies T, Blanck G, Bresnahan M, Sands J, Strominger JL. A new cluster of genes within the human major histocompatibility complex. Science 1989; 243:214–7.
136. Beutler B, Cerami A. Cachectin: more than a tumor necrosis factor. N Engl J Med 1987; 316:379–85.
137. Ranges G, Zlotnik A, Espevik T, Dinarello CA, Cerami A, Palladino MA Jr. Tumor necrosis factor alpha/cachectin is a growth factor for thymocytes: synergistic interactions with other cytokines. J Exp Med 1988; 167:1472–8.
138. Dayer J-M, Beutler B, Cerami A. Cachectin/tumor necrosis factor stimulates collagenase and prostaglandin E_2 production by human snyovial cells and dermal fibroblasts. J Exp Med 1985; 162:2163–8.
139. Dinarello CA, Cannon JG, Wolff SM, et al. Tumor necrosis factor (cachectin) is an endogenous pyrogen and induces production of interleukin 1. J Exp Med 1986; 163:1433–50.
140. Pober JS Jr, Gimbrone MA, Lapierre LA, et al. Overlapping patterns of activation of human endothelial cells by interleukin 1, tumor necrosis factor, and immune interferon. J Immunol 1986; 137:1893–6.
141. Berkow RL, Wang D, Larrick JW, Dodson RW, Howard TH. Enhancement of neutrophil superoxide production by incubation with recombinant human tumor necrosis factor. J Immunol 1987; 139:3783–91.
142. She Z-W, Wewers MD, Herzyk DJ, Sagone AL, Davis WB. Tumor necrosis factor primes neutrophils for hypochlorous acid production. Am J Physiol 1989; 257:L338–45.
143. Tracey KJ, Beutler B, Lowry SF, et al. Shock and tissue injury induced by recombinant human cachectin. Science 1986; 234:470–4.
144. Waage A, Halstensen A, Espevik T. Association between tumour necrosis factor in serum and fatal outcome in patients with meningococcal disease. Lancet 1987; 1:355–7.
145. Wewers MD, Rinehart JJ, She Z-W, et al. Tumor necrosis factor infusions in humans prime neutrophils for hypochlorous acid production. Am J Physiol 1990; 259:L276–82.
146. Beutler B, Tkacenko V, Milsark I, Krochin N, Cerami A. Effect of gamma interferon on cachectin expression by mononuclear phagocytes: reversal of the lps d (endotoxin resistance) phenotype. J Exp Med 1986; 164:1791–6.
147. Han J, Thompson P, Beutler B. Dexamethasone and pentoxifylline inhibit endotoxin-induced cachectin/tumor necrosis factor synthesis at separate points in the signaling pathway. J Exp Med 1990; 172:391–4.
148. Mathison JC, Virca GD, Wolfson E, Tobias PS, Glaser K, Ulevitch RJ. Adaptation to bacterial lipopolysaccharide controls lipopolysaccharide-induced tumor necrosis factor production in rabbit macrophages. J Clin Invest 1990; 85:1108–18.
149. Sehgal PB, May LT, Tamm I, Vilcek J. Human β_2 interferon and B-cell differentiation factor BSF-2 are identical. Science 1987; 235:731–2.
150. Van Snick J. Interleukin 6: an overview. Annu Rev Immunol 1990; 8:253–78.
151. Shirakawa F, Chedid M, Suttles J, Pollok BA, Mizel SB. Interleukin 1 and cyclic AMP induce kappa immunoglobulin light-chain expression via activation of an NF-kappaB-like KNA-binding protein. Mol Cell Biol 1989; 9:959–64.
152. Osborn L, Kunkel S, Nabel GJ. Tumor necrosis factor alpha and interleukin 1 stimulate the human immunodeficiency virus enhancer by activation of the nuclear factor kappaB. Proc Natl Acad Sci U S A 1989; 86:2336–40.
153. Mizel SB. The interleukins. FASEB J 1989; 3:2379–88.
154. Baggiolini M, Walz A, Kunkel SL. Neutrophil-activating peptide-1/interleukin 8, a novel cytokine that activates neutrophils. J Clin Invest 1989; 84:1045–9.

155. Djeu JY, Matsushima K, Oppenheim JJ, Shiotsuki K, Blanchard DK. Functional activation of human neutrophils by recombinant monocyte-derived neutrophil chemotactic factor/IL-8. J Immunol 1990; 144:2205–10.
156. Detmers PA, Lo SK, Olsen-Egbert E, Walz A, Baggiolini M, Cohn ZA. Neutrophil-activating protein 1/interleukin 8 stimulates the binding activity of the leukocyte adhesion receptor CD11b/CD18 on human neutrophils. J Exp Med 1990; 171:1155–62.
157. Matsushima K, Morishita K, Yoshimura T, et al. Molecular cloning of a human monocyte-derived neutrophil chemotactic factor (MDNCF) and the induction of MDNCF mRNA by interleukin 1 and tumor necrosis factor. J Exp Med 1988; 167:1883–93.
158. Strieter RM, Kunkel SL, Showell HJ, et al. Endothelial cell gene expression of a neutrophil chemotactic factor by TNF alpha, LPS, and IL-1 beta. Science 1989; 243:1467–9.
159. Maestrelli P, Tsai J-J, Cromwell O, Kay AB. The identification and partial characterization of a human mononuclear cell-derived neutrophil chemotactic factor apparently distinct from IL-1, IL-2, GM-CSF, TNF and IFN-gamma. Immunology 1988; 64:219–25.
160. Martinet Y, Rom WN, Grotendorst GR, Martin GR, Crystal RG. Exaggerated spontaneous release of platelet-derived growth factor by alveolar macrophages from patients with idiopathic pulmonary fibrosis. N Engl J Med 1987; 317:202–9.
161. Raines EW, Dower SK, Ross R. Interleukin-1 mitogenic activity for fibroblasts and smooth muscle cells is due to PDGF-AA. Science 1989; 243:393–6.
162. Pierce GF, Mustoe TA, Lingelbach J, Masakowski VR, Gramates P, Deuel TF. Transforming growth factor beta reverses the glucocorticoid-induced wound-healing deficit in rats: possible regulation in macrophages by platelet-derived growth factor. Proc Natl Acad Sci U S A 1989; 86:2229–33.
163. Stiles AD, D'Ercole AJ. The insulin-like growth factors and the lung. Am J Respir Cell Mol Biol 1990; 3:93–100.
164. Rom WN, Basset P, Fells GA, Nukiwa T, Trapnell BC, Crystal RG. Alveolar macrophages release an insulin-like growth factor I-type molecule. J Clin Invest 1988; 82:1685–93.
165. Assoian RK, Komoriya A, Meyers CA, Miller DM, Sporn MB. Transforming growth factor-beta in human platelets: identification of a major storage site, purification, and characterization. J Biol Chem 1983; 258:7155–60.
166. Assoian RK, Fleurdelys BE, Stevenson HC, et al. Expression and secretion of type beta transforming growth factor by activated human macrophages. Proc Natl Acad Sci U S A 1987; 84:6020–4.
167. Postlethwaite AE, Keski-Oja J, Moses HL, Kang AH. Stimulation of the chemotactic migration of human fibroblasts by transforming growth factor beta. J Exp Med 1987; 165:251–6.
168. Khalil N, Bereznay O, Sporn M, Greenberg AH. Macrophage production of transforming growth factor beta and fibroblast collagen synthesis in chronic pulmonary inflammation. J Exp Med 1989; 170:727–37.
169. Mackiewicz A, Ganapathi MK, Schultz D, et al. Transforming growth factor β_1 regulates production of acute-phase proteins. Proc Natl Acad Sci U S A 1990; 87:1491–5.
170. Tsunawaki S, Sporn M, Nathan C. Comparison of transforming growth factor-beta and a macrophage-deactivating polypeptide from tumor cells: differences in antigenicity and mechanism of action. J Immunol 1989; 142:3462–8.
171. Hart PH, Whitty GA, Piccoli DS, Hamilton JA. Synergistic activation of human

monocytes by granulocyte-macrophage colony-stimulating factor and INF-gamma: increased TNF-alpha but not IL-1 activity. J Immunol 1988; 141:1516–21.

172. Haq AU, Rinehart JJ, Maca RD. The effect of gamma interferon on IL-1 secretion of in vitro differentiated human macrophages. J Leukoc Biol 1985; 38:735–46.
173. Eden E, Turino GM. Interleukin-1 secretion by human alveolar macrophages stimulated with endotoxin is augmented by recombinant immune (gamma) interferon. Am Rev Respir Dis 1986; 133:455–60.
174. Ucla C, Roux-Lombard P, Dayer J-M, Mach B. Interferon gamma drastically modifies the regulation of interleukin 1 genes by endotoxin in U937 cells. J Clin Invest 1990; 85:185–91.
175. Collart MA, Belin D, Vassalli J-D, de Kossodo S, Vassalli P. Gamma interferon enhances macrophage transcription of the tumor necrosis factor/cachectin, interleukin 1, and urokinase genes, which are controlled by short-lived repressors. J Exp Med 1986; 164:2113–8.
176. Gerrard TL, Siegel JP, Dyer DR, Zoon KC. Differential effects of interferon-alpha and interferon-gamma on interleukin 1 secretion by monocytes. J Immunol 1987; 138:2535–40.
177. Frendl G, Beller DI. Regulation of macrophage activation by IL-3. I. IL-3 functions as a macrophage-activating factor with unique properties, inducing Ia and lymphocyte function-associated antigen-1 but not cytotoxicity. J Immunol 1990; 144:3392–9.
178. Frendl G, Fenton MJ, Beller DI. Regulation of macrophage activation by IL-3. II. IL-3 and lipopolysaccharide act synergistically in the regulation of IL-1 expression. J Immunol 1990; 144:3400–10.
179. Bachwich PR, Chensue SW, Larrick JW, Kunkel SL. Tumor necrosis factor stimulates interleukin-1 and prostaglandin E_2 production in resting macrophages. Biochem Biophys Res Commun 1986; 136:94–101.
180. Nawroth PP, Bank I, Handley D, Cassimeris J, Chess L, Stern D. 1986; Tumor necrosis factor/cachectin interacts with endothelial cell receptors to induce release of interleukin 1. J Exp Med 1986; 163:1363–75.
181. Meltzer MS, Oppenheim JJ. Bidirectional amplification of macrophage-lymphocyte interactions: enhanced lymphocyte activation factor production by activated adherent mouse peritoneal cells. J Immunol 1977; 118:77–82.
182. Baumgartner JD, Heumann D, Gerain J, Weinbreck P, Grau GE, Glauser MP. Association between protective efficacy of anti-lipopolysaccharide (LPS) antibodies and suppression of LPS-induced tumor necrosis factor α and interleukin 6. Comparison of 0 side chain-specific antibodies with core LPS antibodies. J Exp Med 1990; 171:889–96.
183. Schroder J-M, Persoon NLM, Christopers E. Lipopolysaccharide-stimulted human monocytes secrete, apart from neutrophil-activating peptide 1/interleukin 8, a second neutrophil-activating protein: NH_2-terminal amino acid sequence identity with melanoma growth stimulating activity. J Exp Med 1990; 171:1091–100.
184. Houde M, Arora DJS. Stimulation of tumor necrosis factor secretion by purified influenza virus neuraminidase. Cell Immunol 1990; 129:104–11.
185. Arend WP, Welgus HG, Thompson RC, Eisenberg SP. Biological properties of recombinant human monocyte-derived interleukin 1 receptor antagonist. J Clin Invest 1990; 85:1694–7.
186. Laurenzi MA, Persson MAA, Dalsgaard C-J, Haegerstrand A. The neuropeptide substance P stimulates production of interleukin 1 in human blood monocytes: activated cells are preferentially influenced by the neuropeptide. Scand J Immunol 1990; 31:529–33.

CHAPTER 20

CYTOKINE BIOLOGY AND TRANSPLANTATION

Darrell A. Campbell, Jr., Kenneth McCurry, Lisa Colletti, and John M. Ham

The University of Michigan Medical School
Ann Arbor, Michigan

INTRODUCTION

The science of transplantation has leapfrogged from fond hope to practical reality in only a few decades. Success rates are high because technical problems have been overcome and because powerful immunosuppressive drugs have been developed. The major problem remaining relates to the lack of specificity of the immunosuppressive approach. Because immunity is nonspecifically depressed after transplantation, infectious complications are common and patient death from sepsis continues to occur.

Focusing immunosuppression on the antiallograft response specifically requires improved understanding of the rejection process. The last decade has seen a definition of the sequential immunological events that take place following transplantation. At the risk of oversimplification, these events include the presentation of foreign antigen, antigen recognition by host cells, clonal expansion of alloreactive cells, and cell killing itself. The much more recent development of cytokine biology, described in this text, has begun to refine the understanding of how and why these sequential events actually occur. This information can be tied to the development of immunosuppressive strategies more specific to antiallograft immunity, since inhibitors of antibodies to specific cytokines already exist and are constantly being developed. Interruption of a specific step in the immunological cascade by such a treatment may well abort a meaningful rejection response.

The discussion that follows is intended to relate what is known about cytokine biology to the science of transplantation. Clearly, the area is in its infancy and the next few years are certain to see an explosion of related information involving other cytokines not mentioned or cytokines yet to be discovered. Probably the most significant omission from this review is any mention of regulatory cytokine effects that would act to downregulate inflammation and could possibly be used to great advantage in transplantation. Such information is not available at present but undoubtedly will be in future years.

INTERLEUKIN-1

The proximal location of IL-1 in the cascade of immunological events leading to allograft rejection makes it likely that interventions designed to inhibit or alter IL-1 activity would have profound effects on this process. Somewhat surprisingly, very little documentation of the role of IL-1 in clinical transplantation has been accomplished. This is the result of several problems. First, a sensitive and specific assay for IL-1 effects has not been available until relatively recently (1). Second, many of the involved cytokines, including IL-1, have broadly overlapping activities that makes definition of a specific IL-1 effect difficult. Finally, the clinical transplant recipient receives a virtual pharmacopeia of immunosuppressive agents, many of which would be certain to blunt or eliminate IL-1 effects.

Despite these limitations, preliminary evidence suggests that interference with IL-1 effects could be of benefit in the transplant setting. The general view of activation of the immune response to alloantigen holds that foreign antigen must be presented to recipient T cells, primarily of the T_H (T helper) subclass, in the presence of metabolically active lymphoid cells capable of producing IL-1. The "two signals," antigen and IL-1, cause activation of T_H with subsequent release of soluble mediators, particularly IL-2 and interferon-γ (IFN-γ), capable of driving clonal expansion of T suppressor-cytotoxic subset. In keeping with this view, strategies to inhibit IL-1 effects are expected to impair antigen presentation.

Recently, Fanslow et al. described interesting experiments that were able to specifically examine the relative importance of IL-1 in the process of allograft rejection (2). A solubilized receptor for IL-1, recognizing both IL-1α and IL-1β, was administered systemically to rat recipients of heterotopic heart allografts. Heart allograft survival was substantially prolonged, and the effect was reversed by administration of exogenous IL-1. The mechanism involved is unclear, but the enhancing effect of the solubilized receptor was lost if administered 1 day following heart grafting, indicating a proximal location for IL-1 effects. In other nontransplant experiments, the specificity of the effect was examined. Administration of solubilized IL-1 receptor did not appear to prevent specific sensitization, but it was not clear whether the number of specifically sensitized cells encountered were changed by IL-1R administration. Possibly specific sensitization preceded normally but administration of IL-1R blocked the ability of sensitized cells to produce IL-2 and thus to undergo clonal expansion. An explanation of the inability of the administered IL-1R to block specific sensitization could lie in the overlapping activities of other cytokines. Particularly IL-6, but also IL-4 and granulocyte-macrophage colony-stimulating factor (GM-CSF) (3), are known to function at the level of T cell activation and could have allowed antigen recognition in the absence of IL-1 activity.

In addition to its important role in antigen presentation, IL-1 functions to upregulate immune responsiveness in vitro and thus could theoretically play an important role in the in vivo development of the antiallograft response. Thus, IL-1 is known to enhance natural killer (NK) activity (4), enhance monocyte-mediated cytotoxicity (5), enhance IL-2-induced ADCC (6), and promote the induction of T cell-mediated cytotoxic responses (7), all mechanisms known to participate in the rejection process. Furthermore, IL-1 plays an important role in recruitment of various cell types. Early data suggested that IL-1 had direct chemotactic activity for T cells (8), but a more current view is that IL-1 functions indirectly in T cell recruitment via its effect on upregulation of IL-8 activity, IL-8 being acknowledged as a potent chemoattractant for T cells as well as monocytes (9). Cellular recruitment to the allograft could also be an IL-1-related function by way of IL-1-induced upregulation of adhesion molecules on vascular endothelium (10).

Important information about the in vivo role that IL-1 plays in rejection was recently provided by Ford et al. (11). In these investigations a sponge matrix allograft model was used to delineate the role of certain cytokines in the process of allograft rejection. In this model the sponge matrix, either untreated or injected with syngeneic or allogeneic spleen cells, was evaluated for the presence of cytokines and the character of infiltrating cells. Typically in such a model anti-MHC (major histocompatibility complex) immunity is detected 5–7 days following placement of the graft. In this setting, antiallograft immunity was characterized by an initial high level of tumor necrosis factor (TNF) at day 3, at a time when IL-1 activity was low, but with a subsequent 10-fold increase in IL-1 activity by day 5, at a time when specifically sensitized alloreactive T cells began to appear in the sponge allograft. Subsequently, the number of cells infiltrating the allograft increased dramatically. Interestingly, IL-1 activity was not detectable in serum at a time of peak intragraft IL-1 levels. The heightened IL-1 reactivity in the graft was not the result of increased numbers of cells in the graft because peak IL-1 activity (days 5–8) preceded peak cellular infiltration by several days. Also, it did not seem likely that the IL-1 activity measured was actually IL-2 activity measured in a cellular proliferation assay since no IL-2 activity was noted using an IL-2-specific bioassay. These observations suggest that TNF is an early intragraft signal for upregulation of IL-1 activity, IL-1 subsequently acting to augment intragraft immune processes and to recruit additional cells.

Such elegant studies have not been performed in humans for obvious reasons, but there is in vivo evidence that IL-1 participates in allograft rejection in clinical transplantation. As any intern on a transplant service knows, fever is a prominent clinical feature of allograft rejection, often preceding clinical rejection by 1–3 days. IL-1 is a potent inducer of fever, formerly referred to as endogenous pyrogen (12). Serum IL-1 levels have been found to be elevated in transplant recipients coincident with fever, just before and in association with clinical renal transplant rejection (13). IL-1 levels were found to be elevated 4 days before the clinical development of rejection in human recipients of hepatic allografts (14).

In summary, IL-1 is increasingly recognized as an important participant in the process of allograft rejection both at the very early level of antigen presentation and at later stages of effector cell activity. Glucocorticoids, long the mainstay of the immunosuppressive regimen, are known to inhibit IL-1 release from macrophages (15), but the extent to which this accounts for their effectiveness is not known. Soluble IL-1 receptor or antibodies recognizing IL-1α or β may be able to focus more specifically on IL-1 effects, but any such strategy must account for the overlapping activities of other cytokines as well.

TUMOR NECROSIS FACTOR

Many in vitro and in vivo observations attest to the general proinflammatory nature of the TNF molecule. Only recently has the degree to which these effects influence the success or failure of organ allografts become apparent. The observations to be described have documented that TNF can be found in serum or tissue of allograft recipients and also indicate that specific antibody therapy directed at TNF can significantly influence the intensity of the rejection process. From these observations it seems likely that TNF has been underappreciated as an important participant in the rejection process.

A very important effect of TNF in the process of allograft rejection is the upregulation of the immunogenicity of the transplanted tissue. Thus, cultured human endothelial cells exhibited a ninefold augmentation of HLA-A and B class I determinant expression after exposure to recombinant human TNF (16). Similarly, TNF was found to enhance expression of class II determinants on cultured human pancreas enriched for islet cells in combination with IFN-γ, whereas neither cytokine alone had such an effect (17). Cultured human umbilical vein endothelial cells showed enhanced expression of class II determinants when exposed to IFN-γ (18). Antigen expression was further augmented by TNF but only when TNF was added to culture after cell exposure to INF-γ. These observations indicate that both TNF and IFN-γ act alone, or more often synergistically in vitro, to augment the antigenicity of exposed tissue. Given the profound impact of TNF and IFN-γ on antigen expression, it is tempting to assume that TNF and IFN-γ account for the marked increase in expression of class I and class II antigens that has been noted on allografted tissue during episodes of allograft rejection (19). Some evidence that this is in fact the case has been obtained from in vivo transplant studies in which prior administration of antibody to IFN-γ and TNF was found to inhibit antigen expression on allografted tissue. Stevens et al. pretreated rhesus monkeys with cross-reactive monoclonal antibody to human TNF, IFN-γ, or both and evaluated the effect of such antibodies on the course of allogeneic skin transplants (20). Animals receiving both antibodies demonstrated prolonged survival with reduced MHC class I and class II antigen expression, judged immunohistochemically. Interestingly, neither antibody alone produced such an effect.

Additional mechanisms by which TNF could augment the process of allograft rejection involve direct or indirect cytotoxic effects on targeted allogeneic cells. Local release of TNF could theoretically have a direct cytotoxic effect, since in vitro recombinant TNF is known to mediate cytotoxicity of cultured vascular endothelial cells, as well as a wide variety of tumor target cells (21). Indirectly, TNF acts to augment the cytotoxic properties of a variety of cell types, all of which are known to be involved in the rejection process. The development of T cell-mediated cytotoxicity is enhanced by in vitro exposure to TNF (22), as is macrophage-mediated cytotoxicity (23) and neutrophil superoxide anion production (24). Thus TNF could enhance the rejection process by acting to increase the immunogenicity of allografted cells and also by enhancing cytotoxic mechanisms directed at the allografted cells.

The recruitment of appropriate cells to the site of the allograft is a critical element of the rejection process that could be mediated by TNF effects. The accumulation of cells in the allograft is presumably accomplished via mechanisms that influence migration of cells, that is, chemotactic effects, as well as mechanisms that alter the adhesiveness of cells for vascular endothelium once attracted to the allograft. TNF has been extensively studied in this regard. As was previously mentioned, TNF has chemotactic effects for various cell types but, at least in humans, acts only indirectly via upregulation of IL-8 activity (9). TNF clearly influences the adhesiveness of cells for vascular endothelium, the first cell type to be encountered by host responders. In regard to neutrophils, the increased adhesiveness to endothelial cells may be the result of increased expression of neutrophil receptors for endothelium (25) or increased expression of endothelial cell receptors for neutrophils (26).

With regard to T cell adhesiveness for endothelial cells, TNF acts to upregulate endothelial cell receptors for T cells, such as intracellular adhesion molecule 1 (ICAM-1) (CD54) (27) and VCAM-1 (inducible cell adhesion molecule) (28). These adhesive molecules bind to LFA-1 (29) and Ag-4, respectively, on T cells (30). The TNF effects on T cell adhesiveness are enhanced by IFN-γ and IL-4, but interestingly, neutrophil adhesiveness induced by TNF is not enhanced by IFN-γ or IL-4 (31). These observations may be of importance in explaining the relative preponderance of T cells at the site of the allograft relative to neutrophils.

As mentioned in the earlier section involving IL-1, the sponge matrix allograft model was very useful in linking some of the in vitro observations about cytokine effects to in vivo conditions mimicking allograft rejection. One of the most interesting findings in this experimental setting was the early appearance of TNF. TNF was found in the sponge allograft at day 3 after implantation, before any of the other measured cytokines. The elevated levels of TNF could theoretically be the result of an initial monocyte interaction with foreign antigen, since monocytes are known to be potent sources of TNF. This possibility is supported by in vitro mixed lymphocyte culture data in which it was shown that cocultivation of allogeneic cells resulted in the early release of TNF into media (32). After day 3, levels of IL-1 and GM-CSF were found to increase in the sponge matrix, which in turn preceded the influx of a large number of specifically sensitized T cells and monocytes. Thus, in the sponge matrix allograft model TNF appears to play an early and pivotal role in the induction of subsequent immune events involving the release of other cytokines and the appearance of large numbers of cytotoxic effector cells.

That TNF is involved in allograft rejection on a clinical level has been suggested by investigations in which the serum of renal transplant patients was examined serially for the appearance of TNF (33). Patients undergoing episodes of acute allograft rejection showed substantial increases in serum immunoreactive TNF levels, occasionally occurring 1–2 days before the diagnosis of clinical rejection was made. A similar observation was made when liver transplant recipients were studied. Busuttil et al. evaluated the sera of 50 consecutive patients undergoing liver transplantation (34). Peak levels of TNF-α were found at the time of clinical diagnosis of rejection, and elevated levels were detected 1–2 days before diagnosis. Interestingly, an important distinction could be made in the ultimate clinical success by evaluating the peak TNF level in the first week posttransplant: those with ultimate rejection had substantially higher peak TNF levels than those with long-term graft success.

If TNF is importantly involved in orchestrating the rejection of an allograft, it seems likely that the prior administration of anti-TNF antibody would act to enhance transplant survival. This has been shown to be the case. Busuttil et al. treated rats undergoing allogeneic heterotopic heart transplantation with anti-TNF antiserum on a daily basis (35). These animals showed significantly prolonged transplant survival compared to controls. The effect was even more marked when subtherapeutic levels of cyclosporine were administered concomitantly. Interestingly, the number of graft-infiltrating lymphocytes was markedly reduced in anti-TNF–treated animals. The mechanism of action of anti-TNF antibody (Ab) suppression of allograft rejection is not clear. Since TNF-α is known to upregulate class I HLA determinant expression and TNF-α can be found locally early after exposure to alloantigen, anti-TNF Ab could act to inhibit TNF-induced upregulation of antigen recognition, that is, prevent increased immunogenicity. Alternatively, TNF-related effector functions could be inhibited by anti-TNF Ab. Some insight into this issue was recently provided by Imagawa et al., who administered a monoclonal anti-TNF Ab to rat recipients of cardiac allografts 4 days after implantation of the graft, at a time when rejection was well underway both grossly and histologically (36). In this model graft acceptance was substantially prolonged by such treatment. Addition of antibody recognizing TNF-β (LT) caused further prolongation of allograft survival. In this model, reversal of established rejection suggests a more direct role of anti-TNF antibody in influencing effector functions as opposed to the earlier antigen recognition events.

In addition to the relatively novel immunosuppressive approach using antibody to TNF, it is possible that a very commonly used immunosuppressive drug, cyclosporine, exerts an immunosuppressive effect by inhibition of serum TNF bioactivity. As is discussed in the next section, cyclosporine is thought to act principally by inhibition of IL-2 production. Recently it has been shown, however, that in vitro or in vivo pretreatment with cyclosporine blocks supernatant or serum TNF bioactivity in response to LPS challenge but does not appear to block TNF gene expression or the appearance of cell-bound TNF (37,38). If TNF is an important soluble "messenger" molecule in the rejection process, cyclosporine could exert an important immunosuppressive effect by blocking the production of extracellular TNF.

The information reviewed, that TNF acts to increase immunogenicity of cells, that it acts to augment many immune functions in vitro that it is found in association with clinical transplant rejection, and that antibody to TNF causes prolongation of allograft survival, argues strongly that TNF plays a prominent role in the transplant setting and that future immunosuppressive agents involving inhibition of TNF effects would likely be successful. No clinical transplant studies have been done in which patients were given anti-TNF antibody, but such an antibody suitable for human use is now available and has been used in other clinical settings. The experimental data at hand seem to support pursuit of this new therapeutic strategy.

Ischemia and Reperfusion Injury

Ischemia with subsequent reperfusion is inherent to the transplant process. An interesting question is whether events occurring at the time of reperfusion of the new transplant would result in cytokine release and, if so, if the cytokines released would then have effects on activation of allograft responsiveness, as was previously discussed. This sequence of ischemia and reperfusion leading to rejection may effectively be blocked by strategies aimed at inhibition of cytokine activity. In fact, it seems clear in the renal transplant area that grafts with evidence of more severe ischemic injury at the time of revascularization, manifested by poor early function, have reduced 1 year survival rates and increased rejection, a finding consistent with this hypothesis, if one assumes that more severe injury would result in more enhanced cytokine activity (39).

Our findings in a rat model of graded left lobar hepatic ischemia suggest that TNF is released following reperfusion of the ischemic liver lobe and that the more severe ischemia and reperfusion injury results in greater TNF release (40). Although not yet entirely confirmed, it seems plausible that the ischemia and reperfusion injury affects macrophages, cells that have a vast potential for TNF production. The liver is the largest single repository for cells of this type, in the form of Kupffers cells. TNF release was seen in the suprahepatic inferior venocaval blood as soon as 30 minutes following ischemia and reperfusion of the liver and generally peaked at 1.5–2 following ischemia and reperfusion. This time course is consistent with what is known about macrophage TNF release after other stimuli: early release, peaking at 2 h, with a subsequent sharp falloff (41). Although we began this discussion by considering the effect of ischemia and reperfusion on subsequent immune activation, in these studies involving very severe ischemia and reperfusion with marked TNF release into the circulation, the effect was to cause prompt pulmonary interstitial edema with hemorrhage and death of the animals. The morbidity seemed likely due to TNF effects, since heterologous antibody to TNF given before ischemia and reperfusion prevented the capillary "leak" findings, as assessed by [^{125}I] albumin washout studies (42). It was not clear whether the effect was mediated by neutrophils. Neutrophil accumulation was seen in lungs 1 h following ischemia and reperfusion, but anti-TNF antibody only partially abrogated the increase while profoundly protecting against increased capillary permeability. Further studies are underway to examine this relationship more thoroughly.

Our findings regarding TNF activity and ischemia and reperfusion of the liver in the rat model have been extended to include clinical liver transplantation. In this area the donor liver is removed, packed in ice for up to 24 h, and then transplanted to the patient with end-stage liver failure. This process occasionally results in severe ischemic injury to the liver and subsequent multiple organ failure. We have been able to document TNF release in the right atrial blood of recipients within 1 h of revascularization (43). Although in the rat model TNF release did not seem related to lipopolysaccharide (LPS) activity in the portal blood, in clinical cases LPS may well augment TNF release on the basis of ischemia and reperfusion, since LPS is known to be present in the circulation just before transplantation in the anhepatic phase (44). In any case, it seems possible that some of the severe pulmonary injury seen following transplantation of the ischemic liver could be the result of unwanted TNF activity consequent to the procedure.

Clinically, the TNF activity may have immune effects as well. In one case, the initial TNF activity after transplantation was associated with a subsequent appearance of IL-8 mRNA in peripheral blood buffy coat cells as assessed by northern blot analysis. The IL-8 activity may have occurred as the result of TNF, since in vitro TNF is known to be a potent upregulator of IL-8 activity. It seems likely that given the extensive nature of TNF biological activity an initial marked release of TNF systemically would have far-reaching consequences for the ultimate success or failure of the transplant procedure.

INTERLEUKIN-2

IL-2 production occurs when the T helper subset of T cells is presented with foreign alloantigen and IL-1. Antigen presentation takes place via internalization and subsequent expression of soluble foreign class II determinant by host macrophages, in which case an MHC restriction exists, or by presentation of foreign class II determinants on immunogenic allografted cells themselves, in which case no MHC restriction is involved. In either case interaction of antigen with the T_H antigen receptor complex results in elevation of cytosolic Ca^{2+} (45), and interaction of IL-1, either cell bound (α), or secreted (β) with the IL-1 receptor (IL-1R), results in activation of protein kinase C (46). These final intracellular signals result in IL-2 production. The subsequent clonal expansion of alloreactive cells is largely dependent upon IL-2, thus making IL-2 itself and the interaction of IL-2 with its receptor (IL-2R) the logical target of therapeutic interventions designed to limit clonal expansion.

A potent inhibitor of IL-2 generation is the fungal endecapeptide cyclosporine. The clinical science of transplantation has been completely transformed by the introduction of this drug. Success in renal transplantation increased to 80% 1 year graft survival from approximately 50% in previous years, primarily as the result of the introduction of cyclosporine into clinical practice (47). Liver transplantation and heart transplantation evolved from the experimental stage to clinical reality with 80–90% success 1 year following transplantation (47). Although cyclosporine has important effects on other cytokines, the success of the drug seems related to a more effective reduction in IL-2 levels, particularly compared to glucocorticoids, which have a measurable but modest effect in this regard (48,49). Thus, patients receiving prednisone-azathioprine as an immunosuppressive regimen showed 13.6% reduction in IL-2 production after exposure of their cells to phtohemagglutinin (PHA) compared to control, but patients receiving prednisone-cyclosporine or cyclosporine alone showed 40.6 and 36.8% inhibition, respectively (49). Six patients experiencing drug-resistant allograft rejection were found to have unimpaired IL-2 responsiveness in the posttransplant period.

Although a potent inhibitor of IL-2 generation, cyclosporine does not appear to inhibit the expression of IL-2R on antigen-activated cells (50), nor does it interfere with antigen binding to the T cell antigen receptor (51). Thus, the simplest view of the immunosuppressive effect of cyclosporine is that the drug acts to limit circulating IL-2, the fuel for clonal expansion.

FK506 is a newer drug structurally dissimilar to cyclosporine that also exerts its immunosuppressive effect via a very potent inhibition of IL-2 production (52). Like cyclosporine, FK506 also acts to inhibit MLR reactivity (53), the generation of cytotoxic lymphocytes (54), and the production of interferon-γ (52) but at concentrations 100-fold lower than those required by cyclosporine (55). Evidence suggests that FK506 binds to a different intracellular protein than cyclosporine (56) but one that has a very similar functional role, since the immune functions inhibited by FK506 and cyclosporine are virtually identical (55). FK506 does not inhibit IL-2R expression except at very high doses, similar to cyclosporine. The critical role of IL-2 in the development of the immune response is underscored by the observation that the two most potent inhibitors of IL-2 production, cyclosporine and FK506, are also the most effective immunosuppressive drugs available.

Concomitant with antigen presentation at the level of macrophage T_H, the suppressor-cytotoxic subset of T cells is exposed to foreign class I determinant. The antigen-T cell receptor interaction generates the expression of the IL-2R, an event that provides a distinguishing marker for the "activated" T cell (hence the designation of IL-2R as the Tac antigen) (57). By analogy to in vitro mixed lymphocyte culture studies, only 2% of allogeneic lymphocytes are expected to become "activated" in response to alloantigen, leaving 98% of cells in the resting condition. Because IL-2 has no effect on the non-IL-2R–bearing, "resting" population but provides a profound impetus for clonal expansion to cells bearing IL-2R, a selective expansion of alloantigen reactive cells rapidly develops when IL-2 binds to IL-2R (57). In a practical sense expression of IL-2R by T cells is helpful in the clinical management of transplant patients, since shed IL-2R is easily measurable in the systemic circulation and levels rise markedly before and in association with acute rejection episodes (58).

The selective nature of IL-2R expression on antigen reactive cells has been exploited with the development of recent immunosuppressive strategies. Waldmann et al. first described the production of a mouse IgG_{2a} monoclonal antibody recognizing the human IL-2R (anti-Tac) (59). Recent studies have shown that antigen interaction with the T cell antigen receptor results in expression of a cell surface high-affinity IL-2R composed of a 55 kD glycosylated polypeptide, recognized by anti-Tac, and an additional 75 kD IL-2 binding peptide (60). In the resting state the 55 kD polypeptide and 75 kD polypeptide demonstrate low and medium antibody binding affinity, respectively (61), but with antigen recognition cell surface assembly of the two polypeptides occurs, resulting in a single high-affinity IL-2R. Anti-Tac recognizes the 55 kD peptide and is thought to prevent assembly (62).

Numerous animal studies have documented the effectiveness of focused inhibition of IL-2R activity as an immunosuppressive approach. Anti-Tac antibody was first demonstrated to inhibit rejection of murine cardiac allografts in 1985 by Kirkman et al. (63). Volk et al. were able to prevent graft-versus-host disease across a strong histocompatibility barrier by in vivo administration of AMT-13, a monoclonal antibody recognizing the 55 kD IL-2 receptor (64). Subsequently, anti-Tac was shown to delay unmodified renal allograft rejection in cynolmolgus monkeys (65). Curiously, in this model the addition of cyclosporine did not result in additional protection from rejection.

Kirkman et al. recently reported the results of a clinical prospective randomized trial evaluating the results of anti-Tac antibody in renal transplant recipients (66). Patients received anti-Tac (20 mg/day for 10 days) prophylactically in combination with low-dose cyclosporine, azathioprine, and prednisone. Control patients did not receive anti-Tac but received a high dose of cyclosporine. Of importance was the early finding that cyclosporine was absolutely required concomitantly with anti-Tac; 4 of the first 5 patients treated without cyclosporine showed vigorous rejection. In combination with low-dose cyclosporine, anti-Tac antibody administration resulted in a lower incidence of rejection episodes within the first 10 days and caused delay in the interval to the first rejection episode but overall did not influence actuarial 1 year patient or graft survival. Detailed flow cytometric evaluation demonstrated a moderately reduced percentage of T cells bearing IL-2R, the significance of which is unknown.

Cantarovich et al. studied a rat, rather than mouse IgG_{2a} monoclonal antibody (33.B3.1) also recognizing human IL-2R (67). Patients received the antibody daily for 14 days in conjunction with standard immunosuppression. Of 30 patients tested, only one experienced rejection within the first 30 days, and these results compared favorably to other patients receiving antithymocyte globulin (ATG), a broadly reactive heterologous antibody preparation recognizing all mature T cells. In contrast to the report from Kirkman et al. using a mouse IgG_{2a} monoclonal antibody, cyclosporine was not required as an additional agent when the rat 33.B3.1 was used, possibly the result of relatively increased steroid administration. In contrast to prophylactic use, rat anti-IL-2R administered at the time of acute rejection was ineffective in reversing established rejection (68). One might hypothesize that a previously expanded clone of alloreactive cells, in contrast to newly activated cells, might respond to different cytokines capable of causing clonal proliferation, such as IL-6 and IFN-γ.

A cyclosporine requirement, either concomitant with IL-2R antibody (anti-Tac) or subsequent to anti-Tac administration (33.B3.1) seems clear-cut in clinical studies. Because it is an important clinical issue, animal models have been used for detailed investigations of the mechanisms accounting for this synergy. A priori, one might expect that a simple additive effect of decreased IL-2 production and blockade of IL-2R explained the observed results. In a rat model of renal transplantation, however, the explanation was considerably more complex (69). Renal allografts transplanted into uremic allogeneic hosts showed a modestly improved survival with ART-18 alone (mouse antirat IL-2R mAB) and marginal improvement in survival with a very small (0.75 mg/kg) dose of cyclosporine alone. Combination therapy, however, resulted in markedly prolonged survival. When the transplanted organ from single-therapy recipients were examined, graft-infiltrating cells positive for IL-2R and capable of producing TNF, IFN-γ, and IL-2 were found. Such cells could not be identified in the transplanted organs of animals receiving combination therapy. In adoptive transfer studies nonspecific suppressor cells capable of prolonging graft survival themselves were isolated from renal allografts of combined therapy rats. Moreover, donor-specific suppressor cells were isolated from the spleens of such animals. The mechanisms by which suppressor cells develop in the model is completely unknown.

Whatever the mechanism involved in rats or in humans, the two clinical trials have at least demonstrated that monoclonal antibodies to IL-2R can be safely administered to humans and that they have an immunosuppressive effect. However, results using conventional therapy in transplantation are already at a level that the IL-2R antibody approach has not had an incremental beneficial effect. Certainly this type of therapy has not produced tolerance or completely prevented rejection. It is possible that IL-2R Ab prophylaxis is somewhat safer than broadly reactive antibodies used for the same purpose by virtue of its selective effect on subpopulations of T cells, but larger numbers of patients are required for study before this can be established. The field will not remain static, however, and the clinical reports evaluated should probably be considered only as promising initial attempts at selective immunotherapy.

One of the issues potentially limiting the effectiveness of the murine monoclonal Ab to IL-2R is that neither mouse nor rat IgG_{2a} fix human complement effectively and consequently do not kill the targeted cell. In this sense these monoclonal antibodies function only transiently by binding to IL-2R. Strom recently suggested that because rat IgG_{2b} rather than 2a antibodies fix human complement well, they could theoretically be used more effectively to kill the targeted IL-2R-bearing cell, an approach that is at present untested (70). Another strategy has been to fuse the gene for IL-2 with the gene for a segment of diphtheria toxin (71). The hybrid gene product is recognized by IL-2R. In contrast to monoclonal antibodies recognizing IL-2R, which are not internalized by the cell, the IL-2–toxin conjugate is internalized and cell death occurs. Elimination of the clone of alloreactive cells entirely could theoretically produce a permanent, tolerant effect. Clinical studies utilizing this innovative approach will provide interesting information in this regard. Another approach using a similar strategy has been to link anti-Tac monoclonal antibody with the β-emitting ^{90}Y (72). This hybrid antibody-cytotoxic agent was effective in prolonging xenografted heart survival in a primate model. Similarly, Cavazzana-Calvo et al. used a ricin A chain toxin linked to 33.B3.1 anti-IL-2R antibody to selectively deplete host bone marrow cells of alloreactive T cells grown in MLC (73). Alloreactivity of the remaining cells to a third party was unimpaired, indicating the selectivity of the approach.

A final potential limitation on the use of murine monoclonal Ab to IL-2R is that human hosts rapidly develop antimouse or antirat antibody, usually idiotypic, which inhibits effectiveness. In the initial report from Kirkman et al. using anti-Tac antibody, 7 of 10 patients tested developed antimouse antibody (66). Two very different strategies are in development that could obviate this problem. First, a chimeric or "humanized" monoclonal antibody has been developed that contains a specific mouse hypervariable region but is otherwise of human derivation. This Ab recognizes human IL-2R; presumably antibody formation to this molecule would be reduced (74). An approach using protein engineering has also been utilized to interfere with normal IL-2–IL-2R interaction (75). An IL-2 variant molecule was created that would bind to the IL-2 receptor, but because of a change in the α-helix portion of the molecule, it would not initiate growth promotion signals. Development of an IL-2 antagonist is a fascinating approach to the problem of immunosuppression that could obviously avoid problems associated with the development of antibodies to murine monoclonal antibodies.

INTERLEUKIN-6

Interleukin-6 is a cytokine with many diverse biological functions, including roles in hematopoiesis, immune function, and acute-phase responses. Elevated systemic levels of IL-6 have been found in such disease states as rheumatoid arthritis, multiple myeloma, and systemic lupus erythematosus. Recently, IL-6 has also been suggested to have a role in allograft rejection following transplantation.

IL-6 was originally identified as a T cell-derived lymphokine capable of inducing antibody production in B-cells and as such was referred to as B cell stimulatory factor 2 (BSF-2). Several other substances, hybridoma growth factor (HGF), interferon-β_2 (IFN-β_2), and hepatocyte stimulating factor (HSF), named for their effects, were subsequently found to have identical cDNA sequences as BSF-2 and the IL-6 designation was proposed (76). IL-6 appears to have many biological roles and is produced by a multitude of cell lines, including fibroblasts, endothelial cells, Kupffer's cells, B cells, T cells, and hepatocytes (77,78). A variety of stimuli induce IL-6 production, including the cytokines tumor necrosis factor-α and interleukin-1, as well as lipopolysaccharide and a variety of other substances. The biological effects of IL-6 include stimulating proliferation of IL-6-dependent B cell hybridoma lines (the basis for the biological assay of IL-6), stimulation of quiescent stem cells, and production of the acute-phase response, including stimulation of acute-phase protein production by hepatocytes, induction of fever, and stimulation of the release of adrenocorticotropic hormone (ACTH) (77). This list is by no means exhaustive, and these and other roles of IL-6 are discussed in other chapters of this text.

The role of IL-6 in allograft rejection has not been extensively evaluated. In vitro studies have shown that IL-6 is involved in T cell proliferation and activation as well as B cell differentiation. IL-6 receptors are expressed on the surface of resting T cells (79), and it appears that IL-6 is required to move T cells from G_0 to G_1 of the cell cycle, where they become responsive to IL-2 (77). The induction of IL-2 responsiveness seems to occur via IL-6-mediated stimulation of IL-2 receptor expression (77). IL-6 has also been described to be a factor necessary for the in vitro induction of cytotoxic T lymphocytes (79). Such in vitro data suggest that IL-6 could play a prominent role in critical processes involved in rejection related to cytotoxic T cell clonal expansion and B cell proliferation with development of alloantibody.

Several human clinical studies have attempted to evaluate the role of IL-6 in transplantation. Van Oers et al. (80) showed that healthy volunteers and preoperative patients with end-stage renal failure have low circulating levels of IL-6. Following renal transplantation, there was a marked increase in IL-6 levels in serum and the appearance of IL-6 in the urine within 1 day with a subsequent decrease to the normal range within 2–3 weeks in uncomplicated cases. Serum and urinary levels of IL-6 increased substantially during episodes of rejection, with the earliest increase occurring 2 days before the development of clinical signs or symptoms. Similar elevations of IL-6 were seen, however, in a series of patients undergoing abdominal gynecological procedures, suggesting that the IL-6 response may be a nonspecific response to stress or inflammation.

Yoshimura et al. (81) also evaluated the role of IL-6 in the context of clinical renal transplantation. Four groups of patients were evaluated: those with a stable clinical course following transplantation, without evidence of rejection or infection, those with rejection but no infection, those with infection but no rejection, and those with cyclosporine nephrotoxicity and neither rejection or infection. Determination of serum IL-6 levels showed elevation under conditions of infection or rejection but, like the previous study, low levels in stable patients. Because the IL-6 levels were low in patients with cyclosporine nephrotoxicity, the IL-6 level was useful in distinguishing acute rejection from cyclosporine nephrotoxicity, an occasionally vexing clinical problem.

Whether IL-6 is a central mediator of the rejection process or plays a less critical role is not yet understood. By analogy to the TNF and IL-2 literature, this type of question is best investigated using monoclonal antibodies specific for the molecule in question. With regards to IL-6 and transplantation, this has not yet occurred but will certainly be done in the near future as various appropriate antibody molecules become available. Recently it was noted that antibody to IL-6 protected against lethality induced by cecal ligation and puncture (82). Because of the many described in vitro activities of IL-6 relevant to immune responses, it may well be that anti-IL-6 antibody could produce an ameliorating effect on the rejection process as well.

INTERLEUKIN-8 AND RANTES

The rapidly expanding pool of information about cytokine biology and the appearance of cytokines at sites of antiallograft activity bring into focus a very important question: what are the important molecular communications that result in the rapid influx of T cells and monocytes into the allograft? Information about specific mechanisms might lead to specific therapies capable of interrupting or blunting the rejection process. TNF-α and IL-1 appear in the allograft early and have been reported to have potent chemoattractant properties. As was recently described, however, the in vivo chemoattractant effects of either cytokine are not reproducible in vitro, suggesting that they act indirectly. IL-8, formerly referred to as neutrophil chemotactic factor (NCF) and identical to T cell chemotactic factor (TCF) produced by endothelial cells, fibroblasts, and monocytes, is known to have important effects on neutrophils and T cells migration and is inducible by both TNF-α and IL-1 (83). Thus IL-8 could play an important role in directing lymphocyte traffic into the interstices of the offending allograft in response to TNF and IL-1.

Very little information about IL-8 in clinical transplantation exists. However, our group has produced initial results indicating IL-8 involvement in a rejecting renal allograft. In this case, a 7-year-old child developed multiple episodes of drug-resistant rejection after receiving a maternal donor-related renal allograft. After removal of the graft, in situ hybridization studies were done using a cDNA probe for IL-8. In this case, there was intense IL-8 activity in glomerular cells. Further work by Schmouder et al. (84) demonstrated the capacity for renal tubular epithelial cells to induce IL-8 (85) with appropriate stimulation. Additionally, an ELISA was developed and used to demonstrate IL-8 activity in the urine of patients with rejecting renal allografts. Because IL-8 has potent chemoattractive properties for T cells, it could be an important element in the recruitment of host cells to the sites of the transplant. At the current level of understanding, IL-8 attracts T cells of all types but at manyfold lower concentrations than required to recruit neutrophils (86).

The Rantes cytokine, a product of the same supergene family as IL-8, has been recently shown to have important selective effects on the recruitment of monocytes and certain types of T cells, but not neutrophils. Thus, although IL-8 recruits neutrophils and T cells, Rantes recruits monocytes but not neutrophils and T cells of the memory (VCHL-1^+) phenotype only. The latter cells are of particular interest to the transplant community since they have profound cytotoxic potential compared to nonmemory T cells, and are capable of vigorous cytokine production on antigenic challenge (87,88). Like IL-8, Rantes attracts lymphocytes at manyfold lower concentrations (100 to 200-fold) than are required to recruit neutrophils and monocytes. Thus, the relative abundance of T cells and paucity of neutrophils and monocytes during the early stages of allograft rejection do not rule out involvement of these cytokines in the rejection process, since a single concentration phenomenon could be involved.

REFERENCES

1. Conlon PJ. A rapid biologic assay for the detection of interleukin-1. J Immunol 1983; 131:1280–2.
2. Fanslow WC, Sims JE, Sassenfeld H, et al. Regulation of alloreactivity in vivo by a soluble form of the interleukin-1 receptor. Science 1990; 248:739–42.
3. Ho S, Abraham RT, Nilson A, Handwerger BS, McKean DJ. Interleukin 1 mediated activation of interleukin 4 (IL-4) producing T lymphocytes. Proliferation by IL-4 dependent and IL-4 independent mechanisms. J Immunol 1987; 139:1532–40.
4. Herman J, Dinarello CA, Kew MC, Rabson AR. The role of interleukin 1 (IL-1) in tumor-NK cell interactions: correction of defective NK cell activity in cancer patients by treating target cells with IL-1. J Immunol 1985; 135:2882–6.
5. Onozaki K, Matsushima K, Kleinerman ES, Saito T, Oppenhein JJ. Role of interleukin-1 in promoting human monocyte-mediated tumor cytotoxicity. J Immunol 1985; 135:314–20.
6. Eisenthal AVI, Rosenberg SA. The effect of various cytokines on the in vitro induction of antibody-dependent cellular cytotoxicity in murine cells. J Immunol 1989; 142:2307–13.
7. Farrar WL, Mizel SB, Farrar J. Participation of lymphocyte activating factor (interleukin 1) with induction of cytotoxic T cell responses. 1980; J Immunol 124: 1371–7.
8. Miossec P, Yu C, Ziff M. Lymphocyte chemotactic activity of human interleukin-1. J Immunol 1984; 133:2007–11.
9. Larsen CG, Anderson AO, Appella E, Oppenheim JJ, Matsushima K. The neutrophil-activating protein (NAP-1) is also chemotactic for T lymphocytes. Science 1989; 243:1464–6.
10. Cavender DE, Haskard DO, Joseph B, Ziff M. Interleukin-1 increases the binding of human B and T lymphocytes to endothelial cell monolayers. J Immunol 1986; 136:203–7.

11. Ford HR, Hoffman RA, Wing EJ, Magee DM, McIntryre LA, Simmons RL. Tumor necrosis factor, macrophage colony-stimulating factor, and interleukin-1 production within sponge matrix allografts. Transplantation 1990; 50:460–6.
12. Dinarello CA Cannon JG, Mier JW, et al. Multiple biological activities of human recombinant interleukin-1. J Clin Invest 1986; 77:1734–9.
13. Maury CPJ, Teppo AM. Serum immunoreactive interleukin-1 in renal transplant recipients. Transplantation 1988; 45:143–7.
14. Tilg H, Vogel W, Aulitzky WE, et al. Evaluation of cytokines and cytokine-induced secondary messages in sera of patients after liver transplantation. Transplantation 1990; 49:1074–80.
15. Snyder DS, Uranve ER. Corticosteroids inhibit murine macrophage Ia expression and IL-1 production. J Immunol 1982; 129:1803–5.
16. Collins T, Lapierre LA, Fiers W, Strominger JL, Pober JS. Recombinant human tumor necrosis factor increases mRNA levels and surface expression of HLA-A, B antigens in vascular endothelial cells and dermal fibroblasts in vitro. Proc Natl Acad Sci U S A 1985; 83:466.
17. Pujol-Borrell R, Todd I, Doshi M, et al. HLA class II induction in human islet cells by interferon-γ plus tumor necrosis factor or lymphotoxin. Nature 1987; 326:305–6.
18. Leeuwenberg JFM, van Damme J, Meager T, Jeunhomme TMAA, Buurman W. Effects of tumor necrosis factor on the interferon-γ-induced histocompatibility complex class II antigen expression by human endothelial cells. Eur J Immunol 1988; 18:1469–72.
19. Hall BM, Duggin GG, Phillips J. Increased expression of HLA-DR antigens on renal tubular cells in renal transplant: relevance to the rejection response. Lancet 1984; 2:247–51.
20. Stevens HP, van der Kwast TH, van der Meide PH, Vuzevski VD, Buurmen WA, Jonker M. Synergistic immunosuppressive effects of monoclonal antibodies specific for interferon-gamma and tumor necrosis factor alpha. A skin transplantation study in the rhesus monkey. Transplantation 1990; 50:856–61.
21. Sato N, Goto T, Haranaka K, et al. Actions of tumor necrosis factor on cultured vascular endothelial cells: morphologic modulation, growth inhibition and cytotoxicity. J Natl Cancer Inst 1986; 76:1113–21.
22. Ranges GE, Figari IS, Espevik T, Palladino MA Jr. Inhibition of cytotoxic T cell development by transforming growth factor-beta and reversal by recombinant tumor necrosis factor-alpha. J Exp Med 1987; 166:991.
23. Philip R, Epstein LB. Tumor necrosis factor as immunomodulator and mediator of monocyte cytotoxicity induced by itself, gamma-interferon, and interleukin-1. Nature 1986; 323:86–9.
24. Klebanoff SJ, Vadas MA, Harlan JM, et al. Stimulation of neutrophils by tumor necrosis factor. J Immunol 1986; 136:4220–5.
25. Gamble JR, Harlan JM, Klebanoff S, Vadas MA. Stimulation of the adherence of neutrophils to umbilical vein endothelium by human tumor necrosis factor. Proc Natl Acad Sci U S A 1985; 82:8667–71.
26. Pohlman TH, Stannes KA, Beatty PG, Ochs HD, Harlan JM. An endothelial cell surface factor(s) induced in vitro by lypopolysacharide, interleukin-1 and tumor necrosis factor-α increases neutrophil adhesiveness by a CDw18-dependent mechanism. J Immunol 1986; 136:4548–53.
27. Dustin ML, Springer TA. Lymphocyte function associated antigen-1 (LFA-1) interaction with intercellular adhesion molecule-1 (ICAM-1) is one of at least three mechanisms for lymphocyte adhesion to cultured endothelial cells. J Cell Biol 1988; 107:321.

28. Osborn L, Hession C, Tizard R, et al. Direct expression cloning of vascular cell adhesion molecule 1, a cytokine-induced endothelial protein that binds to lymphocytes. 1989; Cell 59:1203–11.
29. Marlin SD, Springer TA. Purified intercellular adhesion molecule-1 (1CAM-1) is a ligand for lymphocyte function associated antigen 1 (LFA-1). 1987; Cell 51:813–9.
30. Elices MJ, Osborn L, Takada Y, et al. VCAM-1 on activated endothelium interacts with the leukocyte integrin VLA-4 at a site distinct from the VLA-4/fibronectin binding site. 1990; Cell 60:577–84.
31. Thornhill H, Wellicome SM, Mahiouz DL, Lanchbury JSS, Kyan-Aung V, Haskard D. Tumor necrosis factor combines with IL-4 or IFN-γ to selectively enhance endothelial cell adhesiveness for T cells. J Immunol 1991; 146:592–8.
32. Shalaby MR, Espevik T, Rice GC, et al. The involvement of human tumor necrosis factors alpha and beta in the mixed lymphocyte reaction. J Immunol 1988; 141:499–503.
33. Maury CPJ, Teppo AM. Raised serum levels of cachectin/tumor necrosis factor α in renel allograft rejection. J Exp Med 1987; 166:1132–7.
34. Imagawa DK, Millis JM, Olthoff KM, et al. The role of tumor necrosis factor in allograft rejection. I. Evidence that elevated levels of tumor necrosis factor-alpha predict rejection following orthotopic liver transplantation. Transplantation 1990; 50:219–25.
35. Imagawa DK, Millis JM, Olthoff KM. The role of tumor necrosis factor in allograft rejection. II. Antibody therapy against tumor necrosis factor-alpha and lymphotoxin enhances cardiac allograft survival in rats. Transplantation 1990; 50:189.
36. Imagawa DK, Millis JM, Seu P, et al. The role of tumor necrosis factor in allograft rejection. III. Evidence that anti-TNF antibody therapy prolongs allograft survival in rats with acute rejection. Transplantation 1991; 51:57–62.
37. Nguyen DT, Eskandari MK, DeForge LE, et al. Cyclosporin A modulation of tumor necrosis factor gene expression and effects in vitro and in vivo. J Immunol 1990; 144:3822–8.
38. Remick DG, Nguyen DT, Eskandari MK, Strieter RM, Kunke SL. Cyclosporine A inhibits TNF production without decreasing TNF mRNA levels. Biochem Biophys Res Commun 1989; 161:551–5.
39. Dawidson I, Coorpender L, Drake D, et al. Intraoperative albumin improves the outcome of cadaver renal transplantation. Transplant Proc 1987; 19:4137–9.
40. Colletti L, Remick D, Burtch G, Kundel S, Strieter R, Campbell DA Jr. Role of tumor necrosis factor-α in the pathophysiologic alterations after hepatic ischemia/reperfusion injury in the rat. J Clin Invest 1990; 85:1936–43.
41. Remick DG, Strieter RM, Lynch JP, Nguyen D, Eskandari M, Kinkel SL. In vivo dynamics of murine tumor necrosis factor-alpha gene expression. Kinetics of dexamethasone-induced suppression. Lab Invest 1989; 60:766–71.
42. Colletti L, Burtch G, Remick D, et al. Production of tumor necrosis factor-α and the development of a pulmonary capillary injury folowing hepatic ischemia/reperfusion. Transplantation 1989; 49:268–73.
43. Unpublished.
44. Yokoyama I, Todo S, Mijata T, Selby R, Tzakis AG, Starzl TE. Endotoxemia and human liver transplantation. Transplant Proc 1989; 21:3833–41.
45. Palacios R. Mechanism of T cell activation: role and functional relationship of HLA-DR antigens and interleukins. Immunol Rev 1982; 63:73–110.
46. Robb RJ, Munck A, Smith KA. T cell growth factor receptors. Quantitation, specificity, and biological relevances. J Exp Med 1981; 154:1455–74.
47. Annual Report of the U.S. Scientific Registry for Organ Transplantation and the Organ Procurement and Transplantation Network. VC DHHS.
48. Polacios R, Sugawara I. Hydrocortisone abrogates proliferation of T cells in auto-

logous mixed lymphocytes reaction by rendering the interleukin-2 producer T cells unresponsive to interleukin-1 and unable to synthesize the T cell growth factor. Scand J Immunol 1982; 15:25–31.
49. Yoshimura N, Kahan BD. Pharmacodynamic assessment of the in vivo cyclosporine effect on interleukin-2 production by lymphocytes in kidney transplant recipients. Transplantation 1985; 40:661–6.
50. Miyawaki T, Yachie A, Ohzeki S, Nagaoki T, Taniguchi N. Cyclosporin A does not prevent expression of Tac antigen, a probable TCGF receptor molecule, on mitogen-stimulated human T cells. J Immunol 1983; 130:2737–42.
51. Kahan BD. Pharmocokinetics and pharmacodynamics of cyclosporine. Transplant Proc 1989; 21:9–15.
52. Kino T, Hatanaka H, Miyata S, et al. FK-506, a novel immunosuppressant isolated from a *Streptomyces*. II. Immunosuppressive effect of FK-506 in vitro. J Antibiot (Tokyo) 1987; 40:1256–65.
53. Kino T, Inamura N, Sakai F, et al. Effect of FK-506 on human mixed lymphocyte reaction in vitro. Transplant Proc 1987; 19:36–9.
54. Sawada S, Suzuki G, Kawase Y, Takaku F. Novel immunosuppressive agent, FK 506. In vitro effects on the cloned T cell activation. J Immunol 1987; 139:1797–803.
55. Johansson A, Moller E. Evidence that the immunosuppressive effects of FK506 and cyclosporine are identical. Transplantation 1990; 50:1001–7.
56. Siekierka JJ, Hung SH, Poe M, Lin CS, Sigal NH. A cytosolic binding protein for the immunosuppressant FK506 has peptidyl-prolyl isomerase activity but is distinct from cyclophilin. Nature 1989; 341:755–7.
57. Waldmann TA. The structure, function, and expression of interleukin-2 receptors on normal and malignant T cells. Science 1986; 232:727–32.
58. Colvin RB, Fuller TC, Mackeen L, Kung PC, Ip SH, Cosimi AB. Plasma interleukin-2 receptor levels in renal allograft recipients. Clin Immunol Immunopathol 1987; 43:273–6.
59. Uchiyama T, Broder S, Waldmann TA. A monoclonal antibody (anti-Tac) reactive with activated and functionally mature human T cells. I. Production of anti-Tac monoclonal antibody and distribution of Tac^+ cells. J Immunol 1981; 126:1393–7.
60. Tsudo M, Kozak RW, Goldman CK, Waldmann TA. Demonstration of a non-Tac peptide that binds interleukin-2: a potential participant in the multichain interleukin-2 receptor complex. Proc Natl Acad Sci U S A 1986; 83:9694–8.
61. Robb RJ, Greene WC, Rusk CM. Low and high affinity cellular receptors for interleukin-2. Implications for the level of Tac antigen. J Exp Med 1984; 160:1126–46.
62. Wang HM, Smith KA. The interleukin-2 receptor. Functional consequences of its bimolecular structure. J Exp Med 1987; 66:1055–69.
63. Kirkman RL, Barrett LV, Gaulton GN, Delley BE, Ythier A, Strom TB. Administration of an anti-interleukin 2 receptor monochonal antibody prolongs cardiac allograft survival in mice. J Exp Med 1985; 162:358–62.
64. Volk HD, Brocke S, Osawa H, Diamantstein T. Effects of in-vivo administration of a monoclonal antibody specific for the interleukin-2 receptor on the acute graft-versus-host reaction in mice. Clin Exp Immunol 1986; 66:126–31.
65. Reed, MH, Shapiro ME, Strom TB, et al. Prolongation of primate renal allograft survival by anti-Tac, an anti-human IL-2 receptor monoclonal antibody. Transplantation 1989; 47:55–9.
66. Kirkman RL, Shapiro ME, Carpenter CB, et al. A randomized prospective trial of anti-Tac monoclonal antibody in human renal transplantation. Transplantation 1991; 51:107–13.
67. Cantanovich D, LeMauff B, Hourmant P, et al. Prophylactic use of a monoclonal antibody (33B3.1) directed against interleukin-2 receptor following human renal transplantation. Am J Kidney Dis 1988; 11:101–6.

68. Cantanovich D, LeMauff B, Hourmant M. Anti-interleukin-2 receptor monoclonal antibody with treatment of ongoing acute rejection episodes of human kidney graft—a pilot study. Transplantation 1989; 47:454–7.
69. Ueda H, Hancok WW, Cheung YC, Diamantstein T, Tilney NL, Kupiec-Weglinski JW. The mechanism of synergistic interaction between anti-interleukin 2 receptor monoclonal antibody and cyclosporine therapy in rat recipients of organ allografts. Transplantation 1990; 50:545–50.
70. Strom TB. Summary: today's biotechnology and tomorrow's antirejection therapy. Am J Kidney Dis 1988; 11:163–5.
71. Murphy JR, Kelley VE, Strom TB. Interleukin 2 toxin: a step toward selective immunomodulation. Am J Kidney Dis 1988; 11:159–62.
72. Cooper MM, Robbins RC, Goldman CK, et al. Use of yttrium-90-labeled anti-Tac antibody in primate xenograft transplantation. Transplantation 1990; 50:760–5.
73. Cavazzana-Calvo M, Fromont C, LeDeist F, et al. Specific elimination of alloreactive T cells by an anti-interleukin-2 receptor B chain-specific immunotoxin. Transplantation 1990: 50:1–7.
74. Queen C, Schneider WP, Selick HE, et al. A humanized antibody that binds to the interleukin-2 receptor. Proc Natl Acad Sci U S A 1989; 86:10029–33.
75. Landgraf B, Smith KA, Gadski R, Ciardelli TL. Structural significance of the C-terminal amphiphilic helix of interleukin-2. J Biol Chem 1989; 264:816–22.
76. Brakenhoff JP, deGroot ER, Evers R, Pannekoek H, Aarden LA. Molecular cloning and expression of hybridoma growth factor in *Escherichia coli.* J Immunol 1987; 139:4116–21.
77. Van Snick J. Interleukin-6: an overview. Annu Rev Immunol 1990; 8:253–78.
78. Wolvekamp MC, Marquet RL. Interleukin-6: historical background, genetics and bilogical significance. Immunol Lett 1990; 24:1–9.
79. Okada M, Kitahara M, Kishimoto S, Matsuda T, Hirano T, Kishimoto T. IL-6/BSF-2 functions as a killer helper factor in the in vitro induction of cytotoxic T cells. J Immunol 1988; 141:1543–9.
80. Van Oers MHJ, van der Heyden AAPAM, Aarden LA. Interleukin-6 (IL-6) in serum and urine of renal transplant recipients. Clin Exp Immunol 1988; 17:314–9.
81. Yoshimura N, Oka T, Kahan BD. Sequential determinations of serum interleukin 6 levels as an immunodiagnostic tool to differentiate rejection from nephrotoxicity in renal allograft recipients. Transplantation 1991; 51(1):172–6.
82. Starnes HF, Pearce MK, Tewari A, Yim JH, Zou JC, Abrans JS. Anti-IL-6 monoclonal antibodies protect against lethal *Escherichia coli* infection and lethal tumor necrosis factor-α challenge in mice. J Immunol 1990; 145:4185–91.
83. Matsushima K, Larsen CG, DuBois G, Oppenheim J. Purification and characterization of a novel monocyte chemotactic and activating factor produced by a human myelomonocytic cell line. J Exp Med 1989; 169:1485–90.
84. Schmouder R. Unpublished observation.
85. DeForge LE, Remick DG. Sandwich ELISA for detecting program quantities of interleukin-8. Immun Invest 1991; 20:89–97.
86. Schall TJ, Baco K, Toy KJ, Goeddel DV. Selective attraction of monocytes and T lymphocytes of the memory phenotype by cytokine Rantes. Nature 1990; 347:669–70.
87. Sanders ME, Makgoba MW, Shaw S. Human naive and memory cells: reinterpretation of helper-inducer and suppressor-inducer subsets. Immunol Today 1988; 9:195–8.
88. Budd RC, Cerottini JC, MacDonald HR. Selectively increased production of interferon-gamma by subsets of Lyt-2^+ and L3T4^+ T cells indentified by expression of Pgp-1. J Immunol 1987; 138:3583–6.

CHAPTER 21

CYTOKINES AND RHEUMATIC DISEASES

Deborah DeMarco

Temple University Hospital
Philadelphia, Pennsylvania

Robert B. Zurier

University of Massachusetts Medical Center
Worcester, Massachusetts

INTRODUCTION

Joint inflammation in rheumatoid arthritis (RA) and other diseases with associated chronic arthritis is characterized by the presence of lymphocytes and monocyte-derived macrophages in a hyperplastic synovium. The reasons cells invade the synovium and synovial cells proliferate in RA patients have not been defined. Experimental evidence indicates that products exported by monocytes, macrophages, lymphocytes, and platelets help regulate synovial cell proliferation and take part in cartilage degradation and bone resorption. Factors specifically chemotactic for particular cells (monocytes, lymphocytes, and neutrophils) have also been identified in several cell types. These cytokines interact in a complex and poorly understood manner. For example, interleukin-1 (IL-1) and tumor necrosis factor (TNF) are each capable of inducing the production of their respective molecules as well as each other, and IL-1 and IL-6 act in synergy to induce T cell proliferation. This self-amplification network may play an important role in sustaining a pathological process. Normally, inhibitors of these cytokines serve to modify their activities. The delicate balance is not preserved in the rheumatic diseases. In this chapter we review the association of a variety of cytokines with rheumatic disease in general and inflammatory arthritis in particular.

INTERLEUKIN-1

Long before the diverse biological activities of IL-1 were recognized, IL-1-like factors (i.e., pyrogens) were reported (1) to be present in synovial fluids from patients with inflammatory arthritis. It was subsequently shown (2) that IL-1-like activity stimulated bone resorption in vitro by a mechanism independent of prostaglandin synthesis by the bone cells. In addition, IL-1-like activity induces proteoglycan resorption in cartilage explants (3).

Substantial experimental evidence now exists to support the view that IL-1 is an important mediator in the development of synovitis. Injection of IL-1 into rabbit knee joints initiates both a transient acute arthritis and a chronic synovitis (4–6). Increased IL-1 activity has been demonstrated in synovial fluid (SF) from patients with rheumatoid arthritis, osteoarthritis (OA), and other forms of synovitis (7–11). Duff et al. (12) also found increased expression of the IL-1 gene in synovial cells from OA and RA patients, observations that also suggest that IL-1 is important in the initiation and/or progression of arthritis. DiGiovine et al. (13) and Duff et al. (14) showed that monosodium urate (MSU) crystals stimulate both blood monocytes and adherent synovial cells to release IL-1 activity. The MSU-induced IL-1-containing supernatant was then shown to stimulate the long-term growth of human synovial fibroblast lines in vitro.

Mean plasma levels of IL-1β were increased significantly in a group of 51 RA patients compared to 21 healthy age-matched controls (15). The increased plasma IL-1β levels in these patients correlated with disease activity as measured by the Ritchie articular index (16), pain score, and erythrocyte sedimentation rate.

The role of IL-1 in the destructive arthritis seen in many connective tissue diseases appears due in large part to its effects on bone and cartilage. For example, osteoclast activating factor (OAF), a soluble factor produced by peripheral blood mononuclear cells that leads to bone resorption, has amino acid sequence homology with human IL-1β (17). IL-1 is now considered one of the most potent OAFs known. It increases bone resorption by stimulation of mediators from the synovium and by its systemic effects. Pettipher et al. (5) showed that injection of IL-1 into rabbit knees induced the accumulation of polymorphonuclear leukocytes and mononuclear cells in the joint space and loss of proteoglycan from the articular cartilage. Injections of endotoxin, which also stimulated leukocyte accumulation, had no effect on proteoglycan loss, suggesting a direct effect for IL-1 in erosive arthritis. Dayer et al. (18–21) showed that IL-1-stimulated adherent synovial cells, dermal fibroblasts, chondrocytes, and bone-derived cells produce increased amounts of collagenase and prostaglandin E_2 (PGE_2). IL-1 also stimulates osteoblasts to release macrophage colony-stimulating factor (M-CSF) in a dose-dependent manner (22). Thus IL-1 may potentiate bone resorption by increasing the number of available osteoclast precursors.

Cartilage destruction, associated with irreversible degradation of proteoglycan and collagen in joints of RA patients, is mediated by the combined activities of proteases and collagenase derived from the proliferative synovial lining (pannus). There is evidence that plasminogen activator (PA), a serine protease that converts plasminogen into the active protease plasmin, may also be involved in cartilage destruction in RA. PA has been found in increased amounts in synovial fluid from RA patients (23); cartilage proteoglycan is degraded by plasmin (24), and plasmin has also been shown to activate collagenase (25), neutral proteoglycanase (26), complement (27), and kininogen (27), all of which are produced by the synovium in inactive forms. Mochan and his colleagues (23) showed that addition of human IL-1 to cultured human synovial cells caused a 30- to 40-fold increase in cell-associated and extracellular PA activity. Further, the IL-1 present in mononuclear cell-conditioned medium stimulates synovial cells to produce PA. Thus, the catabolic activity of IL-1 in cartilage and bone very likely contributes to joint tissue injury, leading to deforming arthritis in RA and perhaps in other connective tissue diseases as well.

In addition to the role it plays in stimulating synovial cells to produce inflammatory mediators, the interaction of IL-1 with endothelial cells (EC) also contributes to the acute and chronic inflammation seen in rheumatic disease. IL-1 activates human endothelial cells in vitro to synthesize and release PGI_2 and PGE_2, both potent vasodilators (28). In RA, the synovial tissue—the development of which is dependent on certain functions of the synovial endothelial cells (29)—is infiltrated with a variety of mononuclear cells. For example, IL-1 alters endothelial cell plasma membranes so that binding of blood lymphocytes and monocytes to endothelial cells is increased. IL-1, which is also a potent lymphocyte chemotactic factor, perpetuates the lymphocytic infiltrate in synovium by causing increased lymphocyte movement through the postcapillary venule.

IL-1 also stimulates increased endothelial cell procoagulant activity and increased production of plasminogen activator inhibitor (30). These factors may contribute to development of vasculitis in connective tissue disease by activating the clotting cascade, decreasing blood flow, and increasing the numbers of leukocytes and platelets in affected tissue. IL-1 also induces endothelial cell proliferation and neovascularization. Production of type IV collagen, the type found in vascular basement membranes (31), is also increased by IL-1. The basement membrane thickening in RA synovial vessels is heterogeneous: transition areas are most dense, with wide distribution of lymphocytes, macrophages, and plasma cells. However, the lining is minimal in lymphocyte-rich areas containing aggregates of mainly T helper cells (31).

Several drugs used in the treatment of arthritis may exert their beneficial effects via modulation of IL-1 activity. Corticosteroids and cyclosporine A, both of which generally down-regulate immune responses, suppress IL-1 secretion (32–34).

INTERLEUKIN-2

IL-2, first described as a T cell growth factor (35), is a 15,000 D glycoprotein produced by T cells of helper phenotype in response to antigenic and mitogenic stimuli (36). IL-2 represents an important lymphokine in the initiation and regulation of cell-mediated immune responses; its production is stimulated by accessory cells via the secretion of IL-1. By binding to high-affinity receptors, IL-2 supports the proliferation of stimulated T cells (37), B lymphocytes (38), and natural killer (NK) cells (39). In addition, IL-2 stimulates the production of interferon-γ (IFN-γ) (40), augments the reactivity of cytolytic T cells, NK cells (41), and monocytes (42), and is essential for the induction of lymphokine-activated killer cells (43). Human T lymphocytes can be activated by interaction with different stimuli, such as antigens, mitogenic lectins, and antibodies directed to cell surface membrane structures, and best characterized of which are the CD3-TCR complex and the CD2 (T11, sheep E receptor) protein (44,45). During activation, T cells acquire a number of cell surface glycoproteins, some of which (IL-2, transferrin and insulin receptors, 4F2 and EA.1 antigens) appear early, even before DNA synthesis; others (HLA-DR, CB.1, Ta-1, TLiSA1, T10, and

VLA-1) appear later (46–53). The activation process also stimulates the production and secretion of IL-2 (54), which is accompanied by the upregulation of the Tac (CD25) antigen (55) and the ultimate expansion of sensitized T lymphocytes (56). The progressive loss of high-affinity IL-2 receptors leads to termination of T cell growth in vitro.

Activated T cells appear to have a central role in the pathogenesis of many autoimmune and inflammatory diseases. Although measurements of IL-2 in RA patients have produced conflicting results (57), excessive production of IL-2, as well as B cell activation and high levels of soluble IL-2 receptors, have been observed in these patients (58,59) and in patients with multiple sclerosis (MS) (60) and systemic lupus erythematosus (61). IL-2-responsive activated T cell clones have been described at the site of tissue injury in patients with RA (62,63), MS (64), and pulmonary sarcoidosis (65). Thus, downregulation of IL-2-dependent T cell proliferation may be a useful therapeutic maneuver in these patients. Indeed, gold sodium thiomalate, in concentrations attainable during chrysotherapy for RA, significantly inhibits the proliferative responses of cultured human T cells stimulated by IL-2 (66). Because IL-2 is immunostimulatory, antibodies directed against IL-2 receptors have been proposed as potential immunosuppressive therapy. Antibodies specific for the IL-2 receptor may prove to be protective in conditions of aberrant immune function, such as systemic lupus erythematosus (67). On the other hand, the immunostimulatory functions of IL-2 may allow its use as therapy in immunocompromised patients. Further research is necessary to sort out an appropriate clinical role for IL-2.

INTERLEUKIN-3

IL-3 is one of a group of cytokines known as colony-stimulating factors. These cytokines have the ability to stimulate the development of many cell types, including granulocyte and macrophage colony formation in bone marrow cultures (68,69), as well as growth of mast cells and T and B lymphocytes. IL-3 is produced predominantly by activated T cells so that IL-1, which is important in T cell proliferation and differentiation, may play a role in its production.

Factors with IL-2-like activity that can induce proliferation of IL-3-dependent murine cell lines have been isolated from inflamed joints (70). It has recently been determined, however, that there is a high degree of species specificity for IL-3 and message for human IL-3 is not detectable in RA synovial tissue (71). It is therefore unlikely that human IL-3 is responsible for the proliferation observed in the murine cells. Nonetheless, IL-3 produced during immune reactions may serve to recruit additional hematopoietic cells to amplify these responses.

No other role for IL-3 in rheumatic diseases has yet been found. However, other cytokines in this group, such as granulocyte-macrophage CSF (GM-CSF), which is discussed later, may in fact be involved in the development of arthritis.

INTERLEUKIN-4

IL-4, initially known as B cell stimulatory factor 1, is produced by some activated T cells (72). It acts on resting B cells to increase their expression of class II major histocompatibility complex molecules (73), augments the proliferation of activated

B cells (74), and is involved in isotype differentiation in lipopolysaccharide (LPS)-stimulated murine B cells (75,76). These B cells exhibit markedly increased production of IgG_1 and IgE when stimulated with LPS in the presence of IL-4.

Although originally thought to influence B cells only, IL-4 affects T cells as well. IL-4 enhances T cell proliferation directly (77) and promotes proliferation induced by exposure to costimuli (78). The effects of IL-4 on T cells occur by several different mechanisms, including direct stimulation of resting cells into the cell cycle, enhancement of IL-2 production, and induction of high-affinity IL-2 receptors (79). The capacity of IL-4 to stimulate proliferation of $CD4^+$ and $CD8^+$ cells may be enhanced by IL-1 (80). Whereas induction by IL-4 of expression of class II major histocompatibility complex (MHC) antigens on B cells and B cell synthesis of IgG_1 and IgE are both blocked by exposure of cells to interferon-γ (IFN-γ) (80), the stimulatory effect of IL-4 on T cells is not influenced by IFN-γ (81).

In a study by Fay (82), IL-4 activity was found in all synovial fluids from 37 RA patients but in none from patients with other types of synovitis, such as Reiter's disease, trauma, or psoriasis. Although its precise role in autoimmune disease has not been defined, IL-4 may be important in T-B cell interactions, such as antigen presentation (83), local immunoglobulin secretion, and recruitment of new T cells to the ongoing inflammatory process (77). Also, there is some evidence that IL-4 may act to restrain inflammation under certain conditions. For example, macrophages that normally produce IL-1, tumor necrosis factor α, and PGE_2 when exposed to LPS and IFN-γ do not produce these factors if IL-4 is also present (84).

INTERLEUKIN-5

The biological role of IL-5 in humans has not been defined, although murine IL-5, with which it shares about 70% sequence homology, acts as an eosinophil differentiation factor and a B cell growth factor. IL-5 was identified initially in supernatants from concanavalin A (ConA)-stimulated murine lymphocytes as a factor capable of causing B cells either to differentiate into antibody-producing cells or to undergo proliferation in the absence of T cells (85,86). It was therefore called T cell replacing factor (TRF) or B cell growth factor (BCGF) II. It was later determined that IL-2 and IL-4 were components of TRF (87), but IL-5 was found to be distinct both biochemically and functionally from these other lymphokines (88–90). Whereas IL-4 acts on resting cells, IL-5 influences cells only after they have been activated. It is not yet clear whether IL-5 receptors are present on cells in the resting state, but available evidence suggests that their appearance is cell cycle dependent.

Murine IL-5 is clearly capable of inducing the expression of high-affinity IL-2 receptors on thymocytes (91) and of inducing B cell differentiation with resultant antibody secretion (92–95), but functional studies of human recombinant IL-5 (rhIL-5) are few in number and are controversial. Purified rhIL-5 exhibits potent eosinophil colony-stimulating activity (96,97). However, although initial cloning studies showed that IL-5 had weak but definite TRF activity (98) and increased the activity of IgG- and IgM-producing cells, subsequent studies

(97) did not demonstrate human B cell proliferation or differentiation, even after B cells were activated by a variety of stimulants. Other laboratories (99) have shown B cell stimulatory effects, but less pure preparations of rhIL-5 were used.

Although the effects of IL-5 in humans remain controversial, the strong B cell proliferative and differentiative functions shown in murine cell lines suggest a role for IL-5 in the pathogenesis of autoimmune diseases characterized by autoantibody production. It is possible that the activity of IL-5 as well as the panel of BCGFs may be different in humans and mice and raises the possibility that the mouse may not be the best model for study of the human antibody response.

INTERLEUKIN-6

IL-6, also known as interferon-β_2, B cell stimulating factor 2, and hepatocyte stimulating factor, is a glycoprotein derived from a wide variety of cell types, including T and B cells, fibroblasts, macrophages, monocytes, endothelial cells, and certain tumor cells (80). Normal cells do not produce IL-6 unless stimulated to do so (100,101). Gene transcription of IL-6 is enhanced by IL-1 and to a lesser extent by tumor necrosis factor, platelet-derived growth factor (PDGF), and IFN-β_1. Lipopolysaccharide also increases IL-6 mRNA synthesis in fibroblasts. The multiple effects of IL-6 are usually seen only in the presence of stimuli (such as IL-1), and IL-6 mediates its effects via the same receptor as type 1 IFN (i.e., IFN-α and IFN-β_1).

IL-6 is produced during immune responses and has marked effects on the growth and differentiation of B and T lymphocytes. The stimulation of T cells by IL-6 involves the induction of IL-2 receptors, which converts the T cells to an IL-2-responsive state. IL-1 and IL-6 are strongly synergistic in the induction of T cell proliferation (102,103).

IL-6 probably plays a role in the induction and propagation of the inflammatory response, since the hepatocyte (a major source of acute-phase proteins) is a major target for IL-6 (104). Stimulation by IL-6 of acute-phase protein release from liver, coupled with its effects as a pyrogen, suggest that IL-6, together with IL-1, is responsible for many of the systemic signs and symptoms observed in connective tissue diseases, including fever, weight loss, leukocytosis, and elevated erythrocyte sedimentation rate (ESR).

Another important function of IL-6 is to induce activated B lymphocytes to terminally differentiate into immunoglobulin-producing plasma cells (105,106). IL-6 may therefore be involved in rheumatoid factor (RF) production. Increased levels of IL-6 have been observed in supernatants from tumor cells associated with autoimmunity, suggesting an important role for IL-6 in autoimmune diseases (107,108). Tumors often associated with autoantibody production, such as cardiac myxoma, cervical carcinoma, and bladder cell carcinoma, produce large amounts of IL-6 (108).

Waage and colleagues (109) found concentrations of IL-6 in serum and synovial fluid to correlate with the activity of inflammatory arthritis. This group studied paired samples of serum and synovial fluid from seropositive and seronegative RA patients as well as synovial fluid only from patients with psoriatic arthritis, Reiter's syndrome, and traumatic synovitis. They found that the level of IL-6 in synovial fluid correlated with the ESR in patients with inflammatory disease and that the median level of IL-6 was higher in patients with inflammatory arthritis than in those with a traumatic etiology, although this difference was not statistically significant.

Guerne and colleagues (110) showed that IL-6 is produced spontaneously by synovial cells in culture and that IL-1, TNF-α, and lymphotoxin (TNF-β) augment its synthesis. They found very high levels of IL-6 in synovial fluid obtained from patients with inflammatory synovitis. This synovial cell-derived IL-6 was able to induce hybridoma-plasmacytoma proliferation as well as immunoglobulin and acute-phase protein synthesis. They also showed that IL-6 is present in rheumatoid synovium in much higher concentrations than either IL-1 or TNF-α, suggesting an important role for this cytokine in the hypergammaglobulinemia and RF production seen in RA. However, the levels of IL-6 found in seropositive RA are comparable to those found in seronegative RA and psoriatic arthritis, both of which exhibit hypergammaglobulinemia but not autoantibodies. IL-6 may therefore act as a general stimulus for antibody synthesis rather than an inducer of specific autoantibodies.

TUMOR NECROSIS FACTOR

Tumor necrosis factor, a polypeptide product of stimulated macrophages, and the closely related TNF-β (lymphotoxin) produced by activated T lymphocytes were named for their ability to lyse tumor targets (111–114). These cytokines cause hemorrhagic necrosis of certain tumors by destruction of neovasculature. An historical perspective as well as a description of the isolation, characterization, and cloning of TNF are provided by Kunkel et al. (115).

TNF-α and β share a common receptor (116) and are coded for by genes that are located on chromosome 6 near the MHC locus (117). They share 50% amino acid sequence homology and stimulate many of the same functional activities. Administration of TNF in experimental models leads to a syndrome indistinguishable from that of endotoxic shock, suggesting that TNF is the direct mediator of organ dysfunction seen in this disorder (118,119).

TNF has several clearly defined activities related to patients with arthritis and chronic rheumatic diseases, including development of constitutional symptoms, increased bone resorption, stimulation of enzyme release from synovial cells, stimulation of fibroblast growth, and effects on cell-cell interactions important in the immune response.

Several groups have found TNF activity in serum of patients with inflammatory arthritis, such as RA, reactive arthritis, ankylosing spondylitis, and gout (120–122). TNF activity has also been found in children with Kawasaki disease (123) and in adults with scleroderma (124). At least one group (122) showed that RA patients with TNF-α present in serum and synovial fluid had higher sedimentation rates and synovial fluid leukocyte counts than RA patients without elevated TNF.

TNF, like IL-1, acts as a potent endogenous pyrogen (125), inducing a biphasic fever response. The initial temperature elevation is mediated by a direct effect on the hypothalamus; the secondary response is caused by augmentation of IL-1 production (125). Release of acute-phase proteins is also stimulated by TNF. TNF is likely responsible in part for another systemic reaction seen in chronic inflammatory diseases: cachexia with muscle wasting. TNF suppresses the expression of mRNA that codes for lipogenic enzymes, thereby inducing lipolysis (126). TNF administration to animals results in depletion of protein stores (127) with subsequent muscle wasting.

In RA, bone resorption occurs in areas adjacent to the inflamed synovial pannus. Although the mechanisms of bone destruction are probably several, it is likely that TNF produced locally by macrophages in pannus plays a major role. TNF is a potent stimulus to bone resorption in vitro (128–132). It stimulates osteoclasts directly by a mechanism that is not prostaglandin mediated, since indomethacin has no effect on the process (132). TNF-α stimulates synoviocyte PGE_2 and collagenase production (133,134); it also stimulates osteoblasts to release PGE_2 and M-CSF (135). TNF suppression of bone formation by osteoblasts leads to decreased intracellular alkaline phosphatase and reduced synthesis of collagen and noncollagen matrix proteins (128). These activities all contribute to loss of bone and cartilage in RA.

TNF-α and TNF-β, as well as IL-1α and IL-1β increase the amount of hyaluronic acid (HA) secreted by human synovial fibroblasts (136). The effect is inhibited by indomethacin, suggesting a prostaglandin-mediated mechanism. Increased levels of HA, a glycosaminoglycan that has structural and regulatory functions in connective tissues, have been found in synovial fluid and serum from patients with RA (137). Also, rheumatoid synovial cells in culture produce greater amounts of HA than synovial cells from normal controls (138). Although the significance of increased HA in RA patients is not clear, it has been postulated that this is one alteration in synovial cell properties that helps to explain the invasive nature of the pannus in RA (139). There also may be a positive feedback (amplification) loop established by the TNF-induced increase in HA levels. HA stimulation of IL-1 production by human monocytes (140) may help explain the increased amounts of IL-1 found in rheumatoid pannus. Synergy between IL-1 and TNF-α, known to be important in rheumatoid synovium, has been shown in the induction of prostaglandin synthesis by lung fibroblasts (141) and in osteoclast-mediated bone resorption (142). Firestein and Zvaifler (143) noted that IL-1 and TNF-α together are more potent stimulators of synovial cell proliferation than either alone.

Finally, in such diseases as OA and RA, TNF may also cause destruction of articular cartilage. Shinmei et al. (144) studied the effects of IL-1 and TNF on collagenase and caseinase production by and proteoglycan release from human articular cartilage. They showed that IL-1 and TNF caused increased proteoglycan release and increased production of metalloproteinases leading to destruction of articular cartilage.

Some activities of TNF may protect the host. In addition to inducing fever, TNF stimulates human neutrophils to produce oxygen free radicals and potentiates their ability to kill pathogens (145). Acting synergistically with interferon (IFN-γ), TNF enhances leukocyte phagocytosis and antibody-dependent cellular cytotoxicity (146). Thus, whereas TNF contributes to organ dysfunction, it also augments the host immune status and promotes the inflammatory response. This heightened immune response may be beneficial or harmful depending on the location of the TNF produced. For example, the interaction of TNF with endothelium results in suppression of proteins important in maintaining a patent vasculature. This may be useful in tumor lysis, or it may be harmful, leading to vasculitis associated with some of the rheumatic diseases.

INTERLEUKIN-8

IL-8, also known as neutrophil chemotactic factor and neutrophil activating factor, is a tissue-derived cytokine secreted by several different cell types, including human peripheral blood mononuclear cells, fibroblasts, epithelial cells, and hepatocytes stimulated by IL-1α, IL-β, and TNF-α. Monocytes, alveolar macrophages, and endothelial cells can also be induced by lipopolysaccharide to secrete IL-8. Watson et al. (147) have also shown that rhIL-1-stimulated human synovial cells in culture express an activity in their supernatant that stimulates neutrophils, as assessed by an increase in neutrophil free calcium concentration and chemokinesis. They termed this activity polymorphonuclear leukocyte stimulating factor (PSF). In addition, human synovial cells stimulated by IL-1α and IL-1β express mRNA for IL-8 (148).

Although IL-8 is a recently discovered cytokine, it has already been implicated in several rheumatic disorders. Schroeder and Christopher (149) demonstrated IL-8 in psoriatic plaques. These lesions also contain high levels of IL-1, which could be the stimulus for IL-8 production. IL-8 is probably involved in arthritis since, as discussed earlier, it has been shown that IL-1-stimulated synovial cells express the gene for IL-8 and produce a neutrophil activating factor. The exact role of IL-8 in arthritis and other inflammatory diseases is not known, but since neutrophils are a major source of cartilage-degrading enzymes, at least one role for IL-8 may be in the cartilage degradation commonly seen in these disorders. IL-1 and TNF are considered the major cytokines responsible for destruction of articular cartilage by virtue of their ability to liberate proteoglycans and metalloproteinases from the synovial pannus. IL-1 stimulation of synovial cell IL-8 may provide an additional mechanism by which IL-1 causes cartilage destruction in inflammatory arthritis.

INTERFERON-γ

Interferons, the first cytokines discovered, have a wide range of biological activity. Three major groups of interferons are known: IFN-α, produced by leukocytes, and IFN-β, produced by fibroblasts, were formerly known as type I interferons. These cytokines are secreted in response to stimulation by virus or double-stranded RNA. IFN-γ (type II), produced primarily by mitogen- or antigen-stimulated T lymphocytes (150), shares only 10% structural homology with IFN-α and IFN-β and it has a different cell surface receptor. This group of cytokines has antiviral and antiproliferative activities, which is why they have been used as anticancer agents. All three are immunoregulatory, but IFN-γ is the most active in this regard. Although IFN-γ is the focus of this discussion, it must be realized that there may be synergy between the various interferons. Most of the work that relates to the rheumatic diseases has focused on IFN-γ.

IFN-γ has diverse effects on immune responses, and it interacts with other lymphokines in either a synergistic or an antagonistic manner: IFN-γ augments B cell-stimulating lymphokines and increases antibody production but antagonizes the effects of IL-1 on connective tissue by inhibiting collagen synthesis (151–153). The main functions of IFN-γ appear to be stimulatory. It induces the appearance of new surface markers associated with differentiation, and it enhances the proliferation of T lymphocytes and probably natural killer cells (154); IFN-γ also enhances the expression of class I and class II MHC antigens (155). The effects on class II MHC antigens are seen in a number of cell types, including myelomonocytic cells, lymphoid cells, mast cells, endothelial cells, fibroblasts, neuronal cells, melanocytes, and melanoma cells (156).

In summary, IFN-γ plays a pivotal role in host defense. After antigenic stimulation, T cells activated by IL-2 produce IFN-γ, which then influences their response as well as their interactions with B cells. Although much work has been done with IFN-γ in rheumatic diseases, especially RA and scleroderma, controversy remains about its role in the pathogenesis of these disorders.

Several investigators have assessed IFN-γ in peripheral blood mononuclear cells from patients with RA and other rheumatic diseases (157–160). In 1979, Hooks et al. found (160) "immune" interferon (now known as IFN-γ) in sera of patients with systemic lupus erythematosus (SLE), RA, scleroderma, and Sjögren's syndrome. A positive correlation between serial IFN titers, clinical disease activity, and serological activity (complement levels and anti-ds-DNA antibodies) was observed in the lupus patients. Cesario et al. (161) detected IFN from 11 of 84 synovial fluid samples and 10 of 84 simultaneous serum samples of patients with RA, SLE, seronegative spondyloarthritis, pseudogout, and unclassified arthritis; the highest titers were identified in RA patients. IFN activity was not identified in synovial fluids from patients with gout, disseminated gonococcal infection, or degenerative arthritis. No relationship was found between serum and synovial fluid levels of IFN; in fact, it was uncommon for IFN to be found in both body fluids simultaneously, suggesting local production of IFN in the joint space. More recently, several groups have found decreased or defective production of IFN-γ from peripheral blood mononuclear cells in patients with SLE and RA (158,162). Reuter's group found (162) that patients with active disease produced significantly less IFN-γ than those who were in remission. Firestein and Zvaifler (163,164) postulated that IFN-γ was the primary macrophage activating factor in synovial tissue and synovial fluid because the phenotype of synovial fluid monocytes resembled that of peripheral blood monocytes exposed to IFN-γ. However, when they measured synovial fluid and synovial fluid monocytes by sensitive radioimmunoassay (RIA), very little IFN-γ was identified, suggesting that activation of synovial fluid monocytes occurs by other mechanisms.

Despite these controversies, several observations suggest the possibility that IFN-γ is beneficial in RA. Although RA is a disease of unknown etiology, polyclonal B lymphocyte activation has been identified in the synovial tissue, synovial fluid, and peripheral blood of these patients (165,166) and IFN-γ inhibits the activation of B lymphocytes by the Epstein-Barr virus (EBV) (167). Also, IFN-γ decreases IgM synthesis by EBV-sensitized B lymphocytes from patients with RA (168). Additionally, many investigators believe that despite an increase in the number of activated T lymphocytes in peripheral blood and in synovium of RA patients, at least some of these lymphocytes may be defective in that they exhibit decreased production of IL-2 and IFN-γ (169,170). Finally, decreased NK activity has been reported in patients with active RA (171), and IFN-γ has been shown to enhance NK activity (154). These activities of IFN-γ prompted several clinical trials in RA patients. Firestein et al. (172) evaluated the effects of IFN-γ on 12 patients with active RA during a 12 week open trial: 9 patients were unchanged clinically and only 2 had 50% improvement. Surprisingly, parenteral IFN-γ failed to increase DR on peripheral blood monocytes from the RA patients. Since this was the first time parenteral IFN-γ had been evaluated, the dose given may not have been sufficient to produce the anticipated results.

Veys et al. (173), in a double-blind trial of 6 months duration, evaluated the effects of subcutaneous IFN-γ compared to placebo in 22 RA patients. Although all clinical parameters tested showed a trend in favor of the treatment group, only the tender joint score improved significantly. No serious adverse effects were observed. The authors concluded that the optimal regimen for using IFN-γ had not been established and that further double-blind studies using this agent in a larger number of patients were needed.

In 1989, Cannon et al. (174) completed a 12 week, double-blind, randomized, prospective, placebo-controlled trial of recombinant human (rh)IFN-γ for the treatment of RA; 54 patients received rhIFN-γ and 51 received placebo. A total of 42 patients in each group completed the study, and some clinical improvement occurred in both groups of patients. Although the improvement with IFN-γ was greater than that observed in the placebo group, the differences were not statistically significant.

IFN-γ has also been evaluated as therapy for systemic juvenile rheumatoid arthritis (JRA) in a small, open study involving nine severely ill children who did not respond to conventional therapy (175). Of nine patients seven improved, but as in the adult studies, changes in clinical parameters were not statistically significant.

In addition to the trials in RA, the use of IFN-γ has been studied in scleroderma. The pathogenesis of scleroderma remains uncertain, but histopathological examination reveals excessive fibroblast activity with collagen deposition in numerous organs (176). There is at present no satisfactory treatment for scleroderma. IFN-γ, because of its ability to inhibit collagen production by normal human dermal fibroblasts (177) and by scleroderma dermal fibroblasts (151), was evaluated in an open trial of 6 months duration involving 10 patients (178); 9 patients completed the study. After the 6 month treatment period, significant improvement (compared to baseline) was observed in total skin score, maximal mouth opening, range of motion of wrists and elbows, grip strength, functional index, dysphagia, and creatinine clearance. No serious side effects were observed, but a significant decrease in blood and leukocyte counts and peripheral blood lymphocytes were noted. The study had several limitations, including the small sample size and the open, uncontrolled design. Also, some degree of spontaneous regression in dermal sclerosis may occur in some patients, making evaluation of any drug difficult in this disease. Despite these reservations, IFN-γ may be useful in the treatment of scleroderma. However, a large double-blind, controlled trial must be done.

TRANSFORMING GROWTH FACTOR-β

Transforming growth factor β (TGF-β) was first isolated from human platelets and is made by almost all cell types. It was originally identified in an assay that measured the ability of TGF-β to enhance the growth of fibroblasts in soft agar.

The terms "multifunctional" or "pleiotropic" have been applied to TGF-β because it stimulates the proliferation of some cells, especially cells from connective tissue, while inhibiting the proliferation of others, such as lymphocytes and epithelial cells. This cytokine also has many other actions that have little relationship to cell growth, such as regulation of collagen synthesis and other molecules of the extracellular matrix. It is especially important during formation of normal tissues in embryogenesis and during response to injury with inflammation and repair. The relationship of TGF-β to the rheumatic diseases has focused on its effects on bone and cartilage, its effects in rheumatoid arthritis, and its potential role in the pathogenesis of scleroderma. TGF-β enhances the proliferation of many cells of mesenchymal origin, including the osteoblast. This cell is important for the formation of new bone during fracture healing and for maintenance of existing bone to prevent osteoporosis. In addition to acting as a mitogen for the osteoblast, TGF-β also stimulates this cell type to produce extracellular matrix proteins. Although little is known about the role of TGF-β in the pathogenesis of bone disease, there is evidence that the estrogen receptor can activate the gene for TGF-β, thus promoting the formation of new bone matrix (179). Therefore, further studies on the role of TGF-β in the modulation of osteoporosis need to be done.

TGF-β has many direct actions on fibroblasts in addition to being a strong chemotactic factor for these cells (180). It has therefore been the subject of much research relating to scleroderma, a disease characterized by collagen overproduction. Skin fibroblasts produce collagens, proteoglycans, and attachment proteins, including fibronectin (181). Lesional cells from scleroderma patients produce more type I and type III collagens, glycosaminoglycans, and fibronectin than matched control cells (182,183). Messenger RNA (mRNA) levels of matrix proteins are elevated in scleroderma (184,185), but fibroblasts from unaffected skin of these patients do not exhibit exaggerated matrix synthesis. It has been shown that TGF-β binds to one or more membrane receptors and, by an as yet unknown mechanism, enhances collagen mRNA expression 5- to 10-fold (185,186). It also enhances formation of fibronectin by increasing transcription of the gene coding for this protein (186).

TGF-β plays another direct role in enhancing the formation of extracellular matrix: it can inhibit the proteolytic degradation of newly formed matrix proteins, by at least two mechanisms. First, TGF-β increases the formation and secretion of protease inhibitors, such as plasminogen activator inhibitor (187), and second, TGF-β reduces the secretion of proteases, including plasminogen activator (187), a thiol protease (188), and a metalloprotease (transin/stromelysin) (189).

The effects of TGF-β on collagen and extracellular matrix formation and fibroblast chemotaxis provide evidence for the probable involvement of TGF-β in systemic sclerosis. The finding that TGF-β activates a collagen gene promoter provides a framework for potential intervention in collagen synthesis at the transcriptional level (186) and may provide an exciting therapeutic advance in the thus far untreatable fibrosing diseases.

Finally, TGF-β probably plays a role in the development of synovial pannus and maintenance of inflammation in rheumatoid arthritis. Several cellular responses known to be mediated by TGF-β may be responsible: fibroblast chemotaxis (180), increased production of extracellular matrix proteins by fibroblasts, which may relate to the increased levels of atypical isoforms of fibronectin that have been found in RA synovial fluid (191,192), and chemotaxis of monocytes and antiproliferative or immunosuppressive effects on T cells (193–195). Fava et al. (196) found TGF-β-like activity in inflammatory synovial fluid, with RA patients having the highest levels. They postulate that activation of latent TGF-β by proteases in the synovial pannus could cause a local increase in active TGF-β leading to perpetuation of the destructive inflammatory process. Research with TGF-β in RA may provide clues to the pathogenesis of inflammatory arthritis.

GRANULOCYTE-MACROPHAGE COLONY-STIMULATING FACTOR

Granulocyte-macrophage colony-stimulating factor is a glycoprotein that has growth-enhancing effects on granulocyte, macrophage, and eosinophil colonies in the bone marrow. It was purified from conditioned medium of a T lymphoblast cell line (197), and a cDNA has been cloned (198). Recombinant GM-CSF has been produced from three cell types: mammalian, yeast, and bacterial. The gene for GM-CSF is located on the long arm of chromosome 5 (198).

GM-CSF is produced in large amounts in response to inflammatory stimuli after activation of the producer cells. T lymphocytes produce GM-CSF when stimulated by antigens, lectins, or IL-2 (198), and monocytes release GM-CSF after stimulation with endotoxin (199). Fibroblasts and endothelial cells are also sources of GM-CSF (200–202). This cytokine is undetectable in the serum with current assays (203). It appears to be produced locally and to become compartmentalized in the extracellular matrix of bone marrow (204).

GM-CSF is considered a multipotential hematopoietic growth factor. In addition to its effects on myeloid precursors in the bone marrow, GM-CSF also causes neutrophil and eosinophil activation (205), induces neutrophil phagocytosis (206), and stimulates the proliferation and activation of monocytes-macrophages. Production of cytokines by monocytes-macrophages is also induced by GM-CSF (207).

As already discussed, cytokines play a critical role in establishing and maintaining the inflammatory response seen in many types of chronic synovitis, such as rheumatoid arthritis. In addition to its role as a hematopoietic growth factor, GM-CSF has recently been found in chronic inflammatory joint effusions from RA patients and in the supernatants of cultured RA synovial tissue (208). GM-CSF may have a dual role in the pathogenesis of RA. It is likely that GM-CSF augments the inflammatory response in RA (and possibly other types of inflammatory synovitis) by inhibiting neutrophil migration out of the joint space (209) and by potentiating neutrophil activation (210,211). GM-CSF also increases the cell surface expression of HLA class II histocompatibility antigens (HLA-DR or Ia molecules) on blood monocytes from normal donors (212). Ia molecules are essential elements in antigen presentation. The synovial lining cells from RA patients express large amounts of Ia on the surface, and monocytes derived from rheumatoid synovial effusions exhibit an activated phenotype with increased expression of HLA-DR and low levels of CD14 (monocyte differentiation antigen) (213).

Identification of GM-CSF at the site of a chronic inflammatory disease like RA marks the first time this cytokine has been implicated in a human disease state.

Variation in Ia expression plays a major role in immune regulation (214). Parenteral administration of GM-CSF to mice augments the primary antibody response due to enhanced function of antigen-presenting cells, including increased la expression (215). Monocytes and macrophages isolated from inflammatory foci resemble GM-CSF-treated monocytes, observations that suggest that local production of GM-CSF may play a role in macrophage activation in disease states (212).

REFERENCES

1. Bodel PT, Hollingsworth JW. Pyrogen release from human synovial cell exudates. Br J Exp Pathol 1968; 49:11–9.
2. Gowen M, Wood DD, Ihrie EJ, McGuire MKB, Russell GG. An IL-1 like factor stimulates bone resorption in vitro. Nature 1983; 306:378–80.
3. Saklatvala J, Curry VA, Sarsfield SJ. Purification to homogeneity of pig monocyte catabolism, a protein that causes cartilage resorption in vitro. Biochem J 1983; 215:385–92.
4. Andreis M, Stastny P, Ziff M. Experimental arthritis produced by injection of mediators of delayed hypersensitivity. Arthritis Rheum 1974; 17:537–51.
5. Pettipher ER, Higgs GA, Henderson B. Interleukin 1 induces leukocyte infiltration and cartilage proteoglycan degradation in the synovial joint. Proc Natl Acad Sci U S A 1986; 83:8749–53.
6. Dingle JT, Page-Thomas DP, King B, Bard DR. *In vivo* studies of articular tissue damage mediated by catabolin/interleukin 1. Ann Rheum Dis 1987; 46:527–33.
7. Ise K, Nakamura S, Ohkawara S, Yoshinaga M. DNA synthesis-potentiating activity on mouse thymocytes of synovial fluid of rheumatoid arthritis patients. Acta Pathol Jpn 1982; 32:491–503.
8. Fontana A, Hengartner H, Weber E, Fehr K, Grob PJ, Cohen G. Interleukin 1 activity in the synovial fluid of patients with rheumatoid arthritis. Rheumatol Int 1982; 2:49–53.
9. Wood DD, Ihrie EJ, Dinarello CA, Cohen PL. Isolation of an interleukin 1-like factor from human joint effusions. Arthritis Rheum 1983; 26:975–83.
10. Hopkins SJ, Humphreys M, Jayson MIV. Cytokines in synovial fluid. I. The presence of biologically active and immunoreactive IL-1. Clin Exp Immunol 1988; 72:422–7.
11. Di Giovine F, Situnavake D, Duff GW. Radioimmunoassay of interleukin 1β in acute and chronic rheumatic diseases. Br J Rheumatol 1987; 26(Suppl 1):34.
12. Duff G, Di Giovine F, Dickens E, Symons J, Wood N, Manson J. Tumor necrosis factor and interleukin 1 in arthritis. Immunobiology 1987; 175:10–1.
13. DiGiovine FS, Malawista SE, Nuki G, Duff GW. Interleukin 1 as a mediator of crystal arthritis. J Immunol 1987; 138:3213–8.
14. Duff GW, Atkins E, Malawista SE. The fever of gout: urate crystals activate endogenous pyrogen production from human and rabbit mononuclear phagocytes. Trans Assoc Am Phys 1983; 96:234–45.
15. Eastgate JA, Wood NC, Di Giovine FS, Symons JA, Grinlinton FM, Duff GW. Correlation of plasma interleukin 1 levels with disease activity in rheumatoid arthritis. Lancet 1988; 2:706–9.
16. Ritchie DM, Boyle JA, McInness JM, Jasani MK, Dalakos TD, Grieveson P, Buchanan WW. Clinical studies with an articular index for the assessment of joint tenderness in patients with rheumatoid arthritis. Q J Med 1968; 37:393–406.

17. Dewhirst FE, Stashenko PP, Mole JE, Tsurumachi T. Purification of human osteoclast activating factor: identity with IL-1β. J Immunol 1985; 135:2562–8.
18. Dayer JM, Breard J, Chess L, Krane SM. Participation of monocyte-macrophages and lymphocytes in the production of a factor that stimulates collagenase and prostaglandin release by rheumatoid synovial cells. J Clin Immunol 1979; 64:1386–92.
19. Mizel SB, Dayer JM, Krane SM, Mergenhagen SE. Stimulation of rheumatoid synovial cell collagenase and prostaglandin production by partially purified lymphocyte activating factor (IL-1). Proc Natl Acad Sci U S A 1981; 78:2473–7.
20. Dayer JM, De Rochemonteix B, Burrus B, Demczuk S, Dinarello CA. Human recombinant interleukin 1 stimulates collagenase and prostaglandin E_2 production by human synovial cells. J Clin Invest 1986; 77:645–8.
21. Dayer JM, Demczuk S. Cytokines and other mediators in rheumatoid arthritis. Springer Semin Immunopathol 1984; 7:387–413.
22. Sato K, Fujii Y, Asano S, et al. Recombinant human IL-1 and β production stimulate mouse osteoblast-like cells (mc 3T3-E_1) to produce macrophage colony stimulating activity and PGE_2. Biochem Biophys Res Commun 1986; 141:285–91.
23. Mochan E, Uhl J, Newton R. Interleukin 1 stimulation of synovial cell plasminogen activator production. J Rheumatol 1986; 13:15–9.
24. Lack CH, Rogers HJ. Action of plasmin on cartilage. Nature 1958; 182:948–9.
25. Werb Z, Mainardi CL, Vater CA, Harris ED. Endogenous activation of latent collagenase by rheumatoid synovial cells. N Engl J Med 1977; 296:1017–23.
26. Vaes G, Eeckhout Y, Lenaers-Claeys G, Francois-Gillet C, Druetz J. The simultaneous release by bone explants in culture and the parallel activation of procollagenase and of a latent neutral proteinase that degrades cartilage proteoglycans and denatured collagen. Biochem J 1978; 172:261–74.
27. Wueppes KK. In: Leporo IH, Wand PA, eds. Inflammation mechanisms and control. New York: Academic Press, 1974:93.
28. Rossi V, Bredviario F, Ghenzzi P, Dejana E, Mantovani A. Prostacyclin synthesis induced in vascular cells by interleukin 1. Science 1985; 229:1174–6.
29. Ziff M. Rheumatoid arthritis—its present and future. J Rheumatol 1990; 17:127–33.
30. Nachman RL, Hajjar KA, Silverstein RL, Dinarello CA. IL-1 induces endothelial cell synthesis of plasminogen activator inhibitor. J Exp Med 1986; 163:1595–600.
31. Iguchi T, Ziff M. Electron microscopic study of rheumatoid synovial vasculature. J Clin Invest 1986; 77:355–61.
32. Bunjes D, Hardt C, Rollingnoff M, Wagner H. Cyclosporin A mediates immunosuppression of primary cytotoxic T cell responses by impairing the release of IL-1 and IL-2. Eur J Immunol 1981; 11:657–61.
33. Snyder DS, Unanue ER. Corticosteroids inhibit murine macrophage la expression and interleukin 1 production. J Immunol 1982; 129:1803–5.
34. Vane J, Botting R. Inflammation and the mechanism of action of antiinflammatory drugs. FASEB J 1987; 1:89–196.
35. Morgan FS. Riscetto FW, Gallo RC. Selective *in vitro* growth of T lymphocytes from normal human bone marrow. Science 1976; 193:1007.
36. Schreier MH, Iscove NN, Tees R, Aarden L, von Boehmer H. Clones of killer and helper T cells: growth requirement, specificity and retention of function in long-term cultures. Immunol Rev 1980; 51:315.
37. Gillis S, Fern M, Ou W, Smith K. T cell growth factor parameters of production and a quantitative microassay for activity. J Immunol 1978; 120:2027.
38. Waldmann TA, Goldman CK, Robb RJ, et al. Expression of interleukin 2 receptors on activated human B cells. J Exp Med 1984; 160:1450–8.
39. Ortaldo JR, Mason AT, Gerard JP, et al. Effects of natural and recombinant human

IL-2 in regulation of IFN-γ production and natural killer activity: lack of involvement of the Tac antigen for these immunoregulatory effects. J Immunol 1984; 133:779.

40. Kasahara T, Hooks JJ, Dougherty SF, Oppenheim JJ. Interleukin-2 mediated immune interferon production by human T cells and T cell subsets. J Immunol 1983; 130:1784.
41. Timonen T, Ortaldo JR, Stadler BM, Bonnard GD, Sharrow SO, Herberman RB. Cultures of purified human natural killer cells growth in the presence of interleukin 2. Cell Immunol 1982; 72:178.
42. Malkovsky M, Loeland B, North M, et al. Recombinant interleukin 2 directly augments the cytotoxicity of human monocytes. Nature 1987; 325:262.
43. Grimm EA, Mazumder A, Rosenberg SA. Lymphokine-activated killer cell phenomenon. Lysis of natural killer-resistant fresh solid tumor cells by interleukin 2-activated autologous human peripheral blood lymphocytes. J Exp Med 1982; 155:1823.
44. Meuer SC, Hussey RE, Canatrell A, et al. Triggering of the T3-Ti antigen receptor complex results in clonal T-cell proliferation through an interleukin 2 dependent autocrine pathway. Proc Natl Acad Sci U S A 1984; 81:1509–13.
45. Meuer SC, Hussey RE, Fabbi M, et al. An alternative pathway of T cell activation: a functional role for the 50 kD T11 sheep erythrocyte receptor protein. Cell 1984; 36:897–906.
46. Fox DA, Hussey RE, Fitzgerald KA, et al. Ta_1, a novel 105 kD human T cell activation antigen defined by a monoclonal antibody. J Immunol 1984; 133:1250–6.
47. Reinherz EL, Meuer S, Fitzgerald KA, Hussey RE, Levine H, Schlossman SF. Antigen recognition by human T lymphocytes is linked to surface expression of the T3 molecular complex. Cell 1982; 30:735–43.
48. Swack JA, Nakatsuji T, Ito K, Tsuji K. Preservation of membrane glycoprotein labile epitopes during western blotting with monoclonal antibodies. Biotechniques 1987; 5:564–671.
49. Morimoto C, Letvin N, Distaso JA, Aldrich WR, Schlossman SF. The isolation and characterization of the human suppressor induced T cell subset. J Immunol 1985; 134:1508–15.
50. Hara T, Fu SM, Hansen JA. Human T cell activation. II. A new activation pathway used by a major T cell population via a disulfide-bonded dimer of a 44 kilodalton polypeptide (9.3 antigen). J Exp Med 1985; 161:1513–24.
51. Moretta A, Pantaleo G, Lopez-Botet M, Moretta L. Involvement of T44 molecules in an antigen-independent pathway of T cell activation. Analysis of the correlations to the T cell antigen-receptor complex. J Exp Med 1985; 162:823–38.
52. Fox DA, Schlossman SF, Reinherz EL. Regulation of the alternative pathway of T cell activation by anti-T3 monoclonal antibody. J Immunol 1986; 136:1945–50.
53. Fleischer B. A novel pathway of human T cell activation via a 103 kD T cell activation antigen. J Immunol 1987; 138:1346–50.
54. Ruscetti FW, Morgan DA, Gallo RC. Functional and morphologic characterization of human T cells continuously grown in vitro. J Immunol 1977; 119:131–8.
55. Welte KA, Androeff MA, Platzer E, et al. Interleukin-2 regulates the expression of Tac antigen on peripheral blood lymphocytes. J Exp Med 1984; 160:1390–403.
56. Smith KA. T-cell growth factor. Immunol Rev 1980; 51:337–57.
57. Emery P, Williamson DJ, MacKay IR. The role of cytokines in rheumatological inflammation. In: Cruse JM, Lewis RE Jr, eds. Concepts in immunology: autoimmunoregulation and autoimmune disease, Vol. 4. Basel: Karger, 1987:143–55.
58. Symons JA, Wood NC, DiGiovini FS, Duff GW. Soluble IL-2 receptors in rheumatoid

arthritis: correlation with disease activity, IL-1 and IL-2 inhibition. J Immunol 1988; 141:2612–8.

59. Warrington RJ. Interleukin 2 abnormalities in systemic lupus erythematosus and rheumatoid arthritis. A role for overproduction of interleukin-2 in human autoimmunity? J Rheumatol 1987; 15:616–20.
60. Merrill JE, Mohlstrom C, Uittenbogaart C, Kermani-Arab V, Ellison GW, Myers LW. Response to and production of interleukin 2 by peripheral blood and cerebrospinal fluid lymphocytes of patients with multiple sclerosis. J Immunol 1984; 133:1931–7.
61. Wolf RE, Brelsford WG. Soluble interleukin-2 receptors in systemic lupus erythematosus. Arthritis Rheum 1988; 31:729–35.
62. Buchan G, Barrett K, Fujita T, Taniguchi T, Maini R, Feldmann M. Detection of activated T cell products in the rheumatoid joint using cDNA probes to interleukin-2 (IL-2), IL-2 receptor and IFN-γ. Clin Exp Immunol 1988; 71:295–301.
63. Stamenkovic I, Stegagno M, Wright KA, et al. Clonal dominance among T-lymphocyte infiltrates in arthritis. Proc Natl Acad Sci U S A 1988; 85:1179–83.
64. Konttinen YT, Bergroth V, Kinnunen E, Nordstrom D, Kouri T. Activated T lymphocytes in patients with multiple sclerosis in clinical remission. J Neurol Sci 1987; 81:133–9.
65. Konishi K, Moller DR, Saltini C, Kirby M, Crystal RG. Spontaneous expression of the interleukin 2 receptor gene and presence of functional interleukin 2 receptors on T lymphocytes in the blood of individuals with active pulmonary sarcoidosis. J Clin Invest 1988; 82:775–81.
66. Wolf RE, Hall VC. Inhibition of in vitro proliferative response of culture T lymphocytes to interleukin-2 by gold sodium thiomalate. Arthritis Rheum 1988; 31:176–81.
67. Kelley VE, Gaulton GN, Hattori M, Ikegami H, Eisenbarth G, Strom TB. Anti-interleukin 2 receptor antibody suppresses murine diabetic insulitis and lupus nephritis. J Immunol 1988; 140:59–61.
68. Nicola NA, Vadas M. Hemopoietic colony-stimulating factors. Immunol Today 1984; 5:76–80.
69. Sieff C. Hematopoietic growth factors. J Clin Invest 1987; 79:1549–57.
70. Firestein GS, Zvaifler NJ. The pathogenesis of rheumatoid arthritis. A critical assessment of the role of autologous stimulation in the perpetuation of rheumatoid synovitis. Rheum Dis Clin North A 1987; 13:447–61.
71. Firestein GS, Xu WD, Townsend K, et al. Cytokines in chronic inflammatory arthritis. I. Failure to detect T cell lymphokines (IL-2 and IL-3) and presence of macrophage CSF-1 and a novel mast cell growth factor in rheumatoid synovium. J Exp Med 1988; 168:1573–86.
72. Howard M, Farrar J, Hilfiker M, et al. Identification of a T cell derived B cell growth factor distinct from interleukin-2. J Exp Med 1982; 255:914–23.
73. Noelle R, Krammer PH, O'Hara J, Uhr JW, Vitetta ES. Increased expression of Ia antigens on resting B cells: an additional role for B cell growth factor. Proc Natl Acad Sci U S A 1984; 81(19):6149–6153.
74. Rabin RM, Mond JJ, O'Hara J, Paul WE. B cell stimulatory factor 1 (BSF-1) prepares resting B cells to enter S phase in response to anti-IgM and lipopolysaccharide. J Exp Med 1986; 164:517–31.
75. Vitetta ES, O'Hara J, Myers CD, Layton JE, Krammer PH, Paul WE. Serologic, biochemical and functional identify of B cell stimulatory factor-1 and B cell differentiation factor for IgG. J Exp Med 1985; 162:1726–31.
76. Coffman RL, O'Hara J, Bond MW, Carty J, Zlotnik A, Paul WE. B cell stimulatory

factor-1 enhances the IgE response of lipopolysaccharide-activated B cells. J Immunol 1986; 136:4538–41.
77. Paul WE. Interleukin 4/B cell stimulatory factor 1: one lymphokine, many functions. FASEB J 1987; 1:456–61.
78. Hu-Li J, Shevach EM, Mizuguchi J, O'Hara J, Mosmann T, Paul WE. B cell stimulatory factor 1 (interleukin 4) is a potent costimulant for normal resting T lymphocytes. J Exp Med 1987; 165:157–72.
79. Mitchell LC, David LS, Lipsky PE. Promotion of human T lymphocyte proliferation by IL-4. J Immunol 1989; 142:1548–57.
80. Mizel SB. The interleukins. FASEB J 1989; 3:2379–88.
81. Paul WE, O'Hara J. B cell stimulatory factor-1/Interleukin 4. Annu Rev Immunol 1987; 5:429–59.
82. Fay AC, Trudgett A, McCrea JD, et al. Detection and partial characterization of human B cell colony stimulating activity in synovial fluids of patients with rheumatoid arthritis. Clin Exp Immunol 1985; 60:316–22.
83. Matis LA, Glimcher LH, Paul WE, Schwartz RH. Magnitude of response of histocompatibility restricted T cell clones is a function of the product of the concentrations of antigen and Ia molecules. Proc Natl Acad Sci U S A 1983; 80:6019–23.
84. Hart PH, Vitti GF, Burgess DR, Whitt GA, Piccoli DS, Hamilton JA. Potential antiinflammatory effects of IL-4: suppression of human monocyte TNF-α, IL-1 and PGE_2. Proc Natl Acad Sci U S A 1989; 86:3803–7.
85. Takatsu K, Tominaga A, Hamaoka T. Antigen induced T cell replacing factor (TRF). J Immunol 1980; 124:2414–22.
86. Swain SC, Dennert G, Warner JF, Dutton RW. Culture supernatants of a stimulated T cell line have helper activity that acts synergistically with IL-2 in the response of B cells to antigen. Proc Natl Acad Sci U S A 1981; 78:2517–21.
87. Swain SL, McKenzie DT, Dutton RW, Tonkonogy SL, English M. The role of IL-4 and IL-5: characterization of a distinct helper T cell subset that makes IL-4 and IL-5 (Th2) and requires priming before induction of lymphokine secretion. Immunol Rev 1988; 102:77–105.
88. Takatsu K, Harada N, Hara Y, et al. Purification and physiochemical characterization of murine T cell replacing factor (TRF). J Immunol 1985; 134:382–9.
89. Swain SL. Role of BCGFII in the differentiation to antibody secretion normal and tumor B cells. J Immunol 1985; 134:3934–43.
90. Swain SL, Howard M, Kappler J, et al. Evidence for two distinct classes of murine B cell growth factors with activities in different functional assays. J Exp Med 1983; 158:822–35.
91. Takatsu, Kikuch Y, Takahasui T, et al. IL-5, a T cell derived B cell differentiation factor also induces cytotoxic T lymphocytes. Proc Natl Acad Sci U S A 1987; 84:4234–8.
92. Pure E, Isaksan PC, Kappler JW, Marrack P, Krammer PH, Vitetta ES. T cell derived B cell growth and differentiation factors. J Exp Med 1983; 157:600–12.
93. Nakanishi K, Malek TR, Smith KA, Hamaoka T, Shevach EM, Paul WE. Both IL-2 and second T cell-derived factor in IL-4 supernatant have activity as differentiation factors in IgM synthesis. J Exp Med 1984; 160:1605–21.
94. Brooks K, Yuan D, Uhr JW, Krammer PH, Vitetta ES. Lymphokine induced IgM secretion by clones of neoplastic B cells. Nature 1983; 302:825–6.
95. Pure E, Isakson C, Takatsu K, et al. Induction of B cell differentiation by T cell factors. J Immunol 1981; 127:1953–8.
96. Clutterbuck E, Shields JG. Gordon J, et al. Recombinant human IL-5 is an eosinophil differentiation factor but has no activity in standard human B cell growth factor assays. Eur J Immunol 1987; 17:1743–50.

97. Campbell HD, Tucker WQ, Hort Y, et al. Molecular cloning nucleotide sequence, and expression of the gene encoding human eosinophil differentiation factor (IL-5). Proc Natl Acad Sci U S A 1987; 84:6629–33.
98. Azuma C, Tanabe T, Konishi M, et al. Cloning of cDNA for human T cell replacing factor (IL-5) and comparison with the murine homologue. Nucleic Acids Res 1986; 14:9149–58.
99. Yokota T, Coffman RL, Hagiwara HH, et al. Isolation and characterization of lymphokine cDNA clones encoding mouse and human IgG enhancing factor and eosinophil colony-stimulating factor activities. Relationship to IL-5. Proc Natl Acad Sci U S A 1987; 84:7388–92.
100. Billiau A, Van Damme J, Ceuppens J, Baroja M. Interleukin-6, a ubiquitous cytokine with paracrine as well as endocrine functions. In: Lymphokine receptor interactions. Eurotext, Ltd., Libby J, ed. London: 1989:133–42.
101. Kishimoto T, Hirano T. Molecular regulation of B lymphocyte response. Annu Rev Immunol 1989; 6:485–512.
102. Elias JA, Trinchieri G, Beck JM, et al. A synergistic interaction of IL-6 and IL-1 mediates the thymocyte-stimulating activity produced by recombinant IL-1-stimulated thymocytes. J Immunol 1989; 142:509–14.
103. Lotz M, Jirik F, Kabouridis P, et al. B-cell stimulating factor 21 interleukin 6 is a co-stimulant for human thymocytes and T-lymphocytes. J Exp Med 1989; 167:1253–8.
104. Gauldie J, Richards C, Harnish D, Landsdorp P, Baumann H. Interferon-β_2/B cell stimulatory factor type 2 shares identity with monocyte-derived hepatocyte-stimulating factor and regulates the major acute phase protein response in liver cells. Proc Natl Acad Sci U S A 1987; 84:7251–5.
105. Hirano T, Taga T, Nakano N, et al. Purification to homogeneity and characterization of human B cell differentiation factor (BCDF or BSF P-2). Proc Natl Acad Sci U S A 1985; 82:5490–4.
106. Yasukawa K, Hirano T, Watanabe Y, et al. Structure and expression of human B cell stimulatory factor-2 (BSF-2/IL-6) gene. EMBO J 1987; 6:2939–45.
107. Bataille R, Klein B. Autoimmune conditions induced by epithelial solid tumors. Rheumatol Int 1987; 7:231–3.
108. Hirano T, Taga T, Yasukawa K, et al. Human B cell differentiation factor defined by an anti-peptide antibody and its possible role in autoantibody production. Proc Natl Acad Sci U S A 1987; 84:228–31.
109. Waage A, Kaufmann C, Espevik T, Husby G. Interleukin-6 in synovial fluid from patients with arthritis. Clin Immunol Immunopathol 1989; 50:394–8.
110. Guerne PA, Zuraw BL, Vaughan JH, Carson DA, Lotz M. Synovium as a source of interleukin-6 in vitro. J Clin Invest 1989; 83:585–92.
111. Coley WB. Contribution of the knowledge of sarcoma. III. The treatment of sarcoma by innoculation with erysipelas, with a report of three recent cases. Ann Surg 1981; 14:199–220.
112. Coley WB. The treatment of malignant tumors by repeated innoculation of erysipelas: With a report of ten original cases. Am J Med Sci 1983; 105:487–511.
113. Coley WB. The therapeutic value of the mixed toxins of the streptococcus of erysipelas and *Bacillus prodigiosus* in the treatment of inoperable malignant tumors with a report of one hundred sixty cases. Am J Med Sci 1986; 112:251.
114. Carswell EA, Old LJ, Kassel RL, Green S, Fiore N, Williamson B. An endotoxin-induced serum factor that causes necrosis of tumors. Proc Natl Acad Sci U S A 1975; 72:3666–70.
115. Kunkel SL, Remick DG, Strieter RM, Larrick JW. Mechanisms that regulate the

production and effects of tumor necrosis factor-α. Crit Rev Immunol 1989; 9:93–117.
116. Aggarwal BB, Essalu TE, Hass PE. Characterization of receptors for human tumor necrosis factor and their regulation by interferon. Nature 1985; 318:665–7.
117. Beutler BA, Milsark IW, Cerami A. Cachectin/tumor necrosis factor: production, distribution and metabolic fate in vivo. J Immunol 1985; 135:3972–7.
118. Beutler BA, Cerami A, Cachectin and tumor necrosis factor as two sides of the same biological coin. Nature 1986; 320:584–8.
119. Beutler BA, Cerami A. The endogenous mediators of endotoxic shock. Clin Res 1987; 35:192–7.
120. Duff G, DiGiovine F, Dickens E, Symons J, Wood D, Manson J. Tumor necrosis factor and interleukin-1 in arthritis. Immunobiology 1987; 175:10–1.
121. DiGiovine FS, Nuke G, Duff GW. Tumor necrosis factor in synovial exudates. Ann Rheum Dis 1988; 47:768–72.
122. Saxne T, Palladino MA, Heinegard D, Tala N, Wollheim FA. Detection of tumor necrosis factor-α but not tumor necrosis factor-β in rheumatoid arthritis synovial fluid and serum. Arthritis Rheum 1988; 31:1041–5.
123. Yone K, Suzuki J, Tsunekawa N, et al. Detection of TNF in blood from patients with Kawasaki syndrome. International conference on TNF and related cytokines (abstract). Immunobiology 1987; 175:D24,106.
124. Andrews BS, Mitrick G, Sarkozi J, Yamamoto RS, Friou G. Serum from patients with scleroderma contains lymphotoxin and tumor necrosis factor-α. Arthritis Rheum 1988; #59 (abstract).
125. Dinarello CA, Cannon JG, Wolff SM, et al. Tumor necrosis factor is an endogenous pyrogen and induces production of interleukin-1. J Exp Med 1986; 163:1433–50.
126. Kawakami M, Pekala PH, Lane MD, Cerami A. Lipoprotein lipase suppression in 3T3-L1 cells by an endotoxin-induced mediator from exudate cells. Proc Natl Acad Sci U S A 1982; 79:912–6.
127. Tracey KJ, Wei H, Manogue KR, et al. Cachecin/TNF induces cachexia, anemia and inflammation. J Exp Med 1988; 167:1211–27.
128. Bertolini DR, Nedwin GE, Bringman TS, et al. Stimulation of bone resorption and inhibition of bone formation *in vitro* by human tumor necrosis factor. Nature 1986; 319–515–8.
129. Stashenko P, Dewhirst FE, Peros WJ, et al. Synergistic action between interleukin-1, tumor necrosis factor and lymphotoxin in bone resorption. J Immunol 1987; 138:1464–8.
130. Tashjian AH, Voelkel EF, Lazzaro M, et al. Tumor necrosis factor-α (cachectin) stimulates bone resorption in mouse calvaria via a prostaglandin-mediated mechanism. Endocrinology 1987; 120:2029–36.
131. Andrews BS, Mirick G, Friou GJ, et al. Effect of colchicine and d-penicillamine on interleukin-1 (IL-1) and IL-1 inhibitors production by human peripheral blood mononuclear cells (PBMC). Arthritis Rheum 1988; 31:S114.
132. Thomson BM, Mundy GR, Chambers TJ. Tumor necrosis factors-α and β induce osteoblastic cells to stimulate osteoclastic bone resorption. J Immunol 1987; 138:775–9.
133. Dayer JM, DeRochemonteix B, Burrus B, Demczuk S, Dinarello CA. Human recombinant IL-1 stimulates collagenase and prostaglandin E_2 production by human synovial cell. J Clin Invest 1986; 77:645–8.
134. Dayer JM, Beutler B, Cerami A. Cachectin/tumor necrosis factor stimulates collagenase and prostaglandin E_2 production by human synovial cells and dermal fibroblasts. J Exp Med 1985; 162:2163–8.

135. Sato K, Kasono K, Fujii YK, Kawakami M, Tsushima T, Shizume K. Tumor necrosis factor-α (cachectin) stimulates mouse osteoblast-like cells (MC 3T3-E1) to produce macrophage colony stimulating activity and prostaglandin E_2. Biochem Biophys Res Commun 1987; 145:323–9.
136. Butler DM, Vitti GF, Leizer T, Hamilton JA. Stimulation of the hyaluronic acid levels of human synovial fibroblasts by recombinant human tumor necrosis factor-α, tumor necrosis factor-β (lymphotoxin), IL-1α and IL-1β. Arthritis Rheum 1988; 31:1281–9.
137. Engstrom-Laurent A, Hallgren R. Circulating hyaluronate in rheumatoid arthritis: relationship to inflammatory activity and the effect of corticosteroid therapy. Ann Rheum Dis 1985; 44:83–8.
138. Dahl IM, Husby G. Hyaluronic acid production *in vitro* by synovial lining cells from normal and rheumatoid joints. Ann Rheum Dis 1985; 44:647–57.
139. Hamilton JA. Hypothesis: In vitro evidence for the invasive and tumor-like properties of the rheumatoid pannus. J Rheumatol 1983; 10:845–61.
140. Hiro D, Ito A, Matsuto K, Mori V. Hyaluronic acid is an endogenous inducer of IL-1 production by human monocytes and rabbit macrophages. Biochem Biophys Res Commun 1986; 140:715–22.
141. Elias JA, Gustilo K, Baeder W, Freundlich B. Synergistic stimulation of fibroblast prostaglandin production by recombinant IL-1 and tumor necrosis factor. J Immunol 1987; 138:3812–6.
142. Stashenko P, Dewhirst FE, Peros WJ, Kent RL, Ago JM. Synergistic interactions between IL-1, tumor necrosis factor and lymphotoxin in bone resorption. J Immunol 1987; 138:1464–8.
143. Firestein GS, Zvaifler NJ. The pathogenesis of rheumatoid arthritis: a critical assessment of the role of autologous stimulation in the perpetuation of rheumatoid synovitis. Rheum Dis Clin North A 1987; 13:447–61.
144. Shinmei M, Masuda K, Kikuchi T, Shimomura Y. Interleukin-1, tumor necrosis factor and interleukin-6 as mediators of cartilage destruction. Semin Arthritis Rheum 1989; 18:27–32.
145. Nawroth PP, Stern DM. Modulation of endothelial cell hemostatic properties by tumor necrosis factor. J Exp Med 1986; 163:740–5.
146. Shalaby MR, Aggarwal BB, Rinderknecht E, Svedersky LP, Finkle BS, Palladino MA. Activation of human polymorphonuclear neutrophil functions by interferon-γ and tumor necrosis factors. J Immunol 1985; 135:2069–73.
147. Watson ML, Westwick J, Fincham NJ, Camp RDR. Elevation of PMN cytosolic free calcium and locomotion stimulated by novel peptides from IL-1-treated human synovial cell cultures. Biochem Biophys Res Commun 1988; 155:1154–1160.
148. DeMarco D, Kunkel SL, Strieter RM, Basha M, Zurier RB. Interleukin-1 induced gene expression of neutrophil activating peptide (IL-8) and monocyte chemotactic peptide in human synovial cells. Brochem Biophys Res Commun 1991; 174:411–416.
149. Schroeder JM, Christophers E. Identification of C5a des arg and an anionic neutrophil-activating peptide (ANAP) in psoriatic scales. J Invest Dermatol 1985; 87:53–8.
150. Youngner JS, Salvin SB. Production and properties of migration inhibitory factor and interferon in the circulation of mice with delayed hypersensitivity. J Immunol 1973; 111:1914–22.
151. Rosenbloom J, Feldman G, Fruendlich B, Jimenez SA. Inhibition of excessive scleroderma fibroblast collagen production by recombinant γ-interferon. Arthritis Rheum 1986; 29:851–6.
152. Jurado A, Carballido J, Griffel H, Hochkeppel HK, Wetzel GD. The immuno-

modulatory effects of interferon-gamma on mature B-lymphocyte responses. Experientia 1989; 45:521–36.
153. Dinarello CA, Mier JW. Current concepts. Lymphokines. N Engl J Med 1987; 317:940–5.
154. Trinchieri G, Perussia B. Immune interferon: A pleiotropic lymphokine with multiple effects. Immunol Today 1985; 6:131–136.
155. Steeg PS, Moore RN, Johnson HM. Oppenheim JJ. Regulation of murine macrophage Ia antigen expression by a lymphokine with immune interferon activity. J Exp Med 1982; 156:1780–93.
156. Wong GHW, Clark-Lewis I, McKimm-Breschkin JL, Harris AW, Schrader JW. Interferon-γ induces enhanced expression of Ia and H-2 antigens on B lymphoid, macrophage, and myeloid cell lines. J Immunol 1983; 131:788–93.
157. Franchimont P, Reuter A, Vrindts-Gevaert Y, et al. Production of tumour necrosis factor-α, interferon-γ and interleukin-2 by peripheral blood mononuclear cells in subjects suffering from rheumatoid arthritis. Scand J Rheumatol 1988; 17:203–12.
158. Stolzenburg T, Binz H, Fontana A, Felder M, Wagenhaeuser F-J. Impaired mitogen-induced interferon γ production in rheumatoid arthritis and related diseases. Scand J Immunol 1988; 27:73–81.
159. Hovdenes J, Gaudernack G, Kvien TK, Hovdenes AB, Egeland T. Mitogen-induced interleukin 2 and gamma interferon production by $CD4^+$ and $CD8^+$ cells of patients with inflammatory arthritides. A comparison between cells from synovial fluid and peripheral blood. Scand J Immunol 1989; 30:597–603.
160. Hooks JJ, Haralampos M, Moutsopoulos MD, et al. Immune interferon in the circulation of patients with autoimmune disease. N Engl J Med 1979; 301:5–8.
161. Cesario TC, Andrews BS, Martin DA, et al. Interferon in synovial fluid and serum of patients with rheumatic disease. J Rheumatol 1983; 10:647–50.
162. Reuter A, Bernier J, Vrindts-Gevaert Y, et al. Production of interferon gamma by peripheral blood mononuclear cells from normal subjects and from patients with rheumatoid arthritis. Clin Exp Rheumatol 1988; 6:347–54.
163. Firestein GS, Zvaifler NJ. Peripheral blood and synovial fluid monocyte activation in inflammatory arthritis. Arthritis Rheum 1987; 30:864–71.
164. Firestein GS, Zvaifler NJ. Peripheral blood and synovial fluid monocyte activation in inflammatory arthritis. I. A cytofluyorographic study of monocyte differentiation antigens and class II antigens and their regulation by γ-interferon. Arthritis Rheum 1987; 30:857–63.
165. Janossy G, Duke O, Poulter LW, Panayi G, Bofill M, Goldstein G. Rheumatoid arthritis: a disease of T lymphocyte-macrophage immunoregulation. Lancet 1981; 2:839–42.
166. Veys EM, Hermanns P, Schindler J, et al. Evaluations of T cell subsets with monoclonal antibodies in patients with rheumatoid arthritis. J Rheumatol 1982; 9:25–9.
167. Lotz M, Tsoukas CD, Fong S, Dinarello CA, Carson DA, Vaughan JH. Release of lymphokines after infection with Epstein-Barr virus in vitro. II. A monocyte-dependent inhibitor of interleukin 1 downregulates the production of interleukin 2 and interferon-γ in rheumatoid arthritis. J Immunol 1986; 136:3643–8.
168. Lotz M, Tsoukas CD, Curd JG, Carson DA, Vaughan JH. Effects of recombinant human interferons on rheumatoid arthritis B lymphocytes activated by Epstein-Barr virus. J Rheumatol 1987; 14:42–5.
169. Kitas GD, Salmon M, Allan IM, Bacon PA. The T cell system in rheumatoid arthritis: activated or defective? Scand J Rheumatol 1988: 76:161–73.
170. Lotz M, Tsoukas CD, Robinson CA, Dinarello CA, Carson DA, Vaughan JH. Basis

for defective responses of rheumatoid arthritis synovial fluid lymphocytes to anti-CD3 (T3) antibodies. J Clin Invest 1986; 78:713–21.
171. Barada FA, O'Brien W, Horwitz DA. Defective monocyte cytotoxicity in rheumatoid arthritis. A correlation with disease activity and reversal by levamisole. Arthritis Rheum 1982; 25:10–6.
172. Firestein GS, Weisman MH, Zvaifler NJ. Parenteral IFN-γ in rheumatoid arthritis (RA): effect on disease activity and peripheral blood monocytes (PM) (abstract). Arthritis Rheum 1987; 30:S115.
173. Veys EM, Mielanats H, Verbruggen G, et al. Interferon gamma in rheumatoid arthritis—a double blind study comparing human recombinant interferon gamma with placebo. J Rheumatol 1988; 15:570–4.
174. Cannon GW, Pincus SH, Emkey RD, et al. Double-blind trial of recombinant γ-interferon versus placebo in the treatment of rheumatoid arthritis. Arthritis Rheum 1989; 32:964–73.
175. Pernice W, Schuchmann L, Dippell J, et al. Therapy for systemic juvenile rheumatoid arthritis with γ-interferon: a pilot study of nine patients. Arthritis Rheum 1989; 32:643–6.
176. LeRoy EC. Scleroderma (systemic sclerosis). In: Kelley WN, Harris ED, Ruddy S, Sledge CB, eds. Textbook of rheumatology. Philadelphia: W.B. Saunders, 1985:1183–205.
177. Jimenez SA, Freundlich B, Rosenbloom J. Selective inhibition of human diploid fibroblast collagen synthesis by interferons. J Clin Invest 1984; 74:1112–6.
178. Kahan A, Amor B, Menkes CJ, Strauch G. Recombinant interferon-γ in the treatment of systemic sclerosis. Am J Med 1989; 87:273–7.
179. Komm BS, Terpening CM, Benz DJ, et al. Estrogen binding, receptor mRNA and biologic response in osteoblast-like osteosarcoma cells. Science 1988; 241:81–4.
180. LeRoy EC. Collagen deposition in autoimmune diseases: the expanding role of the fibroblast in human fibrotic disease. In: Fibrosis. Ciba Foundation Symposium 114. London: Pitman, 1985.
181. LeRoy EC. Connective tissue synthesis by scleroderma skin fibroblasts in cell culture. J Exp Med 1972; 135:1351–62.
182. Uitto J, Bauer EA, Elson AZ. Scleroderma: increased biosynthesis of triple-helical type I and type II procollagens associated with unaltered expression of collagenase by skin fibroblasts in cuture. J Clin Invest 1979; 64:921–30.
183. Kahari VM, Multimaki P, Vuorio E. Elevated pro-alpha $_2$(I) collagen mRNA levels in cultured scleroderma fibroblasts result from an increased transcription rate of the corresponding gene. FEBS Lett 1987; 215:331–4.
184. Varga J, Rosenbloom J, Jimenez SA. Transforming growth factor-β causes a persistent increase in steady state amounts of type I and type III collagen and fibronectin mRNAs in normal human dermal fibroblasts. Biochem J 1987; 247:597–604.
185. Rossi P, Karsenty G, Roberts AB, Roche NS, Sporn MB, DeCrombrugghe B. A nuclear factor 1 binding site mediates the transcriptional activation of a type I collagen promoter by enhancing TGF-β cells. Cell 1988; 52:405–14.
186. Ignotz R, Massague J. TGF-β stimulates the expression of fibronectin and collagen and their incorporation into the extracellular matrix. J Biol Chem 1986; 261:4337–45.
187. Laiho M, Sakesela O, Andreasen PA, Keski-Oja J. Enhanced production and extracellular deposition of the endothelial type plasminogen activator inhibitor in cultured human lung fibroblasts by TGF-β. Cell Biol 1986; 103:2403–10.
188. Chiang CP, Nilsen-Hamilton M. Opposite and selective effects of epidermal growth factor and human platelet TGF-β on the production of secreted proteins by murine 3T3 cells and human fibroblasts. J Biol Chem 1986; 261:10478–81.

189. Matrisian LM, LeRoy P, Rahlmann C, Gesnel MC, Breathrach R. Isolation of the oncogene and epidermal growth factor induced transin gene: complex control in rat fibroblasts. Mol Cell Biol 1986; 6:1679–86.

190. Postlethwaite AE, Keski-Oja J, Moses HL, Kang AH. Stimulation of the chemotactic migration of human fibroblasts by TGF-β J. Exp Med 1987; 165:251–6.

191. Carnemolla B, Cutolo M, Castellanai P, Balza E, Raffanti S, Zardi L. Characterization of synovial fluid fibronectin from patients with rheumatic inflammatory diseases and healthy subjects. Arthritis Rheum 1984; 27:913–21.

192. Carsons SE, Clausen H, Berkowitz E. Expression of a developmentally regulated oncofetal fibronectin epitope in inflammatory synovium. Arthritis Rheum 1988; 31:S22.

193. Kehrl JH, Wakefield LM, Roberts AB, et al. Production of TGF-β by human T lymphocytes and its potential role in the regulation of T cell growth. J Exp Med 1986; 163:1037–50.

194. Kehrl JH, Roberts AB, Wakefield LM. Jakowlew S, Sporn MB, Fauci AS. TGF-β is an important immunomodulatory protein for human lymphocytes. J Immunol 1986; 137:3855–60.

195. Wahl SM, Hunt DA, Wong HL, et al. TGF-β is a potent immunosuppressive agent that inhibits IL-1 dependent lymphocyte proliferation. J Immunol 1988; 140:3026–32.

196. Fava R, Olsen N, Keski-Oja J, Moses H, Plncus T. Active and latent forms of TGF-β activity in synovial effusions. J Exp Med 1989; 169:291–6.

197. Gasson JC. Weisbart RH, Kaufman SE, et al. Purified human GM-CSF: direct action on neutrophils. Science 1984; 226:1339–42.

198. Wong GG, Witek JS, Temple PA, et al. Human GM-CSF molecular cloning of the complementary DNA and purification of the natural and recombinant proteins. Science 1985; 228:810–5.

199. Sieff CA, Niemeyer CM, Mentzer SJ, Faller DV. Interleukin-1, tumor necrosis factor and the production of colony-stimulating factors by cultured mesenchymal cells. Blood 1988; 72:1316–23.

200. Koeffler HP, Gasson J, Ranyard J, Souza L, Shepard M, Meinker R. Recombinant human tumor necrosis factor-α stimulates production of granulocyte-CSF. Blood 1987; 70:55–9.

201. Bagby GC Jr, Dinarello CA, Wallace P, Wagner C, Hefeneider S, McCall E. IL-1 stimulates GM-CSF release by vascular endothelial cells. J Clin Invest 1986; 78:1316–23.

202. Karshanskyi K, Lin N, Adamson JW. Interleukin-1 stimulates fibroblasts to synthesize GM-G-CSF mechanism for the hematopoietic resonse to inflammation. J Clin Invest 1988; 81:92–7.

203. Groopman JE, Molina JM, Scadden DT. Hematopoietic growth factors. N Engl J Med 1989; 321:1449–59.

204. Gordon MY, Riley GP, Watt SM, Greaves MF. Compartmentalization of a hematopoietic growth factor (GM-CSF) by glycosaminoglycans in the bone marrow microenvironment. Nature 1987; 326:4033–405.

205. Vadas MA, Varigos G, Nicola N, et al. Eosinophil activation by colony stimulating factor in man. Metabolic effects and analysis by flow cytometry. Blood 1983; 61:1232–41.

206. Metcalf D. Begley LG, Johnson GR, et al. Biologic properties in vitro of a recombinant human GM-CSF. Blood 1986; 67:37–45.

207. Gabrilove JL. Introduction and overview of hematopoietic growth factors. Semin Hematol 1989; 26:1–4.

208. Xu WD, Firestein GS, Teatle R, Kaushansky K, Zvaifler NJ. Cytokines in chronic inflammatory arthritis. II. GM-CSF in rheumatoid synovial effusions. J Clin Invest 1989; 83:876–82.
209. Gasson JC, Weisbart RH, Kaufman SE, et al. Purified human GM-CSF: direct action on neutrophils. Science 1984; 226:1339–42.
210. Weisbart RH, Golde DW, Clark SC, Wong GG, Gasson JC. Human GM-CSF is a neutrophil activator. Nature 1985; 314:361–3.
211. Fleischmann J, Golde DW, Weisbart RH, Gasson JC. GM-CSF enhances phagocytosis of bacteria by human neutrophils. Blood 1986; 68:708–11.
212. Alvaro-Gracia JM, Zvaifler NJ, Firestein GS. Cytokines in chronic inflammatory arthritis. IV. GM-CSF-mediated induction of class II MHC antigen on human monocytes: A possible role in rheumatoid arthritis. J Exp Med 1989; 170:865–75.
213. Firestein GS, Zvaifler NJ. Down regulation of human monocyte differentiation antigens by gamma interferon. Cell Immunol 1987; 104:343–54.
214. Janeway C, Bottomly K, Babich J, et al. Quantitative variation in Ia antigen expression plays a central role in immune regulation. Immunol Today 1985; 5:99–104.
215. Morrissey PJ, Bressler L, Park LS, Alpert A, Gillis S. GM-CSF augments the primary antibody response by enhancing the functions of antigen-presenting cells. J Immunol 1987; 139:1113–9.

CHAPTER 22

CYTOKINES IN PULMONARY INJURY

Robert M. Strieter, Theodore J. Standiford, Mark W. Rolfe, Joseph P. Lynch III, Andrew P. Metinko, and Steven L. Kunkel

The University of Michigan Medical School
Ann Arbor, Michigan

INTRODUCTION

The lungs are organs uniquely situated within the body, interposed between the host and its environment. The function of the lungs for gas exchange is surpassed by their role in mediating host defense against the moment-to-moment exposure to a hostile environment. The extensive alveolar-capillary membrane composed of both immune and nonimmune cells may be susceptible to inflammatory stimuli via either the inhalational or hematogenous routes. The ability of the lungs to respond to these inflammatory stimuli in either an acute or chronic inflammatory manner is imperative to host survival, yet the lung must maintain its structural integrity to function in gas transfer.

The ability of the lung to generate an acute inflammatory response is necessary to assure the adequate clearance of offending agents. In contrast, the evolution from acute to chronic inflammation is usually secondary to the persistence of the inflammatory stimulus, repeated episodes of acute inflammation, or immune reactions perpetuated by the inability to "process" the inflammatory stimulus. The reasons for the inability to clear certain inflammatory stimuli in the lung remain to be fully delineated. The generation of an acute host response to a virulent bacterial organism is characterized as an exuberant, acute inflammatory reaction. The histological hallmark of this pneumonitis is the presence of a neutrophilic infiltration and exudation of plasma proteins into the lung. This results in either lobar or lobular consolidation. The containment and phagocytosis of the inciting organism heralds the onset of resolution and repair with subsequent tissue remodeling that is necessary to return the lung to normal homeostasis. Thus, if undisturbed, the orchestration of this acute inflammatory process is highly organized, proceeding from an acute host response to resolution and resumption of organ function. In contrast, the establishment of a chronic immune response in the lung is characterized by the histological presence of mononuclear cells, proliferating fibroblasts, angiogenesis, and fibrosis, which are the manifestation of intense cell-mediated reaction(s). The classic form of these chronic inflammatory lesions in the lung is the granulomatous lesion. These granulomatous inflammatory reactions are associated with highly destructive tissue reactions that are often unresponsive to therapeutic intervention. The basic mechanisms that drive either acute or chronic pulmonary inflammation appear to be unique, although the participation of immune and nonimmune cells with the release of reactive oxygen metabolites, lipids, and peptide inflammatory mediators are important in either circumstance. In this review we focus on the potential existence of cytokine networks between immune and nonimmune cells in the lung and how these networks may predispose to pulmonary injury through the elicitation of inflammatory leukocytes.

MEDIATORS OF PULMONARY INFLAMMATION

The cellular events that orchestrate the host's response in pulmonary injury are directed by a complicated network of cell-to-cell communication circuits. These intricate networks are composed of soluble or membrane-bound mediators that provide signaling events through autocrine, paracrine, or hormonal influence(s). The subsequent cellular responses are paramount to the initiation, maintenance, and eventual resolution of the evolving inflammatory lesion. A partial list of host-derived putative mediators associated with acute and chronic inflammation are provided in Tables 1 and 2, respectively. Although acute and chronic inflammation are associated with differing cellular constituents, a substantial overlap and redundancy of host-derived inflammatory mediators may be operative in either circumstance.

In the adult respiratory distress syndrome (ARDS) associated with sepsis and septic shock and multiorgan failure, the list of potential inflammatory mediators is extensive. Among the most intensely investigated mediators are tumor necrosis factor (TNF) and interleukin-1 (IL-1). Although these cytokines are structurally and biochemically different, they have pleiotropic and overlapping functions on many cellular functions involved in the inflammatory response. These cytokines are important in regulating cell-to-cell communication at sites of local inflammation. Furthermore, TNF and IL-1 may be dominant in directing sequential events that are necessary for either the resolution of acute inflammation or for the propagation of a chronic inflammatory response. In contrast, the overzealous production and release of these cytokines may result in devastating effects to the host resulting in significant morbidity and mortality (1). Thus, these host-derived cytokines have a broad spectrum of biological activities and the capacity to mediate many aspects of the inflammatory response. This response may range from either local acute or chronic inflammation to the devastating response of ARDS and multiorgan failure leading to death of the host. For further information regarding the regulation and the role of TNF and IL-1 in mediating cellular and tissue injury, the reader is directed to several comprehensive reviews (2–5) and relevant chapters in this text.

TABLE 1 Host-Derived Acute Inflammatory Mediators

Lipid mediators
Platelet-activating factor
Arachidonic acid metabolites
Reactive oxygen metabolites
Superoxide anion
Hydrogen peroxide
Hydroxyl radical
Singlet oxygen
Peptide mediators
Vasoactive amines
Neutrophil/macrophage proteases
Components of the coagulation and fibrinolytic pathways
Complement cascade
Protein-dependent neutrophil-endothelial cell interaction
Cytokines
Tumor necrosis factor (TNF)
Interleukin-1 (IL-1)
Interleukin-6 (IL-6)
Neutrophil chemotactic factor (IL-8)
Platelet-derived growth factor

The elicitation of immune cells to the site(s) of inflammation is dependent upon an initial leukocyte-endothelial interaction, which is followed by the diapedesis and migration of leukocytes along established chemotactic gradients. Table 3 is a partial list of the leukocyte-dependent and endothelial-dependent adherence proteins that modulate endothelial cell-inflammatory cell interaction

TABLE 2 Host-Derived Chronic Inflammatory Mediators

Lipid mediators
Platelet-activating factor
Arachidonic acid metabolites
Reactive oxygen metabolites
Superoxide anion
Hydrogen peroxide
Hydroxyl radical
Singlet oxygen
Peptide mediators: cytokines
Platelet-derived growth factor
Transforming growth factor β
Transforming growth factor α
Fibroblast growth factors
Epidermal growth factor
Interleukins-1 through 8
Interferon-γ
Monocyte chemoattractant protein-1
Tumor necrosis factors α and β

TABLE 3 Leukocyte- and Endothelial Cell-Dependent Adherence Proteins

Leukocyte dependent
CD11a/CD18 [lymphocyte function-associated antigen 1 (LFA1)]
CD11b/CD18 [macrophage antigen 1 (Mac-1, Mo-1), complement receptor type 3 (CR3)]
CD11c/CD18 [p150,95, complement receptor type 4 (CR4, LeuM5)]
Endothelial cell dependent
ICAM-1 and 2 (intercellular adherence molecule)
ELAM-1 (endothelial-leukocyte adherence molecule)
GMP-140, CD62, or PADGEM (granule membrane protein 140 or platelet activation-dependent granule-external membrane protein)
VCAM-1 (vascular cell adhesion molecule 1)

leading to adherence of specific circulating immune cells to the endothelium. The adherence phenomenon is important in localizing the leukocytes to a specific site of inflammation. This process must be reversible to allow the leukocytes to respond to specific chemotactic gradients and migrate into the inflammatory lesion. The elicitation and adherence of immune cells during the pathogenesis of either acute or chronic inflammation may involve overlapping mediators, yet the signals responsible for the maintenance and resolution appear to be disparate. Therefore, the cellular communication networks that are established during acute inflammation that are ultimately responsible for normal tissue repair are distinctly different from networks involved in the maintenance and resolution of chronic inflammation that may lead to end-stage fibrosis and pulmonary injury.

IMMUNE CELL ELICITATION

Acute Pulmonary Inflammation

The salient feature of acute inflammation and injury in the lung is the presence of intrapulmonary neutrophils. During the initiation phase of acute inflammation, the movement of neutrophils from the pulmonary vascular compartment to interstitium and alveolar space is an early event in the propagation of lung inflammation. Inflammatory stimuli on either side of the alveolar-capillary membrane can induce pulmonary microvascular injury leading to endothelial alterations favoring neutrophil adhesion. Adherent neutrophils under the influence of chemoattractants undergo directed migration along chemotactic gradients to the inflamed area. In the process of recruitment these neutrophils become activated, releasing various proteases and reactive oxygen metabolites culminating in acute lung injury. As the acute inflammatory process changes from the initiation to maintenance and resolution stages, the cellular composition of the inflammatory lesion changes to a predominant mononuclear cell population. Hence, this inflammatory leukocyte elicitation is dynamic, whereby specific chemoattractants are expressed at specific temporal windows of the inflammatory response. In bacterial infection the recruitment of inflammatory leukocytes is potentially mediated by a number of biologically active agents. The more commonly recognized leukocyte chemotactic factors include proteins C5a (6), the lipids platelet-activating factor (PAF) and leukotriene B_4 (LTB_4) (7,8), and the small bacterial peptides fMLP (9).

Recently, several investigations have shed new light on the arena of cytokine-mediated neutrophil recruitment. The in vivo administration of lipopolysaccharide (LPS) results in a rapid elicitation of neutrophils to the lung. This LPS-induced pulmonary neutrophil accumulation appears to peak in 1 h, with the persistence of neutrophils observed beyond 15 h (10). This LPS-elicited neutrophil sequestration in the lung is interesting, since LPS itself is not directly chemotactic for neutrophils in vitro (11). Thus, the in vivo effects of LPS in the recruitment of neutrophils to the lung must depend upon the induction of a de novo chemotactic factor(s). LPS is a polyclonal activator and is a potent stimulus for the production of various cytokines, including interleukin-1 (IL-1) and tumor necrosis factor (2). Initial investigation using LPS-conditioned macrophage media found that either purified TNF or IL-1 was chemotactic for neutrophils (12). In addition, the in vivo administration of either of these cytokines resulted in the elicitation of neutrophils (13). These original findings suggested that LPS-induced neutrophil elicitation was secondary to the induction of either TNF or IL-1. Recent studies, however, have now shown that recombinant TNF and IL-1 are not chemotactic for neutrophils in vitro, yet when administered in vivo have potent chemoattractant activity for these cells (14,15).

This apparent paradox has been clarified by the purification, isolation, cloning, and expression of a novel polypeptide with potent neutrophil-activating and chemotactic properties (16–18). This peptide is relatively stable to heat and enzymatic inactivation and has a molecular weight and isoelectric point of 8 kD and pH 8.5, respectively (14,16–18). Since a number of investigators have simultaneously characterized this peptide, the terminology used to identify this protein has varied in the scientific literature. Names for this factor have included neutrophil-activating factor (NAF) (19), granulocyte chemotactic factor (GCF) (20), monocyte-derived neutrophil chemotactic factor (MDNCF) (17), neutrophil chemotactic factor (NCF) (21,22), and interleukin-8 (IL-8), (16). The last term for this cytokine has been the most widely and appropriately accepted as it is now established that the function of IL-8 extends to other cells other than neutrophils, such as lymphocytes and basophils. In addition to being significantly chemotactic for neutrophils (14,16–22), basophils (23), and lymphocytes (24), IL-8 has also been shown to induce neutrophil superoxide anion production (25), cytosolic Ca^{+2} flux (25), shape change (25), and granule exocytosis (25). On a molar basis, IL-8 is 10 to 100-fold more potent than the bacterially derived chemotactic factor fMLP in directing neutrophil chemotaxis (14,17). In addition, IL-8 is 10 to 100-fold more potent in mediating lymphocyte compared to neutrophil chemotaxis (24). Furthermore, all these neutrophil activation events were found to occur at concentrations between 0.1 and 10 nM and mediated through a process that is both Ca^{2+} and protein kinase C dependent (25). Thus IL-8 may share the same signal transduction system utilized by other neutrophil chemotactic factors, such as C5a, fMLP, LTB_4, and PAF (25). Although IL-8 has properties similar to those of other neutrophil chemotactic factors in terms of neutrophil activation, IL-8 is unique among the neutrophil chemoattractants in its physiocochemical stability to heat, biochemical reduction, detergents, or proteolytic digestion (19). As shown in Table 4, IL-8 possesses a protracted biological half-life compared to C5a, fMLP,

Table 4 Stability of Chemotactic Factors

Chemotaxin	Rate of degradation
C5a	Minutes
PAF	Minutes
fMLP	Minutes
LTB_4	Minutes
IL-8	Hours

PAF, or LTB_4, and a variety of cells have been demonstrated to continually produce IL-8 beyond 24 h.

Although IL-8 is clearly a different polypeptide from either C5a, IL-1, or TNF, it possesses significant amino acid sequence homology with other inflammatory mediators and belongs to a supergene family. As shown in Table 5, IL-8 is a member of an interesting supergene family that includes macrophage inflammatory protein 2 (MIP-2) (26), growth-regulated gene product (GRO) (27)/melanoma stimulating activity (MGSA) (28), platelet factor 4 (PF-4) (29), interferon-γ-inducible protein (γ-IP) (30), chicken v-*srs*-inducible protein (9E3), (31), and the cleavage products of platelet basic protein (32), including connective tissue activating protein (CTAP-III), (33), β-thromboglobulin (34), and neutrophil activating peptide 2 (NAP-2) (35). These peptides possess up to 60% homology with IL-8 at the nucleotide level, and share the absolute conservation of 4 half-cysteine residues (23). The biological activities of these polypeptides have not been fully elucidated, but the cysteine residues of IL-8 form disulfide bridges that are essential for its activity (23). Since IL-8 is both structurally and functionally related to this supergene family and this factor is generated in response to known stimuli (e.g., LPS, TNF, and IL-1), it is reasonable to speculate that the role of IL-8 as a chemoattractant is only one of several potential functions that this cytokine may mediate during an immune response.

During the pathogenesis of an acute pulmonary inflammation, the cellular constituents of this inflammatory lesion are in dynamic evolution. Definitive signals are generated to recruit specific populations of immune and nonimmune cells. Several investigations have shown that IL-8 is chemotactic for either neu-

Table 5 Polypeptide Homologs of IL-8

MIP-2
GRO/MGSA
PF-4
γ-IP
PBP
CTAP-III
β-Thromboglobulin
NAP-2
9E3

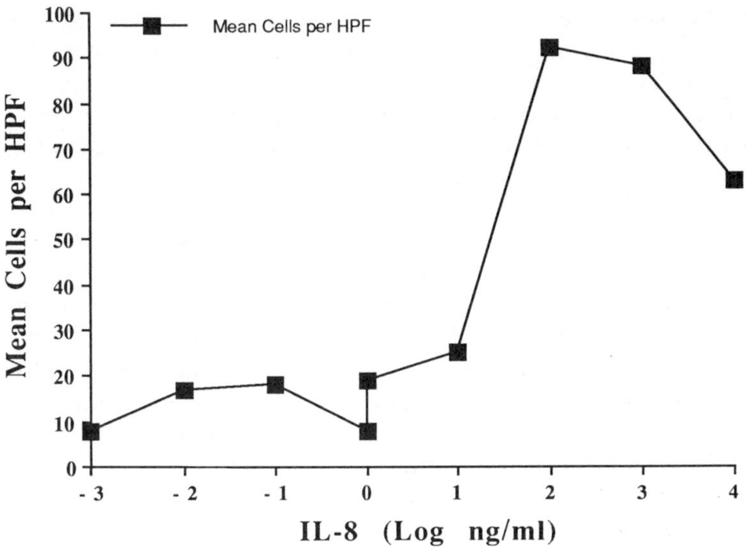

FIGURE 1 IL-8-induced in vitro neutrophil chemotaxis.

trophils or lymphocytes, yet the concentration required for maximal neutrophil migration in vitro is 10- to 100-fold greater than that required for optimal lymphocyte elicitation (24). As shown in Fig. 1, maximal in vitro IL-8-induced chemotactic activity for neutrophils occurs between 1 and 100 ng/ml, with a plateau in neutrophil migration beyond 100 ng/ml. These IL-8 concentrations are compatible with the quantitative levels of IL-8 produced by mononuclear phagocytes, endothelial cells, fibroblasts, and epithelial cells in culture in response to LPS, TNF, or IL-1. Hence, the ability of IL-8 to selectively elicit neutrophils during an acute inflammatory event is related to the magnitude of IL-8 expression in response to physiological concentrations of TNF or IL-1. This selectivity for neutrophil elicitation based on the concentration effect of IL-8 is of great importance, since these cells are often the dominant recruited leukocyte in an acute inflammatory lesion. In contrast, as the acute inflammatory lesion progresses to chronic inflammation, the change in the absolute level of IL-8 may then favor the elicitation of predominantly lymphocytes. The recruitment of neutrophils to the lung is of upmost importance as these phagocytes are often involved in the immunopathology associated with several pulmonary disorders. For example, late-phase asthma, asbestosis, idiopathic pulmonary fibrosis, and the adult respiratory distress syndrome are pulmonary diseases that potentially possess a significant neutrophil component to their histopathology.

The migration of neutrophils from the pulmonary microvascular compartment into the pulmonary interstitium and alveolar space is an important immunopathological consequence, since this process is also accompanied by neutrophil activation. In the setting of enhanced vasodilatation and vascular permeability associated with the initial phases of acute inflammation, neutrophils must first adhere to endothelial cells, followed by diapedesis along established chemotactic gradients. Although the elicitation and activation of neutrophils in the lung are immunopathological events common to a variety of pulmonary diseases, the exact mechanism(s) by which these events occur is still not clear. For an example, the normal differential cell count from bronchoalveolar lavage for individuals who have no underlying pulmonary pathology is less than 1% neutrophils (36). The striking feature of the alveolitis of idiopathic pulmonary fibrosis (IPF), however, is the considerable recruitment of neutrophils into the pulmonary interstitium and alveolar space. Bronchoalveolar lavage of these patients can often yield in excess of 40% neutrophils, yet the relative proportions of other inflammatory cells found in the lungs, including B lymphocytes, T lymphocytes, and alveolar macrophages, are normal (37–39). These findings suggest neutrophil-specific chemotactic factor(s) are potentially responsible for lung parenchymal cell injury. This cellular injury can lead to disorganized repair and end-stage fibrosis. The alveolar macrophage has been extensively studied and incriminated as one of the dominant cellular source of the factor(s) responsible for the influx of neutrophils. IPF and asbestosis are pulmonary disorders that share salient features of pulmonary pathophysiology, clinical symptoms, abnormalities in chest roentgenograms, and histopathology (39,40). In both disease states, alveolar macrophages have been shown to produce a potent neutrophil chemotactic factor. This discovery is of particular importance since both pulmonary disorders are characterized by a predominant neutrophil alveolitis (37–39,41). These findings suggest that a common mechanism may be responsible for the recruitment and activation of neutrophils in these two disparate disease states. The exact identification of these inflammatory mediator(s) and their production by the other cellular constituents of the alveolar-capillary membrane remain to be fully elucidated.

An additional pulmonary disorder with significant systemic manifestations is the adult respiratory distress syndrome (42). The underlying mechanisms operative in ARDS share a common theme of systemic inflammation related to sepsis, shock, trauma, and a host of other inciting causes (43–46). The prominent features of these entities are characterized by the involvement of both cellular and humoral mediators of acute inflammation at the microvascular level (15). The consequence of microvascular injury in the lung is diffuse alveolar-capillary membrane damage resulting in increased vascular permeability leading to extravascular fluid accumulation and augmented intravascular aggregation and transendothelial neutrophil emigration. Although we have progressively gained insight into the pathogenesis of this disease, ARDS remains enigmatic with regard to the mechanism(s) of neutrophil recruitment and activation. The role of complement activation in the pathogenesis or modulation of ARDS remains controversial. Previous studies have shown that the chemotactic and activation factor(s) are neither C5a, C5a-des-arg, a split product of C3, a fragment of fibrinogen, nor a product of fibronectin, as neutralizing antibodies to these proteins failed to alter the chemotactic activity found in the bronchoalveolar lavage fluid of patients with ARDS (47). In addition to neutrophil elicitation in ARDS, several studies have delineated the importance of neutrophil activation. The release of reactive oxygen metabolites and proteolytic enzymes impact on the integrity of surrounding cellular constituents of the alveolar-capillary membrane, resulting in altered pulmonary function. The abnormalities of pulmonary gas exchange

Table 6 IL-8 Production by Cellular Constituents of the Alveolar Capillary Membrane

	Stimulus			
Cell type	LPS	IL-6	TNF	IL-1
Monocytes	++++	—	+++	++++
Endothelial cell	+++	—	+++	++++
Fibroblasts	—	—	+++	++++
Epithelial cells	—	—	+++	++++
Alveolar macrophages	++++	—	+++	++++

in ARDS have correlated with the levels of neutrophil elastase isolated from lavage fluid from patients with this disorder (48). Similarity exists between IPF, asbestosis, and ARDS in their cellular constituents from bronchoalveolar lavage, as the makeup of the bronchoalveolar lavage fluid changes from predominantly alveolar macrophages to a relative or absolute increase in neutrophils. This association of elevated numbers of neutrophils and the preceding pulmonary disorders suggests that these diseases may share a common specific and potent neutrophil chemotactic or activating factor(s).

Our laboratory has examined the mechanism of neutrophil recruitment into the lung by assessing IL-8 production by the major cellular components of the alveolar-capillary membrane. Historically, the alveolar-capillary membrane has been viewed as a barrier for gas exchange, but with the evolution in cellular and molecular biological techniques this concept has dramatically changed. The alveolar-capillary membrane now must be viewed as a dynamic assembly of immune and nonimmune cells that through cytokine networking can result in the expression of a number of bioactive substances, including the potent neutrophil chemotactic activating factor, IL-8. As shown in Table 6, the expression of IL-8 by the major cellular constituents of the alveolar-capillary membrane is stimulus specific. Mononuclear phagocytes and endothelial cells produce IL-8 in response to LPS, TNF, or IL-1, but not to IL-6. In contrast, pulmonary fibroblasts and epithelial cells express IL-8 only in response to specific host-derived signals, such as TNF or IL-1. These findings are significant since cells once thought of as "targets" to TNF and IL-1 can actually participate as effector cells in the production of a potent neutrophil chemoattractant. Furthermore, the scenario for the recruitment of neutrophils to the lung may occur in part as a result of the production of IL-8. Therefore, IL-8 may be present in significant quantities during either local (pneumonia) or systemic inflammation, such as ARDS and multiorgan failure. In Gram-negative pneumonia or sepsis, the release of lipopolysaccharide stimulates alveolar or interstitial macrophages not only to produce IL-8 but to secrete both TNF and IL-1. TNF and IL-1 may act in either an autocrine or paracrine fashion to stimulate contiguous cells to express additional IL-8. This results in recruitment of neutrophils to the pulmonary interstitium or alveolar space. In this anatomic position neutrophil activation and release of reactive oxygen metabolites and proteolytic enzymes culminate in pulmonary parenchymal injury.

Chronic Pulmonary Inflammation

The interactions between cellular and humoral mediators that culminate in leukocyte elicitation and activation in the lung are complex. The accumulation of lymphocytes and monocytes-macrophages with the associated decline in neutrophil elicitation exemplifies the changing composition of immune cells that are recruited during the evolution of the inflammatory process. It is increasingly apparent that the migration of inflammatory cells into the lung is not restricted to novel neutrophil chemotactic factors, as monocyte recruitment is also directed by specific chemoattractant proteins (49,50). Several investigations have demonstrated the production of a monocyte-specific cytokine by a number of nonimmune cells, including fibroblasts (51), smooth muscle cells (52), and endothelial cells (51). This monocyte chemotactic activating peptide has been recently purified, isolated, cloned, and expressed in recombinant form and is referred to as monocyte chemoattractant protein-1 (MCP-1) (49,50). As with IL-8, MCP-1 appears to belong to a similar supergene family of polypeptides (23). The overall amino acid sequence homology between IL-8 and monocyte chemotactic protein are approximately 21% (23,50). MCP-1 is a 15 kD polypeptide derived from a 99 amino acid precursor with characteristic leader sequence of 23 amino acids, with the mature form representing 76 amino acids (23,50). In addition, MCP-1 also functions in activating monocytes. Purified MCP-1 can induce monocyte cytostatic activity for a number of human tumor cell lines (53). Furthermore, MCP-1 can result in the production of superoxide anion and the release of lysosomal enzyme from monocytes in the presence of cytochalasin B (23). As shown in Table 7, MCP-1 also belongs to an unique supergene family of polypeptides that includes macrophage inflammatory protein 1 (54), LD78/pAT464 (55), ACT-2/pAT744 (56), Rantes (57), and TCA-3 (58), and possesses 68% homology at the nucleotide sequence with the murine cell cycle competence gene *JE* (50). In a similar fashion to IL-8, all these proteins have four cysteine residues conserved at the same site, and the disulfide bridges they form are essential for their biological activity (23). In distinction to the IL-8 supergene family of polypeptides, the first two cysteine residues of MCP-1 are adjacent to one another. Interestingly, a major difference exists between MCP-1 and IL-8 in the disparate gene expression of these cytokines by monocytes and alveolar macrophages (59). Both alveolar macrophages and monocytes express IL-8 when stimulated with LPS, TNF, or IL-1, but these cells fail to produce MCP-1 in response to these stimuli (59). However, as shown in Table 8, endothelial cells express MCP-1 mRNA in response to LPS, TNF, or IL-1. In contrast, pulmonary fibroblasts and epithelial cells only express MCP-1 mRNA in response to either TNF or IL-1, but not to

Table 7 Polypeptide Homologs of MCP-1

MIP-1
LD78/pAT464
ACT-2/pAT744
Rantes
TCA-3
JE

TABLE 8 MCP-1 Production by Cellular Constituents of the Alveolar-Capillary Membrane

Cell type	Stimulus			
	LPS	IL-6	TNF	IL-1
Monocytes	—	—	—	—
Endothelial cell	+ + +	—	+ + +	+ + + +
Fibroblasts	—	—	+ + +	+ + + +
Epithelial cells	—	—	+ + +	+ + + +
Alveolar macrophages	—	—	—	—

LPS. Although mononuclear phagocytes do not produce MCP-1, macrophages synthesize a variety of potent monocyte chemotactic factors. These alveolar macrophage-derived polypeptide monocyte chemoattractants include platelet-derived growth factor (60), transforming growth factor β (61), granulocyte-macrophage colony-stimulating factor (62), and fibronectin (63). Thus, during the evolution from acute to chronic inflammation, the elicitation of monocytes to the lung by monocyte chemoattractant(s) may occur via the production of a monocyte chemotaxin by alveolar macrophages or via the expression of MCP-1 by pulmonary nonimmune cells. The MCP-1-induced migration of monocytes into the pulmonary interstitium and alveolar space is therefore dependent primarily upon nonimmune pulmonary cells stimulated by host-derived inflammatory cytokines, such as TNF or IL-1. These findings are relevant to in vivo cytokine networking leading to MCP-1 production. In the context of pulmonary inflammation the activated alveolar or interstitial macrophage in response to an exogenous stimulus (i.e., LPS) can release both TNF and IL-1, which results in the production of MCP-1. These two cytokines act in a paracrine manner to stimulate pulmonary epithelial cells, fibroblasts, and endothelial cells to produce MCP-1. The induction of a specific monocyte chemotactic and activating factor by pulmonary nonimmune cells may prove to be paramount to the elicitation and maintenance phase of chronic inflammation.

Cellular communication via cytokine networks operative between immune and nonimmune cells of the alveolar-capillary membrane may be essential for the generation of inflammation. The subsequent events of these cellular-humoral interactions are pivotal to the initiation and propagation of the inflammatory response leading to pulmonary injury. Both TNF and IL-1 are early response cytokines that not only are necessary for the initiation of acute inflammation but are also required for the persistence of the inflammatory response leading to chronic inflammation. The extent that either TNF or IL-1 participates in a pulmonary immune reaction is unclear. Investigations that have identified two novel chemotactic activating cytokines are exciting. These studies demonstrate that IL-8 and MCP-1 are dependent upon stimulation by either TNF or IL-1. The participation of either of these chemotactic activating cytokines in the inflammatory response may be critical for the orchestration of the directed migration of inflammatory leukocytes into the lung. After arrival to the lung these activated leukocytes induce pulmonary injury through the release of reactive oxygen metabolites and proteolytic enzymes. Current investigation is ongoing to delineate the role of these chemotactic cytokines in mediating specific pulmonary immune responses in health and disease.

ACKNOWLEDGMENTS

This work was supported in part by NIH Grants HL31693, HL35276, HL02401, and DK38149. Additional support was provided by the Council on Tobacco Research and the American Lung Association. Dr. Strieter is an RJR Nabisco Research Scholar.

REFERENCES

1. Larrick JW, Kunkel SL. The role of tumor necrosis factor and interleukin 1 in the immunoinflammatory response. Pharm Res 1988; 5:129–39.
2. Le J, Vilcek J. Tumor necrosis factor and interleukin-1: cytokines with multiple overlapping biological activities. Lab Invest 1987; 56:234–48.
3. Tracy KJ, Lowry SF, Cerami A. Cachectin/TNFα in septic shock and septic adult respiratory distress syndrome. Am Rev Respir Dis 1988; 138:1377–9.
4. Beutler B, Cerami A. Cachetin and tumour necrosis factor as two sides of the same biological coin. Nature 1986; 320:584–9.
5. Sherry B, Cerami A. Cachectin/tumor necrosis factor exerts endocrine, paracrine, and autocrine control of inflammatory responses. J Cell Biol 1988; 107:1269–77.
6. Fernandez HN, Henson PM, Otani A, Hugli TE. Chemotactic response to human C3a and C5a anaphylatoxins. I. Evaluation of C3a and C5a leukotaxis in vitro and under stimulated in vivo conditions. J Immunol 1978; 120:109–19.
7. Braquet P, Touqui L, Shen TY. Perspectives in platelet activating factor research. Pharmacol Rev 1987; 38:97–129.
8. Bray MA, Ford-Hutchinson AW, Smith MJH. Leukotriene B4: an inflammatory mediator in vivo. Prostaglandins 1981; 22:213–9.
9. Showell HJ, Freer RJ, Zigmond SH, et al. Structure-activity relations of synthetic peptides as chemotactic factors and inducers of lysosomal enzyme secretion for neutrophils. J Exp Med. 1976; 143:1154–65.
10. Remick DG, Strieter RM, Lynch JP III, Nguyen D, Eskandari M, Kunkel SL. In vivo dynamics of murine tumor necrosis factor-α gene expression: kinetics of dexamethasone-induced suppression. Lab Invest 1989; 60:766–71.
11. Issekutag A, Bhimji S. Role for endotoxin in the leukocyte infiltration accompanying *E. coli* inflammation. Infect Immun 1982; 36:588–96.
12. Sauder DN, Mounessa NL, Katy SI, Dinarello CA, Gallin JI. The role of leukocyte pyrogen and epidermal cell thymocyte-activating factor in neutrophil chemotaxis. J Immunol 1984; 132:828–37.
13. Becj G, Habicht GS, Benach JL, Miller F. Interleukin-1: a common endogenous mediator of inflammation and the local Schwartzman reaction. J Immunol 1986; 136:3025–34.
14. Yoshmura T, Matsushima K, Oppenheim JJ, Leonard EJ. Neutrophil chemotactic factor produced by LPS-stimulated human blood mononuclear leukocytes: partial characterization and separation from interleukin-1. J Immunol 1987; 139:788–99.
15. Cybulsky MI, Chan MKW, Movat HZ. Acute inflammation and microthrombosis induced by endotoxin, interleukin-1, and tumor necrosis factor and their implication in gram-negative infection. Lab Invest 1988; 58:365–78.
16. Baggiolini M, Walz A, Kunkel SL. Neutrophil-activating peptide-1/interleukin 8, a novel cytokine that activates neutrophils. J Clin Invest 1989; 84:1045–9.

17. Matsushima K, Morishita K, Yoshimura T, et al. Molecular cloning of a human monocyte-derived neutrophil chemotactic factor (MDNCF) and the induction of MDNCF mRNA by interleukin-1 and tumor necrosis factor. J Exp Med 1988; 167:1883–93.
18. Lindley I, Ashauer H, Seifert JM, Lam C, Waltz A, Baggiolini M. Synthesis and expression in *E. coli* of the gene encoding monocyte-derived neutrophil-activating factor: biological equivalence between natural and recombinant neutrophil activating factor. Proc Natl Acad Sci U S A 1988; 85:9199–210.
19. Peveri P, Walz A, DeWald B, Baggiolini M. A novel neutrophil-activating factor produced by human mononuclear phagocytes. J Exp med 1988; 167:1547–59.
20. Van Damme J, Van Beluman J, Opdemakker G, Billian A. A novel, NH_2-terminal sequence-characterized human monokine possessing neutrophil chemotactic, skin reactive, and granulocytosis-promoting activity. J Exp Med 1988; 167:1364–79.
21. Strieter RM, Kunkel SL, Showell HJ, et al. Endothelial cell gene expression of a neutrophil chemotactic factor by TNF-alpha, LPS, and IL-1-beta. Science 1989; 243:1467–9.
22. Strieter RM, Phan SH, Showell HJ, et al. Monokine-induced neutrophil chemotactic factor gene expression in human fibroblasts. J Biol Chem 1989; 264:10621–6.
23. Matsushima K, Oppenheim JJ. Interleukin 8 and MCAF: novel inflammatory cytokines inducible by IL-1 and TNF. Cytokine 1989; 1:2–13.
24. Larsen CG, Anderson AO, Appella E, Oppenheim JJ, Matsushima K. Neutrophil activating protein (NAP-1) is also chemotactic for T lymphocytes. Science 1989; 243:1464–7.
25. Thelen M, Peveri P, Kernen P, Von Tscharner V, Walz A, Baggiolini M. Mechanisms of neutrophil activation by NAF, a novel monocyte-derived peptide agonist. FASEB J 1988; 2:2702–19.
26. Wolpe SD, Sherry B, Juers D, Davatelis G, Yurt RW, Cerami A. Identification and characterization of macrophage inflammatory protein 2. Proc Natl Acad Sci U S A 1989; 86:612–6.
27. Anioswicz A, Bardwell L, Sager R. Constitutive overexpression of growth-regulated gene in transformed Chinese hamster and human cells. Proc Natl Acad U S A 1987; 84:7188–92.
28. Richmond A, Balentien E, Thomas HG, et al. Molecular characterization and chromosomal mapping of melanoma growth stimulatory activity, a growth factor structurally related to beta-thromboglobulin. EMBO J 1988; 7:2025–33.
29. Deuel TF, Keim PS, Farmer M, Heinrikson RL. Amino acid sequence of human platelet factor 4. Proc Natl Acad Sci U S A 1977; 74:2256–8.
30. Luster AD, Unkeless JC, Ravetch JV. Gamma-interferon transcriptionally regulates an early-response gene containing homology to platelet proteins. Nature 1985; 315:672–6.
31. Sugano S, Stoekle MY, Hanafusa H. Transformation by Rous sarcoma virus induces a novel gene with homology to a mitogenic platelet protein. Cell 1987; 49:321–8.
32. Holt JC, Harris ME, Holt AM, Lange E, Henschen A, Niewiarowski S. Characterization of human platelet basic protein, a precursor form of low-affinity platelet factor 4 and β-thromboglobulin. Biochemistry 1986; 25:1988–996.
33. Caster CW, Miller JW, Walz DA. Structural and biological characteristics of connective tissue activating peptide (CTAP-III), a major human platelet-derived growth factor. Proc Natl Acad Sci U S A 1983; 80:765–9.
34. Begg GS, Pepper DS, Chesterman CN, Morgan FJ. Complete covalent structure of human β-thromboglobulin. Biochemistry 1978; 17:1739–44.
35. Wenger RH, Wicki AN, Walz A, Kieffer N, Clemetson KJ. Cloning of cDNA coding

for connective tissue activating peptide III from a human platelet-derived λgtll expression library. Blood 1989; 73:1498–503.

36. The BAL cooperative group steering committee. Bronchoalveolar lavage constituents in healthy individuals, idiopathic pulmonary fibrosis, and selected comparison groups. Am Rev Respir Dis 1990; 141:S175–8.
37. The BAL cooperative group steering committee. Bronchoalveolar lavage constituents in healthy individuals, idiopathic pulmonary fibrosis, and selected comparison groups. Am Rev Respir Dis 1990; 141:S188–92.
38. Hunninghake GW, Gadek JE, Lawley TJ, Crystal RG. Mechanisms of neutrophil accumulation in the lungs of patients with idiopathic pulmonary fibrosis. J Clin Invest 1981; 68:259–68.
39. Hunninghake GW, Kawanami O, Ferrans VJ, Roberts WC, Crystal RG. Characterization of the inflammatory and immune effector cells in the lung parenchyma of patients with interstitial lung disease. Am Rev Respir Dis 1881; 123:407–21.
40. Rebuck AS, Braudi AC. Bronchoalveolar lavage in asbestosis. Arch Intern Med 1983; 143:956–64.
41. Hayes AA, Rose AH, Musk AW, Robinson BW. Neutrophil chemotactic factor release and neutrophil alveolitis in asbestos-exposed individuals. Chest 1988; 94:521–5.
42. McGuire WW, Spregg RG, Cohen AB, Cochran CG. Studies on the pathogenesis of the adult respiratory distress syndrome. J Clin Invest 1982; 69:543–53.
43. Fowler AA, Hamman RF, Good JT, et al. Adult respiratory distress syndrome: risk with common predispositions. Ann Intern Med 1983; 98:593–7.
44. Bell RC, Coalson JJ, Smith JD, Johanson WG. Multiple organ failure and infection in adult respiratory distress syndrome. Ann Intern Med 1983; 99:293–8.
45. Montgomery AB, Stager MA, Carrico CJ, Hudson LD. Causes of mortality in patients with the adult respiratory distress syndrome. Am Rev Respir Dis 1985; 132:485–9.
46. McManus LM, Deavers SI. Platelet activating factor in pulmonary pathobiology. Clin Chest Med 1989; 10:107–17.
47. Parsons PE, Fowler AA, Hyers TM, Henson PM. Chemotactic activity in bronchoalveolar lavage fluid from patients with adult respiratory distress syndrome. Am Rev Respir Dis 1985; 132:490–508.
48. Idell S, Kucich U, Fein A, et al. Neutrophil elastase-releasing factors in the bronchoalveolar lavage from patients with adult respiratory distress syndrome. Ann Rev Respir Dis 1985; 132:1098–109.
49. Furuntani Y, Nomura H, Notake M. Cloning and sequencing of the cDNA for human monocyte chemotactic and activating factor (MCAF). Biochem Biophys Res Commun 1989; 159:249–55.
50. Yoshimura T, Yuhki N, Moore S, Appella E, Lerman M, leonard EJ. Human monocyte chemoattractant protein-1 (MCP-1). Full-length cDNA cloning, expression in mitogen-stimulated blood mononuclear leukocytes and sequence similarity to mouse competence gene JE. FEBS Lett 1989; 244:487–93.
51. Strieter RM, Wiggins R, Phan SH, et al. Monocyte chemotactic protein gene expression by cytokine-treated human fibroblasts and endothelial cells. Biochem Biophys Res Commun 1989; 162:694–700.
52. Valente AJ, Graves DT, Vialle-Valentin CE, Delgado R, Schwartz CJ. Purification of a monocyte chemotactic factor secreted by nonhuman primate vascular cells in culture. Biochemistry 1988; 27:4162–8.
53. Matsushima K, Larsen CG, DuBois GC, Oppenheim JJ. Purification and characterization of a novel monocyte chemotactic and activating factor produced by human myelomonocytic cell line. J Exp Med 1989; 169:1485–90.
54. Wolpe SD, Davatelis G, Sherry B, et al. Macrophages secrete a novel heparin-binding

protein with inflammatory and neutrophil chemokinetic properties. J Exp Med 1988; 167:570–81.
55. Obaru K, Fakuda M, Maeda S, Shimada K. A cDNA clone used to study mRNA inducible in human tonsillar lymphocytes by tumor promoter. J Biochem (Jpn) 1986; 99:885–94.
56. Zipfel PF, Balke J, Irving SG, Kelly K, Siebenlist U. Mitogenic activation of human T cells induces two closely related genes which share structural similarities with a new family of secreted factors. J Immunol 1989; 142:1582–90.
57. Schall TJ, Jonstral J, Dyer BJ, et al. A human T cell-specific molecule is a member of a new gene family. J Immunol 1988; 141:1018–25.
58. Burd PR, Freeman GJ, Wilson SD, et al. Cloning and characterization of a novel T cell activation gene. J Immunol 1987; 139:3126–31.
59. Strieter RM, Chensue SW, Standiford TJ, Basha MA, Showell HJ, Kunkel SL. Disparate gene expression of chemotactic cytokines by human mononuclear phagocytes. Biochem Biophys Res Commun 1990; 166:886–91.
60. Martinet Y, Grom WN, Grotendorst GR, Martin GR, Crystal RG. Exaggerated spontaneous release of platelet-derived growth factor by alveolar macrophages from patients with idiopathic pulmonary fibrosis. N Engl J Med 1987; 317:202–9.
61. Assoian JH, Fleurdelys BE, Stevenson HC, et al. Expression and secretion of type β transforming growth factor by activated human macrophages. Proc Natl Acad Sci U S A 1987; 84:6020.
62. Wang JM, Colella S, Allavena P, Mantovani A. Chemotactic activity of human granulocyte-macrophage colony-stimulating factor. Immunology 1987; 60:439–44.
63. Clark RAF, Wilkner NE, Doherty DE, Norris DA, Howell SE. Cryptic chemotactic activity of fibronectin for human monocytes resides in the 120 kD cell-binding fragment. J Biol Chem 1985; 263:12115–23.

CHAPTER 23

CYTOKINE NETWORKS IN SKIN DISEASE

Brian J. Nickoloff

The University of Michigan Medical School
Ann Arbor, Michigan

INTRODUCTION

The molecular basis for inflammation and immunological reactions in the skin involves cytokines produced by a wide variety of both indigenous and recruited cell types. It is quite fashionable to propose the existence of various cytokine networks in human disease states (1). Based on the responsiveness of isolated cell types in vitro, such as leukocytes, endothelial cells, epithelial cells, and fibroblasts, to stimulation or activation by various lymphokines and monokines, the skin as an organ system has already yielded to the dissection of specific cytokine networks in vivo. Because of its accessibility and the rapid assimilation of molecular probes, immunological advances, and technical breakthroughs, a number of investigative dermatologists have succeeded in mapping a plethora of adhesion molecules, chemotactic factors, and the cytokines capable of modulating their expression in several different skin diseases (2). It is appropriate that the group of polypeptide hormonelike products that were initially termed lymphokines (3), because they were originally thought to be produced only by hematolymphoid cells and selectively interacted only with bone-marrow derived cells, be reconsidered and renamed *cytokines* (4). The term "cytokine" is more appropriate because not only are these proteins and glycoproteins now recognized as being produced by mesenchymal, epithelial, and endothelial cell types, but these molecules can also significantly influence the structure and function of both bone marrow-derived and non–bone marrow-derived cell types. Indeed, it was the early recognition that keratinocytes themselves could produce interleukin-1 (originally termed epidermal cell-derived thymocyte activating factor, ETAF) (5) that helped launch the field of immunodermatology into the forefront of investigative dermatology.

This chapter summarizes these recent discoveries and emphasizes the respective as well as distinctive contribution of epidermal keratinocytes, dermal T cells, macrophages, dendritic cells, and endothelial cells to this exciting and rapidly advancing area of cutaneous immunobiology.

The onset and progression of inflammatory and immune-based processes in the skin require the collaborative interaction between the local, indigenous cell population and the infiltrating, recruited leukocytes. The notion that the skin as a special organ could actually be distinguished from many other organs because of the presence of skin-seeking subsets of T lymphocytes was crystallized in the term "skin-associated lymphoid tissue" by Streilein in 1978 (6) and expanded later by others (7–11). The remarkable similarity in the clinical and histological patterns of cutaneous inflammation for each skin disease (12), in the face of tremendous genetic diversity among dermatological patients, implies the existence of distinctive molecular mediators (13). These soluble molecular mediators include cytokines capable of directing cell-cell communication and are probably responsible for maintaining the fidelity of cellular trafficking for each disease process by modulating the expression of cellular adhesion molecules, chemotactic factors, and growth factors. Since each skin disease possesses a unique constellation of cell-to-cell associations, it should not be surprising to learn that the profile of cytokines and participating cell types, or cytokine network, is relatively disease specific. In the next sections of this chapter we compare and contrast the different cytokine networks in four relatively common skin diseases, with particular emphasis on the pathophysiological significance of these important molecules in allergic contact dermatitis, psoriasis, atopic dermatitis, and mycosis fungoides.

ALLERGIC CONTACT DERMATITIS

When human skin comes in contact with the toxicodendron plant, the waxy catechol-bearing molecules on the leaf surface are transferred to the epidermis, and approximately 1–2 days later, a T cell-mediated inflammatory reaction occurs at such contact points in previously sensitized individuals. Allergic contact dermatitis reactions in the skin are composed of two distinct functional phases, referred to as the inductive or afferent limb, which occurs during the first exposure to the proinflammatory agent, and the elicitation or efferent limb, which occurs during subsequent exposures (14). This immunological reaction is known appropriately as allergic contact dermatitis and has been used to investigate the cellular basis of inflammation in the skin for several decades, following the pioneering work of Landsteiner and Chase in the early 1940s (15). Once an individual is sensitized to the poison ivy antigen, which has been identified as pentadecylcatechol (called urushiol), subsequent exposures produce a rapid, dramatic, and transient series of cellular and molecular alterations in the skin referred to as rhus dermatitis. The urushiol molecule is just one of several dozen or more exogenous contactants believed to act as haptens (i.e., dinitrocholorobenzene, nickel, *p*-phenylenediamine, and others), penetrating the stratum corneum of the epidermis and conjugating to extracellular epidermal proteins before being recognized as "foreign" by the immune system (16).

Conventional dogma has portrayed this immunological delayed-type hypersensitivity phenomena as a result of initial hapten-specific T cell-Langerhans cell interaction (17), with lymphokine production (18) and subsequent epidermal changes, including epidermal injury, edema, and reparative hyperplasia (19). In this schema, the epidermal keratinocytes are viewed wholly as passive targets for this immunological onslaught, with no significant participatory or immunomodulatory capability. Indeed, it has been widely held for many generations that the only role for keratinocytes was to function to maintain the structural integrity of the skin as a protective coat by producing an appropriate environmental barrier. This relatively inert "brick and mortar" model for keratinocytes must now be significantly modified, and the myth that keratinocytes cannot actively participate in the genesis and evolution of cutaneous inflammatory reactions will yield to the experimental results obtained with the last 5 years (20). These new results deal largely with the characterization of the ability of keratinocytes both in vitro, and in vivo to produce an entire spectrum of multifunctional protein cytokine molecules known as interleukins, interferons, adhesion molecules, chemotactic peptides, and growth factors. The keratinocyte must now be added to the growing list of nonhematopoietic cells that can function as an immunocompetent and immunoregulatory cell type.

Based on our recent discoveries to be detailed subsequently, we can actually turn the old dogma completely around by proposing that instead of the keratinocyte being the least important and passive cell in the skin, that it is the most important initiating cell type in allergic contact dermatitis, and that its direct activation by urushiol sets into motion a cascade of cytokines responsible for cellular leukocyte infiltration (21). Our approach to the problem of characterizing the earliest detectable molecular events following topical application of a poison ivy or oak extract has been to perform serial biopsies of skin before clinical changes are detectable and before trafficking of leukocytes begins. We thus initiate our sampling at 4–6 h after application of urushiol and immunostain sequential biopsies over the next 3 weeks, dividing the reaction into three phases (22). Phase I biopsies are obtained during the first 24 h that precede clinical or histological changes. Phase II biopsies are obtained at 48–72 h when the clinical and histological changes are at their maximal levels. Phase III biopsies are obtained at 2–3 weeks following the single application and represent the resolution of this reaction.

In phase I biopsies during the first 4–8 h following topical application of urushiol, even though there no significant light microscopic changes were detectable, the immunohistochemical staining analysis revealed a remarkable series of reproducible changes (22). The antibodies employed included detection of the following molecules: tumor necrosis factor α (TNF-α), interleukin-8 (IL-8), intercellular adhesion molecule-1 (ICAM-1), vascular cell adhesion molecule-1 (VCAM-1), and endothelial leukocyte adhesion molecule-1 (ELAM-1). In the pretreatment normal skin, there was no significant epidermal staining with any of these antibodies, and the only dermal staining was weak endothelial ICAM-1 positivity. The earliest staining change occurred at 4 h, when the lower and midepidermal keratinocytes became positive for TNF-α. By 6–8 h, the superficial and deep vascular plexus contained endothelial cells diffusely positive from ELAM-1 and VCAM-1 and the keratinocytes had focally begun to express

ICAM-1. It should be emphasized that these adhesion molecule inductions occurred subsequent to the keratinocytes expressing detectable TNF-α but before significant movement of leukocytes into the dermis or epidermis.

The keratinocytes were judged to be actually producing TNF-α because the TNF-α immunoreactivity was largely confined to the keratinocytes and TNF-α is the only known cytokine that can simultaneously induce endothelial cells to express ELAM-1 and VCAM-1, as well as stimulating keratinocyte ICAM-1. Furthermore, when purified multipassaged cultured keratinocytes were exposed to urushiol in vitro, the keratinocytes were rapidly induced to produce TNF-α mRNA (23) and protein as detected by northern blot hybridization studies and by using a sensitive and specific bioassay of conditioned culture supernatants. We previously drew attention to the close spatial proximity of basal epidermal keratinocytes and the dermal capillary loop, with the distance separating epithelial cells and endothelial cells approximately 10–20 μm. Thus, we believe it is entirely possible that the epidermal keratinocytes that are directly activated by urushiol to produce TNF-α could, via a paracrine TNF-α-mediated process, stimulate the endothelial cells to produce ELAM-1, VCAM-1, and ICAM-1. The endothelial cell expression of these three leukocyte adhesion molecules would then facilitate the attachment of T cells and monocytes bearing the appropriate complementary ligands to the vessel wall and thereby promote the dermal influx of these mononuclear cells, which occurred in the phase III time period. The infiltrating T cells in rhus dermatitis include both CD4- and CD8-positive subsets (24), which may have distinctive positive and negative regulatory roles (25). However, all the T cells belong to the memory subset (7), which means that they express extremely high levels of various adhesion molecules on their surface (26), which is probably how they gain a selective advantage over their naive T cell counterparts in binding to the endothelial cells (27). The potentially important adhesion molecules include Sialy-Lewis X:ELAM-1 (28–30); VLA-4:VCAM-1 (31); and LFA-1:ICAM-1 (32), which are thought to contribute to lymphocyte migration (33).

Once the T lymphocytes enter the dermis, they have a strong propensity for moving toward the epidermis, which may also require utilization of cell surface adhesion molecule and extracellular matrix receptors (34,35), as well as contact with dermal dendritic cells (36). This directional migration implies the existence of keratinocyte-derived T cell chemotaxins (37,38), and IL-8 was clearly upregulated during this 24–48 h interval and spatially coincided with epidermal T cell influx. IL-8 is a T cell chemotactic factor (38) induced at the mRNA (39,40) and protein level (41) by keratinocytes stimulated by TNF-α. The keratinocyte ICAM-1 expression became stronger and more diffuse in the phase II period, exhibiting excellent spatial colocalization with lymphocyte function-associated antigen-1 (LFA-1)-bearing T cells (21). The dermal and epidermal T lymphocytes belonging to the memory subset (versus naive-type cells) probably produce interferon-γ (IFN-γ), since the surrounding keratinocytes eventually express the class II major histocompatibility antigen, HLA-DR (42,43). Despite the ability of other investigators to isolate urushiol-specific T cell clones from both the peripheral blood and lesional skin of poison ivy patients (44,45), we were unable to detect a clonal population of lymphocytes in either the blood or cutaneous infiltrates using Southern blot analysis of the T cell antigen receptor. Thus, if there is an antigen-specific population of T cells in the skin for either urushiol or nickel (46), it must be present in extremely small numbers (less than 1%). However, the IFN-γ produced by the activated T cells has important consequences for this cytokine network, because IFN-γ can synergize with TNF-α (40) in the stimulation of keratinocytes to produce a variety of important immunoregulatory molecules, including IL-8 and monocyte chemotaxis and activating factor (MCAF) (47). By recruiting more monocytes-macrophages, and activating the indigenous population of other potential antigen-presenting cells, IFN-γ and MCAF can bring about the multicellular complex of "antigen" (i.e., urushiol) in and around keratinocytes, with antigen-presenting cells and the antigen, to amplify the ongoing reaction. The critically important role of dendritic antigen-presenting cells in allergic contact dermatitis cannot be emphasized enough and may include both epidermal and dermal compartments (17,48–52).

During the resolution of the inflammatory reaction, group III biopsies revealed a concomitant dimunition in the expression of epidermal TNF-α, IL-8, and ICAM-1, but the endothelial cells were still expressing ELAM-1 and VCAM-1. There was no significant epidermal population of T cells or monocytes-macrophages, and only a sparse perivascular lymphohistiocytic cell infiltrate remained. The transient expression of ICAM-1 by keratinocytes in vivo is in agreement with our in vitro results in which ICAM-1 expression tended to diminish by day 3 after cytokine stimulation (53). The endothelial cell ELAM-1 expression in our model was somewhat unusual in that it was never associated with any neutrophil efflux (originally ELAM-1 was recognized for its ability to bind neutrophils) (54) and its in vivo persistence contrasts with its transient expression (within 24 h) in vitro. Thus, there may be important differences in the biological properties of endothelial cells when one compares cultured human umbilical vein large-vessel endothelial cells to the microvascular endothelial cells present in the postcapillary venular plexus of the skin.

Taken together, these recent findings indicate that keratinocytes can be directly stimulated by urushiol to produce TNF-α, and this epidermal keratinocyte TNF-α production is then followed by endothelial cell expression of ELAM-1, VCAM-1, and ICAM-1. Moreover, we extended this concept beyond urushiol to also include a centrally important initiating role for keratinocytes as signal transducers involving many other stimuli of cutaneous inflammation, such as croton oil, retinoids, and ultraviolet (UV) light (23). Recently, using a murine model of irritant and allergic contact dermatitis, rapid (within 30 min) induction of keratinocyte TNF-α mRNA was confirmed by another group (55). The orchestration of cellular events and the cytokine network under the control of the epidermal keratinocyte for cutaneous inflammation is shown in Fig. 1.

PSORIASIS

Psoriasis is a common (involving approximately 1–2% of the population) and chronic inflammatory skin disease (56) that features altered keratinocyte maturation (57) and marked keratinocyte hyperplasia (58,59). As was the case for allergic contact dermatitis, previous investigators of psoriasis have suggested that the primary pathophysiologically important cell type involved was the T cell, with the epidermal keratinocytes serving only as targets for T cell-monocyte-macrophage–derived factors (60). The importance of the immune system was signifi-

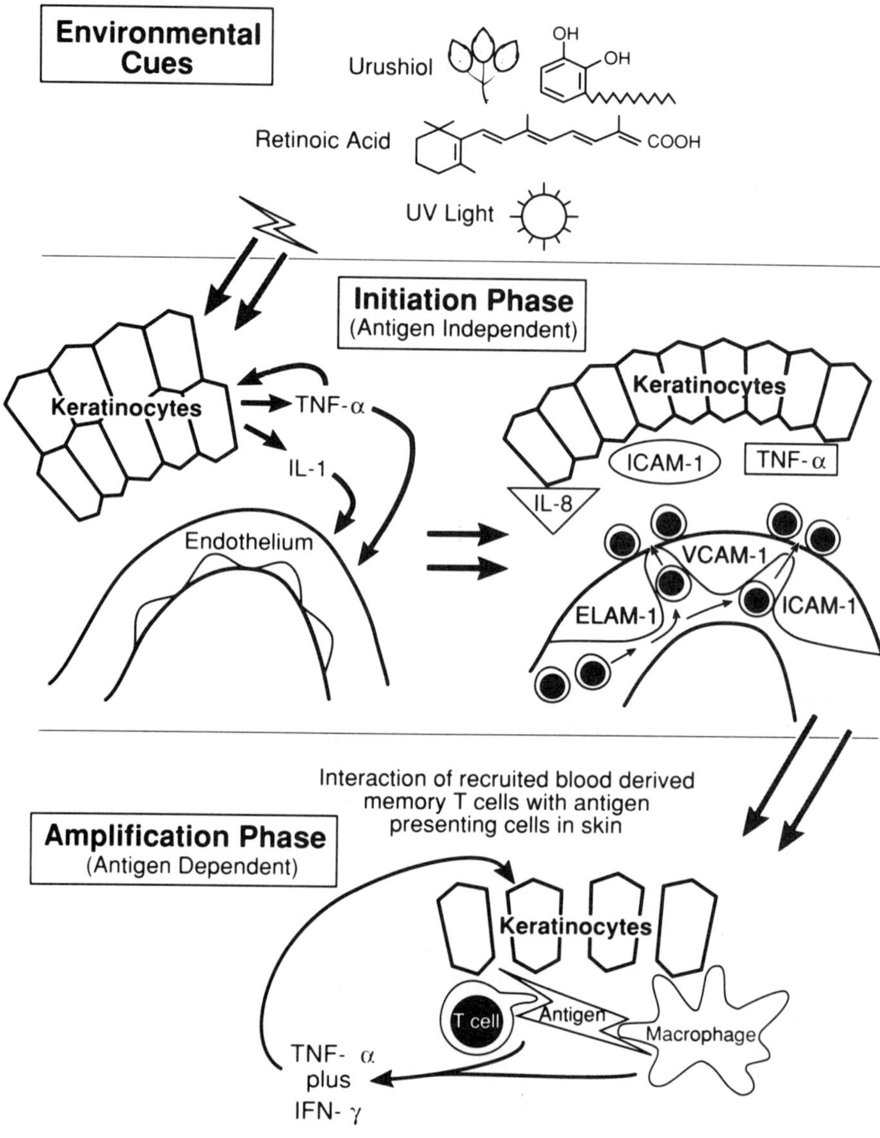

FIGURE 1 Keratinocytes can function as environmental signal transucers converting diverse exogenous stimuli (i.e., urushiol, all-*trans*-retinoic acid, and ultraviolet light) into the production of proinflammatory cytokines (i.e., IL-1 and TNF-α). (Reproduced with permission from Ref. 23.)

cantly advanced by the ability of cyclosporine A and other immunomodulatory therapies to dramatically improve psoriasis (61), but we raised some doubt about this conclusion because cyclosporine A can also directly influence keratinocytes (62). Also, when keratinocytes are isolated from psoriatic lesions and separated from their microenvironment, they continue to exhibit an aberrant phenotype for multiple generations, indicating an inherent abnormality that can be distinguished from the immune cells (63,64). It is therefore still unclear which specific cell type (keratinocyte versus immunocyte) is primarily responsible for the cutaneous alterations of psoriasis (65).

In our approach to the dissection of the cytokine network in psoriasis (65), we were particularly interested in attempting to elucidate the possible molecular link between the overlying epidermal keratinocyte hyperplasia and the infiltrating T cells and monocytes-macrophages. Psoriatic plaques were biopsied and immunostained with the same antibody panel employed in the poison ivy model, and this was supplemented with additional molecular biological probes. In contrast to rhus dermatitis, in which the TNF-α was primarily located in the epidermal keratinocytes, the psoriatic lesional TNF-α was confined almost exclusively to dermal dendrocytes (macrophages) in the papillary dermis and occasional perivascular T cells, epidermal Langerhans' cells, but not keratinocytes. This macrophage-derived TNF-α was thought to be actively produced and secreted because the immediately surrounding keratinocytes were strongly positive for the TNF-α-inducible proteins IL-8 and ICAM-1 (65) and the microvascular endothelial cells were expressing ELAM-1 and VCAM-1 (66). Once again there was excellent spatial colocalization of keratinocytes expressing ICAM-1 and IL-8 with epidermotropic T cell-bearing LFA-1. The importance of LFA-1/ICAM-1 in the epidermal trafficking of T cells in psoriasis is supported by our previous experimental results in which cyclosporine A was injected intralesionally and the first detectable immunological alteration was a reduction in keratinocyte ICAM-1 followed by loss of epidermal T cell influx and eventually resolution of the lesion (67). In this disease, cyclosporine A may be clinically efficacious because it can directly inhibit keratinocyte growth and inhibit IFN-γ (68) and TNF-α production by mononuclear leukocytes (69). The presence of IFN-γ in psoriatic lesions was confirmed by the use of the polymerase chain reaction (PCR). IFN-γ mRNA was detected by PCR in four of five psoriatic lesions (70). This PCR analysis was performed on epidermal sheets prepared by separating the epidermis from the dermis using a rapid sodium chloride heat technique on 6 mm punch biopsy material. After this treatment, which takes only 2–3 minutes, the thin epidermal sheet and the thick dermal fragment can be differentially processed for cellular RNA, allowing mRNA compartmentalization of the cytokines by using northern blots and PCR. Utilizing this strategy, we identified elevated mRNA transcripts in the epidermal sheets for IL-8, ICAM-1, and transforming growth factor α (TGF-α), but not TNF-α, which nicely complemented our protein immunolocalization results. The detection of IFN-γ was particularly important for pathophysiological considerations in psoriasis, because it has recently been observed that intradermal IFN-γ injection can induce lesions in the uninvolved skin of psoriatic patients (71).

The presence of IFN-γ and TNF-α produced by activated T lymphocytes and dermal dendritic macrophages is also important in psoriasis because both cytokines can induce keratinocyte TGF-α production (64,65). The hyperproliferation of keratinocytes has been associated with significantly elevated TGF-α in the psoriatic epidermis (65,72,73), and TGF-α is a major mitogen for keratinocytes. Thus a molecular link could be established that would explain how the infiltrating mononuclear leukocytes, by producing IFN-γ and TNF-α, induced the overlying keratinocyte hyperplasia via TGF-α. Additional components of the cytokine net-

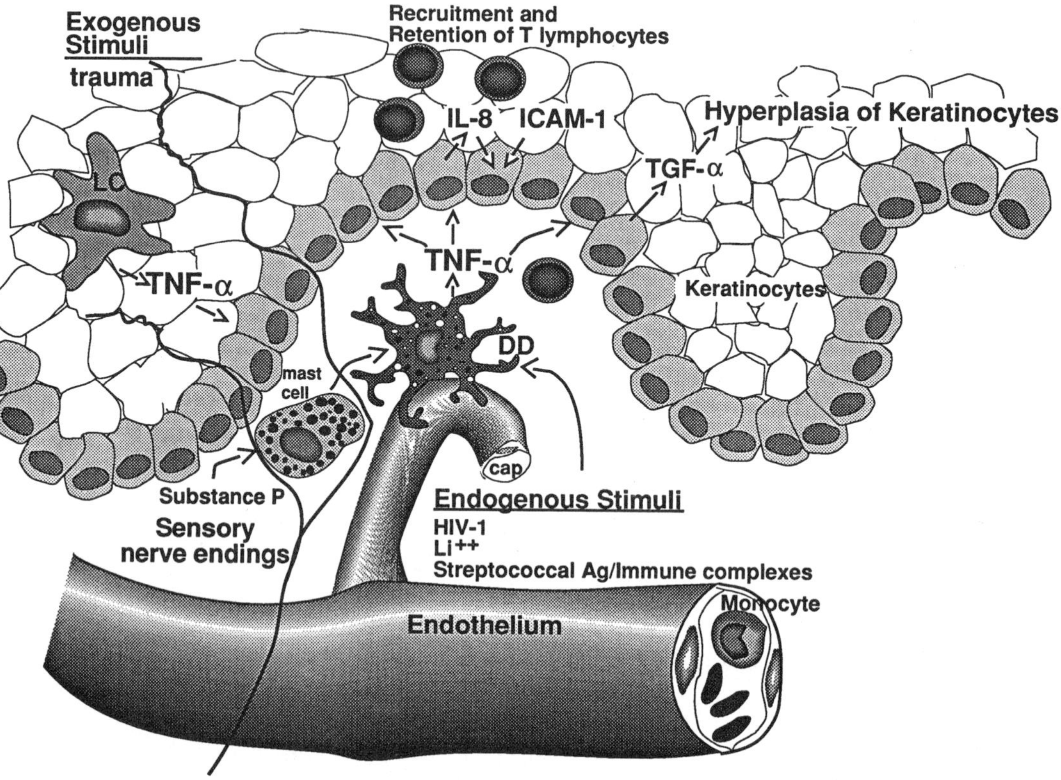

FIGURE 2 Immunoregulatory cytokine network in psoriasis with emphasis on the ability of diverse exogenous as well as endogenous stimuli to activate TNF-α production by dermal dendrocytes. [Reproduced with permission (65).]

work in psoriasis include elevated IL-6 (74), which could have been induced by the TNF-α, as well as increased IL-1α, IL-1β, and IFN-α (75), and inducible protein-10 (IP-10) (76), but not IL-2, IL-4, or GM-CSF (granulocyte-macrophage colony-stimulating factor). Our current dissection of the cytokine network in psoriasis (65), which takes into consideration both exogenous and endogenous triggering stimuli, is shown in Fig. 2.

ATOPIC DERMATITIS

Atopic dermatitis is a pruritic skin disease often associated with other clinical abnormalities, including allergic rhinitis, asthma, and elevated circulating IgE antibodies (77). None of these other systemic abnormalities are associated with psoriasis, but both atopic dermatitis and psoriasis are characterized as chronic, recurring papulosquamous disorders associated with CD4-positive T cell infiltration of the epidermis (78). There are increased numbers of activated mast cells in atopic dermatitis lesions, and IgE deposits are found conspicuously on dermal dendritic cells (79). It has been suggested that this IgE present on the surface of cutaneous dendritic cells may be bound via Fc IgE receptors, and it appears relatively specific for atopic dermatitis because no dermal IgE deposits were seen in 33 other dermatoses (79). It has been recently observed that IgE can bind to two types of Fc receptors found on mast cells, as well as monocytes-macrophages (80). A number of T cell abnormalities are reported in the blood of patients with atopic dermatitis, including impaired CD8 T cell function and decreased capacity to produce IFN-γ (78,81,82). When T cells and T cell clones have been isolated from the blood of atopic dermatitis patients, there has been a disproportionate number of IL-4-producing cells, rather than IFN-γ (83,84). The profile of lymphokines released from T cell clones derived from atopic dermatitis patients specific for the house dust mites (a putative etiological agent in atopic dermatitis) included IL-2 and IL-4, but not IFN-γ (84). This in vitro result has two important clinical correlations with the observed immunological abnormalities observed in atopic dermatitis. First, the increased IL-4 production could be responsible for the elevated IgE levels because IL-4 is a potent inducer of B cell IgE antibody production (85). Second, IFN-γ can suppress IL-4 production and the lack of IFN-γ production may be contributory to the elevated IL-4 levels (85,86).

In the mouse, CD4-positive T cells can be functionally subdivided into two types: Th1 cells, which produce IFN-γ and IL-2 upon stimulation, and Th2 cells, which produce IL-3 and IL-4, but not IFN-γ (87). Based on our previous comments, we postulate that the primary CD4-positive T cell type in allergic contact dermatitis and psoriasis is the Th1 type, whereas in atopic dermatitis the cytokine network involves a substantial contribution by Th2 lymphocytes. In atopic dermatitis, the increased IL-3 and IL-4 may be responsible for mast cell accumulation (i.e., IL-3) and activation (i.e., IL-4). Also, IL-4 can upregulate the Fc receptors for IgE on lymphocytes and monocytes-macrophages including Langerhans' cells (88). Moreover, as the interplay among T cell subsets and cytokines has been further investigated, it has become more apparent that there are reciprocal interactions: for example, IL-4 can suppress IFN-γ production, and vice versa. In a somewhat paradoxical way (compared to psoriasis), investigators have taken advantage of the ability of IFN-γ to suppress IL-4 production by administering IFN-γ systemically to atopic dermatitis patients with clinical improvement (89). In this study, 22 patients with severe atopic dermatitis with elevated IgE levels were given daily subcutaneous injections of IFN-γ (between 0.01 and 0.1 mg/m^2), and although there was no significant reduction in serum IgE levels during the 6 week treatment period, total clinical severity showed improvement ($p < 0.01$).

Another important consideration in atopic dermatitis is that like psoriasis, cutaneous lesions can be exacerbated by stress (77,90). Several neuropeptides have been identified in nerve fibers of normal human skin (91). In psoriasis there are increased numbers of substance P-containing intraepidermal free nerve endings (92), and in atopic dermatitis there was also prominent immunohistochemical staining of substance P nerve fibers, neuropeptide Y-positive dendritic epidermal cells, and an absence of somatostatin nerves (93). These neuropeptides may be important in generating an acute inflammatory release since substance P is a potent mast cell degranulator (which could produce histamine, accounting for the intense pruritus of atopic dermatitis) (94) and because several different neuropeptides are now recognized as potent immunomodulatory agents (95). Also, substance P can induce keratinocytes to release IL-1 and GM-CSF, which could contribute to the local inflammatory response (96). Indeed the entire field of psychoneuroimmunology as it applies to the skin is being actively pursued by a number of investigative dermatologists.

Taken together, the current pathophysiological pathway operative in atopic dermatitis includes a schema in which these patients display a hyperresponsiveness to a variety of ingested foods, contact with dust mites, colonization by staphylococcus, or inhaled allergens (77), which can be exacerbated by stress, and the inflammatory and immunological mediators include the active participation of T cell subsets that preferentially produce IL-4 over IFN-γ.

MYCOSIS FUNGOIDES

Mycosis fungoides is a common type of cutaneous T cell lymphoma (10). It is characterized by a malignant proliferation of CD4+ T lymphocytes (helper-inducer subset), which initially involves the skin as erythematous patches and progresses to infiltrative plaques and tumor nodules. In many cases, there is ultimately involvement of lymph nodes, visceral organs, and the blood with generalized erythrodema (i.e., Sézary syndrome) (10,97). In the earliest phases of this lymphoma, the malignant T cells display a remarkable tendency to infiltrate into the epidermis. With tumor progression, however, the epidermotropic tendency of the T cells is lost, and this lack of epidermal trafficking has been suggested to be related to the development or emergence of clinically aggressive subclones of malignant T cells (10). To probe the immunobiology of cutaneous T cell lymphoma and to compare and contrast the cytokine network involving malignant versus benign T cell trafficking in the skin, several studies have been performed in mycosis fungoides patients.

The first question that has been asked involves whether the malignant T cell in mycosis fungoides infiltrates and binds to epidermal keratinocytes via an LFA-1/ICAM-1 pathway (98). In both patch and plaque state disease, there is excellent colocalization between LFA-1 expressing CD4+ T cells and epidermal keratinocyte ICAM-1 positivity (99,100). With more advanced disease states, however, epidermal keratinocyte ICAM-1 expression is markedly diminished (100) and is almost completely absent in patients with the nonepidermotropic, Sézary syndrome (101). In no cases of cutaneous T cell lymphomas has there been any loss of expression of LFA-1 by the T cells, which is in contrast to extracutaneous high-grade lymphomas in which LFA-1 expression is absent (102). The next question that was posed centered around explaining why the epidermis was devoid of ICAM-1 in these Sézary syndrome skin biopsies. When the malignant CD4+ T cells were isolated from the blood of a patient who had greater than 90% atypical lymphocytes, these T cells were found to be unable to produce IFN-γ either constitutively or after stimulation by concanavalin A or phytohemagglutinin A (101). The reason for the inability of these nonepidermotropic malignant T cells to produce IFN-γ is unclear, although it is possible that important stimulatory signals transduced by interaction with keratinocytes was sufficiently absent in the skin of these patients to contribute to this aberrant phenotype. Support for this concept is derived from the observation that in mycosis fungoides, only the T cells in the epidermis, not the dermis, are positive for the cell cycle-associated antigen, Ki-67 (103). The dermal T cells in mycosis fungoides were Ki-67 negative, which indicates that they are in the G_0 phase of the cell cycle. Since cytokine production by T cells (i.e., IFN-γ) is strictly limited to the early portions of the G_1 phase, it may not be too surprising to observe lack of IFN-γ production by nonepidermotropic, non–cell-cycling population of T cells. Obviously, much more work remains to confirm this hypotheses with the addition of more patients and elucidation of the precise molecular interactive mechanisms by which resting T cells are stimulated by their entry into the epidermal compartment.

The distinctive ability of the epidermal and upper dermis in mycosis fungoides to influence T cell activation and proliferation has been studied by measuring both the quality and quantity of cytokines, as well as examining the dendritic cell network present in lesional skin. The cytokine profile of cytokines in the skin exudate of mycosis fungoides lesions was obtained by placing a collection chamber over gently abraded normal and lesional skin and analyzing the exudative fluid for the presence of soluble amounts of IL-1, IL-2, IL-6, TNF-α, IFN-γ, and GM-CSF. The cytokine assays included a variety of different bioassays, enzyme-linked immunosorbent assay (ELISA), and radioimmunoassay (104). IL-6, which is capable of activating T cells and inducing their directional migration (105), was found to be significantly elevated in mycosis fungoides. However, more of the other measured cytokines were elevated using this sampling technique and assay conditions. The cytokine network in mycosis fungoides is still relatively undefined, and the participating role of these molecules in the pathophysiology of this interesting and complex disease process awaits additional studies. The inability to detect TNF-α in the plaques of mycosis fungoides lesion was somewhat surprising because the keratinocytes express ICAM-1 and the microvascular endothelial cells express ELAM-1 and VCAM-1 (106). As previously mentioned in our discussion on psoriasis, the endothelial ELAM-1 and VCAM-1 expression was associated with a perivascular collection of TNF-α-containing dermal dendrocytes (64). Indeed, in some cases it may be clinically difficult to distinguish a plaque of psoriasis versus mycosis fungoides, and we recently observed that there is a dense upper dermal network of dendritic macrophages in both diseases (106,107).

Using both the immunoreactivity for factor XIIIa and Thy-1, skin lesions of mycosis fungoides contain an incredibly dense array of dendritic cells, which form a continuous cellular network throughout the papillary dermis (106). These Thy-1-positive cells also costained for VCAM-1, ICAM-1, and Leu M3 but were negative for CD1 and S-100. The factor XIIIa-positive dermal dendrocytes isolated from psoriatic plaques have been found to be strong antigen-presenting cells (108), and it is possible that these cells, by their shear density and immunological capacity, play an important role in the pathophysiology of mycosis fungoides.

SUMMARY

The skin, not only the largest organ of the body, but also uniquely positioned at the external environmental interface, must be able to produce both antigen-independent inflammatory reactions as well as antigen-dependent immunological responses. Cytokines produced by indigenous and recruited cells within the skin are important contributors to both inflammatory reactions and immunological responses. The sharing of identical cytokines between acute inflammatory reactions and more chronic or delayed-type immunological responses causes some conceptual confusion and necessitates revision of previous molecular mediators. In the past, chemical mediators of the acute inflammatory reaction included amines (i.e., histamine and epinephrine), kinins, complement components, and various poorly defined protein and tissue extract "factors" (109). Somewhat more recently, experimental and clinical studies of the pathogenesis of inflammation have been focused on a different group of nonprotein mediators, including prostaglandins, leukotrienes, and oxygen radicals and ions. Currently, the inflammatory cascade of mediators that has largely replaced the aforementioned molecular studies principally involves adhesion molecule glycoproteins and cytokines. In contrast to previous tissue extracts and "factors," recombinant biotechnology has provided investigators with a host of purified protein molecules that can be used to understand and explain the classic manifestations of inflammation, such as hemodynamic changes, permeability changes, margination, emigration, chemotaxis, and phagocytosis. Moreover, many immunological phenomena, such as autoimmunity, memory, organ-specific trafficking, and tolerance, can also be understood in terms of cytokine networks and adhesion molecules expressed by T lymphocytes, antigen-presenting cells, thymic epithelial cells, endothelial cells, keratinocytes, and other cells.

To illustrate the need to expand our perspective regarding the importance of specific molecular mediators of inflammation, as just discussed, let us briefly focus on the mast cell. Traditionally it has been suggested that mast cell degranulation and histamine release (mediated by substance P) could account for the axon reflex and the induction of hyperemia, pruritus, and plasma extravasation when "noxious" agents are applied topically to the skin. In addition to histamine, mast cells and mast cell lines have recently been found to contain such cytokines as TNF-α and TNF-α-like molecules (110,111). When small biopsies of normal skin are treated with mast cell-degranulating agents, such as substance P or morphine sulfate, the endothelial cells were induced to express ELAM-1 (112). This ELAM-1 induction may contribute to the adhesion and recruitment of leukocytes into the skin at the point of contact between the skin and the mast cell degranulatory agent. Thus, the TNF-α produced locally could serve as a cytokine-directed cell communication signal between the postcapillary venular endothelial cells and either acute inflammatory cells (i.e., neutrophils) or circulatory immunocompetent leukocytes (i.e., T cells, monocytes-macrophages, and dendritic cells). Based on the excitement and rapid progress in this particular area of investigative dermatology, there can be little doubt that in the 1990s there will be many other examples elucidated to demonstrate important links between neurocutaneous peptides, cytokines, adhesion molecules, and both bone marrow and non–bone marrow-derived dermal and epidermal cell types.

Finally, it should be emphasized that not only do cytokine networks provide an important molecular basis for inflammatory reactions and immune responses within the skin (96), but the skin itself can produce cytokines that have a systemic impact on the immune system and neuroendocrine system, as well as on the central nervous system. For example, following a severe sunburn, not only does the skin become intensely erythematous, but the sunbather subsequently experiences fever, malaise, and several other untoward systemic acute-phase responses.

These noncutaneous effects are probably mediated in part by keratinocyte-derived IL-1, because increased IL-1 can be detected in the serum following acute phototoxicity (113) and IL-1 is responsible for many acute-phase pathogenetic responses (114). However, some of these IL-1 effects may also be mediated by keratinocyte-derived IL-6 and/or TNF-α, since these particular cytokines have many overlapping functional effects (115). Another example of how skin-derived cytokines can have extracutaneous effects involves ultraviolet radiation and systemic immunomodulation. Following ultraviolet radiation, experimental animals have a depressed ability either to initiate or to propagate various types of immune reactions. It has been proposed by Daynes and coworkers that the postultraviolet radiation increase in serum IL-1 induces the hypothalamus and pituitary gland to produce elevated levels of adrenocorticotropin (ACTH), which leads to increased glucocorticosteroids and other immunomodulatory hormones, such as dehydroepiandrosterone and vitamin D_3 derivatives (116,117). These glucocorticosteroids have a differential effect on T cell subsets, such that lymphokines produced by Th1 cells (Il-2 and IFN-γ) are reduced, whereas Th2 cells increase their IL-4 production.

In conclusion, this chapter has reviewed the currently known cytokine networks operative within the skin of four different cutaneous disorders. The microenvironmental cellular constituents, their respective ability to respond to various inciting agents, and their anatomic position, cytokine production capability, and diversity were emphasized. The ability of keratinocytes to initiate cutaneous inflammation in response to a diversity of low-molecular-weight components by producing larger molecular weight cytokine polypeptides indicates the need to reassess the importance of this epidermal constituent. A role for cutaneously derived cytokines in both acute inflammatory reactions, as well as in immune-based responses both within the skin and beyond the skin, was presented. Clearly, many links exist between cytokines, adhesion molecules, chemotactic factors, neuropeptides, and immunomodulatory hormones, and the skin is an excellent organ to investigate further the delicate balance between positive and negative multifactorial communication networks necessary to achieve homeostasis in response to an incredibly diverse array of environmental stimuli. As shown in Fig. 1, the potential environmental cues capable of inducing cutaneous inflammation include physical agents, such as ultraviolet irradiation, plant wax compounds, such as urushiol, and a host of low-molecular-weight chemicals, such as all-*trans*-retinoic acid or phorbol ester derivatives. Several lines of investigation have indicated that the epidermis can serve as the ultimate signal transducer in which keratinocytes directly respond to these diverse stimuli by producing proinflammatory cytokines. These cytokines and the subsequent cytokine network that results from such stimulation will continue to intrigue investigative skin biologists for many years to come (118).

ACKNOWLEDGMENTS

This work was supported by NIH Grants AR38957, AR40065, and AR01823. The author thanks and acknowledges the following collaborators who have actively participated in the laboratory research partially reviewed in this manuscript: Drs. R. Mitra, J. Barker, C. Griffiths, G. Karabin, T. Stoof, V. Sarma, L. Stoolman, and V. Dixit.

REFERENCES

1. Balkwill FR, Burke F. The cytokine network. Immunol Today 1989; 10:299–304.
2. Nickoloff BJ, Griffiths CEM, Barker JNWN. The role of adhesion molecules, chemotactic factors, and cytokines in inflammatory and neoplastic skin disease—1990 update. J Invest Dermatol (Suppl) 1990; 94:151–7.
3. Dumonde DC, Wolstencroft RA, Panayai GS, Mathew M, Morley J, Howson WT. Lymphokines: nonantibody mediators of cellular immunity generated by lymphocyte activation. Nature 1969; 224:38–47.
4. Paul WE. Lymphokine nomenclature. Immunol Today 1988; 9:366–7.
5. Sauder DN, Carter C, Katz SI, Oppenheim JJ. Epidermal cell production of thymocyte activating factor (ETAF). J Invest Dermatol 1982; 79:34–9.
6. Streilein JW. Lymphocyte traffic, T-cell malignancies and the skin. J Invest Dermatol 1978; 71:167–71.
7. Chin W, Hay JB. A comparison of lymphocyte migration through intestinal lymph nodes, subcutaneous lymph nodes, and chronic inflammatory sites in sheep. Gastroenterology 1980; 79:1231–8.
8. Daynes RA, Spangrude GJ, Roberts LK, Krueger GG. Regulation by the skin of lymphoid cell recirculation and localization properties. J Invest Dermatol 1985; 85:145–205.
9. Tigelaar RE. Lymphocyte traffic and the skin. Dermatol Clin 1985; 3:569–85.
10. Knobler RM, Edelson RL. Cutaneous T cell lymphoma. Med Clin North Am 1986; 70:109–38.
11. Nickoloff BJ. Adhesion molecules and inflammatory cell migration pathways in the skin. In: Bos J, Skin immune system Boca Raton, FL: CRC Press, 1990: 49–71.
12. Ackerman AB. Histologic diagnosis of inflammatory skin diseases. Lea and Febiger, Philadelphia, 1987.
13. Nickoloff BJ, Griffiths CEM. Abnormal cutaneous topobiology: the molecular basis for dermatopathological mononuclear cell patterns in inflammatory skin disease. J Invest Dermatol (Suppl) 1990; 95:128–31.
14. Baer RL. The mechanisms of allergic contact dermatitis. In: Fisher AA, ed. Contact dermatitis, 3rd ed. Philadelphia: Lea and Febiger, 1986:1–8.
15. Landsteiner R, Chase MW. Experiments on transfer of cutaneous sensitivity to simple chemicals. Proc Soc Exp Biol Med 1942; 49:688–90.
16. Eisen HN. Hypersensitivity to simple chemicals. In: Lawrence HS, ed. Cellular and humoral aspects of the hypersensitive states. New York: Lawrence HS, ed. Hoeber-Harper Inc., 1959:89–122.
17. Silberberg-Sinakin I, Gigli I, Baer RL, Thorbecke GJ. Langerhans cells: role in contact hypersensitivity, and relationships to lymphoid dendritic cells and to macrophages. Immunol Res 1980; 53:203–52.
18. Thestrup-Pedersen K, Larsen CG,Ronnevig J. The immunology of contact dermatitis. Contact Dermatitis 1989; 20:81–92.
19. Hartman A, Hoedemaekr J, Nater JP. Histological aspects of DNCB sensitization and challege tests. Br J Dermatol 1976; 94:407–16.
20. Streilein JW. Skin associated lymphoid tissue (SALT): the next generation. In: Bos JD, ed. Skin immune system. Boca Raton, FL: CRC Press, 1989:25–48.
21. Griffiths CEM, Nickoloff BJ. Keratinocyte intercellular adhesion molecule-1 (ICAM-1) expression precedes dermal T lymphocyte infiltration in allergic contact dermatitis (rhus dermatitis). Am J Pathol 1989; 135:1045–53.
22. Griffiths CEM, Barker JNWN, Kunkel S, and Nickoloff BJ. Induction, distribution and dimunition of leukocyte adhesion molecules (ELAM-1, VCAM-1, ICAM-1), a

T cell chemotaxin (IL-8) and modulatory cytokine in allergic contact dermatitis (Rhus dermatitis) Br J Dermatol 1991; 124:519–526.

23. Barker JNWN, Mitra RS, Griffiths CEM, Dixit VM, Nickoloff BJ. Keratinocytes as initiators of inflammation: a unifying explanation for the diverse array of environmental stimuli to produce cutaneous inflammation. Lancet 1991; 337:211–214.
24. Gawkrodger DJ, McVittie E, Ross JA, Hunter JAA. Phenotypic characterization of the early cellular responses in allergic and irritant contact dermatitis. Clin Exp Immunol 1986; 66:590–8.
25. Gocinski BL, Tigelaar RE. Roles of CD4$^+$ and CD8$^+$ T cells in murine contact sensitivity revealed by in-vivo monoclonal antibody depletion. J Immunol 1990; 144:4121–8.
26. Sanders ME, Makgoba MW, Shaw S. Human naive and memory T cells. Immunol Today 1988; 9:195–9.
27. Pitzalis C, Kingsley G, Haskard D, Panayi G. The preferential accumulation of helper-induce T lymphocytes in inflammatory lesions: evidence for regulation by selective endothelial and homotypic adhesion. Eur J Immunol 1988; 19:1397–404.
28. Lowe JB, Stoolman LM, Nair RP, Larsen RD, Berhend TL, Marks RM. ELAM-1 dependent cell adhesion to vascular endothelium determined by a transfected human fucosyltransferase cDNA. Cell 1990; 63:475–84.
29. Phillips ML, Nudelman E, Gaeta FCA, et al. ELAM-1 mediates cell adhesion by recognition of a carbohydrate ligand, Sialyl-Le X. Science 1990; 250:1130–2.
30. Walz G, Aruffo A, Kolanus W, Bevilacqua M, Seed B. Recognition by ELAM-1 of the Sialy-Le X determinant on myeloid and tumor cells. Science 1990; 250: 1132–5.
31. Osborn L, Hession C, Tizzard R, et al. Direct expression cloning of vascular cell adhesion molecule-1, a cytokine-induced endothelial protein that binds to lymphocytes. Cell 1989; 59:1203–11.
32. Dustin ML, Springer TA. Lymphocyte function-associated antigen-1 (LFA-1) interaction with intercellular adhesion molecule-1 (ICAM-1) is one of at least three mechanisms for lymphocyte adhesion to cultured endothelial cells. J Cell Biol 1988; 107:321–31.
33. Stoolman LM. Adhesion molecules controlling lymphocyte migration. Cell 1989; 56:907–10.
34. Shiohara T, Moriya N, Gotoh C, et al. Differential expression of lymphocyte function associated antigen 1 (LFA-1) on epidermotropic and non-epidermotropic T-cell clones. J Invest Dermatol 1989; 93:804–8.
35. Hemler ME. Adhesive protein receptors on hematopoietic cells. Immunol Today 1988; 9:109–13.
36. Wilkinson PC, Higgins A. OKT3-activated locomotion of human blood lymphocytes: a phenomenon requiring contact of T cells with Fc receptor-bearing cells. Immunology 1987; 60:445–51.
37. Ternowitz T, Thestrup-Pedersen K. Epidermis and lymphocyte interactions during a tuberculin skin reaction. II. Epidermis contains specific lymphocyte chemotactic factors. J Invest Dermatol 1986; 87:613–6.
38. Larsen CG, Anderson AO, Appella E, Oppenheim JJ, Matsushima K. The neutrophil-activating protein (NAP-1) is also chemotactic for T lymphocytes. Science 1989; 243:1464–7.
38. Shiohara T, Moriya N, Gotoh C, Gomi T, Nagashima M. In vitro migration of L3T4$^+$ cloned T cells to epidermis. Possible role for keratinocyte-derived factors. J Invest Dermatol 1989; 92:360–5.
39. Larsen CG, Anderson AO, Oppenheim JJ, Matsushima K. Production of interleukin-

8 by human dermal fibroblasts and keratinocytes in response to interleukin-1 or tumor necrosis factor. Immunology 1989; 68:31–6.

40. Barker JNWN, Sarma V, Mitra RS, Dixit VM, Nickoloff BJ. Marked synergism between tumor necrosis factor-alpha and interferon-gamma in regulation of keratinocyte-derived adhesion molecules and chemotactic factors. J Clin Invest 1990; 85:605–8.
41. Barker JNWN, Jones ML, Mitra RS, et al. Modulation of keratinocyte-derived interleukin-8 which is chemotactic for neutrophils and T lymphocytes. J Immunol 1991; 139:869–876.
42. Wood GS, Volterra AS, Abel EA, Nickoloff BJ, Adams RM. Allergic contact dermatitis: novel immunohistologic features. J Invest Dermatol 1986; 87:688–92.
43. Barker JNWN, Ophir J, MacDonald DM. Products of class II major histocompatibility complex gene regions are differentially expressed on keratinocytes in cutaneous disease. J Am Dermatol 1988; 19:667–72.
44. Kalish RS, Morimoto C. Quantitation and cloning of human urushiol specific peripheral blood T cells: isolation of urushiol specific supressor T cells. J Invest Dermatol 1989; 92:46–52.
45. Kalish RS, Johnson KL. Enrichment and functions of urushiol (poison ivy) specific T-lymphocytes in lesions of allergic contact dermatitis to urushiol. J Immunol 1990; 145:3706–13.
46. Sinigaglia F, Scheidegger D, Garotta G, Scheper R, Pletscher M, Lanzavecchia A. Isolation and characterization of Ni-specific T-cell clones from patients with Ni-contact dermatitis. J Immunol 1985; 135:3929–35.
47. Barker JNWN, Jones ML, Swenson CL, et al. Monocyte chemotaxis and activating factor production by keratinocytes in response to IFN-γ. J Immunol 1991; 4:1192–7.
48. Stingl G, Katz S, Clement L, Green I, Shevach E. Immunologic function of Ia-bearing Langerhans cells. J Immunol 1978; 121:2005–12.
49. Streilein JW, Bergstresser PR. Langerhans cell function dictates induction of contact hypersensitivity or unresponsiveness to DNFB in Syrian hamsters. J Invest Dermatol 1981; 77:272–7.
50. Res P, Kapsenberg ML, Bos JD, Steikema F. The crucial role of human dendritic antigen presenting cell subsets in nickel-specific T-cell proliferation. J Invest Dermatol 1987; 88:550–4.
51. Steinman R, Inaba K. Immunogeneity: role of dendritic cells. Bioessays 1989; 10:145–52.
52. Streilein JW. Antigen presenting cells in the induction of contact hypersensitivity in mice: evidence that Langerhans cells are sufficient but not required. J Invest Dermatol 1989; 93:443–8.
53. Griffiths CEM, Esmann J, Fisher GJ, Voorhees JJ, Nickoloff BJ. Gamma interferon differentially modulates keratinocyte expression of HLA-DR and intercellular adhesion molecule-1 (ICAM-1): evidence for a protein kinase C-dependent and independent pathway. Br J Dermatol 1990; 122:333–42.
54. Bevilacqua MP, Pober JS, Wheeler ME, Cotran RS, Gimbrone MA. Interleukin-1 acts on cultured vascular endothelium to increase the adhesion of polymorphonuclear leukocytes, monocytes and related cell lines. J Clin Invest 1985; 76:2003–11.
55. Piquet PF, Grau GE, Hauser C, Vassalli P. Tumor necrosis factor is a critical mediator in hapten-induced irritant and contact hypersensitivity reactions. J Exp Med 1991; 173:673–679.
56. Krueger GG, Bergstresser PR, Lowe NJ, Voorhees JJ, Weinstein GD. Psoriasis. J Am Acad Dermatol 1984; 11:937–47.

57. Bernard BA, Robinson SM, Vandaele S, Mansbridge JN, Darmon M. Abnormal maturation pathway of keratinocytes in psoriatic skin. Br J Dermatol 1985; 112:647–53.
58. Weinstein GD, Frost P. Abnormal cell proliferation in psoriasis. J Invest Dermatol 1968; 50:254–8.
59. Cox AJ, Watson W. Histological variation in lesions of psoriasis. Arch Dermatol 1972; 106:503–6.
60. Valdimarsson H, Barker BS, Jonsdottir I, Fry L. Psoriasis: a disease of abnormal keratinocyte proliferation induced by T lymphocytes. Immunol Today 1986; 7:256–9.
61. Fry L. Immunointervention in skin disorders. J Autoimmun 1988; 1:593–601.
62. Nickoloff BJ, Fisher GS, Mitra RS, Voorhees JJ. Additive and synergistic antiproliferative effects of cyclosporine A and gamma interferon on cultured human keratinocytes. Am J Pathol 1988; 131:12–8.
63. Baker BS, Powles AV, Valdimarsson H, Fry L. An altered response by psoriatic keratinocytes to gamma interferon. Scand J Immunol 1988; 28:735–40.
64. Nickoloff BJ, Mitra RS, Elder JT, Fisher GJ, Voorhees JJ. Decreased growth inhibition by recombinant gamma interferon is associated with increased production of transforming growth factor-alpha in keratinocytes cultured from psoriatic lesions. Br J Dermatol 1989; 121:161–74.
65. Nickoloff BJ, Karabin GD, Barker JNWN, et al. Cellular localization of interleukin-8 and its inducer-tumor necrosis factor-alpha in psoriasis. Am J Pathol 1991; 158:129–40.
66. Nickoloff BJ, Griffiths CEM. Lymphocyte trafficking in psoriasis: a new perspective emphasizing the dermal dendrocyte with active dermal recruitment mediated via endothelial cells followed by intraepidermal activation. J Invest Dermatol 1990; 95:35–7.
67. Ho V, Griffiths CEM, Gupta A, et al. Intralesional cyclosporine A. The treatment of psoriasis: a clinical, immunologic and pharmacokinetic study. J Am Acad Dermatol 1990; 22:94–110.
68. Abb J, Abb H. Effect of cyclosporin on human keukocyte interferon production. Selective inhibition of gamma inteferon synthesis. Transplant Proc 1983; 15:2380–2.
69. Remick DG, Ngugyen DT, Eskanderl ME, Streiter RM, Kunkel SL. Cyclosporin A inhibits TNF production without decreasing TNF mRNA levels. Biochem Biophys Res Commer 1989; 161:551–5.
70. Barker JNWN, Karabin GD, Stoof T, et al. Detection of gamma interferon mRNA in psoriatic epidermis by polymerase chain reaction. J Derm Sci 1991; 2:106–11.
71. Fierlbeck G, Rasner G, Muler G. Psoriasis induced at injection site by recombinant gamma interferon. Arch Dermatol 1990; 126:351–5.
72. Gottlieb AB, Chang CK, Posnett DN, Fanelli B, Tam JP. Detection of transforming growth factor alpha in normal, malignant, and hyperproliferative human keratinocytes. J Exp Med 1988; 167:670–5.
73. Tarbitt ML, Akhurst RJ, White SJ, Mackie RM. Localization of elevated transforming growth factor-alpha in psoriatic epidermis. J Invest Dermatol 1990; 95:229–32.
74. Grossman M, Krueger J, Yourish D, et al. Interleukin 6 is expressed in high levels in psoriatic skin and stimulates proliferation of cultured human keratinocytes. Proc Natl Acad Sci USA 1989; 86:6367–71.
75. Gearing AJH, Fincham NJ, Bird CR, et al. Cytokines in skin lesions of psoriasis. Cytokine 1990; 2:68–75.
76. Krueger JG, Krane JF, Carter DM, Gottlieb AB. Role of growth factors, cytokines and their receptors in the pathogenesis of psoriasis. J Invest Dermatol (Suppl) 1990; 94:135–40.
77. Hanifin JM. Atopic dermatitis. J Am Acad Dermatol 1982; 6:1–13.

78. Lever R, Turbitt M, Sanderson A, Mackie R. Immunophenotyping of the cutaneous infiltrate and of the mononuclear cells in the peripheral blood in patients with atopic dermatitis. J Invest Dermatol 1987; 89:4–7.
79. Barker JNWN, Allern VA, MacDonald DM. Surface bound immunoglobulin E on antigen presenting cells in cutaneous tissue of atopic dermatitis. J Invest Dermatol 1988; 90:177–221.
80. Spiegelberg HL. Fc receptors for IgE and interleukin-4 induced IgE and IgG_4 secretion. J Invest Dermatol (Suppl) 1990; 94:49–52.
81. Leung DYM, Wood N, Dubey D, Rhodes AR, Geha RS. Cellular basis of defective cell-mediated lympholysis in atopic dermatitis. J Immunol 1983; 130:1678–82.
82. Rheinhold U, Pawelec G, Wehrmann W, Herold M, Kreggsel HW. Immunoglobulin E and immunoglobulin G subclass distribution in-vivo and relationship to in-vitro generation of interferon-gamma and neopterin in patients with severe atopic dermatitis. Clin Res Allergy 1986; 4:67–86.
83. Brown MA, Li SH, Chan SC, Hanifin J. Interleukin 4 mRNA expression by normal and atopic T lymphocytes (abstract). Clin Res 1989; 37:406.
84. Wiererger EA, Snuek M, Grout C, et al. Evidence for compartmentalization of functional subsets of $CD4^+$ lymphocytes in atopic dermatitis. J Immunol 1990; 144:4651–60.
85. Snapper CM, Paul WE. Interferon-γ and B cell stimulatory factor-1 reciprocally regulate Ig isotype production. Science 1987; 236:944–6.
86. Hernzel FP, Sadick MD, Holaday BJ, Coffman RL, Locksley RM. Reciprocal expression of interferon-γ and interleukin 4 during the resolution or progression of murine leishmaniasis. J Exp Med 1989; 169:59–72.
87. Mosmann TR, Coffman RL. TH1 and TH2 cells: different patterns of lymphokine secretion lead to different functional properties. Am Rev Immunol 1989; 7:146–62.
88. Bieber T, Rieger A, Neuchrist C, et al. Induction of FcεR2/CD23 on human epidermal Langerhans cells by recombinant interleukin 4 and γ-interferon. J Exp Med 1989; 170:309–14.
89. Boguniewicz M, Jaffe HS, Izu A, et al. Recombinant gamma interferon in treatment of patients with atopic dermatitis and elevated IgE levels. Am J Med 1990; 88:365–70.
90. Farber EM, Nickoloff BJ, Fraki J. Stress, symmetry and psoriasis: the possible role of neuropeptides. J Am Acad Dermatol 1986; 14:305–11.
91. Wallengren J, Ekman R, Sundler F. Occurrence and distribution of neuropeptides in the human skin. Acta Derm Venereol (Stockh) 1987; 67:185–92.
92. Naukkarinen A, Farber EM, Nickoloff BJ. Quantification of cutaneous nerves and their substance P content in psoriasis. J Invest Dermatol 1989; 92:126–9.
93. Pincelli C, Fantini F, Massimi P, Girolomoni G, Seidenari S, Giannetti A. Neuropeptides in skin from patients with atopic dermatitis: an immonohistochemical study. Br J Dermatol 1990; 122:745–50.
94. Hagermark O, Hokfelt T, Pernow B. Flare and itch induced by substance P in human skin. J Invest Dermatol 1978; 71:233–7.
95. Goetzl EJ, Chernov T, Renold F, Pagan D. Neuropeptide regulation of the expression of immediate hypersensitivity. J Immunol 1985; 135:8025–55.
96. Ansel J, Perry P, Brown J, et al. Cytokine modulation of keratinocyte cytokines. J Invest Dermatol (Suppl) 1990; 94:101–7.
97. Lutzner M, Edelson R, Schein P, Green I, Kirkpatrick C, Ahmed A. Cutaneous T cell lymphomas: the Sezary syndrome, mycosis fungoides, and related disorders. Ann Intern Med 1975; 83:534–52.
98. Nickoloff BJ, Lewinsohn DM, Butcher EC, Krensky AM, Clayberger C. Recombinant

gamma interferon increases the binding of peripheral blood mononuclear leukocytes and a Leu 3+ T lymphocyte clone to cultured keratinocytes and to a malignant squamous carcinoma cell line that is blocked by antibody against the LFA-1 molecule. J Invest Dermatol 1988; 9:17–22.

99. Griffiths CEM, Voorhees JJ, Nickoloff BJ. Characterization of intercellular adhesion molecule-1 and HLA-DR expression in normal and inflamed skin: modulation by recombinant gamma interferon and tumor necrosis factor. J Am Acad Dermatol 1989; 20:617–29.
100. Vejlsgaard GL, Ralfkiaer E, Aunstorp C, Czajkowski M, Marlin SD, Rothlein R. Kinetics and characterization of intercellular adhesion molecule-1 (ICAM-1) on keratinocytes in various inflammatory skin lesions and malignant cutaneous lymphomas. J Am Acad Dermatol 1989; 20:782–90.
101. Nickoloff BJ, Griffiths CEM, Baadsgaard O, Voorhees JJ, Hanson CA, Cooper KD. Markedly diminished epidermal keratinocyte expression of intercellular adhesion molecule-1 (ICAM-1) in Sezary syndrome. JAMA 1989; 261:2217–21.
102. Clayberger C, Medeiros LJ, Link MP, Krensky A. Absence of cell surface LFA-1 as a mechanism of escape from immunosurveillance. Lancet 1987; 2:533–6.
103. Nickoloff BJ, Griffiths CEM. Intraepidermal but not dermal T cells are positive for a cell-cycle associated antigen (Ki-67) in mycosis fungoides. Am J Pathol 1990; 136:261–6.
104. Lawlor F, Smith NP, Camp RDR, et al. Skin exudate levels of interleukin 6, interleukin 1 and other cytokines in mycosis fungoides. Br J Dermatol 1990; 123:297–304.
105. VanDamme J. Biochemical and biological properties of human HPGF/IL-6. Ann N Y Acad Sci 1989; 557:104–12.
106. Fivenson D, Krull EA, Nickoloff BJ. Thyl+ dermal dendrocytes in mycosis fungoides (abstract). Clin Res 1990; 38:835.
107. Cerio R, Griffiths CEM, Cooper KD, Nickoloff BJ, Headington JT. Characterization of dermal dendritic cells with factor XIIIa in normal and inflamed skin. Br J Dermatol 1989; 121:421–32.
108. Nickoloff BJ, Griffiths CEM. Isolation and characterization of dermal dendrocytes from psoriatic plaques (abstract). Clin Res 1989; 37:969.
109. Wilhelm DL. The mediation of increased vascular permeability in inflammation. Pharmacol Rev 1962; 14:251–69.
110. Young JD, Liu CC, Butler G, Cohn ZA, Galli SJ. Identification, purification, and characterization of a mast cell-associated cytolytic factor related to TNF. Proc Natl Acad Sci U S A 1987; 84:9175–81.
111. Stoffen M, Abboud M, Potter GK, Yung YP, Moore MA. Presence of tumor necrosis factor or a related factor in human basophil/mast cells. Immunology 1989; 66:445–52.
112. Matis WL, Larker RM, Murphy GF. Substance P induces the expression of an endothelial-leukocyte adhesion molecule by microvascular endothelium. J Invest Dermatol 1990; 94:492–6.
113. Ansel JC, Luger TA, Green I. Fever and increased serum IL-1 activity as a systemic manifestation of acute photoxicity in New Zealand white rabbits. J Invest Dermatol 1987; 89:32–7.
114. Dinarello CA. Interleukin-1 and the pathogenesis of acute phase response. N Engl J Med 1984; 311:1413–7.
115. Akira S, Hirano T, Taga T, Kishimoto T. Biology of multifunctional cytokines: IL-6 and related molecules (IL-1 and TNF). FASEB J 1990; 4:2860–7.
116. Araneo BA, Dowell T, Moon HB, Daynes RA. Regulation of murine lymphokine production in-vivo. J Immunol 1985; 143:1737–44.

117. Daynes RA, Araneo BA, Dowell TA, Huang K, Dudley D. Regulation of murine lymphokine production in-vivo. III. The lymphoid tissue microenvironment exerts regulatory influences over T-helper cell functions. J Exp Med 1990; 171:979–96.
118. Nickoloff, BJ. The cytokine network in psoriasis. Arch Dermatol 1991; 127:871–84.

CHAPTER 24

USE OF RECOMBINANT CYTOKINES IN CANCER THERAPY

Charles W. Taylor and Evan M. Hersh

Arizona Cancer Center
University of Arizona
Tucson, Arizona

INTRODUCTION

Immunological and biological approaches to cancer therapy are rapidly becoming established as important modalities in addition to surgery, radiotherapy, and chemotherapy. Biological therapy modifies host cellular and molecular immunological defense mechanisms and alters the proliferation and differentiation of tissues to enhance the host's ability to eradicate tumor cells.

Using recombinant DNA technology, the complementary DNA (cDNA) sequences for most known cytokines have been cloned and expressed. Thus, recombinant cytokines are available for clinical use and have revolutionized the modern approach to cancer immunotherapy research. The first recombinant cytokine produced using this technology and placed into clinical trials in the early 1980s was interferon-α (IFN-α). Subsequently, interleukin-2 (IL-2), tumor necrosis factor (TNF), and colony-stimulating factors (CSFs), such as granulocyte-macrophage CSF (GM-CSF) and granulocyte CSF (G-CSF), were developed and evaluated for therapeutic activity in cancer patients. More recently, a number of the other recombinant interleukins, including IL-1, IL-3, and IL-4, have entered clinical trials. The focus of this review is on these and other more recently described cytokines and their postulated or proven roles in cancer therapy. The use of cytokines in cancer therapy involves not only their direct or indirect antitumor effects as single agents but also the activity of cytokine and chemotherapy drug combinations. Cytokines may act in synergy with chemotherapy drugs (IL-2 and cyclophosphamide) or may decrease drug toxicity (GM-CSF combined with myelosuppressive drugs).

Effects of Cytokines on the Immune System

Cytokines are proteins secreted by diverse cell types in response to specific stimuli. In part they are the products of activated host defense cells and mediate heterogeneous biological responses, allowing "communication" between the components of the immune system. Both the cellular and humoral arms of the immune system are modulated by cytokines. The proliferation and differentiation of a number of cell types (T cells, B cells, hematopoietic cells, and macrophages) are generally increased. However, cytokines and growth factors with negative growth regulatory effects (transforming growth factor β, TGF-β) are also found. In addition, cellular mechanisms of antitumor activity, such as tumor-specific cytotoxic T lymphocytes (CTL) or nontumor-specific lymphokine-activated killer (LAK), cells can be enhanced or activated. Antibody production and function are enhanced via effects on B cell proliferation and differentiation and antibody-dependent cell-mediated cytotoxicity (ADCC).

Principles of Cancer Therapy with Cytokines

The initial hope that single recombinant cytokines would result in a major tumor response was generally not realized. Cytokines interact with each other in complex regulatory networks of positive and negative feedback control. A single cytokine may cause the release of one or more other cytokines in a cascade sequence. Rational attempts at cancer therapy with cytokines require thoughtful insight during the preclinical testing and subsequent design of clinical trials. Appropriate in vitro and animal models should be used to establish a rationale for antitumor cytokines as single agents, in combination with other cytokines, or in combination with other modalities, such as chemotherapy drugs. Appropriately designed clinical trials can then test hypotheses based on the preclinical models.

The end point of most clinical trials using standard chemotherapy drugs is antitumor response. Antitumor activity is certainly a goal of biological therapy, but appropriately designed trials should collect additional information regarding immune modulation to test the original hypotheses. For example, if a cytokine is expected to activate a cellular antitumor mechanism, attempts should be made to obtain relevant clinical specimens from patients entered on the clinical trial, test for immune cell activation in vitro, and correlate with the patient's antitumor response.

Unfortunately, many of the initial attempts at cancer therapy using cytokines were relatively ineffective. A number of factors may be responsible, including irrelevance of the animal or in vitro models to patients with cancer, incorrect hypotheses, and complicating host factors, such as large tumor burden, host immunoincompetence, and poor clinical performance status.

The goal of classic cancer chemotherapy drug trials was to administer the maximum tolerated dose (MTD) of a given agent based on the generally correct assumption that a larger drug dose would result in a large fractional cell kill and therefore greater antitumor efficacy. Because of the complex interactions of cytokines with the immune system, this concept may not equally apply to biological agents, and the concept of optimum biological dose (OBD) has arisen. The OBD is the dose of cytokine that optimizes a biological parameter operationally chosen from preclinical models or previous clinical trials. The MTD may not be equal to the OBD. Specifically, a dose lower than the MTD may give optimal immunomodulation for a given parameter. At the MTD the immunomodulation may be the same or even less than at the OBD. Furthermore, the toxicity may be greater. This further clarifies the need for a rationale developed from preclinical studies that can be tested and verified or disproven in clinical trials.

COLONY-STIMULATING FACTORS

The human hematopoietic colony-stimulating factors are proteins that regulate the growth and differentiation of blood elements, including neutrophils, basophils, eosinophils, monocytes, red blood cells, platelets, and lymphocytes. The CSFs are defined by their ability to support the in vitro growth of individual and combinations of specific blood elements. Their effects may be at the level of the pluripotent stem cell (capable of self-renewal and may become committed to various differentiation pathways) and at the level of progenitor cells (cells with limited self-renewal potential that are more restricted to specific pathways of differentiation). The first hematopoietic CSF to be described was erythropoietin. During the past few years the ability to study these agents and use them therapeutically was enhanced dramatically by their production as recombinant molecules. We discuss the therapeutic potential of interleukin-1, interleukin-3, granulocyte-macrophage CSF, granulocyte CSF, macrophage CSF (M-CSF), and erythropoietin (EPO) (Table 1) (1–3).

Interleukin-1

Interleukin-1 has heterogeneous biological effects. It increases the production of hepatic acute-phase reactants, reduces vascular resistance, induces fever, an-

TABLE 1 Colony-Stimulating Factors

Colony-stimulating factors	Cells of origin	Types of hematopoietic cells affected
Granulocyte-macrophage colony-stimulating factor	T lymphocytes, endothelial cells	Granulocytes, monocytes-macrophages, eosinophils
Granulocyte colony-stimulating factor	Macrophages, fibroblasts	Granulocytes
Erythropoietin	Kidney cells	Erythroid cells
Interleukin-1	Macrophages, endothelial cells, B lymphocytes, fibroblasts, epithelial cells	Granulocytes, monocytes-macrophages, megakaryocytes
Interleukin-3	T lymphocytes	Granulocytes, erythrocytes, monocytes-macrophages, megakaryocytes
Macrophage colony-stimulating factor	Fibroblasts, monocytes, endothelial cells	Monocytes-macrophages

orexia, and the release of other cytokines, including IL-2 and IL-3, and activates macrophages, natural killer (NK) cells, T cells, and B cells (4). The hematological effects of IL-1 include stimulation of proliferation of neutrophils, macrophages, and megakaryocytes (5). In addition, IL-1 can synergize with other CSFs, including GM-CSF and IL-3, to augment bone marrow colony-stimulating activity (6–8).

Recombinant IL-1 recently entered clinical trials as a single agent. In a study by Crown et al., seven patients with colon cancer consecutively received IL-1β alone, followed by chemotherapy with 5-fluorouracil (5-FU) alone, followed by 5-FU combined with IL-1β in consecutive cycles of therapy (9). Five patients developed a two- to threefold increase in white blood cell count, and one patient developed an increase in platelets. Toxicities were tolerable and included fever and chills, headache, nausea and vomiting, and mild hypotension.

Other clinical trials of IL-1 in combination with chemotherapeutic agents and/or other cytokines and colony-stimulating factors are underway or planned.

Interleukin-3

Interleukin-3 is also known as multi-CSF for its ability to effect the proliferation and differentiation of early hematopoietic progenitor cells and thus enhance the production of red blood cells, white blood cells, and platelets (10,12,13). Thus, IL-3 may have clinical utility either as a single agent or in combination with other CSFs, such as GM-CSF. Potential clinical settings in which IL-3 will be used are similar to those in which the other CSFs have been studied and include high-dose chemotherapy with and without bone marrow transplantation and various states of bone marrow failure.

Clinical trials of recombinant IL-3 have recently been initiated in patients with bone marrow failure (14,15). Kurzrock et al. studied 15 patients with pancytopenia due to aplastic anemia, myelodysplastic syndrome, or previous chemotherapy for malignancy (15). Of 13 evaluable patients, 4 developed substantial hematological responses, including increased granulocytes, reticulocytes, platelets, and eosinophils. Treatment was generally well tolerated, with side effects including mild fever and transient headaches. More severe side effects were occasionally seen and included persistent headaches and development of pleural effusions.

Granulocyte-Macrophage Colony-Stimulating Factor

Granulocyte-macrophage colony-stimulating factor is a glycoprotein (approximate molecular weight 22 kD) capable of stimulating the in vitro proliferation and differentiation of granulocyte, monocyte, eosinophil, and to a lesser degree erythroid progenitors (16–18). In clinical trials the predominant effect of recombinant GM-CSF is to increase numbers of mature neutrophils and eosinophils and, to a lesser degree, monocytes. The ability of leukocytes to eradicate infectious organisms might be enhanced by the effects of GM-CSF on neutrophil oxidative metabolism (19).

A common dose-limiting side effect of cancer chemotherapeutic agents is bone marrow suppression resulting in neutropenia, anemia, and thrombocytopenia. Perhaps the most serious and potentially lethal aspect of myelosuppression is the neutropenia that, when severe (less than 500 absolute neutrophils per mm^3), results in an increase in the incidence of severe or life-threatening infections.

Furthermore, transfusions of red blood cells and platelets are readily available and capable of at least temporarily overcoming chemotherapy-induced anemia and thrombocytopenia. However, white blood cell transfusions are much more difficult to administer and much less effective. Therefore, the use of GM-CSF or other CSFs in association with cancer chemotherapy drugs to prevent or decrease the severity and/or duration of chemotherapy-induced neutropenia is an exciting new approach to cancer therapy.

Antman et al. studied recombinant GM-CSF in 16 patients with metastatic sarcoma who received chemotherapy consisting of doxorubicin, ifosfamide, and dacarbazine (20). Leukocyte counts were documented during the first cycle of chemotherapy in which GM-CSF was administered following the chemotherapy drugs and compared with the second cycle of chemotherapy (no GM-CSF). With the first cycle of therapy neutropenia was less severe (mean nadir 1.0 versus 0.45×10^9 cells per liter) and of shorter duration (3.5 versus 7.4 days). Although in most clinical studies the major effect of GM-CSF is on white blood cells, occasionally multi-lineage responses are observed resulting in increases in platelet and reticulocyte counts (21).

A role for GM-CSF is also developing in bone marrow transplantation. In this setting, potentially lethal doses of cytotoxic chemotherapeutic agents are delivered, the primary toxicity of which is myelosuppression. GM-CSF has been used in this setting to accelerate bone marrow recovery (22–25). Brandt et al. studied 19 patients with breast cancer or malignant melanoma treated with high-dose combination chemotherapy (cyclophosphamide, cisplatin, and carmustine) followed by autologous bone marrow transplantation (22). The patients were treated with a 14 day continuous intravenous infusion of GM-CSF beginning 3 h after the bone marrow was reinfused. The leukocyte recovery in these patients was compared with 24 historical control patients. Patients receiving the highest dose of GM-CSF had significantly higher leukocyte counts 2 weeks after transplantation than the historical controls (3120 ± 1744 versus 863 ± 645 cells per μl). Both groups of patients developed severe neutropenia, but the duration was shorter in the GM-CSF-treated group. After GM-CSF was discontinued leukocyte counts dropped, indicating that the effects of GM-CSF were short-lived and longer treatment may be necessary.

GM-CSF has been effective in other clinical conditions associated with low white blood cell counts, including the acquired immunodeficiency syndrome (AIDS) (26), myelodysplastic syndromes (27), aplastic anemia (28), and chronic severe neutropenia (29).

GM-CSF has been administered by continuous or intermittent intravenous infusion or subcutaneous injection in doses up to 500 $\mu g/m^2$/day (20,21,30,31). GM-CSF treatment is generally well tolerated, but at high doses constitutional symptoms (fever and chills, myalgias, fatigue, and headache), bone pains, and pleural or pericardial effusions may occur.

Granulocyte Colony-Stimulating Factor

Granulocyte colony-stimulating factor has a more restricted hematopoietic cell specificity than GM-CSF. G-CSF primarily effects the neutrophil lineage of differentiation (32). Similar to GM-CSF, recombinant G-CSF has been used in clinical settings of chemotherapy with or without bone marrow transplantation (33–36).

Gabrilove et al. treated 27 patients with transitional cell carcinoma of the bladder using a chemotherapy regimen of methotrexate, doxorubicin, vinblastine, and cisplatin (33). G-CSF was administered before and after the first but not the second cycle of chemotherapy and resulted in a significant increase in neutrophil counts, a decrease in days of antibiotic use, and a decrease in mucositis.

Sheridan et al. administered G-CSF to patients with hematological malignancies treated with high-dose chemotherapy followed by autologous bone marrow transplantation (35). Compared to historical controls, the G-CSF-treated patients had an earlier white blood cell recovery and fewer days of antibiotic therapy.

Macrophage Colony-Stimulating Factor

Macrophage CSF was previously known as colony-stimulating factor 1. M-CSF regulates the growth of the macrophage-monocyte cell lineage (37,38) and enhances the ability of macrophages to release oxygen reduction products (39). M-CSF has potential antitumor activity via the increased cytotoxicity of M-CSF-activated macrophages and monocytes within the tumor.

M-CSF purified from human urine has previously been used clinically (40–42). In these studies, M-CSF resulted in hematopoietic stimulation via its ability to induce monocytes to release factors with colony-stimulating activities. Indeed, this preparation had a protective effect against granulocytopenia after chemotherapy (42).

Recombinant human M-CSF is now available and has entered phase I clinical trials. The results of these studies have not yet been published. Recombinant M-CSF has been shown to enhance monocyte tumoricidal activity against WEHI 164 cells (43). Thus, it will be of interest to study this agent in patients with malignancies.

In summary, the CSFs, via their ability to stimulate the bone marrow, will likely revolutionize cancer chemotherapy. It logically follows that a shorter duration of bone marrow suppression after chemotherapy or bone marrow transplantation could decrease the incidence of infection and the number of hospital days and increase patient survival. In addition, by being able to give more cycles of chemotherapy on time and at full dose, a larger fractional tumor cell kill should be achieved. These beneficial end points have yet to be proven, but randomized clinical trials designed to test for these are currently underway. Furthermore, the direct cytotoxic activity of some CSFs (e.g., IL-1 and M-CSF), alone or in combination with chemotherapy drugs, is also being tested in current clinical trials. Finally, the role of the CSFs in the pathogenesis and/or therapy of the leukemias, which have an apparent block in the maturation of early hematopoietic cells, is being studied and may potentially provide new targets for therapy (2).

Erythropoietin

Erythropoietin is a stimulating factor for red blood cell production and is normally produced by the kidney. Patients with end-stage renal disease commonly have moderate to severe anemias. The mechanisms of anemia in these patients are complex, but EPO deficiency plays a significant role. Recombinant EPO was first evaluated clinically in this setting.

Eschbach et al. treated 25 anemic patients with end-stage renal disease with recombinant EPO (44). Dramatic increases in hematocrit and decreased red blood cell transfusion requirements were observed. Associated with the increase in hematocrit, many EPO-treated end-stage renal disease patients develop worsening hypertension, which is perhaps related to the increased blood volume (44,45). Thus, it is recommended that in these patients EPO doses be adjusted to allow a gradual increase in hematocrit with close attention to the patient's blood pressure.

The beneficial effects of EPO in patients with end-stage renal disease include decreased transfusion requirements and thus a decreased risk of transfer of infectious agents and a decreased risk of iron overload. In addition, the quality of life parameters of energy and physical activity in patients receiving EPO is increased at 6 and 10 months after initiation of therapy (46).

Chronic anemias are also commonly seen in cancer patients, especially those receiving chemotherapy. Clinical trials of EPO in this setting have recently been initiated (47,48). It is not clear that cancer patients suffer from EPO deficiency. Endogenous EPO levels may be normal or elevated in anemic cancer patients. However, 47.4% of the cancer patients in a study by Ludwig et al. responded to EPO therapy with an increase in hemoglobin (48). Further clinical trials of EPO in cancer patients are in progress.

INTERFERONS

Antitumor Mechanisms

There are three major categories of interferons: IFN-α, IFN-β, and IFN-γ. IFN-α and IFN-β share many but not all biological properties, are together referred to as type I IFNs, and are acid stable (49). IFN-γ, or type II IFN, is acid labile. IFN-α and IFN-β have relatively more direct antiproliferative effects and IFN-γ has a relatively wider spectrum of immunomodulatory effects, but there is much overlap among the activities of the three IFNs. All three recombinant IFNs have been tested in clinical trial in patients with malignancy. IFN-α is the most thoroughly evaluated and is active in some hematological malignancies as well as certain solid tumors.

The IFNs have antiviral, anticellular (cytotoxic and cytostatic), and immunomodulatory effects. After binding to a specific cell surface receptor (type I IFNs share the same cell surface receptor but type II IFN binds to a distinct receptor), gene activation occurs and results in the synthesis or modification of a number of proteins, such as 2′,5′-oligoadenylate synthetase (50) and class I and II major histocompatibility (MHC) proteins, and release of other cytokines, such as TNF and IL-2 (51). Certain IFN-induced proteins result in an inhibition of cellular protein synthesis that contributes to the antiviral and antitumor activities of the IFNs (52).

Cytokines released by IFN stimulation of immune cells may indirectly contribute to its antitumor mechanism. IFNs also have indirect antitumor effects via augmentation of cellular cytotoxicity of natural killer cells, macrophages, or lymphokine-activated killer cells (53,54), modulation of MHC class I and II expression to enhance immune recognition of tumor cells (55), and augmentation of ADCC by enhancement of Fc receptor expression on tumor cells (54). However, Salmon et al. demonstrated a direct antiproliferative effect of IFN-α in the human tumor colony-forming assay (HTCA) (56). These potential activities can be tested in laboratory and clinical trials. Thus, clinical specimens of peripheral blood and fresh tumor specimens from patients to be treated with IFNs can be evaluated in vitro for their level of cellular cytotoxicity, histocompatibility and tumor antigen expression, Fc receptor expression, and so on. Correlations between in vitro activity and clinical response can then be made.

Therapy of Hematological Malignancies with Interferon-α

Hairy Cell Leukemia

In June 1986, IFN-α was approved by the Food and Drug Administration (FDA) as treatment for hairy cell leukemia and thus represented the first recombinant cytokine approved for the treatment of human cancer. Hairy cell leukemia is a chronic, usually B cell lymphoid malignancy that results in pancytopenia, splenomegaly, and susceptibility to recurrent infections due to deficits in cell-mediated immunity. The usual treatment for hairy cell leukemia was splenectomy, which resulted in improved hematological parameters. Only 10% of patients had long-lasting benefit (57,58).

In 1984, Quesada et al. reported the original trials of IFN-α in hairy cell leukemia using partially purified material obtained from the supernatants of activated leukocytes (59,60). Of the initial 22 patients treated, 82% developed a complete or partial remission. Recombinant IFN-α (rIFN-α) subsequently became available from three commercial sources: rIFN-α2b, Schering Corporation; rIFN-αA, Hoffmann-La Roche; and rIFN-α2c, Boehringer Ingelheim. Several phase II studies in patients with hairy cell leukemia were initiated using rIFN-α (Table 2) (61–66). A total of 116 patients were treated in these studies; 64% had previously undergone splenectomy. The overall response rate was 91%, including complete, partial, and minor responses. A relatively small number of patients achieved a true complete remission, defined as normalization of all peripheral blood elements, resolution of organomegaly, and no residual peripheral blood or bone marrow hairy cells. However, patients with less than a complete remission still had significant benefit via improvement in hematological parameters and a decreased incidence of infections.

The doses of rIFN-α effective in hairy cell leukemia are low and well tolerated. Two commonly used regimens are 3×10^6 units daily or 2×10^6 units/m^2, three times weekly. In a large multicenter trial of 212 patients receiving 2×10^6 units/m^2, three times weekly, only 16% of patients had symptoms classified as grade 3 (severe) or higher (life-threatening) (67). The most common side effect noted was flulike symptoms, which occurred in 96% of patients. Trials of very low dose IFN-α (0.2×10^6 units/m^2) have been performed. The IFN was very well tolerated but less effective (68,69).

It is clear that hairy cell leukemia responds to relatively low, well-tolerated doses of IFN-α, but the optimal duration of therapy is less well defined. Patients commonly receive therapy for up to 1 year, and some patients relapse when IFN

Table 2 Activity of Recombinant Interferon-α in Malignant Diseases

Tumor type	No. patients studied	Overall response rate (%)	Range of responses (%)	References
Hairy cell leukemia	116	91[a]	78–100	61–65
Chronic myelogenous leukemia	153	51[b]	14–63	77–80
Favorable histology non-Hodgkin's lymphoma	40	50[c]	44–54	83, 84
Kaposi's sarcoma	150	36[c,d]	35–38	90, 91
Renal cancer	248	16[c]	0–26	93–96
Malignant melanoma	226	18[c]	6–30	97–102

[a] Complete, partial, and minor remissions.
[b] Complete hematological remission.
[c] Complete, partial remissions.
[d] High-dose interferon-α.

therapy is discontinued. In a study by Golomb et al., 20% of patients relapsed after 12 or 18 months of therapy (70). In another study by Berman et al. there was a 48% relapse rate in 23 patients who completed 2 years of IFN-α therapy (71). Patients commonly respond to reinitiation of IFN therapy, however. Considering that IFN therapy beyond 1 year significantly increases toxicity, it is reasonable to discontinue IFN therapy after 1 year.

Until recently, rIFN-α was thought to be the most effective therapy for hairy cell leukemia. However, 2′-deoxycoformycin (Pentostatin), an inhibitor of adenosine deaminase, has successfully been used to treat hairy cell leukemia. It may result in a higher percentage of complete remissions and fewer relapses after discontinuation of therapy compared to IFN-α (72,73). Randomized studies comparing IFN-α and 2′-deoxycoformycin are currently underway.

Chronic Myelogenous Leukemia

Chronic myelogenous leukemia (CML) is a chronic myeloproliferative disorder. The cytogenetic hallmark of CML is the Philadelphia chromosome (Ph^1). This reciprocal translocation of genetic material from the long arm of chromosome 22 to chromosome 9 results in the juxtaposition of the *c-abl* onogene with the breakpoint cluster region (bcr) (74). This region of DNA codes for a tyrosine protein kinase that may be involved in cellular growth processes.

Most patients with CML present with indolent disease and persist in a chronic phase for a median of 3–4 years. During this time they have few symptoms but may have an elevated white blood cell count that shows a spectrum of immature to mature cells. The majority of patients eventually enter an accelerated or acute blast crisis phase, treatment of which is very difficult.

Partially purified preparations of leukocyte IFN-α were initially observed in the early 1980s to be effective at lowering the elevated white blood cell counts (75) and platelet counts (76) in CML patients. A number of studies were subsequently reported using rIFN-α in the treatment of the chronic phase of CML

(Table 2) (77–80). In a study by Kantarjian et al., 44 patients received rIFN-α at a dose of 5 × 10^6 units/m^2 daily. A complete hematological remission (defined as complete normalization of peripheral blood counts and complete disappearance of all disease-related signs and symptoms) was observed in 61% of the patients. Furthermore, 39% of patients had suppression of the Ph^1 chromosome. Complete suppression of the Ph^1 chromosome was confirmed in a limited number of patients by Southern blot analyses employing a 3′ breakpoint probe (81).

The mechanism of action of IFN against CML cells is unknown. However, Rosenblum et al. found a decreased IFN-α induction of the enzyme 2′,5′-oligoadenylate synthetase in patients who did not respond clinically, indicating this enzyme may be a marker for response and the molecular level at which the drug acts (82).

These results are encouraging, but the long-term follow-up of the patients continues. It is currently unknown if the Ph^1 chromosome suppression seen in a small number of patients will be long lasting. Furthermore, the ability of rIFN-α to alter the natural history of CML and prevent progression to the accelerated or acute blastic phases is unknown. rIFN-α is not active in patients who have progressed to the accelerated or acute blastic phase of the disease.

Non-Hodgkin's Lymphoma

Despite the name, favorable histology non-Hodgkin's lymphoma is generally not curable using standard chemotherapeutic drugs. However, it is "favorable" in that the natural history is relatively long and is, at least initially, indolent. The IFNs are active in this disease. Foon et al. observed a 54% response rate in 24 patients with low histological grade non-Hodgkin's lymphomas using a relatively high dose of rIFN-α (50 × 10^6 units/m^2, three times weekly) (83). In contrast, only 1 of 7 (14%) of patients with high-grade lymphomas (more aggressive clinically, but potentially curable with chemotherapy) had a partial response. Recently, O'Connell et al. treated 16 patients with favorable histology non-Hodgkin's lymphoma using IFN-α at a dose of 12 × 10^6 units/m^2, three times weekly (84). A 44% response rate (1 CR and 6 PR) was observed. The median time to progression of disease was in excess of 26 weeks. Thus, rIFN-α appears to have moderate activity in patients with low-grade, favorable histology non-Hodgkin's lymphomas. The effects on the natural history of the disease and survival are unknown. Studies of rIFN-α in combination with chemotherapy for initial therapy are in progress. Other trials are underway using rIFN-α as maintenance after reduction of tumor burden with standard chemotherapy.

rIFN-α also has activity against mycosis fungoides (MF) and the Sézary syndrome (SS). These lymphoid malignancies primarily affect the skin but can have late internal organ dissemination. Kohn et al. treated 24 patients with advanced, refractory MF or SS using IFN-α at 10 × 10^6 units/m^2 on day 1 and 50 × 10^6 units/m^2 days 2–5, every 3 weeks (85). One complete and six partial responses were observed for an overall response rate of 29%. The response rate was less than the 45% response rate observed in an earlier study from the same group using a more continuous, high dose of IFN-α (50 × 10^6/m^2, three times weekly) (86). However, the 95% confidence intervals of the response rates ranged from a 13% superiority of intermittent to a 44% superiority of continuous, three times weekly IFN-α. The optimal dose and schedule of rIFN-α for MF and SS remains unclear.

Therapy of Solid Tumors with Interferon-α

Kaposi's Sarcoma

A second indication for rIFN-α approved by the FDA is Kaposi's sarcoma (KS) associated with the acquired immunodeficiency syndrome. Up to 30% of AIDS patients develop KS (87). The clinical course of these patients may be one of multiple skin tumors and/or internal organ dissemination in association with the other manifestations of AIDS. Pulmonary and gastrointestinal are the main visceral sites of involvement. Vinblastine and doxorubicin have some activity in AIDS-associated KS (60–85% response rate) (88). However, the responses are usually only partial and of short duration. Also, they occur mainly in patients with limited cutaneous disease.

The antiviral, antiproliferative, and immunomodulatory effects of the IFNs served as an adequate rationale for their study in patients with AIDS-associated KS. In an early report by Krown et al., 5 of 12 patients had objective responses (89). Interestingly, natural killer cell activity in these patients increased in response to rIFN-α therapy but did not significantly correlate with antitumor response.

Two large multicenter studies confirmed the effectiveness of rIFN-α in AIDS-associated KS. Volberding et al. reported the combined experiences of the University of California at San Francisco (UCSF) and at Los Angeles (UCLA) (90). An overall response rate of 35% was observed in 114 men. Real et al. reported the Memorial Sloan-Kettering Cancer Center experience (91). A 38% response rate was observed in 36 patients who received a dose of 36×10^6 units compared to a 3% response rate in 39 patients who received 3×10^6 units rIFN-α.

In summary, rIFN-α is an active agent in AIDS-associated KS. Although higher doses appear to be more effective, they also result in significantly more toxicity. The immune parameters tested in these patients did not consistently improve or consistently correlate with antitumor response. The antitumor activity of rIFN-α in this disease is more likely related to its direct antiproliferative effects. Furthermore, despite the antitumor response, these patients suffer the other potential manifestations of AIDS and survival is not prolonged.

Renal Cancer

The only proven effective therapy for renal cancer is nephrectomy before local or distant spread. Treatment of patients with metastatic disease using standard chemotherapy drugs, such as vinblastine, is largely ineffective. Response rates to single agents are in the range of 9–15% (92). A variety of doses and schedules of rIFN-α have been used to treat patients with advanced renal cancer (93–96). Response rates varied from 6 to 29%, and most were partial responses (Table 2).

There is some evidence to support a dose-response effect for IFN-α in renal cancer. In a randomized study, Quesada et al. observed a 29% response rate in patients who received 20×10^6 units/m^2 daily versus no responses in patients randomized to receive 2×10^6 units/m^2 (94). However, toxicity was generally more severe and persisted longer in the high-dose treatment group.

In summary, the response of renal cancer to IFN-α is only modest, and a survival benefit has not been demonstrated. The search for more effective treatments for this disease using cytokines alone and in combination with other cytokines or chemotherapeutic drugs continues.

Malignant Melanoma

Curative treatment for advanced metastatic disease is not available, and patients with surgically removable disease have the best chance for cure. rIFN-α had modest activity in a number of phase II studies (Table 2) (97–102) in which a total of 226 patients were evaluated. Complete plus partial response rates varied from 6 to 30%, and most of the responses were partial.

In summary, IFN-α has some clinical activity in patients with metastatic melanoma. However, a definite impact on the overall outcome of these patients has not been proven.

Interferons-β and -γ

Interferons-β and -γ have entered clinical trials (103,104). The activities of IFN-β are very similar to those of IFN-α. As discussed earlier, IFN-γ has relatively more immunomodulatory effects. It has been studied in combination with the chemotherapy drug doxorubicin, and the combination was found to result in enhanced cytotoxicity via an effect on macrophages (105). Considering its immunomodulatory effects, there is good rationale for studying IFN-γ in the adjuvant setting after treatment with chemotherapy, radiotherapy, or surgery has significantly decreased tumor bulk (106). Such trials are in progress.

Interferon in Combination with Other Agents

Interferon-α as a single agent has been thoroughly evaluated in most malignant tumor types. Combination studies of interferon plus other cytokines or chemotherapeutic drugs are underway. The rationale for combination studies includes immunomodulation or biochemical interaction between the two agents, resulting in synergistic antitumor activity or additive independent mechanisms of cytotoxicity but different toxicities, allowing combination therapy without additive toxicity. Two recent trials are of particular note.

Wadler et al. reported a clinical trial of 5-fluorouracil combined with IFN-α (107). A group of 30 patients with advanced colon cancer received 5-FU (750 mg/m^2) daily for 5 days followed by weekly intravenous injections. rIFN-α at 9×10^6 units subcutaneously was administered three times weekly. Among 17 previously untreated patients, 13 (76%) achieved an objective response. However, no major responses were observed in 13 previously treated patients. Considering the usual 15–30% response rate of 5-FU alone in metastatic colon cancer and the negligible activity of IFN-α alone, the results of this combination are encouraging. A randomized trial is required to define the role of IFN-α plus 5-FU compared to 5-FU in metastatic colorectal cancer.

Rosenberg et al. recently reported a trial of IFN-α combined with IL-2 in patients with advanced cancer (108). A group of 94 patients received IFN-α at 3 or 6×10^6 units/m^2 in conjunction with IL-2 at 1, 3, or 4.5×10^6 units/m^2. Both agents were administered intravenously every 8 h for 5 consecutive days followed by repeated cycles after a 10 day rest period. A total of 35 patients with renal cancer and 39 patients with melanoma were treated, and objective responses (complete plus partial remissions) were achieved in 31 and 33%, respectively. There was increased antitumor activity at the higher dose levels of each agent. Synergistic toxicities were not observed. These results await further confirmation in a prospective randomized trial comparing the combination with each of the agents alone.

INTERLEUKIN-2

Interleukin-2 and Lymphokine-Activated Killer Cells

Lotze and coworkers reported in 1981 that peripheral blood mononuclear cells (PBMC) from normal individuals and cancer patients could be activated in vitro to demonstrate lytic activity against fresh and cultured tumor cells (109). The cells with lytic activity were referred to as lymphokine-activated killer cells. In the next few years studies of LAK cell therapy were undertaken in murine models (110). Lymphoid cells were removed, incubated in vitro with IL-2, and transferred in vivo for antitumor therapy (adoptive immunotherapy). Optimal antitumor activity in the murine models required very high doses of IL-2 before and after adoptive LAK cell transfer. LAK cells plus IL-2 were more effective than IL-2 alone. This provided the rationale for combined IL-2 plus LAK cells in the early clinical trials, but the superiority of LAK/IL-2 over IL-2 alone has not been proven in cancer patients.

The antitumor activity of LAK cells appears to be distinct from that of cytotoxic T lymphocytes (CTL) and NK cells. The lytic activity is not HLA restricted, and a broad range of tumor types are susceptible. However, LAK cells are not a unique cell type but rather an activity that arises from an activated population of NK cells. Recent evidence suggests that the LAK phenomenon may be mediated by IL-2-activated populations of CD56-positive, CD3-negative (111), and CD16-positive NK cells (112). Furthermore, CD56-positive LAK cells can be isolated from patients receiving IL-2 (113).

Using the principles learned from the murine models, Rosenberg and his colleagues at the National Cancer Institute (NCI) reported in 1985 the first clinical trial of IL-2 plus LAK cells in patients with advanced cancer (114) with a follow-up report in 1987 (115). A group of 49 patients with advanced cancer were treated with IL-2 alone and 108 with IL-2 plus LAK cells. The treatment regimen was very complicated and included removal of large numbers of PBMC via leukapheresis, in vitro incubation with IL-2, and adoptive transfer of activated cells back to the patients in conjunction with further IL-2 in vivo. Complete plus partial remission rates were 33% in renal cancer and 23% in malignant melanoma for LAK cells plus IL-2 therapy.

This innovative approach to cancer immunotherapy generated both excitement and controversy. The antitumor activity was impressive considering the advanced chemotherapy-refractory nature of the tumors. However, significant toxicity, including hypotension, weight gain, renal insufficiency, and hepatotoxicity, were observed, and four patients died of toxicity.

Because of the complexity and toxicity of this regimen, the IL-2/Lymphokine

Activated Killer Cell Extramural Working Group was established with the goal of testing the feasibility and confirming the activity of this regimen in centers outside the NCI. Six extramural centers observed complete and partial remissions in 16% of renal cancer and 19% of malignant melanoma patients (116,117). With better pretreatment screening of patients for cardiac and respiratory problems, severe toxicity was decreased. However, most patients still experienced a "capillary leak" syndrome with transient multiorgan failure.

The toxicities of IL-2 may be severe or life-threatening (118–122). Most prominent is a capillary leak syndrome and increased vascular permeability resulting in hypotension, tachycardia, prerenal azotemia, respiratory distress, and weight gain. The clinical signs and symptoms are similar to those seen in septic shock. However, all the manifestations of IL-2 toxicity may not be secondary to increased vascular permeability. There is a direct renal effect with decreased renal prostaglandin synthesis (123) and a direct cardiac effect (decreased left ventricular function) (118). The majority of the toxicities resolve within 24–48 h after discontinuation of therapy.

Following these initial reports, studies were designed using alternative IL-2 regimens with the hope of decreasing toxicity (Table 3). A regimen of low-dose

TABLE 3 Interleukin-2 Regimens Used in Cancer Therapy

				Response (%)	
Author (reference)	Regimen	IL-2 schedule	No. patients	Renal cancer	Melanoma
Rosenberg et al. (115)	IL-2 alone	Every 8 h bolus	37	5	31
Sosman et al. (127)	IL-2 alone	Continuous infusion or bolus	23	18	0
Rosenberg et al. (115)	IL-2/LAK	Every 8 h bolus	62	33	23
West et al. (126)	IL-2/LAK	Continuous infusion	16	50	50
Eberlein et al. (124)	IL-2/LAK	Every 8 h bolus	20	50	50
Dutcher et al. (117)	IL-2/LAK	Every 8 h bolus	36	—	19
Fisher et al. (116)	IL-2/LAK	Every 8 h bolus	35	16	—
Rosenberg et al. (141)	CTX[a] IL-2, TIL	Every 8 h bolus	20	—	55
Kradin et al. (143)	IL-2/TIL	Continuous infusion	20	29	23
Mitchell et al. (144)	CTX[a]/IL-2	Daily bolus	24	—	25

[a] Cyclophosphamide.

IL-2 (compared to the high doses administered in the NCI studies) was found to be active and less toxic (124). Another approach to IL-2 therapy involves the use of a continuous infusion. Thompson et al. found maximum immunomodulatory effects (as measured by rebound lymphocytosis) when IL-2 was administered by a 24 h continuous intravenous infusion as opposed to the same dose given as a 2 h infusion or in three daily divided doses (125). West et al. treated 48 patients with advanced cancer with IL-2 as a continuous infusion over 5 days. An overall 32.5% partial remission rate was observed in patients with varied tumor types, including 3 of 6 renal cancer patients and 5 of 10 melanoma patients (126). This schedule may also be associated with significant dose-dependent toxicity.

Sosman et al. treated 23 patients with metastatic carcinoma using IL-2 alone as a 96 h continuous intravenous infusion, a single daily bolus injection, or a combination of these schedules (127). Of 17 patients with metastatic renal cancer, 3 developed partial remissions. The toxicity was acceptable, with no patients requiring therapy for hypotension.

The need for LAK cells in addition to IL-2 has been questioned. IL-2 administration to cancer patients results in LAK cell generation in vivo, but there is a poor correlation between in vitro LAK cell activity of the PBMC from these patients and their clinical response to IL-2 therapy (128) (see also Ref. 214). Recent studies indicate other cytokines with potential for direct and indirect antitumor activity, such as TNF and IFN-γ, are released during IL-2/LAK cell therapy (129). Furthermore, immunopathological examination of tumors from patients responding or not responding to IL-2 or IL-2/LAK cell therapy reveals infiltration with T cells rather than cells with NK markers (130). These observations led to therapy using so-called tumor-infiltrating lymphocytes. TIL are distinct from LAK cells and have more antitumor activity.

Tumor-Infiltrating Lymphocytes

Tumor-infiltrating lymphocytes (TIL) isolated from human renal cancer, melanoma, and lung cancer have been shown to have in vitro lytic activity against autologous tumors (131–133). TIL are distinct from LAK in a number of respects. They are predominantly T lymphocytes (CD3 and CD8 positive) and result in tumor lysis in a MHC-restricted manner (131–134). However, TIL with autologous tumor specificity are seen primarily in melanoma (135). TIL cultures from other tumors, such as breast, ovarian, liver, and head and neck cancers, often have nonspecific lytic activity (136–140). After incubation with IL-2 TIL are 50–100 times more potent than LAK cells at mediating lysis of established tumor in murine models (134).

Based on these observations, clinical trials of TIL were initiated. Rosenberg et al. treated 20 patients with metastatic melanoma with 3×10^{10}–75×10^{10} TIL, obtained in smaller numbers from tumor biopsies and expanded in culture with IL-2 for 4–8 weeks (141). All patients were pretreated with a single dose of cyclophosphamide and received concurrent IL-2 in conjunction with infusions of activated TIL. One complete and eight partial responses were observed in 15 patients who were previously untreated with IL-2. Two partial remissions were observed in 5 patients who previously failed IL-2 therapy. The toxicity was associated with the IL-2 and similar to previous observations. Indium^{111}-labeled TIL were found to localize preferentially to tumor as opposed to normal tissues (142).

Kradin et al. reported a similar study (143) in which 13 patients with melanoma, 7 with renal cancer, and 8 with non–small cell lung cancer were treated with TIL and IL-2. Response rates of 29 and 23% were seen in patients with renal cancer and melanoma.

These results are encouraging, but patients must have surgically accessible tumor, must be in good physical condition to tolerate IL-2, and must be able to wait 4–8 weeks for the in vitro culture of TIL before therapy.

Interleukin-2 in Combination with Other Agents

IL-2 has been combined with other treatment modalities in an attempt to enhance antitumor activity and/or reduce toxicity. Mitchell et al. used low-dose IL-2 (3.6×10^6 units/m^2 daily for 5 days on 2 consecutive weeks) preceded by a single low dose of cyclophosphamide (350 mg/m^2) (144). Of 24 evaluable patients with advanced melanoma, 6 had remissions (1 complete and 5 partial). The activity was similar to that of IL-2 plus LAK cells; however, the toxicity was less and the regimen could be administered on an outpatient basis. The rationale for this regimen was based on the ability of cyclophosphamide to selectively deplete a suppressor T cell population hypothesized to downregulate in vivo LAK cell generation (145,146).

Clinical trials of IL-2 combined with interferon-γ have also been initiated. The rationale for these studies involves enhancement of LAK cell activity by IFN-γ pretreatment of the tumor cells (147). In a phase I trial, Taylor et al. treated 37 patients with advanced cancer using sequentially administered IFN-γ (0.1 or 0.25 mg/m^2) and IL-2 ($2–4 \times 10^6$ CETUS units/m^2) (148). Complete and partial remissions were observed in 1 patient with renal cancer and 1 with malignant melanoma.

There is evidence for enhanced or synergistic antitumor activity by combining IL-2 with tumor necrosis factor (149), IL-4 (150), or tumor-specific antibodies (151). Clinical trials of these combinations have been or soon will be initiated. Data on them are not yet available.

THERAPEUTIC POTENTIAL OF OTHER INTERLEUKINS

Interleukins may be defined as factors (proteins) secreted by cells in response to specific stimuli that function to signal between and mediate functions of the cells of the immune, hematopoetic, and other systems. Most interleukins were previously known by other names that described their biological activities (e.g., interleukin-4 was previously known as B cell stimulatory factor 1). By current convention, new cytokines are given an interleukin designation when the amino acid sequence of the human molecule has been elucidated. New interleukins are being described, some of which will have therapeutic potential for cancer (Table 4).

Table 4 The Interleukins

Interleukin	Cells of origin	Targets	Activities with relevance to cancer therapy
IL-1	Macrophages, endothelial cells, lymphocytes, fibroblasts, epithelial cells	Macrophages, B and T lymphocytes, endothelial cells, fibroblasts, thymocytes, neutrophils, hepatocytes	Promotes hematopoiesis, cytostatic or cytotoxic for some tumor cells
IL-2	T lymphocytes	T and B lymphocytes, macrophages	LAK cell induction, enhanced cytotoxicity of TIL
IL-3	T lymphocytes	Granulocytes, erythrocytes, macrophages, megakaryocytes	Promotes hematopoeisis
IL-4	T lymphocytes	T and B lymphocytes, hematopoietic cells, macrophages, mast cells	Synergy with IL-2 for LAK cell, induction, enhanced CTL activity
IL-5	T lymphocytes	Eosinophils	Unknown
IL-6	Fibroblasts, T lymphocytes	B lymphocytes, plasma cells, T lymphocytes, fibroblasts	Autocrine growth factor for myeloma cells
IL-7	Bone marrow stromal cells	Pre- and pro-B lymphocytes	Unknown
IL-8	Endothelial cells	Endothelial cell-neutrophil interaction	Unknown
IL-9	T lymphocytes	T lymphocytes, erythroid cells	Promotes hematopoiesis

Interleukin-4

The first biological activity associated with interleukin-4 was its ability to act in conjunction with antiimmunoglobulin antibodies to stimulate resting mouse B cells to enter *S* phase. Based on this activity it was initially termed B cell stimulatory factor 1 (BSF-1) (152). Subsequently, IL-4 was found to have pleiotropic biological activities, including B cell growth promotion, T cell growth promotion, enhanced MHC class II expression on B cells, mast cell growth promotion, enhanced synthesis of IgG_1 and IgE, IgG class switching, enhanced Fc receptor expression on B cells, and as a costimulant in conjunction with colony-stimulating factors for hematopoietic cells (153–161).

The effects of IL-4 on the development and/or activity of cytotoxic T cells and LAK cells are of interest for cancer therapy. Widmer et al. reported that IL-4 can stimulate antigen-specific cytotoxic T lymphocytes (CTL) (162,163). This has therapeutic potential for cancer in the setting of tumor cell vaccines. Because of immunosuppression associated with their malignancies, most cancer patients respond poorly to autologous or allogeneic tumor cell vaccines. IL-4 could be used as an adjuvant in this setting to enhance CTL activation.

The effects of IL-4 on the generation and activity of LAK cells have also been investigated. There is a different effect of IL-4 on LAK cells in murine versus human systems. In mouse cells IL-4 augments LAK induction and activity (164,165). In human cells IL-4 inhibits IL-2-induced LAK cell generation (166). However, IL-4 can enhance LAK activity if lymphocytes are preactivated in vitro or in vivo with IL-2 (150). IL-4 alone does not produce LAK activity and can inhibit LAK cell induction if cells are exposed to IL-4 before IL-2.

These observations provide a rationale for cancer therapy combining IL-2 and IL-4. Optimal cytolytic activity would be induced by treating patients with IL-2 followed by IL-4. Phase I clinical trials of recombinant human IL-4 and combination studies of IL-2 and IL-4 are in progress.

Interleukin-5

IL-5 was previously known as eosinophil differentiation factor. The human gene for IL-5 has recently been cloned and expressed (168). Its only known activity is on the eosinophil differentiation pathway (168) enhancing eosinophil function (169). Further studies of the role of IL-5 in hypereosinophilia (eosinophilic leukemia, parasitic infections, and malignancies) are underway. A role for IL-5 in cancer therapy is yet to be defined.

Interleukin-6

Interleukin-6 (IL-6) was previously known as interferon-β_2, B cell differentiation factor 2, or hybridoma growth factor. IL-6 has a spectrum of biological activities that are similar to the effects of IL-1 and TNF (170–172).

Of relevance to cancer therapy is the ability of IL-6 to function as a hybridoma growth factor and as an autocrine growth factor for multiple myeloma cells. Hybridomas are produced by the fusion of B cells with myeloma cells and their subsequent cloning for the production of monoclonal antibodies. IL-6 can promote the growth of some hybridomas and might be capable of replacing feeder cell layers previously used to promote hybridoma growth (173,174).

Recently, IL-6 was found to be a growth factor in multiple myeloma. Asaoku et al. found that the in vitro proliferative response to IL-6 was greater in patients with early as opposed to those with later stages of multiple myeloma (175). In contrast, Zhang et al. found that myeloma cells from patients with more advanced disease responded better to IL-6 (176). It appears that at least some clinical cases of multiple myeloma are dependent upon IL-6 for continued proliferation and that this represents a pathway of autocrine growth stimulation, which, if interrupted, could result in tumor regression. Another approach involves the use of IL-6 conjugated to *Pseudomonas* exotoxin (167). Myeloma cells that express the IL-6 receptor were susceptible to lysis by the conjugate, whereas normal IL-6 receptor-negative cells were not affected. Thus, IL-6 may have a role in the clinical therapy of multiple myeloma.

Finally, recombinant human IL-6 was recently shown to have myeloid leukemic cell differentiation activity (177). Thus, IL-6 may also have a role in the therapy of myeloid leukemias and perhaps myelodysplastic syndromes.

Interleukin-7

Recombinant murine interleukin-7 (IL-7) was recently cloned from a stromal cell line (178). IL-7 promotes the growth of early B cell precursors (pre-B cells and pro-B cells) (179,180). A role for IL-7 in cancer therapy has yet to be defined. However, it is feasible that IL-7 may play a role in the pathogenesis of B cell malignancies, such as the non-Hodgkin's lymphomas.

Interleukin-8

The factor previously known as leukocyte adhesion inhibitor was recently re named interleukin-8 (IL-8) (181). Recombinant human IL-8 was recently cloned and expressed (181). Its actions are primarily antiinflammatory as it inhibits the adhesion of leukocytes to endothelial cells. IL-8 appears to act antagonistically to proinflammatory cytokines, such as IL-1 and TNF. A role for IL-8 in cancer therapy is yet to be defined.

Interleukin-9

The gene for human interleukin-9 (IL-9) has been cloned and expressed (182). The regulation and functions of IL-9 are actively being studied. IL-9 supports the growth of erythroid progenitors (burst-forming units-erythroid, BFU-E) (183). A role for IL-9 in cancer therapy has not been defined.

TUMOR NECROSIS FACTOR

Antitumor Mechanisms

In the late 1800s Coley studied the antitumor activity of bacterial toxins (184). These preparations were referred to as "Coley's mixed toxins." Occasional tumor regressions were observed in patients (185). More recent observations indicated that toxic bacterial cell wall components (endotoxin) elicited a serum activity capable of tumor necrosis (186). This activity became known as tumor necrosis factor.

TNF is produced primarily by activated monocytes-macrophages. It has a number of biological effects, including immune regulation, mediation of inflammation, metabolic effects (e.g., lipid metabolism via effects on lipoprotein lipase), and antitumor activity (187–193).

TNF inhibits the growth of a number of human and murine tumor cells (188,189). Direct antitumor mechanisms of TNF have been proposed, including direct DNA damage (190), activation of phospholipases, which may result in the generation of free oxygen radicals (191), and activation of proteases (192).

TNF also has immunomodulatory properties. Talmadge et al. demonstrated that TNF is able to activate macrophages, augment allogeneic mixed lymphocyte responses, and serve as an adjuvant for tumor vaccines (194). Furthermore, TNF was found to inhibit neutrophil and monocyte migration (195). Patients treated with TNF develop a marked, transient neutropenia and monocytopenia shortly after receiving TNF (195) and have decreased NK cell activity (196).

Clinical Trials of Tumor Necrosis Factor as a Single Agent

The gene for human TNF has been cloned and expressed (197,198), and clinical trials of recombinant human TNF have been initiated. In these trials TNF has been administered by various doses, routes, and schedules (Table 5). Thus far, very little antitumor activity has been observed. However, the majority of the studies have been phase I and early phase II clinical trials in which patients with advanced cancer refractory to all other forms of therapy have been treated.

Given the short plasma half-life of TNF following intravenous (IV) injection (10–20 minutes) it would be of interest to administer TNF as a continuous infusion. Spriggs et al. performed a phase I study in which recombinant TNF was administered as a 24 h intravenous infusion (199). Interestingly, plasma levels of TNF were maximal at 3 h and continued to decline despite continued infusion of TNF for up to 24 h. This failure to achieve a steady state indicates that TNF may alter its own metabolism or alter volume of distribution via its vascular effects.

TABLE 5 Clinical Trials of Recombinant Human Tumor Necrosis Factor

Author (reference)	TNF dose	Route	Schedule	No. patients	Response	
					Complete	Partial
Creaven et al. (208)	1–48 × 10^4 units/m^2	1 h, IV infusion	Every 3 weeks	29	0	0
Spriggs et al. (191)	4.5–645 μg/m^2	24 h, IV infusion	Every 3 weeks	50	0	1
Creagen et al. (209)	5–200 μg/m^2	30 minutes IV infusion	Days 1–5 every 3 weeks	27	0	1
Jakubowski et al. (210)	5–200 μg/m^2	IM	Days 1–5 every 2 weeks	19	0	0
Wiedenmann et al. (211)	40–400 μg/m^2	24 h, IV infusion	Once or twice weekly	15	0	0
Zamkoff et al. (212)	5–150 μg/m^2	SC	Days 1–5 every other week	9	0	0
Lenk et al. (213)	683–956 μg/m^2	30–60 minutes IV	Every other week	22	0	0
Feinberg et al. (200)	5–250 μg/m^2	30 minutes and 4 h, IV	Days 1–5 every 2 weeks	39	0	0
Sherman et al. (201)	5 × 10^4–3 × 10^5 units/m^2	5 day continuous IV infusion	Every 4 weeks	19	0	0

Toxicities of TNF include constitutional symptoms of fever, chills, headache, and fatigue. In addition, hypotension, nausea and vomiting, diarrhea, hepatic enzyme elevation, and thrombocytopenia and leukopenia have been observed. The most common dose-limiting toxicities are hypotension and constitutional symptoms. The maximum tolerated dose for TNF when given intravenously for up to 5 days varies from 150 to 200 $\mu g/m^2$. In early studies TNF was shown to have effects on lipoprotein metabolism resulting in decreases in high-density lipoprotein (HDL), increases in very low density lipoproteins (VLDL), and increases in triglycerides in the serum (200,201).

Although little antitumor activity was associated with recombinant TNF in the early phase I trials, the major goal of such studies was achieved (i.e., to define the toxicities, biological activities, and tolerable doses, routes, and schedules). The next step in the clinical evaluation of TNF involved combination therapy with other agents.

TNF in Combination with Other Agents

Owen-Schaub et al. demonstrated synergistic cytotoxicity of TNF and IL-2 against fresh human tumors and cell lines (202). Optimal LAK cell function was observed at a 10-fold lower IL-2 concentration when TNF was present, thus providing a rationale for lower dose IL-2 therapy in combination with TNF. Synergy and significant tumor regression in an MCA sarcoma model was observed at TNF and IL-2 doses, which as single agents were nontoxic (203). The sequence of administration may be important, as synergy was optimal when IL-2 was administered before TNF as opposed to TNF before IL-2. Synergy between TNF and IFN-γ has been shown in an animal tumor model (204). Salmon et al. demonstrated TNF sensitivity in 28% of the fresh human tumors they tested in vitro (205). This included sensitivity in 3 of 4 colorectal cancers, 3 of 7 lung cancers, 8 of 28 malignant melanomas, and 3 of 10 endometrial cancers. Exposure of the fresh human tumors to a combination of TNF and IFN-γ reduced the concentration of TNF required for significant antitumor activity by about threefold.

Based on these and other observations, a number of combination clinical trials of TNF and other agents have been initiated. Yang et al. studied 16 patients with advanced non–small cell lung cancer treated with a continuous intravenous infusion of IL-2 and a daily intramuscular injection of TNF for 5 consecutive days (206). In 12 evaluable patients one partial response and three minor responses were observed, and all patients had augmented LAK and NK activities.

Abbruzzese et al. combined TNF and IFN-γ in a phase I clinical trial in patients with advanced gastrointestinal cancer (207). IFN-γ (50–150 $\mu g/m^2$/day) was administered as a daily intramuscular injection on days 1–5. TNF (50–225 $\mu g/m^2$/day) was administered as a 30 minute intravenous infusion every 8 h on days 1–5. No complete or partial responses were observed. However, minor responses were observed in patients with cholangiocarcinoma and pancreatic cancer. The dose-limiting toxicity in this study was hyperbilirubinemia. Transient myelosuppression was also observed.

Recently, the enthusiasm for TNF as a single anticancer agent has diminished. However, combination trials of TNF plus other cytokines or chemotherapy drugs are in progress.

CONCLUSIONS AND FUTURE PROSPECTS

Since the first recombinant cytokines entered cancer clinical trials in the early 1980s, much progress has been made. Based on preclinical rationale, clinical trials of cytokines alone and in combination with other cytokines and/or chemotherapy drugs have been initiated. Significant advances have been made in the clinical therapy of patients with hairy cell leukemia and AIDS-associated Kaposi's sarcoma. Smaller improvements have been observed for patients with chronic myelogenous leukemia, renal cancer, and melanoma. Furthermore, patients receiving standard cancer chemotherapy now have the potential for reduced severity of myelosuppression due to co-administration of the colony-stimulating factors.

In summary, the future of cancer therapy is promising in large part as a result of the availability of recombinant cytokines as therapeutic agents. Beyond their therapeutic potential, however, the study of the production and regulation of cytokines will likely give new insight into the pathogenesis of malignant diseases and thus a realistic future expectation of more effective treatment for all patients with cancer.

REFERENCES

1. Clark SC, Kamen R. The human hematopoietic colony-stimulating factors. Science 1987; 236:1229–37.
2. Morstyn G, Burgess AW. Hemopoietic growth factors: a review. Cancer Res 1988; 48:5624–37.
3. Andreeff M, Welte K. Hematopoietic colony-stimulating factors. Semins Oncol 1989; 16:211–29.
4. Dinarello CA. Biology of interleukin 1. FASEB J 1988; 2:108.
5. Mochizuki DY, Eisenhan JR, Conlon PJ, Larsen AD, Tushinski RJ. Interleukin 1 regulates hemopoietin activity, a role previously ascribed to hemopoietin 1. Proc Natl Acad Sci U S A 1987; 84:5267–71.
6. Gallicchio VS, Watts TD, DellaPuca R. Synergistic action of recombinant-derived murine interleukin-1 on the augmentation of colony stimulating activity on murine granulocyte-macrophage hematopoietic stem cells in vitro. Expl Cell Biol 1987; 55:83–92.
7. Broxmeyer HE, Williams DE, Hangoc G, et al. Synergistic myelopoietic actions in vivo after administration to mice of combinations of purified natural murine colony-stimulating factor 1, recombinant murine interluekin 3, and recombinant murine granulocyte/macrophage colony-stimulating factor. Proc Natl Acad Sci U S A 1987; 84:3871–5.
8. Moore MAS, Warren DJ. Synergy of interleukin 1 and granulocyte colony-stimulating factor: in vivo stimulation of stem-cell recovery and hematopoietic regeneration following 5-fluorouracil treatment of mice. Proc Natl Acad Sci U S A 1987; 84:7134–8.
9. Crown J, Kemeny N, Jakubowski A, et al. Phase I-II trial of recombinant human interleukin-1B (IL-1) in patients (PTS) with metastatic colorectal cancer (MCC) receiving 5-fluorouracil (5FU). Blood 1989; 74:15a (abstract 43).
10. Yang YC, Clarletta AB, Temple PA, et al. Human IL-3 (multi-CSF): identification by expression cloning of a novel hematopoietic growth factor related to murine IL-3. Cell 1986; 47:3–10.
11. Frei E, III, Spriggs D. Tumor necrosis factor: still a promising agent. J Clin Oncol 1989; 7:291–4.

12. Schrader JW. The panspecific hemopoietin of activated T lymphocytes (interleukin-3). Annu Rev Immunol 1986; 4:205–30.
13. Ishibashi T, Burstein SA. Interleukin 3 promotes the differentiation of isolated single megakaryocytes. Blood 1986; 67:1512–4.
14. Ganser A, Lindemann A, Seipelt G, et al. Effect of recombinant human interleukin-3 (rhIL-3) in patients with bone marrow failure. Blood 1989; 74:50a (abstract 177).
15. Kurzrock R, Talpaz M, Salewski E, Gutterman JU. Phase I study of recombinant human interleukin-3 in patients with bone marrow failure. Blood 1989; 74:154a (abstract 572).
16. Metcalf D, Begley CG, Johnson GR, et al. Biologic properties in vitro of a recombinant human granulocyte-macrophage colony-stimulating factor. Blood 1986; 67:37–45.
17. Tomonaga M, Golde DW, Gasson JC. Biosynthetic (recombinant) human granulocyte-macrophage colony-stimulating factor: effects on normal bone marrow and leukemia cell lines. Blood 1986; 67:31–6.
18. Sieff CA, Emerson SG, Donahue RE, Nathan DG. Human recombinant granulocyte-macrophage colony-stimulating factor: a multilineage hematopoietin. Science 1985; 230:1171–3.
19. DiPersio JF, Billing P, Williams R, Gasson JC. Human granulocyte-macrophage colony-stimulating factor and other cytokines prime human neutrophils for enhanced arachidonic acid release and leukotriene B_4 synthesis. J Immunol 1988; 140:4315–22.
20. Antman KS, Griffin JD, Elias A, et al. Effect of recombinant human granulocyte-macrophage colony-stimulating factor on chemotherapy-induced myelosuppression. N Engl J Med 1988; 319:595–8.
21. Vadhan-Raj S, Buescher S, LeMaistre A, et al. Stimulation of hematopoiesis in patients with bone marrow failure and in patients with malignancy by recombinant human granulocyte-macrophage colony-stimulating factor. Blood 1988; 72:134–41.
22. Brandt SJ, Peters WP, Atwater SK, et al. Effect of recombinant human granulocyte-macrophage colony-stimulating factor on hematopoietic reconstitution after high-dose chmotherapy and autologous bone marrow transplantation. N Engl J Med 1988; 318:869–76.
23. Blazar BR, Kersey JH, McGlave PB, et al. In vivo administration of recombinant human granulocye/macrophage colony-stimulating factor in acute lymphoblastic leukemia patients receiving purged autografts. Blood 1989; 73:849–57.
24. Nemunaitis J, Singer JW, Buckner CD, et al. Use of recombinant human granulocyte-macrophage colony-stimulating factor in autologous marrow transplantation for lymphoid malignancies. Blood 1988; 72:834–6.
25. Devereaux S, Linch DC, Gribben JG, McMillan A, Patterson K, Goldstone AH. GM-CSF accelerates neutrophil recovery after autologous bone marrow transplantation for Hodgkin's disease. Bone Marrow Transplant 1989; 4:49–54.
26. Groopman JE, Mitsuyasu RT, DeLeo MJ, Oette DH, Golde DW. Effect of recombinant human granulocyte-macrophage colony-stimulating factor on myelopoiesis in the acquired immunodeficiency syndrome. N Engl J Med 1987; 317:593–8.
27. Vadhan-Raj S, Keating M, LeMaistre A, et al. Effects of recombinant human granulocyte-macrophage colony-stimulating factor in patients with myelodysplastic syndromes. N Engl J Md 1987; 317:1545–52.
28. Vadhan-Raj S, Buescher S, Broxmeyer HE, et al. Stimulation of myelopoiesis in patients with aplastic anemia by recombinant human granulocyte-macrophage colony-stimulating factor. N Engl J Med 1988; 319:1628–34.
29. Ganser A, Ottman OG, Erdmann H, Schulz G, Hoelzer D. The effect of recombinant

human granulocyte-macrophage colony-stimulating factor on neutropenia and related morbidity in chronic severe neutropenia. Ann Intern Med 1989; 111:887–92.

30. Lieschke GJ, Maher D, Cebon J, et al. Effects of bacterially synthesized recombinant human granulocyte-macrophage colony-stimulating factor in patients with advanced malignancy. Ann Intern Med 1989; 110:357–64.
31. Phillips N, Jacobs S, Stoller R, Earie M, Przepiorka D, Shadduck RK. Effect of recombinant human granulocyte-macrophage colony-stimulating factor on myelopoiesis in patients with refractory metastatic carcinoma. Blood 1989; 74:26–34.
32. Souza LM, Boone TC, Gabrilove J, et al. Recombinant human granulocyte colony-stimulating factor: effects on normal and leukemic myeloid cells. Science 1986; 232:61–5.
33. Gabrilove JL, Jakubowski A, Scher H, et al. Effect of granulocyte colony-stimulating factor on neutropenia and associated morbidity due to chemotherapy for transitional-cell carcinoma of the urothelium. N Engl J Med 1988; 318:1414–22.
34. Neidhart J, Mangolik A, Kohler W, et al. Granulocyte colony-stimulating factor stimulates recovery of granulocytes in patients receiving dose-intensive chemotherapy without bone marrow transplantation. J Clin Oncol 1989; 7:1685–92.
35. Sheridan WP, Wolf M, Lusk J, et al. Granulocyte colony-stimulating factor and neutrophil recovery after high-dose chemotherapy and autologous bone marrow transplantation. Lancet 1989; 2:891–5.
36. Bronchud MH, Scarffe JH, Thatcher N, et al. Phase I/II study of recombinant human granulocyte colony-stimulating factor in patients receiving intensive chemotherapy for small cell lung cancer. Br J Cancer 1987; 56:809–13.
37. Stanley ER, Chen DM, Lin HS. Induction of macrophage production and proliferation by a purified colony stimulating factor. Natur 1978; 274:168–70.
38. Stanley ER, Guilbert LJ, Tushinski RJ, Bartelmez SH. CSF-1—a mononuclear phagocyte lineage-specific hemopoietic growth factor. J Cell Biochem 1983; 21:151–9.
39. Wing EJ, Ampel NM, Waheed A, Shadduck RK. Macrophage colony-stimulating factor (M-SCF) enhances the capacity of murine macrophages to secrete oxygen reduction products. J Immunol 1985; 135:2052–6.
40. Komiyama A, Ishiguro A, Kubo T, et al. Increases in neutrophil counts by purified human urinary colony-stimulating factor in chronic neutropenia of childhood. Blood 1988; 71:41–5.
41. Motoyoshi K, Takaku F, Miura Y. High serum colony-stimulating activity of leukocytopenic patients after intravenous infusions of human urinary colony-stimulating factor. Blood 1983; 62:685–8.
42. Motoyoshi K, Takaku F, Maekawa T, et al. Protective effect of partially purified human urinary colony-stimulating factor on granulocytopenia after antitumor chemotherapy. Exp Hematol 1986; 14:1069–75.
43. Sampson-Johannes A, Carlino JA. Enhancement of human monocyte tumoricidal activity by recombinant M-CSF. J Immunol 1988; 141:3680–6.
44. Eschbach JW, Egrie JC, Downing MR, Browne JK, Adamson JW. Correction of the anemia of end-stage renal disease with recombinant human erythropoietin. N Engl J Med 1987; 316:73–8.
45. Adamson JW. The promise of recombinant human erythropoietin. Semin Hematol 1989; 26:5–8.
46. Evans RW, Rader B, Egrie J, Adamson JW, Eschbach HW. Correction of anemia with recombinant human erythropoietin (r-HuEPO) enhances the quality of life of hemodialysis (HD) patients (PTS) (abstract). Kidney Int 1989; 35:246.
47. Oster W, Herman F, Gamm H, et al. Erythropoietin (EPO) for the treatment of

anemia of malignancy due to neoplastic bone marrow infiltration. Blood 1989; 74:51a (abstract 180).
48. Ludwig H, Fritz E, Kotzmann H, Hocker P, Gisslinger H, Barnas U. Erythropoietin treatment for chronic anemia of malignancy. Blood 1989; 74:16 (abstract 44).
49. Rubin BY, Gupta SL. Differential efficacies of human type I and type II interferons as antiviral and antiproliferative agents. Proc Natl Acad Sci U S A 1980; 77:5928–32.
50. Chebath J, Benech P, Hovanessian A, Galabru J, Revel M. Four different forms of interferon induced 2′5′ oligo(a)synthetase identified by immunoblotting in human cells. J Biol Chem 1987; 262:3852–7.
51. Goldstein D, Laszlo J. The role of interferon in cancer therapy: a current perspective. CA 1988; 38:258–77.
52. Revel M. The interferon system in man: nature of the interferon molecules and mode of action. In: Becker Y, ed. Antiviral drugs and interferon. New York: Martinus Nijhoff, 1984:358–433.
53. Paulnock DM, Borden EC. Modulation of immune functions by interferons. In: Reif AE, Mitchell MS, eds. Immunity to cancer. New York: Academic Press, 1985:545–59.
54. Stewart WE, Blanchard DK. Interferons, cytostatic and immunomodulatory effects. In: Reif AE, Mitchell MS, eds. Immunity to cancer. New York: Academic Press, 1985:295–307.
55. Goldstein D, Laszlo J. Interferon therapy in cancer: from imaginon to interferon. Cancer Res 1986; 46:4315–29.
56. Salmon SE, Durie BGM, Young L, Liu RM, Trown PW, Stebbing N. Effects of cloned human leukocyte interferons in the human tumor stem cell assay. J Clin Oncol 1983; 1:217–25.
57. Flandrin G, Sigaux F, Sebahoun G, Bouffette P. Hairy cell leukemia: clinical presentation and follow-up of 211 patients. Semin Oncol 1984; 11:458–71.
58. Golomb HM, Ratain MJ, Vardiman JW. Sequential treatment of hairy cell leukemia: a new role for interferon. In: DeVita VT, Hellman S, Rosenberg SA, eds. Important advances in oncology. Philadelphia: J.B. Lippincott, 1986:311.
59. Quesada JR, Reuben J, Manning JT, Hersh EM, Gutterman JU. Alpha interferon for induction of remission in hairy-cell leukemia. N Engl J Med 1984; 310:15.
60. Quesada JR, Hersh EM, Gutterman JU. Treatment of hairy cell leukemia with alpha interferon. Proc Am Soc Clin Oncol 1984; 3:207.
61. Ratain MJ, Golomb HM, Vardiman JW, Vokes EE, Jacobs RH, Daly K. Treatment of hairy cell leukemia with recombinant $alpha_2$ interferon. Blood 1985; 65:644–8.
62. Jacobs AD, Champlin RE, Golde DW. Recombinant α-2-interferon for hairy cell leukemia. Blood 1985; 65:1017–20.
63. Thompson JA, Brady J, Kidd P, Fefer A. Recombinant alpha-2 interferon in the treatment of hairy cell leukemia. Can Treat Rep 1985; 69:791–3.
64. Huber C, Flener R, Gastl G. Interferon-alpha-2c in the treatment of advanced hairy cell leukaemia. Oncology 1985; 42:7–9.
65. Foon KA, Maluish AE, Abrams PG, et al. Recombinant leukocyte A interferon therapy for advanced hairy cell leukemia. Am J Med 1986; 80:351–6.
66. Quesada JR, Hersh EM, Manning J, et al. Treatment of hairy cell leukemia with recombinant α-interferon. Blood 1986; 68:493–7.
67. Thompson JA, Fefer A. Interferon in the treatment of hairy cell leukemia. Cancer 1987; 59:605–9.
68. Thompson JA, Kidd P, Rubin E, Fefer A. Very low dose α-2b interferon for the treatment of hairy cell leukemia. Blood 1989; 73:1440–3.
69. Gastl G, Werter M, De Pauw B, et al. Comparison of clinical efficacy and toxicity

of conventional and optimum biological response modifying doses of interferon alpha-2C in the treatment of hairy cell leukemia: a retrospective analysis of 39 patients. Leukemia 1989; 3:453–60.

70. Golomb HM, Ratain MJ, Fefer A, et al. Randomized study of the duration of treatment with interferon alfa-2b in patients with hairy cll leukemia. J Natl Cancer Inst 1988; 80:369–73.
71. Berman E, Heller G, Kempin S, Gee T, Tran LL, Clarkson B. Incidence of response and long-term follow-up in patients with hairy cell leukemia treated with recombinant interferon alfa-2a. Blood 1990; 4:839–45.
72. Johnston JB, Eisenhauer E, Corbett WEN, Scott JG, Zaentz SD. Efficacy of 2′-deoxycoformycin in hairy-cell leukemia: a study of the national cancer institute of Canada clinical trials group, J Natl Cancer Inst 1988; 80:765–9.
73. Kraut EH, Bouroncle BA, Grever MR. Pentostatin in the treatment of advanced hairy cell leukemia. J Clin Oncol 1989; 7:168–72.
74. Stam K, Heisterkamp N, Grosveld G, et al. Evidence of a new chimeric bcr/c-abl MRNA in patients with chronic myelocytic leukemia and the Philadelphia chromosome. N Engl J Med 1985; 313:1422–9.
75. Talpaz M, McCredie KB, Mavligit GM, Gutterman JU. Leukocyte interferon-induced myeloid cytoreduction in chronic myelogenous leukemia. Blood 1983; 62:689–92.
76. Talpaz M, Mavligit G, Keting M, Walters RS, Gutterman JU. Human leukocyte interferon to control thrombocytosis in chronic myelogenous leukemia. Ann Intern Med 1983; 99:789–92.
77. Kantarjian HM, Talpaz M, Gutterman J. Biologic therapy of chronic myelogenous leukemia. Oncology 1987; 1:35–40.
78. Niederle N, Kloke O, Osieka R, Wandl U, Opalka B, Schmidt CG. Interferon alpha-2b in the treatment of chronic myelogenous leukemia. Semin Oncol 1987; 14:29–35.
79. Alimena G, Morra E, Lazzarino M, et al. Interferon alpha-2b as therapy for Ph′ positive chronic myelogenous leukemia: a study of 82 patients treated with intermittent or daily administration. Blood 1988; 72:642–7.
80. Werter M, de Witte R, Janssen J, de Pauw B, Haanen C. Recombinant human interferon-alpha induced cytoreduction in chronic myelogenous leukemia. Blut 1988; 56:209–12.
81. Yoffe G, Blick M, Kantargian H, Spitzer G, Gutterman J, Talpaz M. Molecular analysis of interferon-induced suppression of Philadelphia chromosome in patients with chronic myeloid leukemia. Blood 1987; 69:961–3.
82. Rosenblum MG, Maxwell BL, Talpaz M, Kelleher PJ, McCredie KB, Gutterman JU. In vivo sensitivity and resistance of chronic myelogenous leukemia cells to α-interferon: correlation with receptor binding and induction of 2′,5′-oligoadenylate synthetase. Cancer Res 1986; 46:4848–52.
83. Foon KA, Sherwin SA, Abrams PG, et al. Treatment of advanced non-hodgkin's lymphoma with recombinant leukocyte A interferon. N Engl J Med 1984; 311:1148–52.
84. O'Connell MJ, Colgan JP, Oken MM, Ritts RE, Kay NE, Itri LM. Clinical trial of recombinant leukocyte A interferon as initial therapy for favorable histology non-Hodgkin's lymphomas and chronic lymphocytic leukemia; an Eastern Cooperative Oncology Group pilot study. J Clin Oncol 1986; 4:128–36.
85. Kohn EC, Steis RG, Sausville EA, et al. Phase II trial of intermittent high-dose recombinant interferon alpha-2a in mycosis fungoides and the Sézary syndrome. J Clin Ocol 1990; 8:155–60.

86. Bunn PA, Ihde DC, Foon KA. The role of recombinant interferon alpha-2a in the therapy of cutaneous T-cell lymphomas. Cancer 1986; 57:1698–95.
87. Fauci AS, Macher AM, Longo DL, et al. Acquired immune deficiency syndrome: epidemiologic, clinical, immunologic and therapeutic considerations. Ann Intern Med 1984; 100:92–106.
88. Odajnyk C, Franco FM. Treatment of Kaposi's sarcoma: overview and analysis by clinical setting. J Clin Oncol 1985; 3:1277–85.
89. Krown SE, Real FX, Cunningham-Rundles S, et al. Preliminary observations of the effect of recombinant leukocyte A interferon in homosexual men with Kaposi's sarcoma. N Engl J Med 1983; 308:1071–6.
90. Volberding PA, Mitsuyasu RT, Golando JP, Spiegel RJ. Treatment of Kaposi's sarcoma with interferon alpha-2b (INTRON[R]A). Cancer 1987; 59:620–5.
91. Real FX, Oettgen HF, Krown SE. Kaposi's sarcoma and the acquired immunodeficiency syndrome: treatment with high and low doses of recombinant leukocyte A interferon. J Clin Oncol 1986; 4:544–51.
92. Harris DT. Hormonal therapy and chemotherapy of renal cell carcinoma. Semin Oncol 1983; 10:422–30.
93. Sarna G, Figlin R, de Kernion J. Interferon in renal cell carcinoma: the UCLA experience. Cancer 1987; 59:610–12.
94. Quesada JR, Rios A, Swanson D, Trown P, Gutterman JU. Antitumor activity of recombinant-derived interferon alpha in metastatic renal cell carcinoma. J Clin Oncol 1985; 3:1522–8.
95. Umeda T, Niijima T. Phase II study of alpha interferon on renal cell carcinoma. Cancer 1986; 58:1231–5.
96. Kempf RA, Grunberg SM, Daniels JR, et al. Recombinant interferon α-2 (INTRON A) in a phase II study of renal cell carcinoma. J Biol Response Mod 1986; 5:27–35.
97. Creagan ET, Ahmann DL, Green SJ, et al. Phase II study of recombinant leukocyte A interferon (rIFN-αA) in disseminated malignant melanoma. Cancer 1984; 54:2844–9.
98. Creagan ET, Ahmann DL, Green SJ, et al. Phase II study of low-dose recombinant leukocyte A interferon in disseminated malignant melanoma. J Clin Oncol 1984; 2:1002–5.
99. Creagan ET, Ahmann DL, Green SJ, Long HJ, Frytak S, Itri LM. Phase II study of recombinant leukocyte A interferon (IFN-αA) plus cimetidine in disseminated malignant melanoma. J Clin Oncol 1985; 3:977–81.
100. Hersey P, MacDonald M, Hall C, et al. Immunological effects of recombinant interferon alpha-2a in patients with disseminated melanoma. Cancer 1986; 57:1666–74.
101. McLeod GRC, Thomson DB, Hersey P. Recombinant interferon alpha-2a in advanced malignant melanoma. A phase I-II study in combination with DTIC. Int J Cancer (Suppl) 1987; 1:31–5.
102. Legha SS, Papadopoulas NEJ, Plager C, et al. Clinical evaluation of recombinant interferon alpha-2a (Roferon-A) in metastatic melanoma using two different schedules. J Clin Oncol 1987; 5:1240–6.
103. Borden EC, Hawkins MJ, Sielaff KM, Storer BM, Schiesel JD, Smalley RV. Clinical and biological effects of recombinant interferon-β administered intravenously daily in phase I trial. J Interferon Res 1988; 8:357–66.
104. Perez R, Lipton A, Harvey HA, et al. A phase I trial of recombinant human gamma interferon (IFN-γ_{4A}) in patients with advanced malignancy. J Biol Response Mod 1988; 7:309–17.
105. Eppstein DA, Van der Pas MA, Marsh YV, Bruno NA, Kurahara CG. Enhanced

antitumor efficacy of adriamycin in combination with interferon-γ: effects on macrophages. J Interferon Res 1988; 8:263–73.
106. Jaffe HS, Herberman RB. Rationale for recombinant human interferon-gamma adjuvant immunotherapy for cancer. J Natl Cancer Inst 1988; 80:616–23.
107. Wadler S, Schwartz EL, Goldman M, et al. Fluorouracil and recombinant alpha-2a-interferon: an active regimen against advanced colorectal carcinoma. J Clin Oncol 1989p 7:1769–75.
108. Rosenberg SA, Lotze MT, Yang JC, et al. Combination therapy with interleukin-2 and alpha-interferon for the treatment of patients with advanced cancer. J Clin Oncol 1989; 7:1863–74.
109. Lotze MT, Grimm EA, Mazumder A, Strausser JL, Rosenberg SA. Lysis of fresh and cultured autologous tumor by human lymphocytes cultured in T-cell growth factor. Cancer Res 1981; 41:4420–5.
110. Mule JJ, Rosenberg SA. Successful adoptive immunotherapy of established metastases with lymphokine activated killer cells and recombinant interleukin-2. In: Herberman RB, Wiltrout RH, Gorelik E, eds. Immune responses to metastases, Vol. II. Boca Raton, FL: CRC Press, 1987:69–94.
111. Phillips JH, Lanier LL. Dissection of the lymphokine-activated killer phenomenon: relative contribution of peripheral blood natural killer cells and T lymphocytes to cytolysis. J Exp Med 1986; 164:814–25.
112. Itoh K, Tilden AB, Kumagai K, Balch CM. Leu-11$^+$ lymphocytes with natural killer (NK) activity are precursors of recombinant interleukin 2 (rIL 2)-induced activated killer (LAK) cells. J Immonol 1985; 134:802–7.
113. McMannis JD, Fisher RI, Creekmore SP, Braun DP, Harris JE, Ellis TM. In vivo effects of recombinant IL-2. J Immunol 1988; 140:1335–40.
114. Rosenberg SA, Lotze MT, Muul LM, et al. Observations on the systemic administration of autologous lymphokine-activated killer cell and recombinant interleukin-2 to patients with metastatic cancer. N Engl J Med 1985; 313:1485–92.
115. Rosenberg SA, Lotze MT, Muul LM, et al. A progress report on the treatment of 157 patients with advanced cancer using lympholine-activated killer cells and interleukin-2 or high-dose interleukin-2 alone. N Engl J Med 1987; 316:889–97.
116. Fisher RI, Coltman CA, Doroshow JH, et al. Metastatic renal cancer treated with interleukin-2 and lymphokine-activated killer cells. Ann Intern Med 1988; 108:518–23.
117. Dutcher JP, Creekmore S, Weiss GR, et al. A phase II study of interleukin-2 and lymphokine-activated killer cells in patients with metastatic malignant melanoma. J Clin Oncol 1989; 7:477–85.
118. Lee RE, Lotze MT, Skibber JM, et al. Cardiorespiratory effects of immunotherapy with interleukin-2. J Clin Oncol 1989; 7:7–20.
119. Gaynor ER, Vitek L, Sticklin L, et al. The hemodynamic effects of treatment with interleukin-2 and lymphokine-activated killer cells. Ann Intern Med 1988; 109:953–8.
120. Kozeny GA, Nicolas JD, Creekmore S, Sticklin L, Hano JE, Fisher RI. Effects of interleukin-2 immunotherapy on renal function. J Clin Oncol 1988; 6:1170–6.
121. Ognibene FP, Rosenberg SA, Lotze M, et al. Interleukin-2 administration causes reversible hemodynamic changes and left vntricular dysfunction similar to those seen in septic shock. Chest 1988; 94:750–4.
122. Margolin KA, Rayner AA, Hawkins MJ, et al. Interleukin-2 and lymphokine-activated killer cell therapy of solid tumors: analysis of toxicity and management guidelines. J Clin Oncol 1989; 7:486–98.
123. Christiansen NP, Skubitz KM, Nath K, Ochoa A, Kennedy BJ. Nephrotoxicity of

continuous intravenous infusion of recombinant interleukin-2. Am J Med 1988; 84:1072–5.

124. Eberlein TJ, Schoof DD, Jung SE, et al. A new regimen of interleukin 2 and lymphokine-activated killer cells. Arch Intern Med 1988; 148:2571–6.
125. Thompson JA, Lee DJ, Lindgren CG, et al. Influence of dose and duration of infusion of interleukin-2 on toxicity and immunomodulation. J Clin Oncol 1988; 6:669–78.
126. West WH, Tauer KW, Yannelli JR, et al. Constant-infusion recombinant interleukin-2 in adoptive immunotherapy of advanced cancer. N Engl J Med 1987; 316:898–905.
127. Sosman JA, Kohler PC, Hank J, et al. Repetitive weekly cycles of recombinant human interleukin-2: responses of renal carcinoma with acceptable toxicity. J Natl Cancer Inst 1988; 80:60–3.
128. Boldt DH, Mills BJ, Gemlo BT, et al. Laboratory correlates of adoptive immunotherapy with recombinant interleukin-2 and lymphokine-activated killer cells in humans. Cancer Res 1988; 48:4409–16.
129. Gemlo BT, Palladino MA Jr, Jaffe HS, Espevik TP, Rayner AA. Circulating cytokines in patients with metastatic cancer treated with recombinant interleukin 2 and lymphokine-activated killer cells. Cancer Res 1988; 48:5864–7.
130. Cohen PJ, Lotze MT, Roberts JR, Rosenberg SA, Jaffe ES. The immunopathology of sequential tumor biopsies in patients treated with interleukin-2. Am J Pathol 1987; 129:208–16.
131. Itoh K, Tilden AB, Balch CM. Interleukin-2 activation of cytotoxic T-lymphocytes infiltrating into human metastatic melanomas. Cancer Res 1986; 46:3011–7.
132. Rabinowich H, Cohen R, Bruderman I, Steiner Z, Klajman A. Functional analysis of mononuclear cells infiltrating into tumors: lysis of autologous human tumor cells by cultured infiltrating lymphocytes. Cancer Res 1987; 47:173–7.
133. Belldegrun A, Muul LM, Rosenberg SA. Interleukin-2 expanded tumor-infiltrating lymphocytes in human renal cell cancer: isolation, characterization, and antitumor activity. Cancer Res 1988; 48:206–14.
134. Spiess PJ, Yang JC, Rosenberg SA. In vivo antitumor activity of tumor-infiltrating lymphocytes expanded in recombinant interleukin-2. J Natl Cancer Inst 1987; 79:1067–75.
135. Muul LM, Spiess PJ, Director EP, Rosenberg SA. Identification of specific cytolytic immune responses against autologous tumor in humans bearing malignant melanoma. J Immunol 1987; 138:989.
136. Heo DS, Whiteside TL, Kanbour A, Herberman RB. Lymphocytes infiltrating human ovarian tumors. I. Role of Leu-19(NKH1)-positive recombinant IL-2-activated cultures of lymphocytes infiltrating human ovarian tumors. J Immunol 1988; 140:4042.
137. Tagaki S, Chen K, Schwarz R, Iwatsuki S, Heberman RB, Whiteside TL. Functional and phenotypic analysis of tumor-infiltrating lymphocytes isolated from human primary and metastatic liver tumors and cultured in recombinant interleukin-2. Cancer 1989; 63:102.
138. Heo DL, Whiteside TL, Johnson JT, Chen K, Barnes EL, Herberman RB. Long-term interleukin 2-dependent growth and cytotoxic activity of tumor-infiltrating lymphocytes from human squamous cell carcinomas of the head and neck. Cancer Res 1987; 47:6353.
139. Whiteside TL, Miescher S, Hurlimann J, Moretta J, von Fliedner, V. Clonal analysis and in situ characterization of lymphocytes infiltrating human breast carcinomas. Cancer Immunol Immunother 1986; 23:169.
140. Belldegrun A, Muul LM, Rosenberg SA. Interleukin-2 expanded tumor-infiltrating

lymphocytes in human renal cell cancer: isolation, characterization, and antitumor activity. Cancer Res 1988; 48:206.

141. Rosenberg SA, Packard BS, Aebersold PM, et al. Use of tumor-infiltrating lymphocytes and interleukin-2 in the immunotherapy of patients with metastatic melanoma. N Engl J Med 1988; 319:1676–80.

142. Fisher B, Packard BS, Read EJ, et al. Tumor localization of adoptively transferred indium-111 labeled tumor infiltrating lymphocytes in patients with metastatic melanoma. J Clin Oncol 1989; 7:250–61.

143. Kradin RL, Lazarus DS, Dubinett SM, et al. Tumour-infiltrating lymphocytes and interleukin-2 in treatment of advanced cancer. Lancet 1989; 1:577–80.

144. Mitchell MS, Kempf RA, Harel W, et al. Effectiveness and tolerability of low-dose cyclophosphamide and low-dose intravenous interleukin-2 disseminated melanoma. J Clin Oncol 1988; 6:409–24.

145. Berd D, Maguire HC Jr, Mastrangelo MJ. Impairment of concanavalin A-inducible suppressor activity following administration of cyclophosphamide to patients with advanced cancer. Cancer Res 1984; 44:1275–80.

146. Berd D, Maguire HC Jr, Mastrangelo MJ. Potentiation of human cell-mediated and humoral immunity by low-dose cyclophosphamide. Cancer Res 1984; 44:5439–43.

147. Di Raimondo F, LaPushin R, Hersh EM. Synergistic antitumor activity of a sequential combination of IFN-γ and IL-2 activated killer cells against human melanoma cells in vitro. Submitted to J Immunol Immunother.

148. Taylor CW, Chase EM, Hersh EM, et al. A phase I study of the sequential combination of recombinant gamma-interferon (IFNγ) and recombinant interleukin-2 (IL-2) in patients with disseminated malignant disease. Proc Am Soc Clin Oncol 1990; 9:192.

149. Winkelhake JL, Stampfl S, Zimmerman RJ. Synergistic effects of combination therapy with human recombinant interleukin-2 and tumor necrosis factor in murine tumor models. Cancer Res 1987; 47:3948–53.

150. Higuchi CM, Thompson JA, Lindgren CG, et al. Induction of lymphokine-activated killer activity by interleukin 4 in human lymphocytes preactivated by interleukin 2 in vivo or in vitro. Cancer Res 1989; 49:6487–92.

151. Shiloni E, Eisenthal A, Sachs D, Rosenberg SA. Antibody-dependent cellular cytotoxicity mediated by murine lymphocytes activated in recombinant interleukin 2. J Immunol 1987; 138:1992–8.

152. Howard M, Farrar J, Hilfiker M, et al. Identification of a T cell-derived B cell growth factor distinct form interleukin 2. J Exp Med 1982; 155:914.

153. Paul WE, Ohara J. B-cell stimulatory factor-1/interleukin 4. Annu Rev Immunol 1987; 5:429–59.

154. Defrance T, Vanbervliet B, Aubry JP, et al. B cell growth-promoting activity of recombinant human interleukin 4. J Immunol 1987; 139:1135–47.

155. Spits H, Yssel H, Takebe Y, et al. Recombinant interleukin 4 promotes the growth of human T cells. J Immunol 1987; 139:1142–7.

156. Fernandez-Botran R, Sanders VM, Oliver KG, et al. Interleukin 4 mediates autocrine growth of helper T cells after antigen stimulation. Proc Natl Acad Sci U S A 1986; 83:9689–93.

157. Peschel C, Green I, Paul WE. Interleukin-4 induces a substance in bone marrow stromal cells that reversibly inhibits factor-dependent and factor-independent cell proliferation. Blood 1989; 73:1130–41.

158. Hamaguchi Y, Kanakura Y, Fujita J, et al. Interleukin 4 as an essential factor for in vitro clonal growth of murine connective tissue-type mast cells. J Exp Med 1987; 165:268–73.

159. Defrance T, Aubry JP, Rousset F, et al. Human recombinant interleukin 4 induces

Fcε repectors (CD23) on normal human B lymphocytes. J Exp Med 1987; 165:1459–67.

160. Noelle R, Krammer PH, Ohara J, Uhr JW, Vitetta ES. Increased expression of Ia antigens on resting B cells: an additional role for B-cell growth factor. Proc Natl Acad Sci U S A 1984; 81:6149–53.
161. Mosmann TR, Bond MW, Coffman RL, Ohara J, Paul WE. T-cell and mast cell lines respond to B-cell stimulatory factor 1. Proc Natl Acad Sci 1986; 83:5654–8.
162. Widmer MB, Gradstein KH. Regulation of cytolytic T-lymphocyte generation by B cell stimulatory factor. Nature 1987; 326:795–8.
163. Widmer MB, Acres RB, Sassenfeld HM, Grabstein KH. Regulation of cytolytic cell populations from human peripheral blood by B cell stimulatory factor 1 (interleukin 4). J Exp Med 1987; 166:1447–55.
164. Mule JJ, Smith CA, Rosenberg SA. Interleukin 4 (B-cell stimulatory factor 1) can mediate the induction of lymphokine-activated killer cell activity directed against fresh tumor cells. J Exp Med 1987; 166:792–7.
165. Mule JJ, Krosnick JA, Rosenberg SA. IL-4 regulation of murine lymphokine-activated killer activity in vitro: effects of the IL-2-induced expansion, cytotoxicity and phenotype of lymphokine-activated killer effectors. J Immunol 1989; 142:726–33.
166. Spits H, Yssel H, Paliard S, Kastelein R, Figdor C, DeVries JE. IL-4 inhibits IL-2 mediated induction of human lymphokine-activated killer cells but not the generation of antigen-specific cytotoxic T lymphocytes in mixed leukocyte cultures. J Immunol 1988; 141:29–36.
167. Siegall CB, Chaudhary VK, FitzGerald DJ, Pastan I. Cytotoxic activity of an interleukin 6-*Pseudomonas* exotoxin fusion protein on human myeloma cells. Proc Natl Acad Sci 1988; 85:9738–42.
168. Campbell HD, Tucker WQJ, Hort Y, et al. Molecular cloning, nucleotide sequence, and expression of the gene encoding human eosinophil differentiation factor (interleukin 5). Proc Natl Acad Sci U S A 1987; 84:6629–33.
169. Lopez AF, Sanderson CJ, Gamble JR, Campbell HD, Young IG, Vadas MA. Recombinant human interleukin 5 is a selective activator of human eosinophil function. J Exp Med 1988; 167:219–24.
170. Kishimoto T. The biology of Interleukin-6. Blood 1989; 74:1–10.
171. Ramadori G, Van Damme J, Rieder H, zum Buschenfelde KHM. Interleukin 6, the third mediator of acute-phase reaction, modulates hepatic protein synthesis in human and mouse. Comparison with interleukin 1 β and tumor necrosis factor-α. Eur J Immunol 1988; 18:1259–64.
172. Schindler R, Mancilla J, Endres S, Ghorbani R, Clark SC, Dinarello CA. Correlations and interactions in the production of interluekin-6 (IL-6), IL-1, and tumor necrosis factor (TNF) in human blood mononuclear cells: IL-6 suppresses Il-1 and TNF. Blood 1990; 75:40–7.
173. Van Damme J, Opdenakker G, Simpson RJ, et al. Identification of the human 26-kD protein, interferon β2 (IFN β2), as a B cell hybridoma/plasmacytoma growth factor induced by interleukin 1 and tumour necrosis factor. J Exp Med 1987; 165:914–9.
174. Van Damme J, Cayphas S, Opdenakker G, Billiau A, Van Snick J. Interleukin 1 and poly(RI)poly(RC) induce production of a hybridoma growth factor by human fibroblasts. Eur J Immunol 1987; 17:1–7.
175. Asaoku H, Kawano M, Iwato K, et al. Decrease in BSF-2/IL-6 response in advanced cases of multiple myeloma. Blood 1988; 72:429–32.
176. Zhang XG, Klein B, Bataille R. Interleukin-6 is a potent myeloma-cell growth factor in patients with aggressive multiple myeloma. Blood 1989; 74:11–3.

177. Shabo Y, Lotem J, Rubinstein M, et al. The myeloid blood cell differentiation-inducing protein MGI-2A is interleukin-6. Blood 1988; 72:2070–3.
178. Namen AE, Lupton S, Hjerrild K, et al. Stimulation of B cell progenitors by cloned murine interleukin-7. Nature 1988; 333:571.
179. Williams DE, Namen AE, Mochizuki DY, Overell RW. Clonal growth of murine pre-B colony-forming cells and their targeted infection by a retroviral vector: dependence on interleukin-7. Blood 1990; 75:1132–8.
180. Lee G, Namen AE, Gillis S, Ellingsworth LR, Kincade PW. Normal B cell precursors responsive to recombinant murine IL-7 and inhibition of IL-7 activity by transforming growth factor-β. J Immunol 1989; 142:3875–83.
181. Gimbrone MA, Obin MS, Brock AF, et al. Endothelial interleukin-8: a novel inhibitor of leukocyte-endothelial interactions. Science 1989; 246:1601–3.
182. Yang YC, Kelleher K, Ricciardi S, Ciarleta A, Calvetti J, Clark SC. Molecular cloning and characterization of human interleukin-9. Blood 1989; 74:116a (abstract 431).
183. Donahue RE, Yang YC, Paul S, Clark SC. Human interleukin-9 (IL-9) is capable of stimulating erythroid colony formation in vitro. Blood 1989; 74:116a (abstract 432).
184. Coley WB. The treatment of malignant tumors by repeated inoculations of erysipelas: with a report of ten original cases. Am J Med Sci 1893; 105:487–511.
185. Coley-Nauts H, Fowler GA, Bogatko FH. A review of the influence of bacterial infection and of bacterial products (Coley's toxins) on malignant tumors in man. Acta Med Scand (Suppl) 1953; 274(7):29–97.
186. Carswell EA, Old LJ, Kassel RJ, Green S, Fiore N, Williamson B. An endotoxin-induced serum factor that causes necrosis of tumours. Proc Natl Acad Sci U S A 1975; 72:3666–70.
187. Van Der Merwe, PA. Tumour necrosis factor. S Afr Med J 1988; 74:411–7.
188. Sugarman BJ, Aggarwal BB, Hass PE, Figari IS, Palladino MA Jr, Shepard HM. Recombinant human tumor necrosis factor α: effects on proliferation of normal and transformed cell in vitro. Science 1985; 230:943–5.
189. Fransen L, Ruysschaert MR, Van Der Heyden J, Fiers W. Recombinant tumor necrosis factor: species specificity for a variety of human and murine transformed cell lines. Cell Immunol 1986; 100:260–7.
190. Dealtry GB, Naylor MS, Fiers W, Balkwill FT. The effect of recombinant human tumor necrosis factor on growth and macromolecular synthesis of human epithelial cells. Exp Cell Res 1987; 170:428–38.
191. Fiers W, Brouckaert P, Goldberg AL, et al. Structure-function relationship of tumour necrosis factor and its mechanisms of action. CIBA Found Symp 1987; 131:109–23.
192. Ruggiero V, Johnson SE, Baglioni C. Protection from tumor necrosis factor cytotoxicity by protease inhibitors. Cell Immunol 1987; 107:317–25.
193. Tracey KJ, Lowry SF, Cerami A. Cachectin: a hormone that triggers actue shock and chronic cachexia. J Infect Dis 1988; 157:413–20.
194. Talmadge JE, Phillips H, Schneider M, et al. Immunomodulatory properties of recombinant murine and human tumor necrosis factor. Cancer Res 1988; 48:544–50.
195. Schell-Frederick E, Tepass T, Lorscheidt G, Pfreundschuh M, Schaadt M, Diehl V. Effects of recombinant tumor necrosis factor (rHuTNFα) on human neutrophils and monocytes: in vitro, ex vivo and in vivo. Eur J Haematol 1989; 43:286–96.
196. Kist A, Ho AD, Rath U, et al. Decrease of natural killer cell activity and monokine production in peripheral blood of patients treated with recombinant tumor necrosis factor. Blood 1988; 72:344–8.
197. Wang Am, Creasey AA, Ladner MB, et al. Molecular cloning of the complementary DNA for human tumor necrosis factor. Science 1985; 228:149–54.

198. Shirai T, Yamaguchi M, Ito H, et al. Cloning and expression in *Escherichia coli* of the gene of human tumor necrosis factor. Nature 1985; 313:803–6.
199. Spriggs DR, Herman ML, Michie H, et al. Recombinant human tumor necrosis factor administered as a 24-hour intravenous infusion. A phase I and pharmacologic study. J Natl Cancer Inst 1988; 80:1039–44.
200. Feinberg B, Kurzrock R, Talpaz M, Blick M, Saks S, Gutterman JU. A phase I trial of intravenously-administered recombinant tumor necrosis factor-alpha in cancer patients. J Clin Oncol 1988; 6:1328–34.
201. Sherman ML, Spriggs DR, Arthur KA, Imamura K, Frei E III, Kufe KW. Recombinant human tumor necrosis factor adminsitered as a five-day continuous infusion in cancer patients: phase I toxicity and effects on lipid metabolism. J Clin Oncol 1988; 6:344–50.
202. Owen-Schaub LB, Gutterman JU, Grimm EA. Synergy of tumor necrosis factor and interleukin 2 in the activation of human cytotoxic lymphocytes: effect of tumor necrosis factor α and interleukin-2 in the generation of human lymphokine-activated killer cell cytotoxicity. Cancer Res 1988; 48:788–92.
203. Agah R, Malloy B, Sherrod A, Bean P, Girgis E, Mazumder A. Therapy of disseminated NK-resistant tumor by the synergistic effects of recombinant interleukin-2 and tumor necrosis factor. J Biol Response Mod 1988; 7:140–51.
204. Watanabe N, Niitsu Y, Yamauchi N, et al. Antitumor synergism between recombinant human tumor necrosis factor and recombinant human interferon-r. J Biol Response Mod 1988; 7:24–31.
205. Salmon SE, Young L. Scuderi P. Clark B. Antineoplastic effects of tumor necrosis factor alone and in combination with gamma-interferon on tumor biopsies in clonogenic assay. J Clin Oncol 1987; 5:1816–21.
206. Yang SC, Owne-Schaub L, Mendiguren-Rodriguez A, Grimm EA, Hong WK, Roth JA. Combination immunotherapy for non-small cell lung cancer. J Thorac Cardiovasc Surg 1990; 99:8–13.
207. Abbruzzese JL, Levin B, Ajani JA, et al. Phase I trial of recombinant human γ-interferon and recombinant human tumor necrosis factor in patients with advanced gastrointestinal cancer. Cancer Res 1989; 49:4057–61.
208. Creaven PJ, Plager JE, Dupere S, et al. Phase I clinical trial of recombinant human tumor necrosis factor. Cancer Chemother Pharmacol 1987; 20:137–44.
209. Creagan ET, Kovach JS, Moertel CG, Frytak S, Kvols LK. A phase I clinical trial of recombinant human tumor necrosis factor. Cancer 1988; 62:2467–71.
210. Jakubowski AA, Casper ES, Gabrilove JL, Templeton MA, Sherwin SA, Oettgen HF. Phase I trial of intramuscularly administered tumor necrosis factor in patients with advanced cancer. J Clin Oncol 1989; 7:298–303.
211. Wiedenmann B, Reichardt P, Rath U, et al. Phase-I trial of intravenous continuous infusion of tumor necrosis factor in advanced metastatic carcinomas. J Cancer Res Clin Oncol 1989; 115:189–92.
212. Zamkoff KW, Newman NB, Rudolph AF, Young J, Poiesz BJ. A phase I trial of subcutaneously administered recombinant tumor necrosis factor to patients with advanced malignancy. J Biol Response Mod 1989; 8:539–52.
213. Lenk H, Tannenberger ST, Muller U, Ebert J, Shiga T. Phase II clinical trial of high-dose recombinant human tumor necrosis factor. Cancer Chemother Pharmacol 1989; 24:391–2.
214. Ghosh AK, Dazzi H, Thatcher N, Moore M. Lack of correlation between peripheral blood lymphokine-activated killer (LAK) cell function and clinical response in patients with advanced malignant melanoma receiving recombinant interleukin-2. Int J Cancer 1989; 43:410–4.

CHAPTER 25

CYTOKINES AND RENAL DISEASE

Steven N. Emancipator and John R. Sedor

Case Western Reserve University
Cleveland, Ohio

INTRODUCTION

Classic immune mechanisms clearly initiate glomerular injury, but recent evidence has strongly suggested that the intrinsic population of glomerular cells is a key participant in both the restorative and destructive processes that follow renal injury. A number of potential mediators have been studied, but accumulating in vitro and in vivo evidence has implicated several interleukins (IL) and tumor necrosis factor α (TNF-α) as mediators of glomerular injury. Much of the work published to date has focused on the role of the interleukins and TNF-α in the pathogenesis of glomerulonephritis and their interactions with glomerular cells in culture (almost exclusively the glomerular mesangial cell). Cytokine synthesis and release is much less well studied in the pathogenesis of tubulointerstitial disease. In this chapter, we summarize the available in vitro and in vivo evidence demonstrating that inflammatory interleukins and TNF-α are important mediators of glomerulonephritis and describe the published data suggesting that these cytokines may also be important in tubulointerstitial injury.

GLOMERULAR CELLS IN CULTURE

Cytokine Production

The mechanisms underlying progressive glomerular injury are incompletely understood. Recent evidence in vitro strongly suggests that the intrinsic glomerular population perpetuates ongoing glomerular inflammation. We have focused on the mesangial cell because studies describing either the synthesis of the interleukins by or the interactions with other glomerular cells are limited or lacking.

More importantly, mesangial cells occupy a central anatomic position within the glomerulus and are in a pivotal position to orchestrate events underlying glomerular immune injury (1,2). The individual studies of mesangial cell biology, when viewed as an aggregate body of work, provide convincing evidence that mesangial cells are specialized pericytes that not only provide structural support to the glomerulus and control glomerular filtration, functions discussed since the 1920s and 1930s, but also respond to immune reactants, cytokines, and peptides to express new structural and functional characteristics (1,2).

Mesangial cells morphologically resemble smooth muscle cells and contract in response to vasoconstrictor hormones and inflammatory mediators (1,2). Mesangial cells synthesize basement membrane components, including collagen and fibronectin (1,2). These cells also secrete inflammatory mediators, including oxygen radicals, lipoxygenase, and cyclooxygenase products and a neutral protease capable of digesting glomerular basement membrane (1,2). In many instances, such inflammatory mediators have been produced in response to immunological stimuli. We have observed superoxide release (3) and enhanced eicosanoid synthesis (4) by mesangial cells after incubation with immune complexes, effects dependent on the Fc region of antibody. Schlondorff and his associates reported that phagocytosis of serum-treated zymosan is associated with stimulation of lipoxygenase and cyclooxygenase activity, and IgG-opsonized gold stimulates platelet-activating factor (PAF) and increases prostaglandin E_2 (PGE_2) synthesis by mesangial cells (2,5).

Proliferation of mesangial cells has also been demonstrated in response to platelet and macrophage products and is characteristic of many forms of immune-mediated glomerulonephritis (GN) (1,2). Local release within the glomerulus of growth factors and cytokines may be an important pathogenetic determinant of the structural and functional changes associated with glomerular immune injury, at least in part by expanding and activating this population of resident immune effector cells. Studies demonstrating that mesangial cells elaborate growth factors and cytokines, as described later, further emphasize the pivotal role of glomerular mesangial cells in mediating glomerular immune injury. Mesangial cells in culture also express receptors for some of these cytokines, as well as others potentially synthesized by glomerular endothelium, epithelium, or infiltrating cells (1,2). These in vitro studies therefore create a scenario in which the mesangial cell is a key participant in generating and responding to a network of polypeptide cytokines, which are potentially important in the pathogenesis of glomerulonephritis. They also suggest that mesangial cells can be induced to switch from a contractile to a secretory or activated phenotype.

Of all the cytokines, the synthesis of IL-1 by glomerular cells and the actions of IL-1 on glomerular cells has been best studied in a number of laboratories. Lovett and his colleagues originally demonstrated that proliferating cultured rat mesangial cells produced an IL-1-like cytokine, originally termed mesangial cell-derived thymocyte activating factor, which was an endogenous pyrogen (6,7). Both they (8) and we (9) demonstrated concurrently that cultured human and rat mesangial cells, respectively, contain transcripts that comigrate on northern analyses with macrophage IL-1α and IL-1β. The pI and molecular weights of rat and human mesangial cell IL-1 proteins are indistinguishable from those of macrophage IL-1α and IL-1β (8,10). The transcriptional and posttranscriptional regulation of mesangial cell IL-1 biosynthesis is only sketchily understood. Serum, platelet-derived growth factor and epidermal growth factor in combination, complement, and endotoxin (lipopolysaccharide, LPS) appear to increase mesangial cell IL-1 production (10–12). Mesangial cell-derived, as well as monocyte-derived, IL-1α and IL-1β are myristylated after translation (13). Although cultured endothelium derived from other tissues synthesizes IL-1, convincing data demonstrating that either glomerular endothelial cells or epithelial cells express IL-1 mRNA or synthesize IL-1 protein are lacking.

Mesangial cell production of other cytokines has been studied to a more limited degree. Baud and his colleagues demonstrated that tumor necrosis factor is released by mesangial cells upon stimulation by LPS. TNF-α synthesis is regulated by both prostaglandin E_2 and cyclic AMP (14). Three studies have demonstrated that cultured mesangial cells express IL-6 mRNA transcripts and release IL-6 bioactivity in response to LPS IL-6, IL-Iβ, and TNF-α (15,16a,16b).

Cultured mesangial cells secrete a cytokine indistinguishable from granulocyte-macrophage colony-stimulating factor (17), exhibited by the capacity of mesangial cell-conditioned serum-free medium to support the growth of HT-2 cells, but not the IL-2- or IL-4-dependent CTLL-2 line. Proliferation of HT-2 cells was completely blocked by antibody specific for granulocyte-macrophage colony-stimulating factor (GM-CSF). Mesangial cell-derived GM-CSF has a molecular weight of 22–44 kD and a pI of 4.4–5.0 and elutes from a C-18 reversed-phase column at 48–50% acetonitrile. Both northern and in situ hybridization demonstrated GM-CSF transcripts in mesangial cells. Schlondorff and his coworkers have shown that mouse mesangial cells also synthesize colony-stimulating factor 1 (CSF-1) (18). The synthesis of CSF-1 was stimulated by interferon-γ and inhibited by dibutyryl cyclic AMP. The changes in the synthetic rates of CSF-1 were preceded by corresponding changes in the mRNA levels encoding CSF-1.

Since immune injured glomeruli have been shown to produce IL-8 activity in vitro, we recently assessed whether LPS- or cytokine-activated mesangial cells are a source of this activity (19). IL-1α, IL-1β, TNF, and LPS stimulated the release of a neutrophil chemotactic factor from cultured human mesangial cells in our study (19). Despite similar results, another group did not observe IL-8 production in response to IL-8 (19a). Both concentrated and unconcentrated mesangial cell supernatants stimulated directed neutrophil migration under agarose at a level similar to that of the bacterial chemotactic peptide, formyl-methionyl leucyl phenylalanine (FMLP). In contrast, unstimulated mesangial cell-conditioned media and IL-1α, IL-1β, TNF, and LPS in medium alone did not directly induce neutrophil migration. Monoclonal anti-IL-8 antibody significantly inhibited neutrophil chemotaxis. Chemotactic activity was present in the 3–10 kD faction of TNF-stimulated, mesangial cell-conditioned media. S_1 nuclease analyses of total RNA extracted from TNF-stimulated mesangial cells showed a dose- and time-dependent increase in IL-8 mRNA transcripts. The northern analysis of TNF-stimulated mesangial cell RNA identified IL-8 transcripts of mesangial cells that comigrated with the 1.8 kD message in LPS-stimulated human monocytes. Using ^{35}S-labeled oligonucleotide probes, IL-8 mRNA transcripts were demonstrated in the cytoplasm of IL-1- and TNF-stimulated, but not control, mesangial cells. Collectively, these data demonstrate that a chemotaxin highly homologous to IL-8 is produced by cytokine- and LPS-stimulated mesangial cells. Synthesis of a basic 10 kD protein related to the KC/gro family, chemotactic for neutrophils, is induced in a kidney-derived epithelioid cell line as well as in rat glomerular epithelial cells by IL-1β and TNF-α (20,21).

Effects of Cytokines on Cell Metabolism and Function

In addition to synthesizing IL-1, cultured human and rat mesangial cells have IL-1 receptors. Scatchard analysis of mesangial cell binding of radioiodinated IL-1α and IL-1β revealed a single class of high-affinity receptors with a K_d of 5.5×10^{-11} M and approximately 4000 receptors per cell (22). Using RNA-RNA solution hybridization, we demonstrated further that mesangial cells express mRNA transcripts for the T cell–fibroblast-type IL-1 receptor (J. R. Sedor, unpublished observations).

IL-1 induces a variety of biochemical and functional responses in mesangial cells. IL-1 is a comitogen for cultured mesangial cells, in that purified rat IL-1 enhanced the proliferative rates of mesangial cells only in the presence of serum (10,23). To address this issue further, we used a fully defined medium that supports mesangial cell growth. Addition of fibroblast growth factor (FGF) at submitogenic concentrations or IL-1α did not further enhance the proliferation of mesangial cells upon changing from holding to defined medium (24). However, IL-1α and FGF synergistically increased [^{3}H]thymidine incorporation, suggesting that the signaling pathways activated by interleukin-1α alone do not induce cell growth. Stahl and his coworkers recently extended these observations and demonstrated that, although rat recombinant IL-1β is a mesangial cell comitogen, endogenous PGE_2 formation, which is also stimulated by the addition of the cytokine, antagonizes the growth-promoting activities of the cytokine (25). When prostaglandin synthesis was inhibited by indomethacin, interleukin-1β-induced cell proliferation was sevenfold greater compared with interleukin-1 alone. In addition to being a comitogen, both macrophage and mesangial cell-derived interleukin-1 stimulate cultured mesangial cells to generate prostaglandin E_2, to express IL-6 and IL-8 (16b), to synthesize collagen, to enhance interferon-γ-induced class II histocompatability antigens, and to enhance secretion of a glomerular basement membrane-degrading neutral protease (26–29). A recent report has also demonstrated that these cells in culture produce significant amounts of superoxide anion and hydrogen peroxide after exposure to IL-1β (30).

The early transmembrane signaling pathways activating mesangial cells by IL-1 have also been studied in some detail. We initially focused on the phospholipid-derived and ionic signals that may transduce the effects of IL-1 on cultured mesangial cells (24). We demonstrated that IL-1α induces a rapid increase in 1,2-diacylglycerol formation that peaks at 1 minute. Interleukin-1α had no effect on inositol phosphate or cytosolic calcium concentrations, demonstrating that interleukin-1 does not activate an inositol phospholipid-specific phospholipase C. We also found that [^{3}H]phosphorylethanolamine, but not [^{3}H]phosphorylserine or [^{3}H]phosphorylcholine, was maximally elevated at 1 minute in mesangial cells incubated with interleukin-1. Radioactivity incorporated into phosphatidylethanolamine but not phosphatidylcholine was also decreased in interleukin-1-stimulated mesangial cells compared with control at 1 minute.

These data suggest that interleukin-1 activates a phospholipase C in mesangial cells that is predominantly linked to phosphatidylethanolamine. In contrast to other mitogens, interleukin-1 did not alter intracellular pH in mesangial cells (24). Bursten et al. have also shown in cultured mesangial cells rapid interleukin-1-stimulated diacylglycerol formation from phosphatidic acid by phosphatidic phosphohydrolase (31).

The effects of IL-1 on other early transmembrane signaling pathways have also been studied. Pfeilschifter and his colleagues recently demonstrated that IL-1β did not stimulate cyclic AMP formation in incubations as long as 24 h (32) but increased cyclic GMP formation after a long period of 4–8 h (33). Regulation of cell function often involves changes in protein phosphorylation. In vitro, interleukin-1 stimulates the rapid phosphorylation of several membrane proteins, which are 52–55, 46, and 20 kD in size (34). The 46 kD phosphoprotein, which was the most prominently phosphorylated, contained phosphotyrosine when examined by phosphoamino acid analysis. The 52–55 and 20 kD phosphoproteins were alkaline labile and contained phosphoserine. In addition, we recently found that interleukin-1 does not change the phosphorylation state of the putative 80 kD substrate of protein kinase C (J. R. Sedor, unpublished data). Taken together, these studies suggest that interleukin-1 induces an activated mesangial cell phenotype by activating early transmembrane signaling mechanisms that are independent of both protein kinase C and cyclic AMP-dependent protein kinase activation.

The molecular mechanisms by which interleukin-1 induces prostaglandin synthesis by mesangial cells have also been extensively studied. Similar to its effects on other cells, purified rat interleukin-1 induces prostaglandin production by serum-stimulated but not quiescent rat mesangial cells (26). We used this model to study the mechanisms by which recombinant IL-1α enhances cellular prostaglandin synthesis (35). Serum was required for extended mesangial cell prostaglandin formation. Both cycloheximide and actinomycin D inhibited IL-1-induced prostaglandin production. Arachidonate availability is a key determinant of prostaglandin production, and phospholipase A_2 activity directly regulates cellular arachidonate levels. In vitro, phospholipase activity was increased 5- to 10-fold in acid extracts of IL-1-treated cells as measured by arachidonate release from exogenous [^{14}C]arachidonylphosphatidylethanolamine. This phospholipase activity was calcium dependent and inhibited by phospholipase A_2 inhibitors. A sensitive and specific solution hybridization assay demonstrated coordinate, time-dependent induction of nonpancreatic (type II) phospholipase A_2 mRNA transcripts. In whole cells, basal arachidonate release was equivalent in vehicle- and IL-1-primed cells, but vasopressin-stimulated arachidonate release was potentiated two- to threefold by interleukin-1 pretreatment, suggesting that IL-1 may prime cells for increased prostaglandin synthesis by increasing phospholipase A_2 activity. Our data demonstrate that IL-1 induces a nonpancreatic phospholipase A_2 and imply that IL-1 directly stimulates, as well as primes cells for, enhanced prostaglandin synthesis, in part by increasing phospholipase A_2 activity through new enzyme synthesis.

Pfeilschifter and his coworkers also showed that IL-1β-stimulated mesangial cell prostaglandin synthesis requires a cofactor in serum and that IL-1 increased mesangial cell phospholipase A_2 activity (32). They recently characterized the IL-

1-stimulated phospholipase A_2 activity as a nonpancreatic (type II) phospholipase A_2 using immunoblotting (36). The role of different second messenger systems in the regulation or reconstitution of the induction of phospholipase A_2 activity by IL-1 has also been studied (32). These data demonstrate that cytokines specifically induce a nonpancreatic type II phospholipase A_2 in a highly regulated manner that is independent of protein kinase C activation and is potentiated but not reconstituted by cyclic AMP formation.

Epithelial cell responses to IL-1 have been much less extensively studied. Human epithelial cells in culture synthesize collagen IV and release tissue plasminogen activator and plasminogen activator inhibitor in increased amounts after addition of IL-1, relative to normal culture medium (37,38). No other effects of IL-1 on glomerular epithelium have been recognized.

The effects of TNF-α on mesangial cells have been somewhat less well studied than those of IL-1. TNF-α has pleiotropic effects on the mesangial cell in culture. Similar to IL-1, TNF-α potently stimulates prostaglandin production by cultured mesangial cells and induces the synthesis and release of a nonpancreatic (type II) phospholipase A_2 (32,36,39), and promotes IL-8 expression (19,19a). TNF-α also exerts a priming effect on prostaglandin production by mesangial cells (40). TNF-α has been reported to be both mitogenic and cytostatic for mesangial but not glomerular epithelial cells (29,41). TNF-α induces mesangial cell expression of class I histocompatability determinants and synergizes with interferon-γ to increase expression of class II loci (29). Metabolically, mesangial cell oxygen radical production (30), 5′-nucleotidase activity (42), and cGMP (33) are increased by TNF-α. Marsden and Ballermann demonstrated that TNF-α increases mesangial cell cyclic GMP content by inducing the expression of an enzyme involved in the formation of L-arginine-derived nitric oxide, which acts in an autocrine fashion to activate mesangial cell-soluble guanylate cyclase (43).

Camussi and his coworkers have demonstrated that TNF-α induces profound changes in mesangial shape and cytoskeletal organization (44). The early morphological changes, which are evident after 1 h and peak at 3–4 h after TNF stimulation, are fully reversible. The changes in mesangial cell shape occur concomitantly with cytoskeletal rearrangements. Actin distribution changes from a pattern of circumferential peripheral bands associated with centrally oriented stress fibers to a more disorganized pattern of actin microfilaments. Vinculin also disappears at stress fiber endings, which correspond to focal contacts between membrane and substrate. We demonstrated that TNF-α induces the synthesis of a mesangial cell membrane-associated procoagulant activity, which had the characteristics of tissue factor (45).

Similar to other cytokines, the effects of tumor necrosis factor on glomerular epithelial cells and endothelial cells are essentially unstudied. One published account indicates that TNF increases the release of both urokinase and tissue types of plasminogen activator (38); another fails to identify an effect of TNF on glomerular epithelial proliferation (41).

The effects of the other interleukins on mesangial cell function are limited. Subconfluent rat mesangial cells respond to IL-6 stimulation with dose-dependent proliferation (16a). Mesangial cell CSF-1 receptor expression was demonstrated by immunofluorescence with an antireceptor antibody, specific binding of iodinated CSF-1 and expression of CSF-1 receptor mRNA by northern blot analysis

(18). Interestingly, neither GM-CSF nor CSF-1 is mitogenic for mesangial cells (17,18). The effects of these and other cytokines on the glomerular epithelial and endothelial cell are unknown.

GLOMERULAR DISEASE IN VIVO

Cytokine Production

Mice of the MRL strain, homozygous for a lymphoproliferative gene (*lpr/lpr*), develop an autoimmune disease that clinically, serologically, and histologically resembles spontaneous systemic lupus erythematosus in humans. Multiple organs, particularly kidney, joints, and skin, are affected. As these animals age from 12 to 30 weeks, renal function deteriorates progressively and a proliferative glomerulonephritis develops pari passu with a tubulointerstitial nephritis. The content of mRNA encoding IL-1β and TNF in renal cortex and isolated glomeruli increases with advancing age in *lpr/lpr* mice, but this message is absent or much less abundant in age-matched congenic MRL +/+ mice, which lack the lymphoproliferative gene (46–48). Similar alterations are described in NZB/NZW F_1 mice, a genetically distinct spontaneous murine model of lupus (49). Supernatant from glomeruli isolated from diseased *lpr/lpr* mice, but not +/+ or predisease *lpr/lpr* mice, contained detectable IL-1 and TNF bioactivity (46,47). These investigators reported that IL-1α transcripts were undetectable in diseased or predisease *lpr/lpr* mice or age-matched +/+ mice but were present in cultured cells. A novel 1200 base truncated IL-1β transcript was identified.

Autoimmune glomerular disease induced by antibodies specific for the glomerular basement membrane (GBM) is modeled in several species. Although active anti-GBM disease can be induced, passive injection of heterologous anti-GBM is most frequently employed. In this instance, two phases of injury are recognized: one is induced by the heterologous anti-GBM, the other by the autologous antibody specific for the heterologous IgG deposited in the GBM. An accelerated autologous phase can be induced by priming animals with nonspecific heterologous IgG a week before injecting the anti-GBM antibody. Both rabbits and rats with the accelerated autologous model have a necrotizing and crescentic glomerulonephritis. Glomeruli isolated from these animals, when maintained in short-term culture, produce significantly more IL-1 activity than controls (50–53). Anti-IL-1 added to glomerular culture supernatant eliminates thymocyte proliferation activity. Glomeruli from rabbits with a simple heterologous phase produced much lower, but still abnormal, amounts of IL-1, notwithstanding that the rabbits were heavily proteinuric. Culture supernatant from glomeruli isolated from each of three patients with crescentic glomerulonephritis contained IL-1 bioactivity far in excess of that in supernatants from glomeruli isolated from four donor kidneys not deemed suitable for allografting or from one normal kidney (54). The production of active IL-1 increased progressively from 3 to 28 days in culture. Glomeruli isolated from rats with anti-GBM nephritis adhere to plastic cell culture dishes better than normal glomeruli (55). Although this may be an indicator of yet another example of the influence of cytokines on glomerular structure and function, it may also be taken as a caveat in the interpretation of the aforementioned data. To the extent that increased glomerular adhesiveness in culture improves cell yield, this increased adhesiveness may result in parallel increases in the amount of cytokines released into the culture medium.

Immune complex glomerulonephritis induced by immunization and challenge with alloantigens is also associated with enhanced renal cytokine expression. In a model of membranous nephropathy induced in rats by cationized bovine gammaglobulin, enhanced IL-1 mRNA is detectable in the RNA extracted from renal cortex by both northern and ribonuclease protection assays (9). Further study of this model indicates that IL-1β, but not IL-1α, is transcribed. There is increased urinary excretion of IL-1 in the proteinuric phase of chronic serum sickness and of TNF in the progressive renal failure phase (56).

Mesangiopathic glomerulonephritis with predominant IgA deposits, induced in mice by dextran immunization, is associated with phasic expression of IL-1β but no increases in IL-1α or TNF (L. Gesualdo et al., unpublished observations). In the proliferative form of this model, IL-6 mRNA was also detected in renal cortex; none was present in normals or in the form that lacks proliferation. Increased IL-6 activity was detected in the urine of half the patients with mesangial proliferative glomerulonephritis but none of those with minimal change nephrosis or membranous nephropathy (15). Interleukin-6 was demonstrable immunohistochemically in glomeruli only of those patients with mesangial proliferative glomerulonephritis.

Nonimmune glomerular injury also elicits cytokine production. The nephrotoxic drug puromycin aminonucleoside induces nephrosis when injected into rats; the effects are enhanced by concomitant administration of protamine sulfate. Culture supernatants of glomeruli isolated from rats 10 days after injection of both agents contained 60% more IL-1 bioactivity than control rats injected with saline. By 80 days after injection, however, glomeruli from rats given the drugs produced 40% less IL-1 than controls. Although this may be explained on the basis of the increasing glomerulosclerosis observed over this period, the sclerosis was not very severe. Therefore, phasic regulation of IL-1 may be operative in this injury (57). Recently, increased numbers of cells containing IL-1 and TNF were observed immunohistochemically in glomeruli of rats with puromycin aminonucleoside nephrosis (58). Rats deficient in essential fatty acids did not become proteinuric after puromycin injection and lacked IL-1- or TNF-containing cells in their glomeruli. Endotoxemia instigated by injection of LPS also promotes increased renal TNF expression (59).

Effects of Cytokines on Glomerular Structure and Function

Exogenous IL-1 or TNF, when given to NZB/NZW mice, accelerates and increases proteinuria and increases mortality (49). However, decreased TNF production in NZB/NZW mice, ascribed to a genetic alteration, was associated with disease in that replacement therapy with TNF ameliorated renal injury (60). Administration of the experimental immunosuppressive drug OK432 to NZB/NZW mice is associated with increased TNF synthesis and also decreased renal injury, again suggesting that TNF can reduce disease (61). The discrepancies between these experiments in terms of the effects of TNF may be related to the differences in dose and timing and argue that TNF has phasic effects on glomerular inflammation. The increases in renal cortical TNF and interferon-γ observed in MRL/

lpr mice were associated with increased expression of class I and II histocompatibility determinants (48) and intercellular adhesion molecule 1 (62). Doses of cyclosporine reduced renal levels of cytokines and histocompatability antigens in parallel with renal injury, suggesting that increases in the expression of accessory (histocompatibility) determinants are important for pathogenesis.

In accelerated autologous nephrotoxic nephritis, endotoxin (LPS) administered before or with anti-GBM antibody increases the glomerular production of IL-1, measured by bioactivity, and potentiates proteinuria and histological abnormalities, particularly monocyte infiltration and mesangial matrix expansion, when subnephritogenic doses of anti-GBM are given (51). Both antimacrophage and anti-IL-1 antibodies markedly attenuate proteinuria, histological changes, and IL-1 activity, although only antimacrophage antibody abrogates these effects. Interestingly, indomethacin increases recovery of IL-1 activity. Collectively, these data suggest that stimulation of circulating macrophages by LPS potentiates glomerular injury by otherwise innocuous levels of anti-GBM antibody and that this effect is primarily mediated by IL-1. In this system, prostaglandins may attenuate IL-1 production by macrophages in response to LPS or indomethacin may have other effects that synergize to enhance IL-1 production.

In the heterologous phase of anti-GBM nephritis, sequential injections of anti-GBM antibody and LPS in rats, at doses well below those that caused any changes with either agonist alone, resulted in marked glomerular thrombosis and neutrophil influx in association with deposition of anti-GBM within the glomeruli (63). Although most experiments infused anti-GBM first, LPS could be given up to 6 h before anti-GBM for this synergism to occur. Glomerular thrombosis was not evident until 3 h after LPS infusion. Depletion of circulating neutrophils in rats before sequential injection of anti-GBM and LPS markedly reduced glomerular thrombosis, but depletion of platelets had no effect. Since IL-1 promotes adherence of neutrophils to normal isolated glomeruli (64), possibly via increased glomerular intercellular adhesion molecule 1 (ICAM-1) (62), the neutrophil influx was not surprising. The neutrophil-dependent increase in intraglomerular thrombosis, however, suggested the concept that neutrophils are primed by LPS to elicit injury. Neutrophils pulsed in vitro with LPS and then infused into rats previously given anti-GBM lead to striking glomerular thrombosis (63). Both IL-1 and TNF promote adhesion and diapedesis of neutrophils to and through human umbilical vein endothelium in vitro (65). Endothelial protein synthesis is required for the diapedesis and enhanced adhesion of neutrophils, but the effect is specific for neutrophils and the authors cannot exclude the possibility that neutrophils produce a factor that promotes endothelial synthesis of a requisite protein. The authors clearly excluded IL-2, interferon-γ, platelet-derived growth factor, histamine, thrombin, platelet-activating factor, and leukotriene B_4 as critical elements in the interaction between neutrophils and endothelium, but IL-8 may account for this effect (reviewed in Ref. 19).

The effects of LPS appear to be mediated principally by monokines. Human recombinant IL-1β and/or TNF, given to rats 1 h before subnephritogenic doses of anti-GBM, significantly increased albuminuria, glomerular thrombosis, and glomerular neutrophil infiltration and necrosis, as did LPS (66). The two recombinant monokines had similar effects at similar doses and showed synergy when given together. The response to LPS seems to incorporate elements other than

IL-1 and TNF, since LPS promoted thrombosis better than the combination of monokines. None of these stimuli, given 1 h before an equal mass of nonspecific rabbit IgG, had any effect, even at doses 10–100 times those given with rabbit anti-GBM, indicating that the cytokines potentiate antibody-mediated injury but do not elicit injury in and of themselves.

In rabbits, infusion of human recombinant TNF at doses of 800 or 8000 ng/kg body weight per hour induced pancytopenia, conjunctival inflammation, fever, and a neutrophil infiltrate in glomeruli (67). At the higher dose, azotemia developed, interpreted by the authors as acute renal failure. Although no measure of glomerular filtration rate was undertaken, renal plasma flow decreased progressively after 3 h. Of the eight rabbits in this group two also developed fibrin deposition in the glomeruli. Widespread endothelial damage was evident ultrastructurally, but no proteinuria was observed. These changes were not observed when boiled TNF or 0.5 ng/kg/h of LPS was infused, and addition of polymyxin B did not affect the response to TNF. Although infusion of human recombinant IL-1β had little effect itself, syngergism was observed when IL-1β was added to TNF. Interestingly, TNF had no influence when infused into functioning isolated kidneys maintained on extracorporeal perfusion. This suggests that the effects of TNF on the kidney are mediated via extrarenal cells, rather than via a direct action of TNF on endogenous renal cells, at least in this system.

Interleukin-6 also influences the response of glomeruli to injurious stimuli. Transgenic mice bearing copies of recombinant IL-6 genes and expressing increased transcripts had, in addition to increased IgG_1, IgA, and IgM levels, plasma cell infiltrates in the kidney and profound mesangial cell proliferation (15,68).

There is appreciable correlation between intraglomerular cytokine levels and histological evidence of glomerular damage. Increased IL-1β mRNA was present in a model of membranous nephropathy that progresses to glomerulosclerosis but not in a clinically and morphologically similar nonprogressive glomerulonephritis induced in the same strain by a different immunization protocol with the same antigen (9). In murine IgA nephropathy induced by dextran immunization, the levels of IL-1 mRNA estimated by densitometry correlated with the degree of cellularity and particularly with expansion of glomerular matrix, as well as with the clinical signs of renal disease, hematuria and proteinuria (L. Gesualdo et al., unpublished observations). In the form of this model associated with cell proliferation, IL-6 mRNA was also detected, increasing in parallel to the proliferation in glomeruli. No IL-6 mRNA was detected in the similar model that lacks proliferation, or in normals. In patients, it seemed that higher urine levels of IL-6 were associated with progression to glomerulosclerosis (15). Urinary excretion of IL-1 in chronic serum sickness nephritis peaks during the phase of glomerular dysfunction and begins to subside as glomerulosclerosis commences (56). Finally, infusion of IL-1 or IL-6 markedly potentiates urinary abnormalities and glomerular proliferation, matrix expansion and thrombosis in a model of passive IgA nephropathy (69). This model, induced by immune complexes of IgA antiphosphorylcholine antibody and phosphorylcholine-substituted bovine albumin, is characteristically devoid of changes in glomerular function or histology. Hence, IL-1β and/or IL-6, perhaps in concert with other factors, may promote mesangial cell proliferation in glomerulonephritis and may be causally related to glomerulosclerosis. This concept is further supported by the observation that in isolated perfused rat kidneys, IL-1 promoted increases in heparan sulfate proteoglycan synthesis and enhanced proteoglycan catabolism (70).

Cellular Sources and Targets for Cytokines in Glomerular Injury

Most investigators argue that monocytes and/or macrophages within glomeruli are the major, if not exclusive, source of intraglomerular cytokines in glomerulonephritis. In murine lupus nephritis, both mesangial cells and macrophages cultured from glomeruli produce a novel truncated 1200 base transcript that accounts in part for the increase in IL-1 observed in these animals. Mesangial cells and macrophages cultured from predisease or congenic healthy mice lack this novel transcript, as do peritoneal macrophages from diseased mice. The vast majority of this novel transcript, and of 16 kb IL-1β and TNF, is produced by glomerular macrophages, not endogenous mesangial cells (46). Preliminary in situ hybridization indicates that most cells that hybridize to an IL-1 probe are macrophages, both within glomeruli and within tubulointerstitial infiltrates (V.E. Rubin Kelley, personal communication).

Antimacrophage serum injected into rats before administration of anti-GBM prevents the increased adhesiveness, macrophage infiltration, and mesangial hyperplasia and proliferation seen in glomeruli isolated from macrophage-replete rats given anti-GBM (55); prior treatment of rats with antimacrophage serum also eliminates the increase in IL-1 activity in glomeruli after anti-GBM injection (51,52). Although proteinuria is not totally macrophage dependent in rabbits with accelerated autologous anti-GBM nephritis, glomerular IL-1 production is completely eliminated by prior leukocyte depletion. Moreover, macrophages isolated from glomeruli with anti-GBM nephritis produce far more IL-1 than peripheral blood monocytes or elicited peritoneal macrophages and account for essentially all the IL-1 production in glomeruli (53). In patients with necrotizing and crescentic glomerulonephritis, the abundant macrophages infiltrating glomeruli are considered the source of the increased IL-1. Macrophages emigrate from glomeruli in culture and adhere to the culture dishes; thus, they can be separated from the glomeruli. It is the supernatant from the glomerular macrophages that contains most of the bioactive IL-1 (50–54). In chronic serum sickness nephritis, onset of cytokine excretion in the urine correlated with glomerular macrophage infiltration (56).

In toxic nephrosis induced by puromycin aminonucleoside, increased macrophages were recognized in glomeruli, more abundant in the early phases of injury (57). Peak glomerular infiltration by macrophages was associated with peak production of IL-1; endogenous cell growth and glomerular attachment to culture dishes were reduced at this point, inversely varying with the macrophage content of the glomeruli. Intraglomerular cells staining with monoclonal antibody specific for rat monocytes-macrophages, ED-1, coincided with the appearance of cells staining for IL-1 and TNF (58).

Macrophages and monocytes are apparently not the only source of cytokines within injured glomeruli in vivo. Although leukocytes, particularly macrophages, are not increased within renal cortex of mice or humans with IgA nephropathy, there is increased mRNA encoding IL-1β and IL-6 in kidneys of mice with IgA nephropathy (L. Gesualdo et al., unpublished observations) and immunohistochemically demonstrable IL-6 in the mesangium of patients with IgA nephropathy (15). In experimental membranous nephropathy in rats, increased IL-1β mRNA occurs in the absence of an increase in cells bearing common leukocyte antigen in the kidney (9). Preliminary results with in situ hybridization in our laboratory show mesangial cell IL-1 in this model.

Overall, it appears that in diseases characterized by leukocytic infiltration, macrophages are the overriding source of cytokines, but intraglomerular cytokine production by endogenous cells may be enhanced in noninfiltrative diseases. In these noninfiltrative glomerulonephritides, endogenous mesangial cells emerge as the prime source of cytokines. In this context, it is noteworthy that bioactive cytokines have not yet been demonstrated in supernatants from glomeruli isolated from animals or patients with noninfiltrative glomerulonephritis. Particularly when considered in light of the relative paucity of IL-1 and TNF mRNA in cultured mesangial cells compared to cells of monocyte-macrophage lineage, this suggests that the amounts of cytokines within glomeruli differ in different patterns of glomerular disease. Such differences, however, do not presuppose that cytokines are less important in noninfiltrative disease. Indeed, the cytokines may play a more prominent role in disease, particularly in progression to scarring in these diseases, since the injury is less devastating and more chronic overall. The correlations observed to date relating glomerular hypercellularity and matrix expansion to IL-1 and IL-6 levels strongly suggest that the cytokines influence glomerular response to immune stimuli in these diseases.

The targets of cytokines produced in vivo are also uncertain and likely to be multiple. Injection of LPS into rats given subnephritogenic doses of anti-GBM antibody exacerbated disease through neutrophils; depletion of circulating neutrophils prevented glomerular injury consequent upon sequential injection of anti-GBM and LPS (63). Although TNF infusion profoundly affected glomeruli in rabbits, infusion of TNF into isolated rabbit kidneys maintained on extracorporeal perfusion had no effects on renal structure or function. This suggests that TNF activates extrarenal cells to elicit the renal injury observed in the whole-animal experiments (67). Both IL-1 and TNF promote proinflammatory interaction between neutrophils and endothelium independent of IL-2, interferon-γ, platelet-derived growth factor, histamine, thrombin, platelet-activating factor, and leukotriene B4 (65); cytokines, however, promote mesangial cell IL-8 synthesis (19). Hence, endothelial cells and/or neutrophils may prove to be important targets for cytokines in glomerulonephritis. Other cells indigenous to the glomerulus are also responsive to several cytokines (see earlier). Therefore, one can envision several distinct routes by which cytokines influence glomerular structure and function. More information is obviously required to identify major pathways operative in glomerular disease.

TUBULOINTERSTITIAL DISEASE

As is the case for pathogenesis and pathophysiology in general, there is less information regarding the role of cytokines in tubulointerstitial disease than in glomerular disease. Notwithstanding, there is significant evidence to suggest that cytokines are produced in inflammation of the renal parenchyma and that they play a role in interstitial nephritides. We focus here upon those effects unique to the kidney.

Production of Inflammatory Cytokines

The technical capacity to study cytokines in both human and experimental hypersensitivity interstitial nephritis exists, as manifest by the recent study of a soluble antigen-specific helper factor that induces interstitial nephritis (71). Reports of the application of analytical techniques to the study of this prevalent form of tubulointerstitial nephritis to date are just emerging now with the recognition of IL-8 production (71a). One would predict from the following observations, however, that cytokines will ultimately prove critical determinants of functional derangements and long-term course in these diseases.

Infectious interstitial nephritis, modeled in mice, is associated with increased IL-1, IL-6, TNF, G-CSF, and GM-CSF mRNA in renal homogenates from 12 to 72 h after infection as determined by reverse transcription and polymerase chain amplification of the derived cDNA (72). Convalescent animals from 5 to 14 days manifest minimal or no signals, and age-matched controls lacked signal. Translation of increased amounts of IL-6 was documented by the presence of this protein in urine but not serum of infected animals. Curiously, immunohistochemistry implicates the glomerulus rather than the infected tubulointerstitium as the source of this IL-6. Another transcript detected in increased amounts was H400, homologous to IL-8 and associated chemotactic peptides.

In regard to allograft rejection, cortical IL-6 mRNA is increased up to sixfold in seven of eight patients experiencing acute cellular rejection, relative to five normal kidneys and five transplants with stable renal function (73). This message, detected in the tubulointerstitium by in situ hybridization, was also present in the glomeruli and vasculature. The specificity of the signal was confirmed by displacement of radioactive probe by excess unlabeled probe. In the one acutely rejecting patient lacking IL-6, there was increased TNF, which was not seen in the other patients. The authors, noting that TNF stimulates IL-6 production, considered that this patient was in an evanescent phase of rejection.

Although treatment of acute rejection with anti-T cell monoclonal antibody results in detectable TNF, IL-2, and interferon-γ, but not IL-1β, in serum, kidneys were not studied for production of these cytokines, or for any response to the serum content (74,75). Interstingly, renal replacement therapy, including engraftment, is associated with increases in IL-2 and TNF relative to IL-1 in the same patient (74–76).

Effects of Cytokines on Tubulointerstitial Structure and Function

Perhaps the most widely appreciated effect of cytokines on renal tubules relates to the enhanced expression of histocompatibility and cellular adhesion molecules. During rejection and in autoimmune interstitial nephritis, there is a documented increase in tubular expression of ICAM-1 protein and mRNA (62,77) ascribed to the action of IL-1, TNF, and interferon-γ from in vitro studies (62). Although this remains to be documented, it is certainly reasonable, since distinct but overlapping responses to IL-1, TNF, and interferon-γ occur in a variety of cell lineages

(78). TNF and interferon-γ, at least, are also implicated in the increased expression of histocompatibility products in renal tubules, a known concomitant with interstitial nephritis (48,79,80). The capacity for T cells to injure target cells is certainly enhanced by increased expression of histocompatibility products and adhesion molecules on the targets. On the other hand, supernatants from mixed lymphocyte reactions and pure interferon-γ decrease susceptibility of cultured renal tubular epithelial cells to lymphokine-activated killer (LAK) cell-mediated lysis (81).

Cytokines also have direct effects on the metabolism and function of renal tubular cells. Addition of LPS or IL-1 to a murine proximal renal tubular cell line stimulates transcription of TNF and production of membrane-associated TNF activity (82). Both IL-1 and interferon-γ reduce protein synthesis by renal tubular cells in culture, without cytotoxicity. The combination of the two agents was synergistic but was also toxic, resulting in profound disturbances in morphological appearance and increased lactic dehydrogenase release into the supernatant (83). Finally, both IL-1 and TNF promote increased sodium uptake and sodium-dependent glucose transport by proximal renal tubular cells in culture (84–86). Increased urine flow and sodium excretion observed in response to IL-1 is mediated by effects on the distal nephron (medullary collecting duct cells), probably mediated through prostaglandins, since cyclooxgenase inhibitors prevent these effects. Finally, IL-1β, TNF, and TGF-β increase synthesis of endothelin-1 by porcine renal cortical tubular epithelium (87). Interestingly, interferon-γ has less profound influences on all these functions, despite its more conspicuous effect on expression of histocompatability loci and ICAM-1.

OTHER PLEIOTROPIC PROTEINS IMPLICATED IN RENAL DISEASE

Several proteins that fit the broad category of cytokines, but are in fact not members of the family of inflammatory cytokines emphasized in this book, are emerging as important elements in renal pathophysiology. Platelet-derived growth factor (PDGF) is a group of three dimeric proteins: either homodimer or the heterodimer of A or B chains, encoded by separate genes. These molecules, synthesized by macrophages, smooth muscle, endothelial, and glomerular mesangial cells, as well as by platelets, are mitogenic for mesenchymal cells, influence synthesis and degradation of constituents of the extracellular matrix, and possess chemoattractor and vasoconstrictor properties. Recently, increases in the expression of B-chain mRNA in renal cortex and immunohistochemically demonstrable protein in glomerular mesangium was reported in a mouse model of IgA nephropathy; the mRNA content correlated with the severity of clinical signs of glomerulonephritis, such as proteinuria and hematuria, as well as with proliferation and matrix expansion in the glomerular mesangium (88). Increased PDGF expression is evident in another murine model of mesangiopathic glomerulonephritis as well as in human glomerulonephritis (88, 88a). Since PDGF is an autocrine growth factor for mesangial cells and is indeed autoinducing, it is likely an important factor in glomerulonephritis. Moreover, other factors, particularly transforming growth factor β and epidermal growth factor, induce PDGF synthesis and secretion, and anti-PDGF inhibits the effect of these other growth factors on mesangial cells, without evident cross-reactivity (89,90). Thus, PDGF may be an intervening factor in the glomerular response to these other agonists and may therefore occupy a central role in proliferative and matrix synthesis responses to glomerular injury.

Tranforming growth factor β is another pleiotropic protein implicated in glomerular disease. Mesangiopathic glomerulonephritis induced by antibody-mediated mesangial cell lysis is accompanied by an increased glomerular content of TGF-β protein and mRNA, and anti-TGF-β inhibited the associated increase in proteoglycan and fibronectin synthesis (91,92). Anti-GBM nephritis is also accompanied by an increase in renal cortical TGF-β activity inhibitable by anti-TGF-β and by increased mRNA encoding TGF-β. Cultured mesangial cell collagen synthesis, stimulated by supernatants from cultures of diseased but not control glomeruli, was inhibited by anti-TGF-β (93). Endothelial, mesangial, and epithelial cell lines derived from mouse glomeruli bear receptors for TGF-β, and binding of TGF-β to these cells influenced the replication rate and synthesis of collagen and fibronectin (94). Unexpectedly, TGF-β receptors on rat glomerular cells appear to be distinct from those previously described (95). Proteoglycan synthesis by mesangial cells in culture is also regulated by TGF-β (96).

Insulinlike growth factor 1 is synthesized by cultured murine mesangial cells and binds to mesangial, endothelial, and epithelial cells, suggesting paracrine effects of this factor (97–99). However, hyperproduction of insulinlike growth factor 1 does not lead to progressive glomerular sclerosis, as increased production of growth hormone or growth hormone releasing factor does (100). Hypersomatotropism leads to increased production of insulinlike growth factor 1 in renal medullary collecting ducts, associated with hemodynamic abnormalities in rats (101).

Epidermal growth factor (EGF) receptors are present on rat mesangial cells in culture, and binding of this factor causes a sodium-dependent intracellular alkalinization and cell contraction (102). These investigators also reported that intrarenal infusion of epidermal growth factor transiently decreased glomerular filtration rate and renal blood flow in living rats; nephron hemodynamics are apparently altered by mesangial cell contraction. The inhibition of glomerular epithelial cell growth in culture by heparan sulfate is reversed by the addition of EGF (103). Although increased EGF was present in the urine of patients with Schönlein-Henoch nephritis (104), the urine of patients with several other kidney diseases showed decreased EGF content (105). Obviously, this is an area ripe for further investigation.

Infusion of interferon-α or β into neonatal mice delays renal maturation and causes dramatic thickening of the glomerular basement membranes, which appears to be due to increased synthesis by endothelial cells (106), but again does not promote cell proliferation. These factors may be relevant to glomerulosclerosis.

PERSPECTIVES AND PROSPECTS

Taken together, the data reviewed here suggest that local release of interleukins and tumor necrosis factor from either infiltrating inflammatory cells or resident renal cells may be important in the pathogenesis or pathophysiology of inflammatory injury of the kidney. Systemic cytokine production may also increase the incidence or contribute to the severity of renal disease. We focus on the mesangial cell because studies describing either the synthesis of the interleukins by or the interactions with other glomerular cells are limited or lacking. The mesangial cell is an important target for both autocrine and paracrine derived cytokines.

The challenges for the future are clear. How can we best identify altered cytokine production? Do cytokines play a pivotal role in the pathogenesis or progression of renal diseases? How can we establish which cytokines are critical in which diseases? Perhaps most crucial is can the modulation of cytokine effect provide new effective therapies for renal disease? New horizons are emerging from the increasing availability of natural receptor antagonists, antibodies and engineered antibody variable regions specific for cytokines or their receptors, and recombinant truncated soluble receptors that can competitively inhibit the binding of a specific cytokine to its receptor, thereby preventing pathological effects of the cytokines.

The prospect of use of these reagents as pharmaceuticals is indeed intriguing in a field in which no effective therapy exists. However, the prospect of using these agents as analytical tools to probe the contribution of the cytokines to altered function in vitro and in vivo is no less tantalizing. Definition of particular associations of cytokine levels with particular biological responses can be followed rapidly by abrogation of that cytokine's effect with soluble receptor. In this context, we may realize not only the goal of therapy of intractable diseases but of actually understanding the pathophysiology of renal diseases.

REFERENCES

1. Mené P, Simonson MS, Dunn MJ. Physiology of the mesangial cell. Physiol Rev 1989; 69:1347–24.
2. Schlondorff D. The glomerular mesangial cell: an expanding role for a specialized pericyte. FASEB J 1987; 1:272–81.
3. Sedor JR, Carey SW, Emancipator SN. Immune complexes bind to cultured rat glomerular mesangial cells to stimulate superoxide release. J Immunol 1987; 138:3751–7.
4. Knauss TC, Mené P, Ricanati SA, et al. Immune complex activation of rat glomerular mesangial cells: dependence on the Fc region of antibody. Am J Physiol 1989; 257:F478–85.
5. Neuwirth R, Singhal P, Diamond B, et al. Evidence for immunoglobulin Fc receptor-mediated prostaglandin$_2$ and platelet-activating factor formation by cultured rat mesangial cells. J Clin Invest 1988; 82:936–44.
6. Lovett DH, Ryan JL, Sterzel RB. A thymocyte-activating factor derived from glomerular mesangial cells. J Immunol 1983; 130:1796–801.
7. Lovett DH, Sterzel RB, Ryan JL, Atkins E. Production of an endogenous pyrogen by glomerular mesangial cells. J Immunol 1985; 134:670–2.
8. Lovett SH, Larsen A. Cell cycle-dependent interleukin 1 gene expression by cultured glomerular mesangial cells. J Clin Invest 1988; 82:115–22.
9. Werber HI, Emancipator SN, Tykocinski ML, Sedor JR. The interleukin 1 gene is expressed by rat glomerular mesangial cells and is augmented in immune complex glomerulonephritis. J Immunol 1987; 138:3207–12.
10. Lovett DH, Szamel M, Ryan JL, Sterzel RB, Gemsa D, Resch K. Interleukin 1 and the glomerular mesangium. I. Purification and characterization of a mesengial cell-derived autogrowth factor. J Immunol 1986; 136:3700–5.

11. Lovett DH, Haensch GM, Goppelt M, Resch K. Gemsa D. Activation of glomerular mesangial cells by the terminal membrane attack complex of complement. J Immunol 1987; 138:2473–80.
12. Lovett DH, Bursten SL, Gemsa D, Bessler W, Resch K, Ryan JL. Activation of glomerular mesangial cells by gram-negative bacterial cell wall components. Am J Pathol 1988; 133:472–84.
13. Bursten SL, Locksley RM, Ryan JL, Lovett DH. Acylation of monocyte and glomerular mesangial cell proteins. Myristyl acylation of the interleukin 1 precursors. J Clin Invest 1988; 82:1479–88.
14. Baud L, Oudinet JP, Bens M, et al. Production of tumor necrosis factor by rat mesangial cells in response to bacterial lipopolysaccharide. Kidney Int 1989; 35:1111–8.
15. Horii Y, Muraguchi A, Iwano M, et al. Involvement of IL-6 in mesangial proliferative glomerulonephritis. J Immunol 1989; 143:3949–95.
16. Pirotzky E, Delattre RM, Hellegouarch A, et al. Interleukin-6 production by tumor necrosis factor and lipopolysaccharide-stimulated rat renal cells. Clin Immunol Immunopathol 1990; 56:271–9. 16(a). Ruef C, Budde K, Lacy J, Nothemann W, Baumann M, Sterzel RB, Coleman DL. Interleukin 6 is an autocrine growth factor for mesangial cells. Kid Int 1990; 38:249–257. 16(b). Abbott F, Ryan JJ, Ceska M, Matsushima K, Sarraf CE, Rees AJ. Interleukin-1 stimulates human mesangial cells to synthesize and release interleukins 6 and 8. Kid Int 1991; 40:597–605.
17. Budde K, Coleman DL, Lacy J. Sterzel RB. Rat mesangial cells produce granulocyte-macrophage colony-stimulating factor. Am J Physiol 1989; 257:F1065–78.
18. Mori T, Bartocci A, Satriano J, et al. Mouse mesangial cells produce colony-stimulating factor-1 (CSF-1) and express the CSF-1 receptor. J Immunol 1990; 144:4697–702.
19. Kusner DJ, Luebbers EL, Nowinski RJ, Konieczkowski M, King CH, Sedor JR. Cytokine- and LPS-induced synthesis of interleukin-8 from human mesangial cells. Kidney Int 1991; 39: 1240–1248. 19(a). Brown Z, Strieter RM, Chensue SW, Ceska M, Lindley I, Neild GH, Kunkel SL, Westwick J. Cytokine-activated human mesangial cells generate the neutrophil chemoattractant, interleukin 8. Kid Int 1991; 40:86–90.
20. Watanabe K, Konishi K, Fujioka M, Kinoshita S, Nakagawa H. The neutrophil chemoattractant produced by the rat kidney epithelioid cell line NRK-52E is a protein related to the KC/gro protein. J Biol Chem 1989; 264:19559–63.
21. Watanabe K, Nakagawa H. Cytokines enhance the production of a chemotactic factor for polymorphonuclear leukocytes by rat renal glomerular epithelioid cells. Nephron 1990; 54:169–75.
22. Sedor JR, Malone K, Njoku N, Kilian PL, Coe B, Douglas JG. Interleukin-1 binds to both glomerular mesangial and tubular epithelial cells. Clin res 1989; 37:501.
23. Lovett DH, Ryan JL, Sterzel RB. Stimulation of rat mesangial cell proliferation by macrophage interleukin 1. J Immunol 1983; 131:2830–6.
24. Kester M, Simonson MS, Mene' P, Sedor JR. Interleukin-1 generates transmembrane signals from phospholipids through novel pathways in cultured rat mesangial cells. J Clin Invest 1989; 83:718–23.
25. Stahl RAK, Thaiss F, Haberstroh U, Kahf S, Shaw A, Schoeppe W. Cyclooxygenase inhibition enhances rat interleukin 1β-induced growth of rat mesangial cells in culture. Am J Physiol 1990; 259:F419–24.
26. Lovett DH, Resch K, Gemsa D. Interleukin I and the glomerular mesangium. II. Monokine stimulation of mesangial cell prostanoid secretion. Am J Pathol 1987; 129:543–51.
27. Topley N, Floege J, Wessel K. et al. Prostaglandin E_2 production is synergistically

increased in cultured human glomerular mesangial cells by combinations of IL-1 and tumor necrosis factor-α[1]. J Immunol 1989; 143:1989–95.
28. Martin J, Lovett DH, Gemsa D. Sterzel RB, Davies M. Enhancement of glomerular mesangial cell neutral proteinase secretion by macrophages: role of interleukin 1. J Immunol 1986; 137:525–9.
29. Martin M, Schwinzer R, Schellekens H, Resch K. Glomerular mesangial cells in local inflammation. Induction of the expression of MHC class II antigens by IFN-γ. J Immunol 1989; 142:1887–94.
30. Radeke HH, Meier B, Topley N, Floge J, Habermehl GG, Resch K. Interleukin 1-α and tumor necrosis factor-α induce oxygen radical production in mesangial cells. Kidney Int 1990; 37:767–75.
31. Bursten SL, Harris WE, Bomsztyk K, Lovett DL. Interleukin-1 rapidly stimulates lysophosphatidate acyltransferase and phosphatidate phosphohydrolase activities in human mesangial cells: stimulation by interleukin 1. J Biol Chem 1991; 266:20732–20743.
32. Pfeilschifter J, Leighton J, Pignat W, Marki F, Vosbeck K. Cyclic AMP mimics, but does not mediate, interleukin-1- and tumour-necrosis-factor-stimulated phospholipase A_2 secretion from rat renal mesangial cells. Biochem J 1991; 273:199–204.
33. Pfeilschifter J, Schwarzenbach H. Interleukin 1 and tumor necrosis factor stimulate cGMP formation in rat renal mesangial cells. FEB Lett 1990; 273:185–7.
34. Lovett DH, Martin M, Bursten S, Szamel M, Gemsa D, Resch K. Interleukin 1 and the glomerular mesangium. III. IL-1-dependent stimulation of mesangial cell protein kinase activity. Kidney Int 1988; 34:26–35.
35. Nakazato Y, Simonson MS, Herman WH, Konieczkowski M, Sedor JR. Interleukin 1-α stimulates prostaglandin biosynthesis in serum-activated mesangial cells by induction of a non-pancreatic (Type II) phospholipase A_2. J Biol Chem 1991; 266:14119–14127.
36. Schalkwijk C, Pfeilschifter J, Marki F, van den Bosch H. Interleukin-1β, tumor necrosis factor and forskolin stimulate the synthesis and secretion of group II phospholipase A in rat mesangial cells. Biochem Biophys Res Commun 1991; 174:268–75.
37. Torbohm I, Berger B, Schonermark M, Von-Kempis J, Rother K, Hansch GM. Modulation of collagen synthesis in human glomerular epithelial cells by interleukin 1. Clin Exp Immunol 1989; 75:427–31.
38. Iwamoto T, Nakashima Y, Sueishi K. Secretion of plasminogen activator and its inhibitor by glomerular epithelial cells. Kidney Int 1990; 37:1466–76.
39. Baud L, Perez J, Friedlander G, Ardaillou R. Tumor necrosis factor stimulates prostaglandin production and cyclic AMP levels in rat cultured mesangial cells. FEBS Lett 1988; 239:50–4.
40. Pfeilschifter J, Muhl H. Interleukin 1 and tumor necrosis factor potentiate angiotensin II- and calcium ionophore-stimulated prostaglandin E_2 synthesis in rat renal mesangial cells. Biochem Biophys Res Commun 1990; 169:585–95.
41. Hruby ZW, Cybulsky AV, Lowry RP. Effects of tumor necrosis factor on glomerular mesangial and epithelial cells in culture. Nephron 1990; 56:410–3.
42. Savic V, Stefanovic V, Ardaillou N, Ardaillou R. Induction of ecto-5′-nucleotidase of rat cultured mesangial cells by interleukin-1β and tumour necrosis factor-α. Immunology 1990; 70:321–6.
43. Marsden PA, Ballermann BJ. Tumor necrosis factor α activates soluble guanylate cyclase in bovine glomerular mesangial cells via an L-arginine-dependent mechanism. J Exp Med 1990; 172:1843–52.
44. Camussi G, Turello E, Tetta C, Bussolino F, Baglioni C. Tumor necrosis factor

induces contraction of mesangial cells and alters their cytoskeletons. Kidney Int 1990; 38:795–802.

45. Wiggins RC, Njoku N, Sedor JR. Tissue factor production by cultured rat mesangial cells. Stimulation by TNFα and lipopolysaccharide. Kidney Int 1990; 37:1281–5.
46. Boswell JM, Yui MA, Endres S, Burt DW, Kelley VE. Novel and enhanced IL-1 gene expression in autoimmune mice with lupus. J Immunol 1988; 141:118–24.
47. Boswell JM, Yui MA, Burt DW, Kelley VE. Increased tumor necrosis factor and IL-1β gene expression in the kidneys of mice with lupus nephritis. J Immunol 1988; 141:3050–4.
48. Cockfield SM, Ramassar V, Halloran PF. MRL mice with lupus nephritis have enhanced IFN-γ and TNF-α gene expression. Kidney Int 1990; 37:411.
49. Brennan DC, Yui MA, Wuthrich RP, Kelley VE. Tumor necrosis factor and IL-1 in New Zealand black/white mice. Enhanced gene expression and acceleration of renal injury. J Immunol 1989; 143:3470–5.
50. Matsumoto K. Production of interleukin-1 in macrophage cultures from rats with nephrotoxic serum nephritis. Int Arch Allergy Appl Immunol 1988; 87:435–8.
51. Matsumoto K. Interleukin-1 production by lipopolysaccharide-stimulated glomeruli from rats with nephrotoxic serum nephritis. Am J Nephrol 1989; 9:488–94.
52. Matsumoto K, Hatano M. Production of interleukin 1 in glomerular cell cultures from rats with nephrotoxic serum nephritis. Clin Exp Immunol 1989; 75:123–8.
53. Tipping PG, Lowe MG, Holdsworth SR. Glomerular interleukin 1 production is dependent on macrophage infiltration in anti-GBM glomerulonephritis. Kidney Int 1991; 39:103–10.
54. Matsumoto K, Dowling J, Atkins RC. Production of interleukin 1 in glomerular cell cultures from patients with rapidly progressive crescentic glomerulonephritis. Am J Nephol 1988; 8:463–70.
55. Matsumoto K, Hatano M. Effect of antimacrophage serum on the proliferation of glomerular cells in nephrotoxic serum nephritis in the rat. J Clin Lab Immunol 1989; 28:39–44.
56. Noble B, Ren K, Taverne J, et al. Mononuclear cells in glomeruli and cytokines in urine reflect the severity of experimental proliferative immune complex glomerulonephritis. Clin Exp Immunol 1990; 80:281–7.
57. Matsumoto K, Atkins RC. Glomerular cells and macrophages in the progression of experimental focal and segmental glomerulosclerosis. Am J Pathol 1989; 134:933–45.
58. Diamond JR, Pesek I. Glomerular tumor necrosis factor and interleukin 1 during acute aminonucleoside nephrosis. An immunohistochemical study. Lab Invest 1991; 64:21–8.
59. Ulich TR, Guo K, del Castillo J. Endotoxin-induced cytokine gene expression in vivo. I. Expression of tumor necrosis factor mRNA in visceral organs under physiologic conditions and during endotoxemia. Am J Pathol 1989; 134:11–4.
60. Jacob CO, McDevitt HO. Tumour necrosis factor-α in murine autoimmune 'lupus' nephritis. Nature 1988; 331:356–7.
61. Mihara M, Ohsugi Y. The biological response modifier OK-432 (a streptococcal preparation) inhibits the development of autoimmune kidney disease in NZB/W F_1 hybrid mice: possible involvement of tumor necrosis factor. Int Arch Allergy Appl Immunol 1989; 90:37–42.
62. Wuthrich RP, Jevnikar AM, Takei F, Glimcher LH, Kelley VE. Intercellular adhesion molecule-1 (ICAM-1) expression is upregulated in autoimmune murine lupus nephritis. Am J Pathol 1990; 136:441–50.
63. Naruse T, Tsuchida A, Ogawa S, Yano S, Maekawa T. Selective glomerular throm-

bosis in rats induced by combined injections of nephrotoxic antiserum and lipopolysaccharide. J Lab Clin Med 1985; 105:146–56.
64. Samudra K, Mahan JD, McAllister C, Shannon B. Cytokines promote neutrophil (N) adherence to cultured human glomerular cells. Kidney Int 1989; 35:361.
65. Moser R, Schleiffenbaum B, Groscurth P, Fehr J. Interleukin 1 and tumor necrosis factor stimulate human vascular endothelial cells to promote transendothelial neutrophil passage. J Clin Invest 1989; 83:444–55.
66. Tomosugi NI, Cashman SJ, Hay H, et al. Modulation of antibody-mediated glomerular injury in vivo by bacterial lipopolysaccharide, tumor necrosis factor, and IL-1[1]. J Immunol 1989; 142:3083–90.
67. Bertani T, Abbate M, Zoja C, et al. Tumor necrosis factor induces glomerular damage in the rabbit. Am J Pathol 1989; 134:419–30.
68. Suematsu S, Matsuda T, Aozasa K, et al. IgG_1 plasmacytosis in interleukin 6 transgenic mice. Proc Natl Acad Sci U S A 1989; 86:7547–51.
69. Rifai A, Montinaro V, Esparza A. Regulatory peptide factors modulate the glomerular response to IgA immune complexes. In: Sakai H, Sakai O, Nomoto Y, eds. Pathogenesis of IgA nephropathy. Tokyo: Harcourt, Brace, Jovanovich, 1990: 303–17.
70. Kashihara M, Dalecki T, Liu Z, Kanwar YS. Modulation of glomerular basement membrane proteoglycan synthesis by interleukin-1 IL-1 alpha. Kidney Int 1990; 37:418.
71. Hines WH, Mann RA, Kelly CJ, Neilson EG. Induction of the nephritogenic effector T cell repertoire with an antigen-specific T cell cytokine. J Immunol 1990; 144:75–83. 71(a). Schmouder RL, Strieter RM, Wiggins RC, Chensue SW, Kunkel SL. In vitro and in vivo interleukin-8 production in human renal coritical epithelial cells. Kid Int 1992; 41:in press.
72. Rugo H, O'Hanley P, Bishop A, Pearce M, Abrams J, Howard M, O'Garra A. Local cytokine production in a murine model of *E. coli* pyelonephritis (abstract). FASEB J 1990; 4:A2277.
73. Caillat-Zucman S, Vanden Broecke C, Legendre C, et al. Differential in situ expression of cytokine genes in human renal rejection. Transplant Proc 1991; 23:229–30.
74. Abramowicz D, Schandene L, Goldman M, et al. Release of tumor necrosis factor, interleukin-2, and gamma-interferon in serum after injection of OKT3 monoclonal antibody in kidney transplant recipients. Transplantation 1989; 47:606–8.
75. Debets JM, Leunissen KM, van Hooff HJ, van der Linden CJ, Buurman WA. Evidence of involvement of tumor necrosis factor in adverse reactions during treatment of kidney allograft rejection with antithymocyte globulin. Transplantation 1989; 47:487–92.
76. Kimmel PL, Phillips TM, Phillips E, Bosch JP. Effect of renal replacement therapy on cellular cytokine production in patients with renal disease. Kidney Int 1990; 38:129–35.
77. Faull RJ, Russ GR. Tabular expression of intercellular adhesion molecule-1 during renal allograft rejection. Transplantation 1989; 48:226–30.
78. Pober JS, Gimbrone MA Jr, Lapierre LA, et al. Overlapping patterns of activation of human endothelial cells by interleukin 1, tumor necrosis factor, and immune interferon. J Immunol 1986; 137:1893–6.
79. Cockfield SM, Urmson J, Pleasants JR, Halloran PF. The regulation of expression of MHC products in mice. J Immunol 1990; 144:2967–74.
80. Wuthrich RP, Glimcher LH, Yui MA, Jevnikar AM, Dumas SE, Kelley VE. MHC class II, antigen presentation and tumor necrosis factor in renal tubular epithelial cells. Kidney Int 1990; 37:783–92.

81. Kirby JA, Forsythe JL, Simm A, Proud G, Taylor RM. Renal allograft rejection: protection of renal tubular epithelial cells from lymphokine activated killer cell mediated lysis by pretreatment with cytokines. Nephrol Dial Transplant 1989; 4:824–8.
82. Jevnikar AM, Wuthrich RP, Brennan DC, Maslinski W, Glimcher LH, Rubin-Kelley VE. TNFα is expressed on the surface of kidney proximal tubular cells. Transplant Proc 1991; 23:231–2.
83. Maessen JG, Buurman WA, Kootstra G. Direct cytotoxic effect of cytokines in kidney parenchyma: a possible mechanism of allograft destruction. Transplant Proc 1989; 21:309–10.
84. Beasley D, Dinarello CA, Cannon JG. Interleukin-1 induces natriuresis in conscious rats: role of renal prostaglandins. Kidney Int 1988; 33:1059–65.
85. Schreiner GF, Harris KPG, Purkerson ML, Klahr S. Immunological aspects of acute ureteral obstruction: immune cell infiltrate in the kidney. Kidney Int 1988; 34:487–93.
86. Schreiner GF, Kohan DE. Regulation of renal transport processes and hemodynamics by macrophages and lymphocytes. Am J Physiol 1990; 258:F761–7.
87. Ohta K, Hirata Y, Imai T, et al. Cytokine-induced release of endothelin-1 from porcine renal epithelial cell line. Biochem Biophys Res Commun 1990; 169:578–84.
88. Gesualdo L, Pinzani M, Floriano JJ, et al. Platelet derived growth factor expression in mesangial proliferative glomerulonephritis. Lab Invest 1991; 65:160–167. 88(a). Iida H, Seifert R, Alpers CE, Gronwald RGK, Phillips PE, Pritzl P, Gordon K, Gown AM, Ross R, Bowen-Pope DF, Johnson RJ. Platelet-derived growth factor (PDGF) and PDGF receptor are induced in mesangial proliferative nephritis in the rat. Proc Natl Acad Sci (USA) 1991; 88:6560–6564.
89. Jaffer F, Saunders C, Shultz P, Throckmorton D, Weinshell E, Abboud HE. Regulation of mesangial cell growth by polypeptide mitogens. Am J Pathol 1989; 135:261.
90. Silver BJ, Jaffer FE, Abboud HE. Platelet-derived growth factor synthesis in mesangial cells: induction by multiple peptide mitogens. Proc Natl Acad Sci U S A 1989; 86:1056.
91. Okuda S, Languino LR, Ruoslahti E, Border WA. Elevated expression of transforming growth factor-β and proteoglycan production in experimental glomerulonephritis. J Clin Invest 1990; 86:453–62.
92. Border WA, Okuda S, Languino LR, Sporn MB, Ruoslahti E. Suppression of experimental glomerulonephritis by antiserum against transforming growth factor β_1. Nature 1990; 346:371–4.
93. Coimbra T, Wiggins R, Noh JW, Merritt S, Phan SH. Transforming growth factor-β production in anti-glomerular basement membrane disease in the rabbit. Am J Pathol 1991; 138:223–34.
94. MacKay K, Striker LJ, Stauffer JW, Doi T, Agodoa LY, Striker GE. Transforming growth factor-β. Murine glomerular receptors and responses of isolated glomerular cells. J Clin Invest 1989; 83:1160–7.
95. MacKay K, Robbins AR, Bruce MD, Danielpour D. Identification of disulfide-linked transforming growth factor-β_1-specific binding proteins in rat glomeruli. J Biol Chem 1990; 265:9351–6.
96. Border WA, Okuda S, Languino LR, Ruoslahti E. Transforming growth factor-β regulates production of proteoglycans by mesangial cells. Kidney Int 1990; 37:689–95.
97. Conti FG, Striker LJ, Elliot SJ, Andreani D, Striker GE. Synthesis and release of

insulinlike growth factor I by mesangial cells in culture. Am J Physiol 1988; 255:F1214–9.

98. Aron DC, Rosenzweig JL, Abboud HE. Synthesis and binding of insulin-like growth factor I by human glomerular mesangial cells. J Clin Endocrinol Metab 1989; 68:585–91.
99. Conti FG, Elliot SJ, Striker LJ, Striker GE. Binding of insulin-like growth factor-I by glomerular endothelial and epithelial cells: further evidence for IGF-I action in the renal glomerulus. Biochem Biophys Res Commun 1989; 163:952–8.
100. Doi T, Striker LJ, Quaife C, et al. Progressive glomerulosclerosis develops in transgenic mice chronically expressing growth hormone and growth hormone releasing factor but not in those expressing insulinlike growth factor-1. Am J Pathol 1988; 131:398–403.
101. Miller SB, Rotwein P, Bortz JD, et al. Renal expression of IGF I in hypersomatotropic states. Am J Physiol 1990; 259:F251–7.
102. Harris RC, Hoover RL, Jacobson HR, Badr KF. Evidence for glomerular actions of epidermal growth factor in the rat. J Clin Invest 1988; 82:1028–39.
103. Adler S, Eng B. Reversal of inhibition of rat glomerular epithelial cell growth by growth factors. Am J Pathol 1990; 136:557–63.
104. Goodyer PR, Fata J, Goodyer CG. Excretion of epidermal growth factor-like material in acute Henoch-Schonlein purpura nephritis. Pediatr Nephrol 1990; 4:101–4.
105. Mattila AL, Pasternack A, Viinikka L, Perheentupa J. Subnormal concentrations of urinary epidermal growth factor in patients with kidney disease. J Clin Endocrinol Metab 1986; 62:1180–3.
106. Moss J, Shore I, Woodrow D, Gresser I. Interferon-induced glomerular basement membrane and endothelial cell lesions in mice. Am J Pathol 1988; 133:557–63.

CHAPTER 26

TNF-α, PAF, AND INTESTINAL INJURY
Relevance to Necrotizing Enterocolitis

Wei Hsueh, Frank Gonzalez-Crussi,
Michael S. Caplan, and Xiaoming Sun

Northwestern University Medical School
Chicago, Illinois

TUMOR NECROSIS FACTOR-α AND ENDOTOXIN SHOCK

Tumor necrosis factor-α (cachectin, TNF) is a cytokine produced mainly by activated macrophages (1,2). It has many potent proinflammatory actions (reviewed in Refs. 3–5), such as enhancement of chemotaxis (6–8) and phagocytosis (9) by polymorphonuclear leukocytes (PMNs) and macrophages (10); causing release of toxic oxygen intermediates by inflammatory cells (7,9,11–14); activation of endothelial cells (reviewed in Ref. 15), induction of expression of intercellular adhesion molecules (ICAMs) and endothelial leukocyte adhesion molecules (ELAMs) (4,16), increase in endothelial permeability (17), and facilitation of PMN migration across these cells (18,19); induction of procoagulant activity (20,21); induction of other cytokines (5,22–27); and increasing the production of lipid mediators, such as thromboxane, prostaglandins (28–31), leukotrienes (32,33), and platelet-activating factor (PAF) (33–36). When administered in vivo, it produces shock and gastrointestinal injury (37,38). Because (a) TNF induces shock (reviewed in Refs. 1–5, 39 and 40), (b) administration of endotoxin (lipopolysaccharide, LPS) to animals (41–43) and human volunteers (44,45) increases the circulating TNF level, and (c) pretreatment of the animal with anti-TNF prevents LPS-induced shock (46), TNF has been proposed as a pivotal mediator of endotoxin shock.

The mechanism of TNF-induced bowel injury is unknown. It may simply be a consequence of severe splanchnic ischemia secondary to systemic hypotension, or TNF may act alone or in concert with other mediators to directly damage the intestinal epithelial cells. Ischemic bowel necrosis is a complication of septic shock in human patients. It is possible that during sepsis, TNF, a mediator of endotoxin shock, is released systemically or locally in the gut and causes the bowel necrosis. The lamina propria of the intestine contains abundant macrophages, which are believed to be the endogenous source of TNF during endotoxin shock. Recent investigation has shown that Paneth cells in normal murine small intestine contain TNF mRNA that is readily detectable by in situ hybridization (47). However, TNF protein is undetectable in these cells in normal mice. Whether these cells also participate in the production of TNF in endotoxin shock is unclear at present.

PAF AND ENDOTOXIN SHOCK

Platelet-activating factor (PAF-acether) is an endogenous phospholipid mediator that is synthesized and secreted by many cell types, including monocytes, macrophages, PMNs, eosinophils, bone marrow-derived mast cells, endothelial cells, and platelets (for review, see Refs. 48–50). Recently such bacteria as *Escherichia coli* have also been shown to be able to synthesize PAF (51,52). In vitro, PAF aggregates human and rabbit platelets (53,54), is chemotactic for eosinophils (55,56), and activates PMNs to release oxygen radicals (57,58) and lysosomal enzymes (57–60). When injected into animals, PAF has many potent pathophysiological actions (reviewed in Refs. 48, 49, 61, and 62), such as systemic hypotension, pulmonary hypertension, bronchoconstriction, and increased vascular permeability. PAF is proposed as an endogenous mediator of endotoxin shock based on the following evidence: (a) administration of PAF induces shock in animals (reviewed in Refs. 48, 49, 63, and 64), (b) treatment with PAF antagonists prevents endotoxin-induced shock (reviewed in Refs. 64 and 65), and (c) injection of endotoxin stimulates PAF production in vivo (66–68).

PAF AND EXPERIMENTAL ISCHEMIC BOWEL NECROSIS (NECROTIZING ENTEROCOLITIS)

We have developed an experimental model of ischemic bowel necrosis in rats and mice by injecting PAF either into the splanchnic circulation or systemically (69). The pathological features of the experimental disease are similar to those of adult patients with ischemic bowel necrosis or neonates with necrotizing enterocolitis (NEC), both in gross appearance and in pathohistology (Fig. 1) (69). Mild or early bowel injury is found at the tips of the mucosal villi: only superficial loss of epithelium is observed at this stage. When a high dose of PAF is used, which produces prolonged shock, the necrotic change most typically extends throughout the mucosal layer and, in some instances, the entire thickness of the intestine. Priming the animal with a small intravenous (IV) dose of LPS (70 μg/kg) substantially reduces the dose of PAF required to induce bowel necrosis. Thus, LPS and PAF act synergistically to induce bowel necrosis, as well as other systemic symptoms, such as hypotension, hemoconcentration, and leukopenia. LPS alone at this dose is without pathological effect (69).

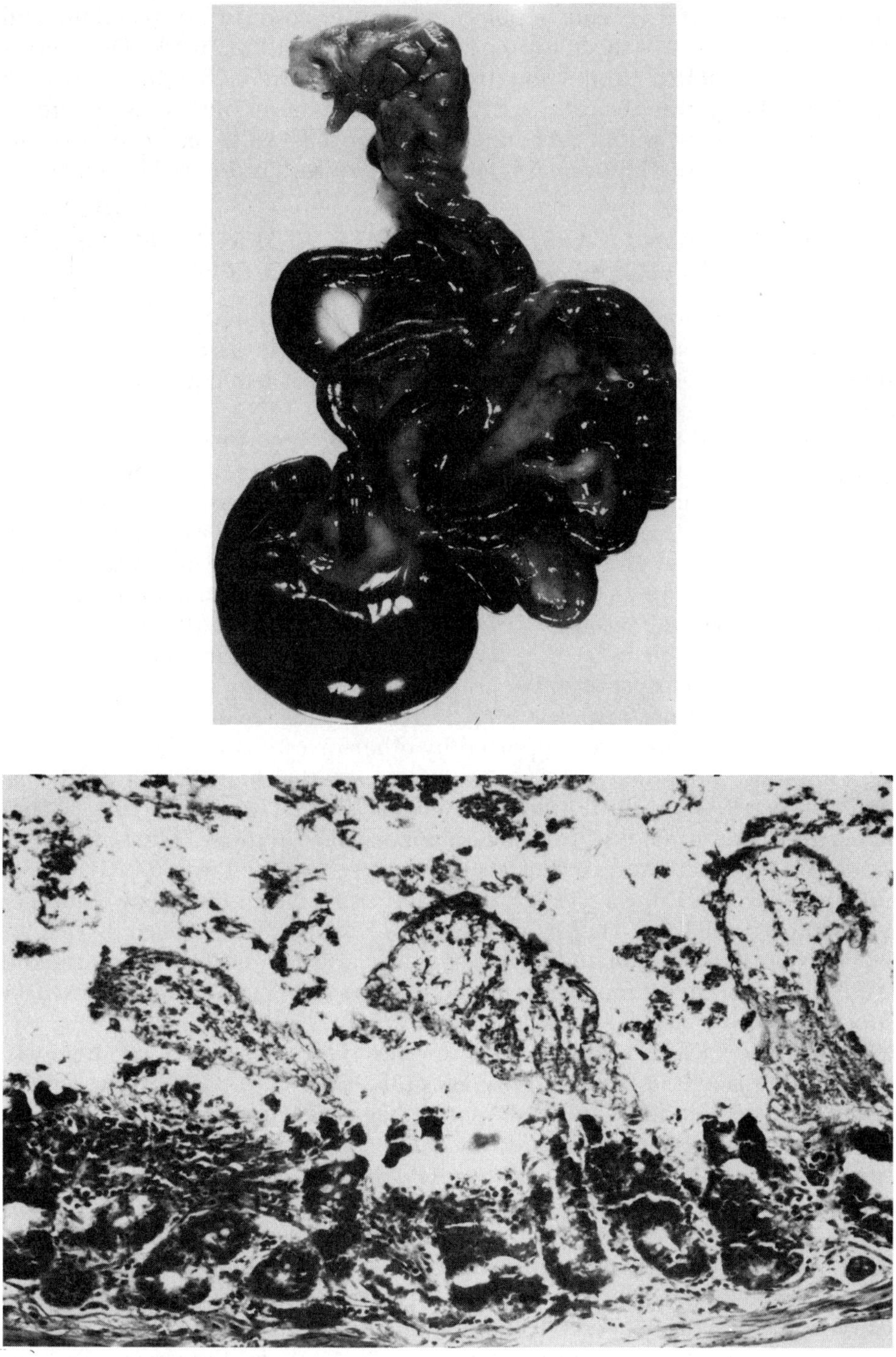

FIGURE 1 Gross and microscopic appearance of small intestine 2 h following intravenous injection of PAF (1-*O*-hexadecyl-2-acetyl-*sn*-glycero-3-phosphocholine; Sigma, St. Louis, MO; 3 μg/kg) into an adult Sprague-Dawley rat.

PAF is probably the key endogenous mediator for bowel injury in endotoxemia (68). This is suggested by the following observations: (a) LPS (2 mg/kg IV) injection increases intestinal PAF production (from control value of 0.13 ± 0.02 ng/g tissue to 2.04 ± 0.44 ng/g) in the rat; (b) LPS at this dose causes mild intestinal injury; and (c) pretreatment with a PAF antagonist, SRI 63-119 (3 mg/kg, Sandoz Research Institute, East Hanover, NJ), prevents LPS-induced bowel injury (68).

INTERACTION OF LPS, TNF, AND PAF, AND ROLE IN THE DEVELOPMENT OF INTESTINAL NECROSIS

Injection of TNF alone induces intestinal injury (37,38), but in our experience the extent and severity of this injury are milder than in lesions resulting from administration of PAF or PAF with LPS. Often, a near lethal dose of TNF must be used to cause severe intestinal damage. However, TNF acts in synergy with either LPS or PAF to induce severe and extensive bowel necrosis (70). To investigate the interaction of LPS and TNF in vivo, we injected recombinant TNF (0.5 mg/kg IV; Genentech, Inc., South San Francisco, CA) together with a low dose of LPS (200 μg/kg) into young male Sprague-Dawley rats and examined the systemic and local effects. We found that all animals treated with LPS and TNF developed severe shock, hemoconcentration, leukopenia, and segmental bowel necrosis, but animals treated with either agent alone at these doses maintained normal blood pressure (Fig. 2) and showed no intestinal injury (70). The leukopenia was also less severe. We also observed a synergy of TNF and LPS on the murine hypotensive response (Fig. 3). Results indicative of synergy between LPS and TNF have also been reported by other investigators (71,72).

An interesting observation in these studies was that both LPS and TNF are able to induce PAF production in the intestinal tissue (70). The effects of these two agents on intestinal PAF production appear to be additive. The bowel injury induced by LPS and TNF can be prevented by pretreatment with a PAF receptor antagonist, SRI 63-119, suggesting that LPS- and TNF-induced bowel injury is mediated by PAF (Table 1) (70). Moreover, systemic effects induced by LPS and TNF, such as hypotension and leukopenia, are also significantly ameliorated by the PAF antagonist, although not entirely reversed (Fig. 2). The increased hematocrit, however, is not affected by this PAF antagonist.

The source of PAF in this model is unclear. TNF causes PAF production in endothelial cells (34,35) and macrophages (35,36) in vitro. Conversely, PAF induces TNF production in cultured macrophages (73) and enhances TNF production by macrophages stimulated by MDP (74). Thus, a vicious cycle of endogenous production of both TNF and PAF could occur after an exogenous injection of LPS and TNF. Furthermore, PAF itself activates the PAF-forming enzyme, acetyltransferase, in macrophages (75). It is possible that a similar phenomenon may also take place in vivo, that is, exogenous PAF administration stimulates endogenous PAF production. This hypothesis is supported by our observation that treatment with PAF antagonists decreases endogenous intestinal PAF formation in response to LPS injection (68). Analysis of the in vivo situation is further complicated by the fact that the experimental animals used in our model are not germ free. Thus, LPS could enter the circulation from the bowel lumen once the initial injury (loss of epithelium) develops. Furthermore, intestinal bac-

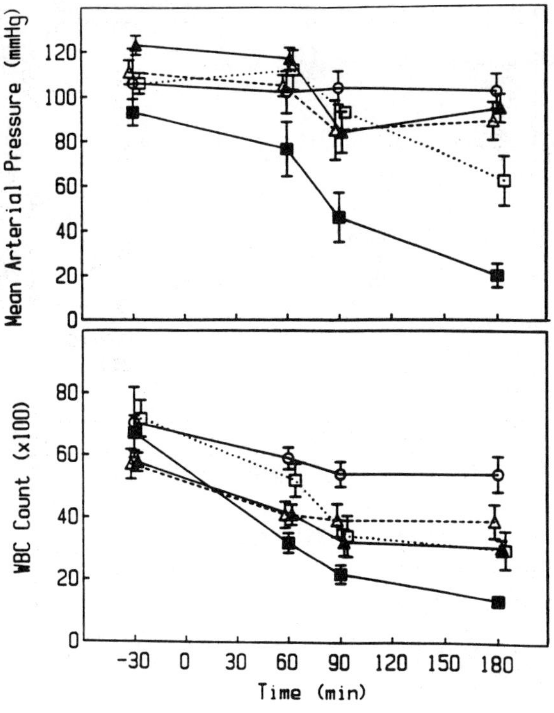

FIGURE 2 TNF- and LPS-induced systemic hypotension and leukopenia in young Sprague-Dawley rats (60–80 g): (open circles) control (n = 5, sham operated); (open triangles) 0.5 mg/kg of TNF injected at time 0 (n = 6); (solid triangles) 200 μg/kg of LPS injected at time 0 (n = 7); (solid squares) 0.5 mg/kg of TNF injected at time 0 + LPS injected at time 60 minutes (n = 5); and (open squares) 5 mg/kg of SRI 63–119 (divided into two doses, injected 20 minutes before TNF and 10 minutes before LPS) + 0.5 mg/kg of TNF, injected at time 0 + LPS injected at 60 minutes (n = 3).

teria have been shown to have the ability to synthesize PAF (51,52). Conceivably, all these factors have a bearing in aggravating the bowel lesion prompted by the synergy between LPS and TNF and between LPS and PAF. Moreover, TNF also acts synergistically with PAF in inducing bowel injury (Table 1) (70). This may explain why the level of endogenously produced PAF is much lower than that required exogenously to induce bowel injury. It should be kept in mind that, contrary to animal experiments in which a single agent is usually administered to induce an inflammatory response, in clinical patients multiple agents are produced. Thus, only minute quantities of LPS, TNF, and PAF are needed to initiate the inflammatory response, but the synergistic actions of these agents and the positive feedback loops may potentiate and perpetuate the response, culminating in tissue injury.

Although LPS and TNF synergize with PAF and with each other in inducing shock and tissue injury, strictly speaking neither of them is a true priming agent, since each, when applied in high dose, has effects similar to those of PAF. We used two methods to "prime" young Sprague-Dawley rats in vivo and found that under these circumstances the response of bowel injury to endotoxemia is ex-

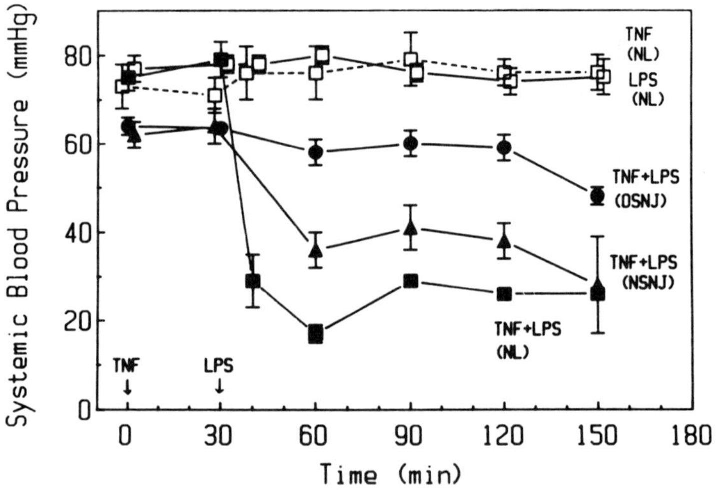

FIGURE 3 Change in systemic blood pressure following injection of TNF (0.2 μg/g), LPS (3 μg/g), or both in normal (C57BL/6J) and complement-deficient (B10.D2/OSNJ) mice: (--□--) C57BL/6J, TNF only (n = 4); (–□–) C57BL/6J, LPS only (n = 4); (■) C57BL/6J with TNF + LPS (n = 8); values from one mouse are presented at 90 minutes and on because of the death of all other mice); (▲) B10.D2/NSNJ, TNF + LPS (n = 11); and (●) B10.D2/OSNJ, TNF + LPS (n = 14).

aggerated (76). These two methods, injection of bacillus Calmette-Guérin (BCG) and intraperitoneal (IP) injection of zymosan, activate mononuclear phagocytes via different mechanisms. The former is T cell dependent, and the latter probably directly activates peritoneal macrophages. In either case, LPS-induced TNF re-

TABLE 1 Synergistic Effects of TNF and LPS and TNF and PAF on Intestinal Injury in the Rat and Its Prevention by PAF Antagonist SRI 63–119

Treatment	No. of animals	Gross lesions[a] (%)	Microscopic necrosis[b]
None	5	0	0
TFN,[c] 0.5 mg/kg	6	0	0
LPS, 200 μg/kg	7	0	0
TNF + LPS	5	35 ± 7	Mild (1), moderate (4)
PAF, 1 μg/kg	3	0	0
TNF + PAF	4	35 ± 4	Mild (1), moderate (3)
SRI 63–119[d] + TFN + LPS	3	0	0

[a] Gross lesions: violaceous, dark, and lusterless areas as percentage of the entire length of small intestine.

[b] Microscopic lesions are graded as previously reported (69). Mild: necrosis is confined to the tips of mucosal villi. Moderate: partial or total loss of villi but necrosis confined to the mucosa.

[c] TNF (5.02×10^7 U/mg, 0.5 mg/kg) was injected intravenously into young Sprague-Dawley rats (60–80 g) 1 h before the intravenous injection of LPS or PAF.

[d] SRI 63–119 was divided into two doses injected 20 minutes before TNF and 10 minutes before LPS.

Table 2 Effects of In Vivo Priming with Zymosan or BCG on LPS (0.5 mg/kg IV)-Induced Hypotention and Tissue Injury in the Rat[a]

Treatment	No. of animals	End BP (mmHg)	Plasma TNF (% killing)	Plasma PAF (ng/ml)	Bowel injury
None	5	102 ± 7.8	0	2.1 ± 0.8	0
LPS	10	73 ± 3.5	55 ± 3.6	8.3 ± 3.2	0 (9), mild (1)
Zymosan[b]	3	98 ± 3.3	<25	1.2 ± 0.5	0
Zymosan + LPS	12	55 ± 4.1	77 ± 2.2	21.4 ± 5.9	0 (4), mild (3), moderate (4)
BCG[c]	3	112 ± 4		0	0
BCG + LPS	11	74 ± 4.4	81 ± 5.7	12.7 ± 7.7	0 (3), mild (8)
SRI 63–441[d] + zymosan + LPS	5	89 ± 7.8			0 (4), mild (1)
SRI 63–441 + BCG + LPS	7	103 ± 2.1			0 (6), mild (1)

[a] Young Sprague-Dawley rats (approximately 100 g body weight) were used. Blood pressure at 3 h following LPS injection is presented. TNF activity is expressed as percentage killing of fibrosarcoma cell line 1591-RE 3.5 (76).
[b] Zymosan (50 mg/kg) was injected IP 24 h before LPS.
[c] BCG (2 × 10^7 organisms IV) was injected 12–15 days before LPS.
[d] SRI 63–441 (5 mg/kg), divided into two doses, 20 minutes before and 30 minutes after LPS administration.

lease is enhanced (Table 2). Interestingly, although in both cases the intestinal injury in response to LPS is aggravated, the systemic manifestation, that is, hypotension, is enhanced only in zymosan-pretreated animals. We do not know why there is no exaggerated systemic response to LPS in BCG-primed animals. Analysis of plasma PAF levels showed an enhanced response to LPS only in zymosan-primed rats (Table 2) (76), suggesting that systemic elevation of PAF may be necessary for the animal to respond to LPS with hypotension. This hypothesis is supported by the observation that pretreatment of the animals with SRI 63-119 (Sandoz Research Institute, East Hanover, NJ), a PAF antagonist, completely abolished the LPS-induced hypotensive response and bowel injury (Table 2). We (77) and Palmantier et al. (78) showed that the PAF-degrading enzyme, acetylhydrolase (79,80), is upregulated in BCG or complete Freund's adjuvant-activated macrophages. It is thus possible that in BCG-primed rats, PAF degradation as well as synthesis are simultaneously upregulated, thereby explaining why the circulating PAF level is not increased in these animals. In a similar mouse model using complete Freund's adjuvant as the priming agent, Remick et al. (81) showed that the TNF level was elevated in the primed mice, and PMN infiltration of the lung developed following LPS injection in these animals. Thus, in vivo priming (which activates the mononuclear phagocytic system to produce TNF) results in exaggerated responses to LPS in multiple organs.

ROLES OF EICOSANOIDS, NOREPINEPHRINE, AND OXYGEN RADICALS

Platelet aggregation, from which PAF originally derived its name, is not uniform in response to PAF in all animal species. Rat platelets are relatively refractory to PAF (69,82), and disseminated intravascular thrombi are not a feature of the pathohistology in our model. Thus, a thromboembolic phenomenon is not the cause of intestinal ischemia and the subsequent tissue necrosis seen in LPS-, TNF-, and PAF-induced bowel injury. Furthermore, neither LPS nor TNF has direct vasoconstricting actions. In addition, PAF itself is a vasodilator when directly applied to vessels (83), and at low doses it elicits a vasodilating response in various vascular beds (84,85). At high dose, however, PAF injection results in a severe and prolonged drop in mesenteric blood flow (85,86). Therefore, it seemed necessary to propose that vasoconstrictors are released following PAF production and that this, in turn, leads to intestinal ischemia. The association of the metabolism of arachidonic acid and PAF in PMNs is well established (reviewed in Ref. 87). It is thus possible that leukotrienes and prostaglandins are released following PAF production. We have shown that leukotriene C_4 (88,89) and norepinephrine (90) are released in vivo as well as from isolated, perfused rat small intestine after PAF injection. Thus, the prolonged splanchnic vasoconstriction in our model is at least in part mediated by these vasoconstricting substances.

After an initial phase of profound hypotension immediately following PAF administration, some branches of the mesenteric artery show gradual reversal of the vasoconstrictive response with partial recovery of the blood flow. Reperfusion is only focal if prolonged shock is observed. [This vascular change affects peripheral vascular territories and can be observed by a stereoscope (91) but may not be detected by monitoring the main superior mesenteric flow with flow probes.] It is possible that focal reperfusion may contribute to the development of necrosis seen at the end point. Since oxygen-derived free radicals are primarily responsible for ischemia and reperfusion injury (92–96), we infused the oxygen free-radical scavenger superoxide dismutase (10 mg/kg) and catalase (10 mg/kg) or pretreated the animal with the xanthine oxidase inhibitor allopurinol (5 mg/kg) before PAF administration. We found that these treatments significantly ameliorate the intestinal injury. When PAF was administered alone, only 50% or less of the small bowel was perfused at the end of the experiment. Pretreatment with allopurinol or superoxide dismutase or catalase significantly improved the extent of perfusion to 65–70% (91). The histological grading of necrosis was also ameliorated. Most animals receiving PAF alone showed necrosis involving the entire mucosa; pretreatment, either with superoxide dismutase or catalase or allopurinol, suppressed the PAF-induced injury or resulted in injury limited to the villous tips (91). These observations suggest a role of oxygen-derived free radicals in the pathogenesis of experimental bowel necrosis.

ROLE OF THE COMPLEMENT SYSTEM

The complement system plays an important role in inflammation, tissue injury, and endotoxin shock. LPS is known to activate complement through the classic and alternative pathways, and activation of the alternative pathway has been

TABLE 3 Lethality and Bowel Injury Induced by TNF and LPS in Normal Mice and Complement-Deficient Mice[a]

Mouse strain	Plasma C5	Inducing agent TNF (μg/g)	Inducing agent LPS (μg/g)	CH100 (U/ml)	Mortality at 2.5 h	Perfused bowel (%)
C57BL/6J	Normal	0	0	18 ± 2	0/6	100
		0	3	16 ± 2	0/4	100
		0.2	0	12 ± 4	0/4	100
		0.2	3	1 ± 1	7/8	13 ± 5
B10.D2/ NSNJ	Normal	0	3		0/3	100
		0.2	0		0/3	100
		0.2	3	2 ± 0	6/11	31 ± 7
B10.D2/ OSNJ	0	0	3		0/3	100
		0.2	0		0/3	100
		0.2	3	0	0/14	80 ± 9

[a] B10.D2/OSNJ mice have no detectable C5 (122).
TFN was injected (IV or intraarterially) 30 minutes before LPS injection (IV).

demonstrated in patients with Gram-negative septicemia (97). Conceivably, the potentiating effect of LPS in our model could be related to activation of the complement system. To investigate the role of in vivo complement activation, we assayed serum CH100 activity in mice in response to injection of various agents (a decrease in CH100 indicates in vivo complement activation). We found that TNF (0.2 μg/g, 2.5 h) does not significantly activate the complement system, LPS (3 μg/g, 2.5 h) mildly activates it, and a combination of the two results in marked complement activation (Table 3) (98). Neither of these two agents by itself causes intestinal necrosis (Table 3). TNF and LPS at these doses have no systemic effect, but combined treatment of TNF followed by LPS resulted in severe shock (Fig. 3), reduction of intestinal perfusion, and bowel injury (Table 3) (98). These observations suggest an association of complement activation with LPS- and TNF-induced bowel injury. To further investigate the role of the complement system, congenitally C5-deficient mice (B10.D2/OSNJ strain) were injected with TNF (0.2 μg/g) followed at 30 minutes by LPS (3 μg/g), and the effects were compared with those observed in C5-sufficient mice treated in the same way (98). Several control mouse strains, B10.D2/NSNJ (having low C3 level), C57BL/10SNJ, and C57BL/6J, were used. The doses mentioned are lethal for normal control mice: 10 of 11 mice died, most of them within 15 minutes, and more than half of the B10.D2/NSNJ mice died. In contrast, all 14 B10.D2/OSNJ (C5-deficient) mice survived (Table 3). C5-deficient mice also show much less severe hypotension (Fig. 3) and less hemoconcentration compared with the control mice (98). This indicates that for shock and bowel injury to develop, an intact complement system, more specifically C5, is required. Although it is not known if C5a or the membrane attack complex, or both, are involved in the mediation of tissue injury, the following evidence suggests that C5a plays a significant role in our model: (a) C5a increases microvascular permeability (99); (b) C5a stimulates TNF production by mononuclear cells (100); (c) pretreatment of rats with F(ab′) fragments of rabbit antirat C5a significantly improves LPS-induced hypotension and hemoconcentration (101); and (d) C5a is required for the development of TNF-induced hemorrhagic necrosis of the skin in mice exposed to bacterial agents (102).

Although the complement system, especially C5, plays an essential role in the TNF- and LPS-induced gut injury, activation of the complement system alone is insufficient to induce bowel necrosis (103). Administration of cobra venom factor, which activates the complement system in vivo, aggravated the hypotension and bowel necrosis induced by PAF and LPS but did not produce intestinal damage by itself, even when the complement level was depleted to 15% of control (103). Therefore, it is likely that other mediators, such as PAF, TNF, or LPS, must act in synergy with activated complement fragments to induce bowel necrosis. In this particular model (98) in complement-sufficient mice, TNF acts as a priming agent, since TNF alone did not cause systemic changes, such as blood pressure, temperature, CH100, or hematocrit. Following LPS administration, the primed system (inflammatory cells and endothelial cells) showed an exaggerated response to LPS. Preliminary experiments showed that PAF may be the essential mediator in this response, since pretreatment with PAF antagonist abrogates both the systemic and local (intestinal) responses to TNF and LPS (104). The activated complement fragments, in synergy with TNF, LPS, and PAF, mediate shock and bowel necrosis.

The observation that congenitally C5-deficient mice are protected from TNF- (0.2 μg/g) and LPS (3 μg/g)-induced shock and tissue injury seems to indicate that C5 is absolutely required for their action. When 0.5 μg/g of TNF was used to prime the animal (with the same LPS dose), however, all animals, C5 deficient or sufficient, developed shock and severe hemoconcentration and died (98). This observation indicates that TNF and LPS induce shock and tissue injury through complement-dependent as well as complement-independent pathways. A high dose of TNF (with LPS) may have a direct effect on the vascular system and inflammatory cells or may release other mediators, independent of the complement system.

NECROTIZING ENTEROCOLITIS: A CLINICAL DISEASE THAT MAY INVOLVE TNF AND PAF

Necrotizing enterocolitis is an acute gastrointestinal disease, primarily of premature infants, with high morbidity and mortality (105,106). In some epidemiological surveys, NEC ranks as the third leading cause of death in children less than 1 year of age, next only to respiratory distress syndrome (RDS) and congenital malformations. This pattern may change in the next decade following widespread use of surfactant therapy for RDS, which dramatically decreases the mortality and morbidity of RDS. NEC occurs predominantly in the first 3 months of life and is characterized by the rapid onset of abdominal distention and tenderness, bloody stools, and the pathognomonic radiographic evidence of pneumatosis intestinalis. Frequently, NEC progresses and affected patients develop shock, disseminated intravascular coagulation, neutropenia, thrombocytopenia, peritonitis, and pneumoperitoneum. Supportive therapy, consisting of fluids, bicarbonate, blood and platelet transfusions, pressors and antibiotics, is often inadequate, leading to surgical exploration, bowel resection, and in 30–50% of cases, death (107,108).

NEC occurs either endemically or as an epidemic in the neonatal intensive care unit. It is generally accepted that an infectious agent may initiate the disease process in the epidemic cases. However, the exact pathogenesis of bowel necrosis remains unclear. Even less is known about the endemic form of NEC. Several risk factors have been implicated. These include prematurity (109), feeding practice (110), hypoxia and intestinal ischemia (111), and infection (112). Prematurity is a consistent feature: more than 95% of NEC cases afflict premature infants (105). More than 90% of NEC patients develop the disease following enteral feedings. However, the cause of the correlation between enteral feeding and development of NEC is not understood. It has been thought to be due to massive proliferation of the intestinal flora following feeding (113) or to the speed or volume of feeding (114,115). Some investigators also believe that maternal milk protects against the development of NEC (116). Very little attention has been paid, heretofore, to the role of inflammatory mediators in this disease. Since the animal model we produced resembles clinical NEC in both gross and microscopic appearance, we hypothesize that LPS, PAF, and TNF may also play important roles in the pathogenesis of NEC in human patients (117,118).

To test our hypothesis and to investigate the role of these inflammatory mediators in NEC, we conducted a pilot study to measure plasma TNF, PAF, and the PAF-specific degrading enzyme acetylhydrolase in 12 patients with NEC and compared the results to 8 age-matched control infants (118). We found that plasma TNF concentrations were significantly higher in NEC patients than in controls (136 ± 75 versus 1.5 ± 0.8 U/ml, $p < 0.05$; Fig. 4). Plasma PAF levels were also higher in NEC patients compared to controls (18.1 ± 3.6 versus 3.1 ± 0.9 ng/ml, $p < 0.01$; Fig. 5), sometimes markedly so. Plasma acetylhydrolase activity (the enzyme critical to PAF regulation) was lower in NEC patients compared to controls (10.6 ± 0.7 versus 23.0 ± 1.4 n mol/ml/minute, $p < 0.01$; Fig. 5). However, there was no correlation between PAF level and the severity of outcome of the disease. Interestingly, although plasma TNF concentrations were higher in NEC patients, there was wide individual variation and the levels did not correlate with the plasma PAF levels or the severity of the disease.

These observations, of course, do not prove that TNF and/or PAF are the primary mediators in the development of NEC. However, demonstration of abnormally high levels of these potent inflammatory mediators, as well as abnormally low activity of the PAF-degrading enzyme in the circulation of NEC patients, compellingly suggest that these mediators participate in the pathogenesis of NEC and may play an important role in its pathophysiology.

Maturation of PAF-Specific Acetylhydrolase: A Role for Developing NEC?

The tissue level of PAF is regulated by a balance between PAF production and PAF degradation. PAF is degraded by an acetylhydrolase present in plasma and most tissues (79) that hydrolyses the acetate moiety to produce the biologically inactive lyso-PAF. Since PAF has a short half-life (80), acetylhydrolase is important in systemic and local PAF regulation. As described earlier, plasma acetylhydrolase

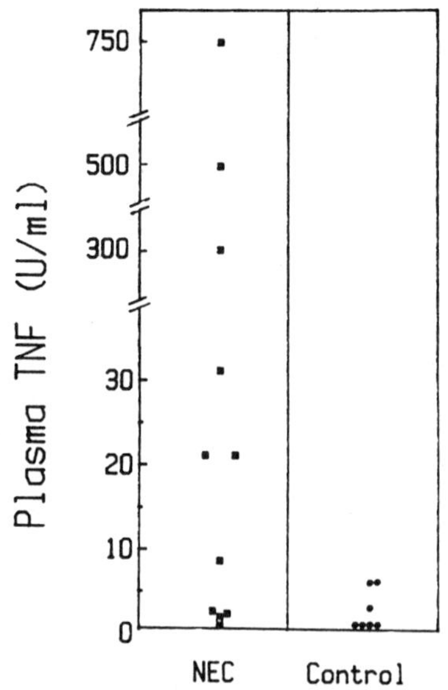

FIGURE 4 Individual plasma TNF values in NEC patients and controls; $p < 0.05$ with Mann-Whitney U test to compare nonparametric group means. (From Ref. 118, with permission from J Pediatr, C. V. Mosby.)

activity was abnormally low in NEC patients and PAF concentration was higher than in controls. Thus, suppressed PAF degradation in NEC patients may be an important causative factor in the pathophysiology of NEC.

Because NEC is a disease so strikingly confined to newborns in the first few

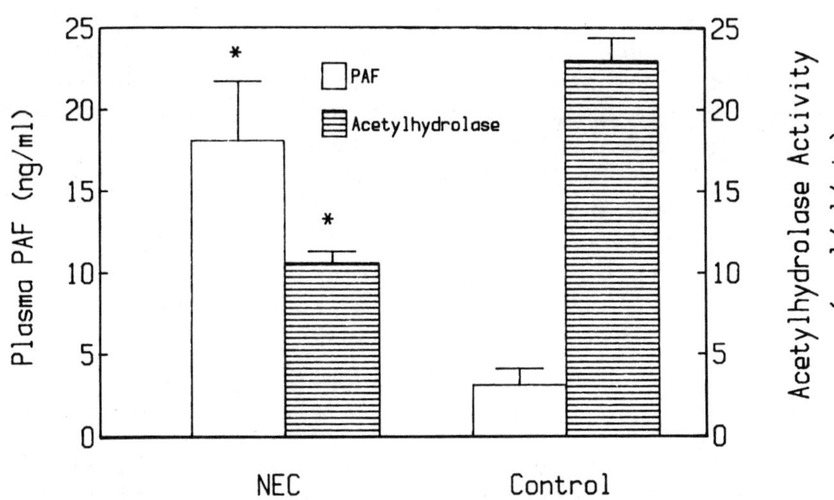

FIGURE 5 Plasma PAF and plasma acetylhydrolase activity in NEC patients and controls. $^*p < 0.01$ compared with control values with two-tailed unpaired Student's *t*-test. (From Ref. 118, with permission from J Pediatr, C. V. Mosby.)

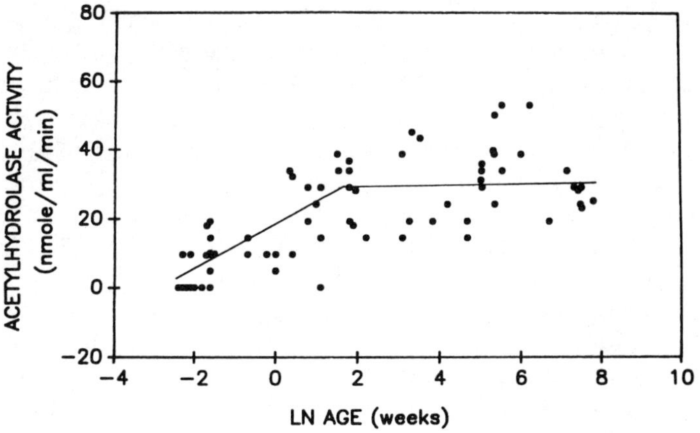

FIGURE 6 Scatter diagram of the effect of the natural logarithm of age on acetylhydrolase activity. The equation for the regression lines are age < 6 weeks, $AH_i = 17.45 + 6.01 \ln age_i$; age > 5 weeks, $AH_i = 26.64 + 0.752 \ln age_i$. (From Ref. 120, with permission from Prostaglandins, Butterworth-Heinemann.)

weeks of life, we investigated human plasma acetylhydrolase activity as a function of age (119). We found that enzyme activity increases linearly with respect to the natural logarithm of age over the first 6 weeks of life, at the end of which it approaches adult values ($r = 0.65$, $p < 0.001$; Fig. 6). We also established that in infants less than 3 weeks of age, acetylhydrolase activity is lower than at all other ages (8.2 ± 1.4 versus 30.0 ± 1.6 nmol/ml/minute, $p < 0.01$). We found no significant differences in acetylhydrolase activity between term or premature newborns (8.6 ± 1.9 versus 7.2 ± 2.4 nmol/ml/minute, respectively; p = NS). These findings suggest that newborns are at increased risk for PAF-related diseases because of a constitutional inability to degrade PAF locally and systemically. Preterm infants are more likely to have hypoxic stress and to develop infections than term neonates. Since bacterial endotoxin (67,68) and hypoxia (120) elicit endogenous PAF production, a suppressed acetylhydrolase activity renders premature infants uniquely susceptible to those diseases in which PAF is likely to be an important mediator. The evidence described here points to NEC as an example of a PAF-related disorder.

PROPOSED MECHANISM FOR THE PATHOGENESIS OF NEC

Ischemic bowel necrosis in adult patients is usually a complication of shock and sepsis, and it is not difficult to conceptualize how the mediators of shock and septicemia, such as TNF, PAF, leukotrienes, and catecholamines, interact with one another and with endotoxin to mediate intestinal ischemia and injury. The pathogenesis of necrotizing enterocolitis in neonates may be an entirely different story. The development of NEC usually precedes sepsis and shock. We hypothesize that the following events may take place in the endemic form of neonatal NEC.

Since the majority of these infants are premature, most of them have experienced some degree of perinatal stress, that is, hypoxia. We have shown that hypoxia induces the initial, mild mucosal damage with loss of superficial epithelium (120). This step involves PAF (120), but not TNF. Upon the first feeding, a large amount of bacteria is introduced into the gastrointestinal tract. In addition, the nutrient facilitates bacterial growth in the intestine. The immature and sometimes impaired mucosal barrier allows entry of the bacterial products, such as LPS, and sometimes bacteria themselves, into the gut tissue, eliciting endogenous production of inflammatory mediators, such as TNF and PAF. [The ability of the digestive system to synthesize TNF is demonstrated by a recent report that showed that the largest proportion of circulating TNF comes from the splanchnic area (121).] In addition, *E. coli* and perhaps other enteral bacteria synthesize PAF (51,52). The amount of these mediators produced may or may not be sufficient to cause shock and/or bowel necrosis in normal infants. The situation may be more serious in selected neonates, who as a result of immaturity or other reasons, are deficient in the PAF-degrading enzyme, acetylhydrolase. As a result, PAF may accumulate and synergize with TNF and/or LPS to produce more PAF and TNF. These agents synergize with each other to activate inflammatory cells and the complement system and act on the vascular system. A vicious cycle of self-perpetuating inflammatory response is then initiated. Other mediators and oxygen radicals are released, and the sympathetic system is activated. The ultimate result is irreversible shock and bowel necrosis.

In the epidemic form of NEC, which also affects term infants, the initial injurious agent may not be hypoxia but an infectious agent, such as virus or bacteria. Viral or bacterial infection causes the initial mucosal damage, and enteral feeding may facilitate the entrance of bacteria and production of inflammatory mediators. The same process as just described is initiated, resulting in shock and bowel necrosis.

ACKNOWLEDGMENT

This work was supported by NIH Grant DK34574.

REFERENCES

1. Beutler B, Cerami A. Cachectin: more than a tumor necrosis factor. N Engl J Med 1987; 316:379–85.
2. Old LJ. Tumor necrosis factor. Science 1985; 230:630–2.
3. Beutler B, Cerami A. Tumor necrosis, cachexia, shock, and inflammation: a common mediator. Annu Rev Biochem 1988; 57:505–18.
4. Tracey KJ, Vlassara H, Cerami A. Cachectin/tumour necrosis factor. Lancet 1989; 1:1122–6.
5. Beutler B, Cerami A. The biology of cachectin/TNF—a primary mediator of the host response. Annu Rev Immunol 1989; 7:625–55.
6. Yonemaru M, Stephens KE, Ishizaka A, et al. Effects of tumor necrosis factor on PMN chemotaxis, chemiluminescence, and elastase activity. J Lab Clin Med 1989; 114:674–81.
7. Figari I, Mori N, Palladino M Jr. Regulating of neutrophil chemotaxis and superoxide production by recombinant tumor necrosis factor-alpha and beta comparison to recombinant interferon-gamma and interleukin-1 alpha. Blood 1987; 70:979–84.

8. Ming WJ, Bersani L, Mantovani A. Tumor necrosis factor is chemotactic for monocytes and polymorphonuclear leukocytes. J Immunol 1987; 138:1469–74.
9. Ferrante A. Tumor necrosis factor alpha potentiates neutrophil antimicrobial activity: increased fungicidal activity against *Torulopsis glabrata* and *Candida albicans* and associated increases in oxygen radical production and lysosomal enzyme release. Infect Immun 1989; 57:2115–22.
10. Hoffman M, Weinberg JB. Tumor necrosis factor-alpha induces increased hydrogen peroxide production and Fc receptor expression, but not increased Ia antigen expression by peritoneal macrophages. J Leuko Biol 1987; 42:704–7.
11. Klebanoff SJ, Vadas MA, Harlan JM, et al. Stimulation of neutrophils by tumor necrosis factor. J Immunol 1986; 136:4220–5.
12. Berkow RL, Wang D, Larrick JW, Dodson RW, Howard TH. Enhancement of neutrophil superoxide production by preincubation with recombinant human tumor necrosis factor. J Immunol 1987; 139:3783–91.
13. Nathan CF. Neutrophil activation on biological surfaces: massive secretion of hydrogen peroxide in response to product of macrophages and lymphocytes. J Clin Invest 1987; 80:1550–60.
14. Laudanna C, Miron S, Berton G, Rossi F. Tumor necrosis factor-alpha/cachectin activates the O_2-generating system of human neutrophils independently of the hydrolysis of phosphoinositides and the release of arachidonic acid. Biochem Biophys Res Commun 1990; 166:308–15.
15. Pober JS. Cytokine-mediated activation of vascular endothelium. Physiology and pathology. Am J Pathol 1988; 133:426–33.
16. Luscinskas FW, Brock AF, Arnaout MA, Gimbrone MA Jr. Endothelial-leukocyte adhesion molecule-1-dependent and leukocyte (CD11/CD18)-dependent mechanisms contribute to polymorphonuclear leukocyte adhesion to cytokine-activated human vascular endothelium. J Immunol 1989; 142:2257–63.
17. Brett J, Gerlach H, Nawroth P, Steinberg S, Godman G, Stern D. Tumor necrosis factor/cachectin increases permeability of endothelial cell monolayers by a mechanism involving regulatory G proteins. J Exp Med 1989; 169:1977–91.
18. Furie MB, McHugh DD. Migration of neutrophils across endothelial monolayers is stimulated by treatment of the monolayers with interleukin-1 or tumor necrosis factor alpha. J Immunol 1989; 143:3309–17.
19. Moser R, Schleiffenbaum B, Groscurth P, Fehr J. Interleukin 1 and tumor necrosis factor stimulate human vascular endothelial cells to promote transendothelial neutrophil passage. J Clin Invest 1989; 83:444–55.
20. McKenna TM, Titius WA. Role of monokines in altering receptor and non-receptor mediated vascular contraction in sepsis. Prog Clin Biol Res 1989; 286:279–303.
21. Bauer KA, ten Cate H, Barzegar S, Spriggs DR, Sherman ML, Rosenberg RD. Tumor necrosis factor infusions have a procoagulant effect on the hemostatic mechanism of humans. Blood 1989; 74:165–72.
22. Brouckaert PG, Libert C, Everaerdt B, Takahashi N, Fiers W. A role for interleukin 1 in the in vivo actions of tumor necrosis factor. Lymphokine Res 1989; 8(3):269–74.
23. Sica A, Wang JM, Colotta F, et al. Monocyte chemotactic and activating factor gene expression induced in endothelial cells by IL-1 and tumor necrosis factor. J Immunol 1990; 144:3034–8.
24. Shalaby MR, Waage A, Aarden L, Espevik T. Endotoxin, tumor necrosis factor-alpha and interleukin 1 induce interleukin 6 production in vivo. Clin Immunol Immunopathol 1989; 53:488–98.
25. Locksley RM, Heinzel FP, Shepard HM, et al. Tumor necrosis factors alpha and

beta differ in their capacities to generate interleukin 1 release from human endothelial cells. J Immunol 1987; 139:1891–5.
26. Dinarello CA, Cannon JG, Wolff SM, et al. Tumor necrosis factor (cachectin) is an endogenous pyrogen and induces production of interleukin 1. J Exp Med 1986; 163:1433–50.
27. Kaushansky K, Broudy VC, Harlan JM, Adamson JW. Tumor necrosis factor-alpha and tumor necrosis factor-beta (lymphotoxin) stimulate the production of granulocyte-macrophage colony-stimulating factor, macrophage colony-stimulating factor, and IL-1 in vivo. J Immunol 1988; 141:3410–5.
28. Dayer JM, Beutler B, Cerami A. Cachectin/tumor necrosis factor stimulates collagenase and prostaglandin E_2 production by human synovial cells and dermal fibroblasts. J Exp Med 1985; 162:2163–8.
29. Endo H, Akahoshi T, Kashiwazaki S. Additive effects of IL-1 and TNF on induction of prostacyclin synthesis in human vascular endothelial cells. Biochem Biophys Res Commun 1988; 156:1007–14.
30. Zavoico GB, Ewenstein BM, Schafer AI, Pober JS. IL-1 and related cytokines enhance thrombin-stimulated PGI_2 production in cultured endothelial cells without affecting thrombin-stimulated von Willebrand factor secretion or platelet-activating factor biosynthesis. J Immunol 1989; 142:3993–9.
31. Kettelhut IC, Fiers W, Goldberg AL. The toxic effects of tumor necrosis factor in vivo and their prevention by cyclooxygenase inhibitors. Proc Natl Acad Sci U S A 1987; 84:4273–7.
32. Huber M, Beutler B, Keppler D. Tumor necrosis factor alpha stimulates leukotriene production in vivo. Eur J Immunol 1988; 18:2085–8.
33. Camussi G, Tetta C, Bussolino F, Baglioni C. Tumor necrosis factor stimulates human neutrophils to release leukotriene B_4 and platelet-activating factor. Induction of phospholipase A_2 and acetyl-CoA:1-alkyl-*sn*-glycero-3-phosphocholine 2-acetyltransferase activity and inhibition by antiproteinase. Eur J Biochem 1989; 182:661–6.
34. Bussolino F, Camussi G, Baglioni C. Synthesis and release of platelet-activating factor by human vascular endothelial cells treated with tumor necrosis factor or interleukin 1 alpha. J Biol Chem 1988; 263:11856–61.
35. Camussi G, Bussolino F, Salvidio G, Baglioni C. Tumor necrosis factor/cachectin stimulates peritoneal macrophages, polymorphonuclear neutrophils, and vascular endothelial cells to synthesize and release platelet-activating factor. J Exp Med 1987; 166:1390–404.
36. Valone FH, Epstein LB. Biphasic platelet-activating factor synthesis by human monocytes stimulated with IL-1-beta, tumor necrosis factor, or IFN-gamma. J Immunol 1988; 141:3945–50.
37. Tracey KJ, Beutler B, Lowry SF, et al. Shock and tissue injury induced by recombinant human cachectin. Science 1986; 234:470–4.
38. Remick DG, Kunkel RG, Larrick JW, Kunkel SL. Acute in vivo effects of human recombinant tumor necrosis factor. Lab Invest 1987; 56:583–90.
39. Tracey KJ, Lowry SF, Cerami A. Cachectin/TNF-alpha in septic shock and septic adult respiratory distress syndrome. Am Rev Respir Dis 1988; 138:1377–9.
40. Remick DG, Kunkel SL. Toxic effects of cytokines in vivo. Lab Invest 1989; 60:317–9.
41. Waage A. Production and clearance of tumor necrosis factor in rats exposed to endotoxin and dexamethasone. Clin Immunol Immunopathol 1987; 45:348–55.
42. Beutler BA, Milsark IW, Cerami A. Cachectin/tumor necrosis factor: production, distribution, and metabolic fate in vivo. J Immunol 1985; 135:3972–7.
43. Mathison JC, Wolfson E, Ulevitch RJ. Participation of tumor necrosis factor in the

mediation of Gram negative bacterial lipopolysaccharide-induced injury in rabbits. J Clin Invest 1988; 81:1925–37.
44. Cannon JG, Tompkins RG, Gelfand JA, et al. Circulating interleukin-1 and tumor necrosis factor in septic shock and experimental endotoxin fever. J Infect Dis 1990; 161:79–84.
45. Michie HR, Manogue KR, Spriggs DR, et al. Detection of circulating tumor necrosis factor after endotoxin administration. N Engl J Med 1988; 318:1481–6.
46. Tracey KJ, Fong Y, Hesse DG, et al. Anti-cachectin/TNF monoclonal antibodies prevent septic shock during lethal bacteraemia. Nature 1987; 330:662–4.
47. Keshav S, Lawson L, Chung LP, Stein M, Perry VH, Gordon S. Tumor necrosis factor mRNA localized to Paneth cells of normal murine intestinal epithelium by in situ hybridization. J Exp Med 1990; 171:327–32.
48. Benveniste J. Paf-acether, an ether phospholipid with biological activity. Prog Clin Biol Res 1988; 282:73–85.
49. Hanahan DJ. Platelet activating factor: a biologically active phosphoglyceride. Annu Rev Biochem 1986; 55:483–509.
50. Snyder F. Biochemistry of platelet-activating factor: a unique class of biologically active phospholipids. Proc Soc Exp Biol Med 1989; 190:125–35.
51. Denizot Y, Dassa E, Kim HY, et al. Synthesis of PAF-acether from exogenous precursors by the prokaryote *Escherichia coli*. FEBS Lett 1989; 243:13–6.
52. Denizot Y, Dassa E, Benveniste J, Thomas Y. Paf-acether production by *Escherichia coli*. Biochem Biophys Res Commun 1989; 161:939–43.
53. McManus LM, Hanahan DJ, Pinckard RN. Human platelet stimulation by acetyl glyceryl ether phosphorylcholine. J Clin Invest 1981; 67:903–6.
54. Sugatani J, Miwa M, Hanahan DJ. Platelet-activating factor stimulation of rabbit platelets is blocked by serine protease inhibitor (chymotryptic protease inhibitor). J Biol Chem 1987; 262:5740–7.
55. Wardlaw AJ, Moqbel R, Cromwell O, Kay AB. Platelet-activating factor. A potent chemotactic and chemokinetic factor for human eosinophils. J Clin Invest 1986; 78:1701–6.
56. Sigal CE, Valone FH, Holtzman MJ, Goetzl EJ. Preferential human eosinophil chemotactic activity of the platelet-activating factor (PAF) 1-0-hexadecyl-2-acetyl-*sn*-glycedryl-3-phosphocholine (AGEPC). J Clin Immunol 1987; 7:179–84.
57. Shaw JO, Pinckard RN, Ferrigni KS, McManus LM, Hanahan DJ. Activation of human neutrophils with 1-0-hexadecyl/octadecyl-2-acetyl-*sn*-glyceryl-3-phosphorylcholine (platelet activating factor). J Immunol 1981; 127:1250–5.
58. Gay JC, Beckman JK, Zaboy KA, Lukens JN. Modulation of neutrophil oxidative responses to soluble stimuli by platelet-activating factor. Blood 1986; 67:931–6.
59. O'Flaherty JT, Wykle RL, Miller CH, et al. 1-0-Alkyl-*sn*-glyceryl-3-phosphoryl-cholines. A novel class of neutrophil stimulants. Am J Pathol 1981; 103:70–9.
60. Dewald B, Baggiolini M. Platelet-activating factor as a stimulus of exocytosis in human neutrophils. Biochim Biophys Acta 1986; 888:42–8.
61. Feuerstein G, Goldstein RE. Effect of PAF on the cardiovascular system. In: Snyder F, ed. Platelet-activating factor and related lipid mediators. New York: Plenum Press, 1987:403–24.
62. Vargaftig BB. Bronchopulmonary pharmacology of PAF-acether. In: Synder F, ed. Platelet-activating factor and related lipid mediators. New York: Plenum Press, 1987:341–53.
63. Feuerstein G, Siren AL. Platelet-activating factor and shock. Prog Biochem Pharmacol 1988; 22:181–90.
64. Handley DA. Platelet-activating factor as a mediator of endotoxin-related diseases. In: Handley DA, Saunders RN, Houlihan WJ, Tomesch JC, eds. Platelet-activating

factor in endotoxin and immune diseases. New York: Marcel Dekker, 1990:451–95.
65. Toth PD. The biological effects of PAF antagonists on endotoxemia. In: Handley DA, Saunders RN, Houlihan WJ, Tomesch JC, eds. Platelet-activating factor in endotoxin and immune diseases. New York: Marcel Dekker, 1990:589–608.
66. Inarrea P, Gomez-Cambronero J, Pascual J, del Carmen Ponte M, Hernando L, Sanchez-Crespo M. Synthesis of PAF-acether and blood volume changes in gram-negative sepsis. Immunopharmacology 1985; 9:45–52.
67. Chang SW, Feddersen CO, Henson PM, Voelkel NF. Platelet-activating factor mediates hemodynamic changes and lung injury in endotoxin treated rat. J Clin Invest 1987; 79:1498–509.
68. Hsueh W, Gonzalez Crussi F, Arroyave JL. Platelet-activating factor: an endogenous mediator for bowel necrosis in endotoxemia. FASEB J 1987; 1:403–5.
69. Gonzalez-Crussi F, Hsueh W. Experimental model of ischemic bowel necrosis. The role of platelet-activating factor and endotoxin. Am J Pathol 1983; 112:127–35.
70. Sun XM, Hsueh W. Bowel necrosis induced by tumor necrosis factor in rats is mediated by platelet-activating factor. J Clin Invest 1988; 81:1328–31.
71. Neilson IR, Neilson KA, Yunis EJ, Rowe MI. Failure of tumor necrosis factor to produce hypotensive shock in the absence of endotoxin. Surgery 1989; 106:439–43.
72. Rothstein JL, Schreiber H. Synergy between tumor necrosis factor and bacterial products causes hemorrhagic necrosis and lethal shock in normal mice. Proc Natl Acad Sci U S A 1988; 85:607–11.
73. Bonavida B, Mencia-Huerta J-M, Braquet P. Effect of platelet activating factor on monocyte activation and production of tumor necrosis factor. Int Arch Allergy Apply Immunol 1989; 88:157–60.
74. Dubois C, Bissonnette E, Rola-Pleszczynski M. Platelet-activating (PAF) enhances tumor necrosis factor production by alveolar macrophages. Prevention by PAF receptor antagonists and lipoxygenase inhibitors. J Immunol 1989; 143:964–70.
75. Doebber TW, Wu MS. Plateledt-activating factor (PAF) stimulates the PAF-synthesizing enzyme acetyl-CoA:1-alkyl-*sn*-glycero-3-phosphocholine O^2-acetyltransferase and PAF synthesis in neutrophils. Proc Natl Acad Sci U S A 1987; 84:7557–61.
76. Sun XM, Hsueh W, Torre-Amione G. Effects of in vivo "priming" on endotoxin-induced hypotension and tissue injury. The role of PAF and tumor necrosis factor. Am J Pathol 1990; 136:949–56.
77. Hursh DM, Hsueh W, Kartha RK. PAF metabolism in resident and activated alveolar macrophages: Role of protein kinase C. Cell Immunol 1990; 130:429–36.
78. Palmantier R, Dulioust A, Maiza H, Benveniste J, Ninio E. Biosynthesis of Paf-acether. XIV. Paf-acether output in murine peritoneal macrophages is regulated by the level of acetylhydrolases. Biochem Biophys Res Commun 1989; 162:475–82.
79. Blank ML, Lee TC, Fitzgerald V, Snyder F. A specific acetylhydrolase for 1-alkyl-2-acetyl-*sn*-glycero-3-phosphocholine (a hypotensive and platelet-activating lipid). J Biol Chem 1981; 256:175–8.
80. Stafforini DM, Prescott SM, McIntyre TM. Human plasma platelet-activating factor acetylhydrolase. Purification and properties. J Biol Chem 1987; 262:4223–30.
81. Remick DG, Strieter RM, Eskandari MK, et al. Role of tumor necrosis factor-alpha in lipopolysaccharide-induced pathologic alterations. Am J Pathol 1990; 136:49–60.
82. Sanchez-Crespo M, Alonso F, Inarrea P, Alvarez V, Egido J. Vascular actions of

synthetic PAF-acether (a synthetic platelet-activating factor) in the rat: evidence for a platelet independent mechanism. Immunopharmacology 1982; 4:173–85.
83. Kasuya Y, Masuda Y, Shigenobu K. Possible role of endothelium in the vasodilator response of rat thoracic aorta to platelet activating factor (PAF). J Pharmacobiodyn 1984; 7:138–42.
84. Chu KM, Gerber JG, Nies AS. Local vasodilator effect of platelet activating factor in the gastric, mesenteric and femoral arteries of the dog. J Pharmacol Exp Ther 1988; 246:996–1000.
85. Siren AL, Feuerstein G. Effects of PAF and BN 52021 on cardiac function and regional blood flow in conscious rats. Am J Physiol 1989; 257:H25–32.
86. Zhang C, Hsueh W. PAF-induced bowel injury: the effects of vasodilators. FASEB J 1990; 4:A346.
87. Wykle R. Interrelationships in the metabolism of platelet-activating factor and arachidonate in neutrophils. In: Snyder F, ed. Platelet-activating factor and related lipid mediators. New York: Plenum Press, 1987:273–82.
88. Hsueh W, Gonzalez Crussi F, Arroyave JL. Release of leukotriene C_4 by isolated, perfused rat small intestine in response to platelet-activating factor. J Clin Invest 1986; 78:108–14.
89. Hsueh W, Gonzalez-Crussi F, Arroyave JL. Platelet activating factor-induced ischemic bowel necrosis: an investigation of secondary mediators in its pathogenesis. Am J Pathol 1986; 122:231–9.
90. Hsueh W, Gonzalez Crussi F, Arroyave JL. Sequential release of leukotrienes and norepinephrine in rat bowel after platelet-activating factor. A mechanistic study of platelet-activating factor-induced bowel necrosis. Gastroenterology 1988; 94:1412–8.
91. Cueva JP, Hsueh W. Role of oxygen derived free radicals in platelet activating factor induced bowel necrosis. Gut 1988; 29:1207–12.
92. McCord JM. Oxygen-derived free radicals in postischemic tissue injury. N Engl J Med 1985; 312:159–63.
93. Granger DN. Role of xanthine oxidase and granulocytes in ischemia-reperfusion injury. Am J Physiol 1988; 255:H1269–75.
94. Grisham MB. Granger DN. Neutrophil-mediated mucosal injury. Role of reactive oxygen metabolites. Dig Dis Sci (Suppl) 1988; 33:6S–15S.
95. McKelvey TG, Hollwarth ME, Granger DN, Engerson TD, Landler U, Jones HP. Mechanisms of conversion of xanthine dehydrogenase to xanthine oxidase in ischemic rat liver and kidney. Am J Physiol 1988; 254:G753–60.
96. Parks DA, Granger DN. Ischemia-induced vascular changes: role of xanthine oxidase and hydroxyl radicals. Am J Physiol 1983; 245:G285–9.
97. Fearon DT, Ruddy S, Schur PH, McCabe WR. Activation of the properdin pathway of complement in patients with Gram negative bacteremia. N Engl J Med 1975; 292:937–40.
98. Hsueh W, Sun X, Rioja LN, Gonzalez-Crussi F. The role of the complement system in shock and tissue injury induced by tumour necrosis factor and endotoxin. Immunology 1990; 70:309–14.
99. Bjork J, Hugli TE, Smedegard G. Microvascular effects of anaphylatoxins C3a and C5a. J Immunol 1985; 134:1115–9.
100. Okusawa S, Yancey KB, van der Meer JWM, et al. C5a stimulates secretion of tumor necrosis factor from human mononuclear cells in vitro. Comparison with secretion of interleukin 1 beta and interleukin 1 alpha. J Exp Med 1988; 168:443–8.
101. Smedegard G, Cui L, Hugli TE. Endotoxin-induced shock in the rat: a role for C5a. Am J Pathol 1989; 135:489–97.
102. Rothstein JL, Lint TF, Schreiber H. Tumor necrosis factor/cachectin. Induction of

hemorrhagic necrosis in normal tissue requires the fifth component of complement (C5). J Exp Med 1988; 168:2007–21.

103. Llausas-Magana E, Hsueh W, Arroyave CM, Arroyave JL, Torre-Amione G, Gonzalez-Crussi F. Cobra venom factor, an activator of the complement system, enhances the bowel necrosis induced by platelet-activating factor. Immunopharmacology 1988; 15:31–8.
104. Hsueh W, Sun XM, Rioja LN. Tumor necrosis factor and endotoxin induced shock and bowel necrosis in mice: role of the complement system and PAF. FASEB J 1990; 4:A1866.
105. Kliegman RM, Fanaroff AA. Necrotizing enterocolitis. N Engl J Med 1984; 310:1093–103.
106. Walsh MC, Kliegman RM. Necrotizing enterocolitis: treatment based on staging criteria. Pediatr Clin North Am 1986; 33:179–201.
107. Ryder RW, Shelton JD, Guinan ME. Necrotizing enterocolitis: a prospective multicenter investigation. Am J Epidemiol 1980; 112:113–23.
108. Kliegman RM, Fanaroff AA. Neonatal necrotizing enterocolitis: a nine year experience. Am J Dis Child 1981; 135:608–11.
109. Wilson R, Kanto WP Jr, McCarthy BJ, et al. Epidemiologic characteristics of necrotizing enterocolitis: a population based study. Am J Epidemiol 1981; 114:880–7.
110. Frantz ID III, L'Heureux P, Engel RR, Hunt CE. Necrotizing enterocolitis. J Pediatr 1975; 86:259–63.
111. Touloukian RJ, Posch JN, Spencer R. The pathogenesis of ischemic gastroenterocolitis of the neonate: selective gut mucosal ischemia in asphyxiated neonatal piglets. J Pediatr Surg 1972; 7:194–205.
112. Kosloske AM, Ulrich JA. A bacteriologic basis for the clinical presentations of necrotizing enterocolitis. J Pediatr Surg 1980; 15:558–64.
113. Brown EG, Ainbender E, Henley WL, Hodes HL. Etiologic role of bacteria and intestinal function. In: Brown EG, Sweet AY, eds. Neonatal necrotizing enterocolitis. New York: Grune & Stratton, 1980:69–100.
114. LaGamma EF, Ostertag SG, Birenbaum H. Failure of delayed oral feedings to prevent necrotizing enterocolitis. Am J Dis Child 1985; 139:385–9.
115. Brown EG, Sweet AY. Preventing necrotizing enterocolitis in neonates. JAMA 1978; 240:2452–4.
116. Pitt J, Barlow B, Heird WC. Protection against experimental necrotizing enterocolitis by maternal milk: role of milk leukocytes. Pediatr Res 1977; 11:906–9.
117. Caplan MS, Hsueh W. Necrotizing enterocolitis: role of platelet activating factor, endotoxin, and tumor necrosis factor. J Pediatr (suppl) 1990; 117:s47–51.
118. Caplan MS, Sun XM, Hsueh H, Hageman JR. Role of platelet activating factor and tumor necrosis factor-alpha in neonatal necrotizing enterocolitis. J Pediatr 1990; 116:960–4.
119. Caplan M, Hsueh W, Kelly A, Donovan M. Serum PAF acetylhydrolase increases during neonatal maturation. Prostaglandins 1990; 39:705–14.
120. Caplan MS, Sun XM, Hsueh W. Hypoxia causes ischemic bowel necrosis in rats: the role of platelet activating factor (PAF-acether). Gastroenterology 1990; 99:979–86.
121. Fong Y, Marano MA, Moldawer LL, et al. The acute splanchnic and peripheral tissue metabolic response to endotoxin in humans. J Clin Invest 1990; 85:1896–904.
122. Erickson RP, Tachibana DK, Herzenberg LA, Rosenberg LT. A single gene controlling hemolytic complement and a serum antigen in the mouse. J Immunol 1964; 92:611–5.

CHAPTER 27

CYTOKINE RECEPTORS

Virginia L. Shepherd

Vanderbilt University and
Veterans Administration Medical Center
Nashville, Tennessee

INTRODUCTION

The term "cytokine" defines a specific set of cell-derived protein mediators that have a wide range of activities on a variety of target cells. In 1979, the term "interleukin" (IL) was first put to use in defining two specific proteins, one of macrophage origin (IL-1) and one of T cell origin (IL-2). Both were able to induce a spectrum of T cell activation events from proliferation to the generation of helper and cytolytic T cells. Since 1979, 10 interleukins and related colony-stimulating factors (CSF) and the macrophage product tumor necrosis factor (TNF) have been described in molecular detail and their genes have been cloned and sequenced. These proteins comprise the group of mediators called cytokines.

An area of intense research involves an understanding of how these cytokines act on their target cells to elicit specific responses. Central to this understanding is the hypothesis that cytokines act through a cell surface receptor and that this interaction is absolutely required for generation of the specific cytokine signal. Receptors for IL-2 were first described in 1981. Since that time, receptors have been identified for interleukins 1, 4, 5, 6, 7, and 8, IL-3 and related colony-stimulating factors, and tumor necrosis factor. Binding studies from many laboratories using radiolabeled ligand have demonstrated that receptor number on the cell surface is low and ligand binds with a relatively high affinity. The low receptor number has hampered receptor purification, although receptors for IL-1, IL-2, and TNF have been isolated. Receptor characteristics were first identified by affinity cross-linking studies, offering some information about molecular size of the receptors involved and, later, supporting the idea that many if not all cytokines interact with a membrane-associated multimolecular complex. To date, the cDNAs encoding the binding subunits of six of the interleukins, granulocyte-macrophage CSF (GM-CSF) and G-CSF, and TNF have been cloned and sequenced.

The receptors for these cytokines fall into a unique class of endocytic, signal-transducing membrane proteins. Similar to the growth factor and hormone receptors, they bind a specific ligand at the cell surface, promote internalization, and generate a signal to the target cell. Unlike their counterparts, the cytokine receptors do not appear to function as protein kinases. This chapter examines the information known about each of the cytokine receptors and how the characteristics of receptor structure and ligand-receptor interaction relate to the mechanism of cytokine action. Early binding studies and cross-linking studies are not covered in detail except when they might have relevance to an understanding of the mechanism of signal generation. It must be emphasized that research into the structure and involvement of receptors in cytokine signal transduction is still in its infancy. As more information becomes available, both at the cellular level and the gene level, we will gain a more complete understanding of how these protein mediators use cell surface receptors to affect the wide range of activities on the variety of cells with which they interact.

CYTOKINE RECEPTOR STRUCTURE

Cell surface receptors have now been identified for all the known cytokines. Binding affinities, cell distribution of receptors, receptor number per cell, and at least some biochemical characteristics have been reported for all these cytokines. The cDNAs for the receptors for IL-1, IL-2, IL-3, IL-4, IL-6, IL-7, G-CSF, GM-CSF, and TNF have been cloned and sequenced (1–16). Within the near future it is expected that the cDNA structure for the IL-5 and IL-8 receptors will be deduced. This section deals with an overview of what is known today concerning the structures of these receptors and a discussion of the similarities and differences among the various receptors. Figure 1 shows a simplified picture of the structures of these receptors, emphasizing orientation within the membrane, superfamily classification, lengths of intracellular and extracellular domains, and common structural features. Data from the molecular cloning studies are summarized in Table 1.

The IL-1 Receptors

IL-1 was originally described as a product of activated macrophages that stimulated proliferation of thymocytes in the presence of lectins or mitogens (reviewed in Refs. 17 and 18). It is now known that IL-1 has multiple biological effects on cells involved in immune or inflammatory responses, including stimulation of lymphocyte differentiation and activation and stimulation of hematopoietic cell growth. In addition, IL-1 has profound proinflammatory effects on a variety of cell types. IL-1 receptors have been identified on all these target cells (19–23). IL-1 is known to exist in at least two forms, designated α and β. The primary structures of IL-1α and IL-1β are known and show low amino acid identity (22–26%) (24). However, both interact with the same cell surface receptor (19,22,25). Information on the structure of IL-1 receptors was first gained through chemical

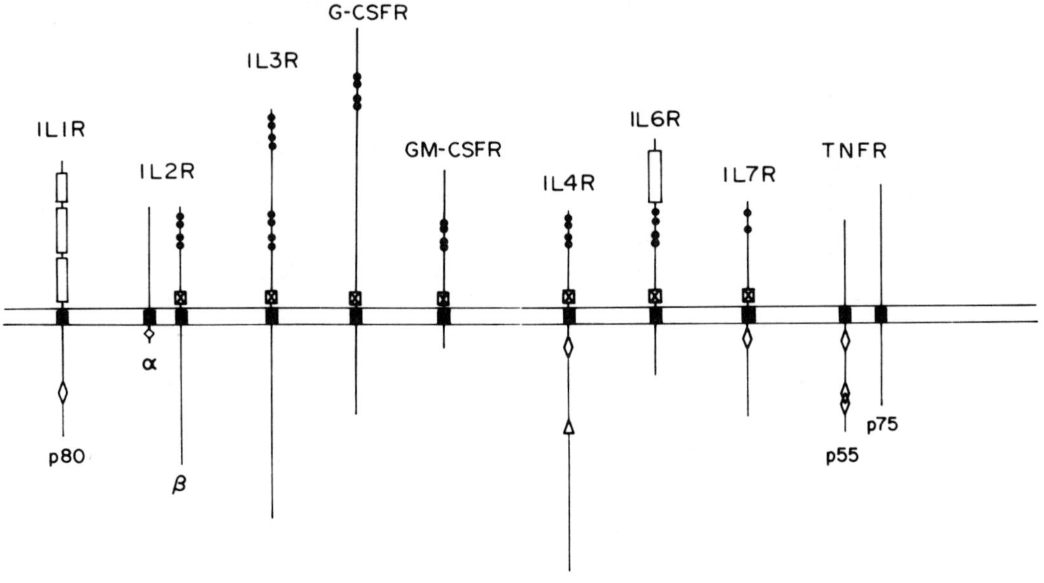

FIGURE 1 Comparison of the membrane-associated cytokine receptors. The protein structures shown are derived from molecular cloning and biochemical data as described in the text. Extracellular domains: the open boxes represent immunoglobulinlike domains; filled circles are the positions of conserved cysteine residues; the squares with the X represent the conserved trp-ser-X-ser-trp sequence. Black boxes within the membrane are the transmembrane region of each receptor. The cytoplasmic domain: open diamonds represent potential kinase acceptor sequences, and the open triangle is a potential protein kinase catalytic sequence.

cross-linking studies. A receptor of 80 kD was identified on T cells and fibroblasts (19,23,25,26) and of 60 kD on virus-transformed B cells (22). Several groups have reported the purification of the 80 kD receptor from a murine cell line (27–29).

Sims et al. (1) cloned and sequenced the murine 80 kD cDNA using expression cloning techniques. The extracellular domain (319 amino acids) is organized into three domains, similar to those of members of the immunoglobulin gene superfamily (30). These domains share a common three-dimensional structure and are suggested to be involved in ligand binding. The cysteines involved in disulfide bonds are highly conserved. The cytoplasmic domain contains the sequence lys-lys-ser-arg, which resembles a protein kinase C acceptor site. The IL-1 receptor from human T cells and fibroblasts (2) has also been cloned and found to be very similar to the murine receptor.

Results from several groups have demonstrated that the IL-1 receptor expressed on B cells has different characteristics than the T cell receptor. Using the pre-B lymphocyte cell line 70Z/3 and the T lymphoid cell line EL-4 6.1 C10, Bomsztyk et al. (31) investigated the structural characteristics of the two receptors. They demonstrated that monoclonal antibodies raised against the T cell receptor did not bind to the 70Z/3 cell receptor. Affinity cross-linking studies showed that IL-1 bound to a receptor of 66 kD on the 70Z/3 line. In addition, the T cell

TABLE 1 Summary of Cytokine Receptor Structural Characteristics[a]

Ligand	Species	Distribution of amino acid residues: Total	Extracellular (number cysteine residues)	TM	Cytoplasmic	Extracellular N-glycosylation sites	Superfamily	Kinase acceptor site	Mature molecular weight (kD)	References
IL-1	Human	552	319 (10)	20	213	7	Ig	Yes	80	1
	Murine	557	319 (10)	21	217	6	Ig	Yes	80	2
IL-2α	Human	251	219 (10)	19	13	2		Yes	55	3–5
IL-2β	Human	525	214 (8)	25	286	4	Hemat	Yes	70	6
IL-3	Murine	856	417 (13)	26	413	2	Hemat	Yes	140	7
G-CSF	Murine	812	601 (17)	24	187	11	Hemat	NR	95–125	8
GM-CSF	Human	378	297 (11)	27	54	11	Hemat	NR	85	9
IL-4	Human	800	207 (7)	24	569	6	Hemat	No	140	10
	Murine	785	208 (7)	24	553	5	Hemat	Yes	140	11
IL-6	Human	449	338 (10)	29	82	5	Ig/Hemat	NR	80	12
IL-7	Human	439	219 (6)	25	195	6	Hemat	NR	75	13
	Murine	439	219 (6)	25	195	3	Hemat	NR	75	13
TNF (p55)	Human	415	172 (22)	23	220	3	NGF-R	NR	55	14, 15
TNF (p75)	Human	439	235 (22)	30	174	2	NGF-R	NR	75	16

[a] Ig, immunoglobulin superfamily; Hemat, hematopoietic superfamily; NGF-R, nerve growth factor receptor superfamily; NR, not reported.

receptor cDNA probe reacted with EL-4 mRNA but not with 70Z/3 mRNA. These results were supported by the work of Chizzonite et al. (32), who concluded that T cells, fibroblasts, and epithelial cells expressed the 80 kD receptor but the IL-1 receptor on pre-B cells, macrophages, and bone marrow cells represented a separate gene product encoding a 60 kD receptor.

The cDNA has not yet been cloned for the p60 IL-1 receptor. The p60 and p80 differ in intracellular delivery of ligand and signal transduction. Since both these functions are presumably controlled by a cytoplasmic domain in the receptor, it might be predicted that more homology will be seen in the extracellular, ligand binding domain than in the intracellular domain. Mizel (17) suggested that IL-1 may use different second messengers in different cells. For example, in both T and B cells, IL-1 action appears to involve a GTP binding protein (33,34), although the second messenger systems in the two cell types are different. It is conceivable that the different receptor structures in T and B cells direct the specific signaling mechanisms and cellular responses.

The IL-2 Receptor

IL-2 is a 14 kD protein produced by activated T cells and originally described as a T cell growth factor. More recent studies have reported that IL-2 also acts on other cells of the immune system, such as B cells, macrophages, and natural killer cells (reviewed in Ref. 35). The IL-2 receptor was the first cytokine receptor to be studied in depth. Monoclonal antibodies raised against stimulated T cells blocked IL-2 binding to and action on activated T cells. The antigen was later identified as a single 55 kD surface glycoprotein called Tac (36–38). In 1984, the protein was purified using immunoaffinity chromatography and the cDNAs were cloned and sequenced (3–5). Only 13 of the 251 total amino acids are cytoplasmic. This domain contains no tyrosines, and even though it contains serine and threonine, phosphorylation of these residues does not alter IL-2 binding (39).

After the p55 chain was characterized, studies from a number of laboratories demonstrated that this chain was not functional in IL-2 internalization or signal transduction and must be associated with other specific membrane components (40–43). Results from binding studies indicated that activated lymphocytes expressed two distinct classes of receptors with different affinities for IL-2 (44–46). Results suggested that the high-affinity binding was responsible for IL-2 action. In addition, only high-affinity receptors could mediate IL-2 internalization (47). From transfection studies using only the p55 cDNA, it was shown that p55 was an IL-2 binding protein. However, the transfected cells, unlike lymphocytes, expressed only low-affinity binding. Sharon et al. and others (48–52) demonstrated that expression of a second IL-2 binding protein, the p70 or β chain, could transform the p55 receptor into the high-affinity form.

In 1989, Hatakeyama et al. (6) reported the cloning of the cDNA for the p70 chain. The protein contains 525 amino acids and does not appear to belong to the Ig superfamily. There are 214 amino acids in the extracellular domain, which contains eight cysteine residues and four potential N-linked glycosylation sites. The cytoplasmic domain (286 amino acids) contains the ala-pro-glu consensus sequence for the catalytic domain of a possible protein kinase. It is rich in proline and serine and has a high acidic amino acid content. These same authors used the p70 cDNA in transfection experiments to study in depth the contribution of each chain to ligand binding. Using a receptor-negative T cell line, a stable p55 T cell-transfected cell, and non-T cells (COS cells), they examined the functional characteristics of each receptor chain. T cells transfected with p55 alone bound IL-2 with low affinity (20 nM). These same cells transfected with p70 alone exhibited an intermediate ligand binding (2 nM). Cells with both cDNAs expressed both high- and low-affinity binding (22 pM and 15 nM). These results demonstrated unequivocally that the p70 chain was directly involved in the formation of a high-affinity receptor complex in association with p55. However, when these same transfections were done in non-T cells, p70 alone was incapable of binding IL-2. When transfected with p55, the high-affinity form was generated. These results were the first suggestion that yet a third component, present only in T cells, was necessary for a functional p70 receptor. This work was followed by affinity cross-linking studies by Colamonici et al. (53). These authors concluded that a 95–110 kD γ subunit was absolutely required for IL-2 binding by p70. Neither p70 nor p95–110 alone bound IL-2. In association with each other, an intermediate-affinity binding was found. They defined the receptor structures involved in IL-2 binding as follows: p55 alone binds IL-2 with low affinity but does not transduce a signal; expression of p70 with the γ subunit results in an intermediate-affinity receptor that responds to IL-2 binding; and, expression of both p70 and p55 results in a high-affinity fully functional receptor. The current model for receptor-chain interaction and corresponding ligand binding affinities is shown in Table 2.

This is the only cytokine receptor to date to be described as a compound receptor consisting of two or more subunits. Regulation of expression of each of these chains can dramatically affect ligand binding and thereby finely regulate the response of target cells to IL-2. This regulation is discussed later.

The IL-3, G-CSF, and GM-CSF Receptors

IL-3, G-CSF, GM-CSF, and M-CSF are members of a family of related cytokines called colony-stimulating factors. They are involved in regulating the survival, proliferation, and differentiation of hematopoietic progenitor cells and also affect many functional activities of mature cells. The following discussion presents data relating to three of these factors, GM-CSF, G-CSF, and IL-3, and other sections

Table 2 IL-2 Receptor Structures

IL-2 receptor subunit	Binding affinity	Signal transduction
p55 (α)	Low (Kd = 20 nM)	No
p70 (β)	None	No
p70/p95–110 (β/γ)	Intermediate (Kd = 2 nM)	Yes
p55/p70 (α/β)	High (Kd = 20 pM)	Yes

limit discussions to IL-3. The CSF-1 or M-CSF receptor has been studied in great detail. One structural feature that distinguishes the CSF-1 receptor from the other cytokine receptors is that the CSF-1 receptor is a member of a family of growth factor receptors that exhibit ligand-induced tyrosine-specific protein kinase activity. A detailed discussion of this receptor is beyond the scope of this chapter, and the reader is referred to the recent review by Sherr (54). The following discussion presents structural and biochemical data for the receptors for IL-3 and G- and GM-CSF.

The IL-3 receptor

IL-3 is a 23–28 kD glycoprotein produced by activated T cells (55). IL-3 has a variety of effects on hematopoietic cells and is a growth factor for certain cell lines (56,57). IL-3 binds to target cells with both high and low affinities (58–61). A number of groups reported a molecular size of 60–70 kD for the murine receptor (58–61), although a higher molecular weight protein (140 kD) was also suggested to be involved in IL-3 binding (59). The relationship of the 70 and 140 kD proteins is not yet known. Itoh et al. (7) recently published the cloning and sequencing of a 140 kD murine IL-3 binding protein. Since this protein binds IL-3 with only low affinity, the authors suggested that the 70 kD protein may be an associated protein involved in signal transduction or in the generation of a high-affinity receptor complex.

The cDNA for the 140 kD murine IL-3 receptor encodes a protein with a total of 856 amino acids. The extracellular portion of 417 residues contains eight cysteine residues and two potential N-glycosylation sites. The cytoplasmic domain (413 amino acids) has a relatively high content of serine and proline, which is similar to the IL-2 p70 receptor. There does not appear to be any consensus sequence for a protein kinase catalytic domain. However, Sorensen et al. (62) reported that IL-3 stimulates tyrosine phosphorylation of the 140 kD receptor, suggesting that the cytoplasmic domain contains a tyrosine kinase acceptor site.

The G-CSF receptor

G-CSF is produced predominantly by macrophages. It is important in the control of proliferation and differentiation of neutrophils, and receptors have been identified in progenitor and mature neutrophils and myeloid cell lines (63–67). There appears to be a single class of high-affinity binding sites with fewer than 2000 sites per cell (63,67,68). Cross-linking studies have suggested that the receptor in WEHI cells has a molecular weight of approximately 150 kD. Fukunaga et al. (8) have reported the cloning and sequencing of the cDNA for a G-CSF binding protein. The mature protein contains a total of 812 amino acids. The extracellular domain (601 amino acids) contains 11 potential N-glycosylation sites and 17 cysteine residues. The cytoplasmic domain (187 amino acids) does not contain a consensus sequence for a protein kinase catalytic domain. This domain also contains a high number of proline and serine residues. Expression of the cDNA in COS cells resulted in a functional receptor that bound G-CSF with the same affinity as the native receptor. However, it is not known if this protein is sufficient to generate a signal in response to G-CSF. Affinity cross-linking experiments using the transfected cells resulted in a receptor molecular weight of 120–150 kD.

The GM-CSF Receptor

GM-CSF is a glycoprotein that acts as a growth and differentiation factor for neutrophils, eosinophils, and macrophages (69). Autoradiographic studies have demonstrated that these cells express low numbers of receptors for GM-CSF (70,71), although there are conflicting reports of whether there is a single high-affinity class (72,73) or both low- and high-affinity binding sites (74). Cross-linking studies have suggested a molecular weight for the receptor on murine cells of 51 kD (74) or 130 kD (72) and for the human receptor of 84 kD (71). Gearing et al. (9) reported the expression cloning of the receptor for human GM-CSF. The mature protein contains a total of 378 amino acids. The expressed protein has a molecular weight of 84 kD by cross-linking experiments. The extracellular domain contains 11 potential N-linked glycosylation sites and 11 cysteine residues. There is no homology to the immunoglobulin superfamily. The relatively short cytoplasmic domain contains no tyrosine kinase domain or obvious kinase acceptor sites. The expressed receptor showed nearly identical low-affinity binding and the same specificity as the receptor on placental membranes. It has not yet been demonstrated that this receptor can mediate GM-CSF action.

The IL-4 Receptor

IL-4 is a T cell product originally described as a B cell growth factor (reviewed in Ref. 75). It has recently been shown that IL-4 also has effects on a wide range of hematopoietic cells as well as nonhematopoietic cells, such as fibroblasts, epithelial cells, and tumor lines. Cells of both hematopoietic and nonhematopoietic origin express a single class of IL-4 receptors with an affinity of approximately 0.1 nM (76–80). Cross-linking studies in murine cells (76,77) showed a single binding protein of 60–75 kD. Subsequent experiments in human cells reported that the IL-4 binding protein was 140 kD (78). Cloning and sequencing of both the murine and human 140 kD IL-4 receptor have been reported (10,11). The murine protein contains a total of 785 amino acids, with 208 amino acids in the extracellular domain. This domain contains five potential N-linked glycosylation sites and seven cysteine residues. The cytoplasmic domain (553 amino acids) contains a threonine at position 298 that may be a protein kinase C phosphorylation acceptor site. This domain is also high in proline and serine and high in acidic amino acid residues, similar to the IL-2 p70 and IL-3 receptors. Transfection of the receptor cDNA into COS cells resulted in expression of an IL-4 binding protein with characteristics similar to that of the natural IL-4 receptor. However, it is not known if this cDNA represents a complete IL-4 receptor that is capable of conferring IL-4 responsiveness when transfected into target cells.

The IL-5 Receptor

IL-5 is a 40–50 kD glycoprotein secreted by activated T cells with effects on both T and B cells (81). Both high- and low-affinity binding sites for IL-5 have been found on B cells (82). From cross-linking studies, a receptor molecular weight of 45–50 kD has been reported (82). Rolink et al. (83) have speculated that a 46 kD protein is the low-affinity IL-5 receptor and that 130 and 140 kD proteins are involved in signal transduction or generation of a high-affinity IL-5 binding complex.

The IL-6 Receptor

IL-6 (B cell stimulatory factor 2) was originally identified as a T cell-derived factor that caused maturation of activated B cells (reviewed in Refs. 84 and 85). It is now established that IL-6 has a wide range of biological activities, including growth and differentiation of B and T cells, stimulation of colony formation in hematopoietic stem cells, induction of neural differentiation, and regulation of acute-phase response. In accordance with the multifunctional properties of IL-6, low numbers of specific IL-6 receptors have been found on a variety of cells (86). Taga et al. (87) demonstrated by affinity cross-linking studies that the cell surface receptor has a molecular weight of 80 kD. The single chain receptor of 80 kD was cloned and sequenced by Yamasaki et al. (12) using expression cloning techniques. The cDNA expressed both high- and low-affinity binding properties similar to those of the naturally expressed IL-6 receptor on U266 cells, a myeloma cell line. The protein consists of an extracellular domain of 357 amino acids and a relatively short cytoplasmic domain of 82 residues. The extracellular portion contains a domain of approximately 90 amino acids that is similar to a domain in the Ig superfamily. Although IL-6 has been shown to be a potent growth factor for myeloma-plasmacytoma cells (86), the IL-6 receptor lacks tyrosine kinase domains in its cytoplasmic portion.

The IL-7 Receptor

IL-7 is a 25 kD protein involved in the regulation of lymphopoiesis (88). Park et al. (89) demonstrated that murine cell lines and primary cells expressed IL-7 receptors, including cells of lymphoid and myeloid origin. The binding of IL-7 to its receptor demonstrated both high- and low-affinity classes. Using a direct expression cloning system, Goodwin et al. (13) reported the cloning of the human and murine IL-7 receptors. Transfection of these cDNAs into COS cells resulted in the expression of receptors that displayed binding properties identical to those of the native receptor. Both the murine and human IL-7 receptors contain 439 amino acids, with an N-terminal, extracellular binding domain of 219 amino acids and a cytoplasmic domain of 195 amino acids. Cross-linking studies demonstrated a receptor molecular weight of 75 kD for the transfected murine receptor; cross-linking of IL-7 to its receptor on 70Z/3 cells showed a second protein at approximately 150 kD. The 75 kD protein is sufficient for IL-7 binding; the higher molecular weight protein may represent an associated protein involved in signal transduction as with the IL-6 receptor.

The IL-8 Receptor

Monocyte-derived neutrophil chemotactic factor (MDNCF or IL-8) is an 8 kD protein produced by stimulated monocytes (90–92). Recent studies have shown specific IL-8 receptors on human neutrophils with a single high-affinity class of binding sites (93). Samanta et al. (94) reported that ligand binding initiates rapid internalization, followed by receptor recycling back to the surface. By affinity cross-linking experiments, a receptor molecular weight of 58 kD has been reported (93,95). It is anticipated that the cDNA for this receptor will soon be available.

The TNF Receptors

Tumor necrosis factor α is a pleiotropic cytokine that is secreted predominantly by macrophages in response to lipopolysaccharide (LPS) (reviewed in Ref. 96). TNF was originally defined by its ability to induce cytolytic or cytotoxic effects in some tumor cells. More recently TNF has been shown to have a variety of effects on other cells, such as endothelial cells, macrophages, fibroblasts, and smooth muscle cells. Virtually all nucleated cells studied express receptors for TNF. Binding in most cases is to a single high-affinity class of receptors, with receptor number varying between 1000 and 5000. A number of reports have suggested varying molecular weights by cross-linking studies for the receptor on transformed cells (97–102). This has been dramatically clarified in the past 2 years with the purification of two TNF receptors from placental tissue and U937 cells (103,104) and the molecular cloning and sequencing of both these receptors (14–16).

Loetscher et al. (14) and Schall et al. (15) simultaneously reported the isolation of the human cDNA for the 55 kD TNF receptor. The extracellular domain (172 amino acids) contains 22 cysteine residues and three potential N-glycosylation sites. There is no similarity to any of the previous described cytokine receptors, nor is there any Ig-like domain. However, there is significant sequence similarity to the nerve growth factor (NGF) receptor, suggesting that this constitutes a third cytokine receptor family. TNF binding induces phosphorylation of a number of cellular proteins (105,106), and the cytoplasmic domain contains a potential kinase acceptor site. However, it is not known if the TNF receptor itself is phosphorylated. The two cloning reports differ slightly in the position of the end of the signal sequence, resulting in a slightly different N-terminal sequence. However, a recent report by Engelmann et al. (107) on the isolation of a soluble form of the receptor from urine (see subsequent discussion) gives an N-terminal sequence for the soluble receptor as asp-ser-val-cys-pro. This agrees with the report by Schall et al. (15), suggesting that this is the start of the mature protein. Smith et al. (16) reported the isolation of the cDNA for the p75 TNF receptor. The N-terminal sequence of this receptor agrees with the N-terminal sequence of the second soluble TNF receptor isolated by Engelmann et al. (107). The extracellular domain (235 amino acids), as with the p55 receptor, is not similar to the Ig superfamily or the other cytokine receptors described previously. However, it also has a high degree of similarity to the NGF receptor and would place this receptor chain also in the NGF receptor family.

Several groups have reported that different cells express differing amounts of the two TNF receptors. Using monoclonal antibodies specific for p55 or p75, Brockhaus et al. (108) reported that Hep 2 cells expressed only the 55 chain, U937 cells expressed predominantly the 75, although some 55 was detected, and HL60 cells expressed both receptors in approximately equal amounts. By affinity cross-linking experiments, Hohmann et al. (109) reported that myeloid cells express predominantly the p75 receptor, but cells of epithelial origin express p55. Preliminary results from our laboratory have demonstrated that U937 clones can be isolated that express either the p55 alone or both p55 and p75 in equal amounts, whereas human monocyte-derived macrophages and rat bone marrow-derived macrophages express only p55 (V. Shepherd, unpublished results).

The existence of two receptors that have different sizes and appear to be somewhat cell specific is very similar to the IL-1 receptor structure. It is probable that these different size receptors for both IL-1 and TNF are indeed cell- and signal-specific. For example, macrophages express the low-molecular weight form of both receptors. The proinflammatory actions of TNF and IL-1 on macrophages, as well as other cells, are similar. It is quite possible that the cytoplasmic domains of the p55 and p60 receptors are similar and interact with a similar intracellular signaling mechanism.

Common Structural Features of the Cytokine Receptors

Close examination of the cytokine receptor structures (Fig. 1 and Table 1) has led to the suggestion that these receptors can be assigned to one of three classes: (a) the immunoglobulin (Ig)-like superfamily (30); (b) a new hematopoietic receptor family (110,111); and (c) a nerve growth factor receptor family.

The Ig Superfamily

The IL-1 and IL-6 receptors have been assigned to the Ig superfamily. These receptors contain the conserved 90 residue extracellular domain that is found in the members of the Ig superfamily. These domains typically possess only minimal amino acid similarity but share a common tertiary structure composed of two β sheets linked by disulfide bonds. Other receptors that also belong to this family include the receptors for platelet-derived growth factor and CSF-1 (30).

The Hematopoietic Receptor Family

Bazan (110) first suggested a new superfamily of growth factor receptors based on sequence homology in their extracellular domains. This group has recently increased and now includes the receptors for IL-2 p70, IL-3, G-CSF, GM-CSF, IL-4, IL-6, and IL-7 and has been called the hematopoietic receptor superfamily (111). Each of these receptors contains a domain with four conserved cysteine residues. There is also a conserved sequence of trp-ser-*X*-ser-trp on the extracellular side of the transmembrane region. Alternatively, little similarity exists in the cytoplasmic domain of these receptors. It has been proposed that the similarities in the extracellular domains relate directly to ligand binding. It has been reported that IL-2, IL-4, and IL-6 have a tertiary structure that is comprised of a helix bundle structure that might then suggest a similar ligand-receptor binding domain (112).

The NGF Receptor Family

Sequencing of the cDNAs for the two TNF receptors revealed that they were not similar to any of the previously reported cytokine receptors but showed striking similarity to the NGF receptor sequence in the extracellular domain (14–16). Also included in this family are CD-40 (113), a B cell surface antigen, and clone 4-1BB (114), a T cell antigen; both these proteins have been suggested as cytokine receptors for unidentified ligands. The extracellular domains of these receptors share a high number of cysteines and other conserved amino acids, including tyrosine, glycine, and proline. The cysteine-rich regions can be resolved into either twofold repeats of 80 amino acids or fourfold repeats of 40 residues. Both NGF and TNF exist as oligomers (16), suggesting that the similar ligand tertiary structure may relate to the corresponding similar extracellular binding domains in the receptors.

It has been suggested for all three classes that similarities in the extracellular domains relate to similar ligand tertiary structure and subsequent receptor-ligand interactions. However, the binding of a cytokine to its receptor is absolutely specific. This specificity in binding may be directed by additional intrachain amino acids that are different among the receptors within each class. Specificity could also be generated by additional domains, such as both an Ig domain and hematopoietic region in the IL-6 receptor, the duplication of the hematopoietic region in the IL-3 receptor, or additional binding proteins, such as the separate p55 IL-2 receptor chain. The dissimilarities in the cytoplasmic regions most likely reflect the specificity of ligand-induced signal transduction. However, intracytoplasmic sequence homologies or motifs will most likely be found that define kinase-association regions, internalization signals, or nuclear translocation signals.

RECEPTOR INVOLVEMENT IN SIGNAL TRANSDUCTION

The mechanisms of how cytokines transduce a signal to a target cell are unknown. The second messenger systems that may be involved have been dealt with in other chapters. The following discussion deals with aspects of receptor structure, receptor-associated proteins, and receptor-mediated ligand internalization that may shed some light on possible signaling mechanisms.

Cytokine-Induced Receptor Phosphorylation

Phosphorylation clearly plays an important role in hormone and growth factor receptor activity. Many of these receptors contain intrinsic tyrosine protein kinase activity. Autophosphorylation as well as cellular kinase-mediated receptor ser/thr phosphorylation regulates the activity of these receptors (reviewed in Ref. 115). Although several of the cytokines have growth-promoting activity, none of the interleukin receptors or TNF receptors have been shown to have intrinsic kinase activity. It has been demonstrated that several cytokine receptors are associated with a cellular protein kinase or have protein kinase C or other kinase acceptor sequences in their cytoplasmic domains that may play a role in signal transduction.

The IL-1 Receptor

Sims et al. (1) reported that the IL-1 receptor cytoplasmic domain contains the sequence lys-lys-ser-arg-arg, which resembles a protein kinase C acceptor site (116). Gallis et al. (117) reported that IL-1 induced rapid ser/thr phosphorylation of its 80 kD receptor on CHO cells. Thus, an early event in IL-1 binding is the activation of a ser/thr protein kinase that results in phosphorylation of the IL-1 receptor as well as a restricted number of cellular proteins (118–120). How this relates to IL-1-mediated cellular events is still unknown.

The IL-2 Receptor

Several groups have reported that IL-2 binding induces tyrosine phosphorylation of a number of cellular proteins (121,122). No tyrosine phosphorylation could be detected in the α chain, and this result was confirmed by the finding from the cDNA sequence that the α chain did not contain a cytoplasmic tyrosine residue (3–5). Subsequently, Ferris et al. (123) reported that IL-2-induced tyrosine kinase activity is mediated through the p70 (β) chain of the IL-2 receptor. Both Asao et al. (124) and Sharon et al. (125) recently demonstrated that one of the proteins that is tyrosine phosphorylated is the β chain of the receptor complex. Neither study could rule out the possibility that the p70 receptor contains kinase activity. However, the cytoplasmic domain does not contain the typical tyrosine kinase consensus sequence (gly-*X*-gly-*X*-*X*-gly) (6). It is more likely that the p70 receptor associates with a cellular tyrosine kinase.

The IL-3 Receptor

Several groups have demonstrated that IL-3 induces rapid tyrosine phosphorylation of a set of cellular proteins (126,127). Sorensen et al. (62) and Isfort et al. (128) demonstrated that one of these proteins is the 140 kD IL-3 receptor. As with the IL-1 and IL-2 receptors, the cDNA sequence indicated no tyrosine kinase consensus sequence. It has therefore been suggested that the receptor associates with a cellular tyrosine kinase.

Receptor-Associated Proteins

From these phosphorylation data and from affinity cross-linking studies, it is becoming increasingly evident that the cytokine receptors actually exist in the membrane in association with one or more cellular proteins. These associated proteins may be involved in signal transduction, in ligand internalization and delivery, or in the production of a functional high-affinity ligand binding domain. A summary of the reported receptor-associated proteins and their proposed functions is presented in Table 3.

TABLE 3 Cytokine Receptor-Associated Proteins

Receptor	Associated proteins	Proposed function	Reference
IL-1R	95	Ser/thr kinase	129
	95, 68, 50, 45	Unknown	129
IL-2R	p95–110/γ	Formation of intermed. K_d receptor with p70	53
	p22	Unknown	130
			130
	p40	Unknown	
IL-5R	130/140	Unknown	83
IL-6R	gp130	Signal transduction	87
IL-7R	150	Unknown	13

The IL-1 Receptor

From these phosphorylation studies, it might be predicted that the IL-1 receptor is associated with a cellular ser/thr protein kinase. Results from cross-linking experiments show a possible 95 kD protein that might be associated with the 80 kD IL-1 receptors. Lewis et al. (129) recently reported that several proteins co-precipitated with the 80 kD receptor of molecular weights of 95, 68, 50, and 45 kD. The involvement of these molecules in IL-1 action remains to be shown.

The IL-2 Receptor

As discussed above, a third subunit in the IL-2-receptor complex has been identified (p95–110, γ) that interacts specifically with the p70 chain to produce the intermediate-affinity receptor. Either p95–110 or p55 is absolutely required for the assembly of a functional IL-2 receptor. In addition, Saragovi and Malek (130) recently reported that additional proteins may be involved. They have suggested a model that incorporates a 22 kD protein complexed through disulfide bonding to p70 and an additional membrane-associated complex of two 40 kD proteins. The role of these additional proteins is not known. From the preceding phosphorylation studies it might be predicted that one of these proteins is an associated tyrosine protein kinase involved in IL-2 action.

The IL-6 Receptor

Taga et al. (86) reported that the 80 kD IL-6 receptor that has been cloned and sequenced appears to be the only surface molecule involved in IL-6 binding. However, IL-6 binding to this receptor induces complex formation between the 80 kD binding protein and an additional membrane-associated glycoprotein, gp130. Mutant IL-6 receptor lacking the transmembrane and cytoplasmic portions can still interact with gp130 and transduce a signal, suggesting that the interaction is between the extracellular domains. The authors concluded that gp130 is involved in IL-6 signal transduction.

Cytokine Internalization and Signal Transduction

Several of the cytokine receptors have been shown from ligand binding and kinetic studies to bind ligand at the surface and then move to an intracellular site (20,47,94,131–135). In several instances, ligand delivery to lysosomes has been demonstrated (134,135). In at least one instance it has been suggested that the receptors recycle to the plasma membrane and are not degraded with their ligands (94). Thus, it appears that the cytokine receptors fall into the category of endocytosis receptors (136). Of interest in the case of any ligand that transduces a signal is the question of whether the ligand must enter the cell to generate a signal. Receptor-mediated endocytosis of cytokines could serve two purposes: first, receptor-ligand interaction at the surface initiates a signal and then the receptor moves the ligand into the cellular lysosomal compartment for degradation and cessation of the signal; or, second, the receptor may bind ligand at the surface and then both receptor and ligand move inside the cell to initiate signaling. The most interesting aspect of the latter hypothesis is that some ligands may be delivered to the nuclear compartment, where they act directly on the transcriptional machinery of the cell. This concept was first proposed for the action of certain growth factors and hormones. Receptors for insulin and epidermal growth factor (EGF) have been localized in the nuclei of various target cells by ligand binding studies (137,138). Intranuclear accumulation of EGF (138), NGF (139), and insulin (137) have also been reported. Delivery of IL-1 and its receptor to the nucleus has been studied extensively. Both Mizel et al. (131) and Qwarnstrom et al. (132) reported that IL-1 receptors mediate internalization of IL-1 at 37°C, and by 6 h a significant amount of the ligand is associated with the cell nucleus. Grenfell et al. (133) reported that the IL-1 found in the nucleus remains intact. In addition, they found specific and saturable binding of IL-1 to intact nuclei. Recently, Curtis et al. (140) demonstrated that IL-1-receptor complexes accumulate in the nucleus, although they detected no nuclear receptors in untreated nuclei. Importantly, they correlated IL-1 translocation to the nucleus with signal transduction. Whether IL-1 receptors exist on isolated nuclei or receptors are translocated from the plasma membrane is not clear. However, it appears that receptor-mediated delivery of IL-1 to a nuclear site of action may play an important role in its signal generation. Finally, it has been suggested that proteins that accumulate in the nucleus contain a specific amino acid sequence that targets them to the nuclear compartment (141). This sequence is not well defined but appears to consist of a sequence rich in basic amino acids and prolines. Sims et al. (2) reported that two such sequences may exist in the IL-1 receptor that could mediate transport to the nucleus.

Little information is known about nuclear translocation for the other receptors. Fujii et al. (134) reported that IL-2 receptors mediate ligand internalization and delivery to lysosomes for degradation. Some IL-2 was detected in the nucleus by light microscopic autoradiography. However, this finding has not been studied further, and the role of translocation of IL-2 to the nucleus is unknown. Finally, although no information on translocation of TNF to the nucleus has been reported, it is interesting to note that NGF is delivered via its receptor to the nucleus. Since the receptors for NGF and TNF belong to the same family, perhaps both contain the nuclear delivery motif for ligand translocation to the nuclear compartment and it might eventually be found that this plays a role in the signal transduction for these ligands.

REGULATION OF CYTOKINE RECEPTOR EXPRESSION

It is apparent that many of these cytokines are integrated into an intricate network and can act in synergy or as inhibitors of other cytokines. This network concept implies coordinated regulation of expression of the cytokines as well as of the expression of their corresponding receptors. In most cases receptor regulation is variable, depending on the physiological state of the target cell, the local concentration of cytokine(s), and the presence of cytokine-secreting cells. The following discussion deals primarily with cytokine receptor regulation by modulators of the immune system. A summary of this regulation is shown in Table 4.

The IL-2 Receptor

IL-2 is the only cytokine receptor that contains two or more binding subunits that coordinately regulate receptor affinity. It has recently been demonstrated

Table 4 Regulation of Cytokine Receptor Expression

Cell type	Receptor	Modulation (agent)	References
Mϕ	IL-2R	↑ (LPS, IFN-γ)	150–152
	IL-4R	↑ (IFN-γ)	153
	IL-6R	↓ (LPS, IL-6, Dex)	157
	TNF	↓ (IFN-γ, LPS, Dex)	163–166
T cells	IL-2R	↑ (IL-1, 2, 5, 6)	143, 144, 149
		↓ (IL-4)	147
	IL-4R	↑ (IL-2, 4, LPS)	154, 155
	TNFR	↑ (IL-2, TNF)	148, 167
B cells	IL-2R	↑ (IL-2, 5)	142, 146
		↓ (IL-4)	142, 146
	IL-4R	↑ (LPS)	154

by several groups that independent regulation of expression of each of these chains has a profound effect on the binding of IL-2 and subsequent signal transduction. IL-2 itself specifically regulates expression of the p55 chain on T and B cells (142–144). Smith (145) and Saito et al. (144) both suggested that this induction ensures that all of the p70 that reaches the cell surface is complexed to p55, resulting in a cell that is always in a "high response mode." Other cytokines appear to regulate IL-2 receptors by interfering with the IL-2 modulation and also independently blocking IL-2 receptor expression. Using a B cell line, Yoshimoto et al. (146) demonstrated that IL-5 can render these cells responsive to IL-2. The first phase is an increase in high-affinity receptor by IL-5 and a modest increase in low-affinity receptors. The second phase is an increase in low-affinity receptor by IL-2 itself. Martinez et al. (147) reported similar results and correlated this inhibition with the ability of IL-4 to block IL-2-induced T cell proliferation.

Regulation of IL-2 receptors on T cells by other cytokines has also been reported. Smith and Cantrell (143) reported that IL-1 increased IL-2 expression in T cells. Scheurich et al. (148) showed that TNF increased IL-2 high-affinity binding. Finally, Le et al. (149) reported that IL-6 and IL-2 act synergistically to enhance thymocyte proliferation. They suggested that this effect could be explained at least in part by an IL-6-induced expression of low-affinity (p55) IL-2 receptors.

Several groups have reported similar IL-2 receptor regulation in monocytes (150–152). Freshly isolated monocytes do not express the p55 IL-2 receptor chain, although they respond to IL-2, presumably through binding to the p70 chain (152). As in B and T cells, when IL-2 binds to monocytes it increases expression of the p55 chain, thereby creating an increased level of high-affinity dimer. Holter et al. (151) also reported that monocyte activation by interferon or bacterial products further increased p55, leading to expression of excess p55 to complex with the p70 to maintain the monocyte in a high response mode.

The IL-4 Receptor

IL-4 has effects on a variety of inflammatory cells. IL-4 receptor regulation has been examined on human and murine B cells and on murine macrophages. Feldman and Finbloom (153) reported that interferon-γ (IFN-γ) increased IL-4 receptor expression on macrophages, but IL-1 and IL-6 had no effect. IL-4 and lipopolysacchoride (LPS) have been reported to be positive regulators of IL-4 receptor expression on resting T and B cells (154), and IL-2 increased IL-4 receptors on activated T cells (155).

The IL-6 Receptor

Dexamethasone increases IL-6 receptor expression on HepG2 cells by stimulating de novo receptor synthesis (156). This could explain the known synergy between glucocorticoids and IL-6 in stimulating the synthesis of acute-phase proteins by HepG2 cells. Bauer et al. (157) reported that an inverse regulation of IL-6 receptors on monocytes and hepatocytes could effectively alter the target cell during immune challenge. Unstimulated monocytes express IL-6 receptors; these receptors are downregulated by LPS, dexamethasone, and IL-6 itself. Alternatively, hepatocytes normally express only low levels of IL-6 receptors and LPS, dexamethasone, and IL-6 increase receptor expression.

The TNF Receptor

A number of laboratories have reported modulation of TNF receptors on transformed cell lines by several agents, such as IFN-γ and phorbol esters (158–162). Very few reports are available on the regulation of TNF receptors on cells of the immune system. Several groups have begun studies of IFN-τ regulation of TNF receptors on macrophages and have reported that, in contrast to the effect on transformed cells, IFN-γ downregulates receptor expression (163–165). LPS and dexamethasone are also negative regulators (Ref. 166 and V. Shepherd, unpublished results). Recent data from our group suggest an IL-1-induced increase in TNF receptor expression alters TNF action in macrophages (165). Finally, lymphocytes are known to respond to TNF and appear to have augmented cytotoxic function after IL-2 stimulation. It has been suggested that this increased response to TNF is due to an increase in TNF receptors induced by IL-2 (167,168).

An understanding of the role of receptors in mediating cytokine responses is still in its infancy. It is presumed that receptors are absolutely necessary for transduction of signals, but it is not known if regulation of receptor expression is an important step in modulating the cellular response to a cytokine. The results presented here are intended to shed some light on this topic and to suggest that receptor regulation in inflammatory cells is particularly relevant to an understanding of how one cytokine affects the action of another. Although circumstantial at present, the evidence supports the idea that synergistic and additive effects of cytokines can be explained by changes in receptor expression.

SOLUBLE CYTOKINE RECEPTORS

The final topic that has received recent attention is the discovery of soluble forms of a number of the cytokine receptors. The role that these soluble products might

TABLE 5 Soluble Cytokine Receptors

Ligand	Intact receptor: Molecular weight (kD)	Intact receptor: N-terminus	Soluble receptor: Molecular weight (kD)	Soluble receptor: N-terminus	Reference
IL-2 (p55)	55	ELCDD		ELCDD	168
IL-4	140	IKVLG	32–41	IKVLG	10
IL-6	80	LAPRR	50	LAPRR	171
TNF	55	DSVCP	27	DSVCP	107
	75	VAFTP	30	VAFTP	107

play in the function of their respective cytokine ligands is discussed here. A summary of the molecular weights of the native and soluble receptors and their relationship to the parent molecule is shown in Table 5.

In 1981, Robb and Kutny (168) reported that activated lymphocytes release a soluble form of the IL-2 p55 chain. This soluble product represented the N-terminal portion of the intact p55 (residues 1–192) and appeared to be the result of a proteolytic clip of the cell surface p55 receptor.

Soluble forms of the IL-4 and IL-7 receptors appear to be the products of alternative mRNA splicing, rather than derived by proteolysis of the receptor at the cell surface. Using northern analyses, Mosley et al. (11) reported that in normal tissue, 5–10% of the IL-4 receptor mRNA is in a truncated form that encodes a secreted form of the intact receptor. Two groups have reported that soluble IL-4 receptors can be detected in biological fluids (169,170), suggesting that production of soluble IL-4 binding proteins plays a physiological role. A clone has also been isolated for a soluble form of the IL-7 receptor (13). When expressed in COS cells, a protein with IL-7 binding capability was secreted.

Recently, Novick et al. (171) reported the purification of a soluble IL-6 receptor from human urine with a molecular weight of approximately 50 kD. The N-terminal sequence of the purified soluble product exactly matched the corresponding sequence of the cloned intact IL-6 receptor. Work from this same group (107) and from Seckinger et al. (172,173) also reported the purification of soluble TNF binding proteins from human urine. In each case, the N-terminal sequences were identical to the intact receptors, and the authors suggested that these soluble forms were products released by proteolysis from the corresponding cell surface receptors. However, it is possible that RNA transcripts that encode these soluble forms exist and that the corresponding cDNAs have not yet been isolated.

All these studies suggest that release or production of soluble cytokine receptors is a general phenomenon. With the availability of both recombinant intact and soluble receptors, a physiological role can be investigated. At present, it is intriguing to speculate that these soluble cytokine receptors serve an immunomodulatory role by binding to their respective cytokines, thereby inhibiting the biological activity.

FUTURE DIRECTIONS

The study of the involvement of receptors in cytokine action is just beginning. Great progress has been made in the past 5 years, from identification of specific receptors to molecular cloning of the genes encoding those receptors. The field is continuing to expand, with new cytokines being identified and receptors with ligands yet to be found. The purpose of this chapter was to identify those areas of most intense research at the current time. Certainly it will be outdated quickly as the field continues to expand. The specific questions that have been addressed are the role of receptors in cytokine signal transduction; the role of receptor-mediated ligand internalization in signaling; and specific structural features of the receptors that might predict how a receptor mediates signal transduction from the cytokine to the cell nucleus. The role of receptors in cytokine communication remains a key question and certainly will continue to be the focus of intense research in the future.

REFERENCES

1. Sims JE, March CJ, Cosman D, et al. cDNA expression cloning of the IL-1 receptor, a member of the immunoglobulin superfamily. Science 1988; 241:585–9.
2. Sims JE, Acres RB, Grubin CE, et al. Cloning the interleukin 1 receptor from human T cells. Proc Natl Acad Sci U S A 1989; 86:8946–50.
3. Leonard WJ, Depper JM, Crabtree GR, et al. Molecular cloning and expression of cDNAs for the human interleukin-2 receptor. Nature 1984; 311:626–30.
4. Nikaido T, Shimizu A, Ishida N, et al. Molecular cloning of cDNA encoding human interleukin-2 receptor. Nature 1984; 311:631–5.
5. Cosman D, Cerretti DP, Larsen A, et al. Cloning, sequence and expression of human interleukin-2 receptor. Nature 1984; 312:768–72.
6. Hatakeyama M, Tsudo M, Minamoto S, et al. Interleukin-2 receptor chain gene: generation of three receptor forms by cloned human α and β chain cDNAs. Science 1989; 244:551–6.
7. Itoh N, Yonehara S, Schreurs J, et al. Cloning of an interleukin-3 receptor gene: a member of a distinct receptor gene family. Science 1990; 247:324–6.
8. Fukunaga R, Ishizaka-Ikeda E, Seta Y, Nagata S. Expression cloning of a receptor for murine granulocyte colony-stimulating factor. Cell 1990; 61:341–50.
9. Gearing DP, King JA, Gough NM, Nicola NA. Expression cloning of a receptor for human granulocyte-macrophage colony-stimulating factor. EMBO J 1989; 8:3667–76.
10. Idzerda RL, March CJ, Mosley B, et al. Human interleukin 4 receptor confers biological responsiveness and defines a novel receptor superfamily. J Exp Med 1990; 171:861–73.
11. Mosley B, Beckmann MP, March CJ, et al. The membrane interleukin-4 receptor: molecular cloning and characterization of secreted and membrane bound forms. Cell 1989; 59:335–48.
12. Yamasaki K, Taga T, Hirata Y, et al. Cloning and expression of the human interleukin-6 (BSF-2/IFN 2) receptor. Science 1988; 241:825–8.
13. Goodwin RG, Friend D, Ziegler SF, et al. Cloning of the human and murine interleukin-7 receptors: demonstration of a soluble form and homology to a new receptor super family. Cell 1990; 60:941–51.
14. Loetscher H, Pan Y-CE, Lahm H-W, et al. Molecular cloning and expression of the human 55 kDa tumor necrosis factor receptor. Cell 1990; 61:351–9.

15. Schall TJ, Lewis M, Koller KJ, et al. Molecular cloning and expression of a receptor for human tumor necrosis factor. Cell 1990; 61:361–70.
16. Smith CA, Davis T, Anderson D, et al. A receptor for tumor necrosis factor defines an unusual family of cellular and viral proteins. Science 1990; 248:1019–23.
17. Mizel SB. The interleukins. FASEB J 1989; 3:2379–88.
18. Mizel SB. Interleukin 1. Biology and molecular biology. In: Poste G, Crooke ST, eds. Cellular and molecular aspects of inflammation. New York: Plenum, 1988: 75–96.
19. Dower SK, Kronheim SR, March CJ, et al. Detection and characterization of high affinity plasma membrane receptors for human interleukin 1. J Exp Med 1985; 162:501–15.
20. Lowenthal JW, MacDonald HR. Binding and internalization of interleukin 1 by T cells. J Exp Med 1986; 164:1060–74.
21. Kilian PL, Kaffka KL, Stern AS, et al. Interleukin-1α and interleukin-1β bind to the same receptor on T cells. J Immunol 1986; 136:4509–14.
22. Matsushima KT, Akahoshi T, Yamada M, Furutani Y, Oppenheim JJ. Properties of a specific interleukin 1 (IL1) receptor on human Epstein-Barr virus-transformed B lymphocytes: identity of the receptor for IL 1α and IL 1β. J Immunol 1986; 136:4496–502.
23. Bird TA, Saklatvala J. Identification of a common class of high affinity receptors for both types of porcine interleukin-1 on connective tissue cells. Nature 1986; 324:263–6.
24. March CJ, Mosley B, Larsen A, et al. Cloning, sequence and expression of two distinct human interleukin-1 complementary DNAs. 1985; Nature 315:641–5.
25. Dower SK, Call SM, Gillis S, Urdal DL. Similarity between the interleukin-1 receptors on a murine T-lymphoma cell line and on a murine fibroblast cell line. Proc Natl Acad Sci U S A 1986; 83:1060–4.
26. Chin J, Cameron PM, Rupp C, Schmidt J. Identification of a high-affinity receptor for native human interleukin 1 β and interleukin 1 α on normal human lung fibroblasts. J Exp Med 1987; 165:70–86.
27. Paganelli KA, Stern AS, Kilian PL. Detergent solubilization of the interleukin 1 receptor. J Immunol 1987; 138:2249–53.
28. Urdal DL, Call SM, Jackson JL, Dower SK. Affinity purification and chemical analysis of the interleukin-1 receptor. J Biol Chem 1988; 263:2870–7.
29. Bird TA, Gearing AJH, Saklatvala J. Murine interleukin 1 receptor. J Biol Chem 1988; 263:12063–9.
30. Williams AF, Barclay AN. Immunoglobulin superfamily—domains for cell surface recognition. Annu Rev Immunol 1988; 6:381–405.
31. Bomsztyk K, Sims JE, Stanton TH, et al. Evidence for different interleukin 1 receptors in murine B- and T-cell lines. Proc Natl Acad Sci U S A 1989; 86:8034–8.
32. Chizzonite R, Truitt T, Kilian PL, et al. Two high affinity interleukin 1 receptors represent separate gene products. Proc Natl Acad Sci U S A 1989; 86:8029–33.
33. Shirakawa F, Yamashita U, Chedid M, Mizel SB. Cyclic AMP—an intracellular second messenger for interleukin 1. Proc Natl Acad Sci U S A 1988; 85:8201–5.
34. Chedid M, Shirakawa F, Naylor P, Mizel SB. Signal transduction pathway for interleukin 1. Involvement of a pertussis toxin-sensitive GTP-binding protein in the activation of adenylate cyclase. J Immunol 1989; 142:4301–6.
35. Smith KA. Interleukin-2: inception, impact and implications. Science 1988; 240:1169–76.
36. Uchiyama T, Broder T, Waldmann TA. A monoclonal antibody (anti-Tac) reactive with activated and functionally mature human T cells. 1. Induction of anti-Tac monoclonal antibody and distribution of Tac$^+$ cells. J Immunol 1981; 126:1393–7.

37. Leonard WJ, Depper JM, Uchiyama T, Smith KA, Waldmann TA, Greene WC. A monoclonal antibody, anti-Tac, blocks the membrane binding and action of human T-cell growth factor. Nature 1982; 300:267–9.
38. Robb RJ, Greene WC. Direct demonstration of the identity of T cell growth factor binding protein and the Tac antigen. J Exp Med 1983; 158:1322–7.
39. Sabe H, Kondo S, Shimizu A, et al. Properties of human IL-2 receptors expressed on non-lymphoid cells by cDNA transfection. Mol Biol Med 1986; 2:379–84.
40. Hatakeyama M, Minamoto S, Uchiyama T, Hardy RR, Yamada G, Taniguchi T. Reconstitution of functional receptor for human interleukin 2 in mouse cells. Nature 1985; 318:467–70.
41. Greene WC, Robb RJ, Svetlik PB, Rusk CM, Depper JM, Leonard WJ. Stable expression of cDNA encoding the human interleukin 2 receptor in eukaryotic cells. J Exp Med 1985; 162:363–8.
42. Kondo S, Shimizu A, Maeda M, Tagaya Y, Yodoi J, Honjo T. Expression of functional human interleukin 2 receptor in mouse T cells by cDNA transfection. Nature 1986; 320:75–82.
43. Robb RJ. Conversion of low-affinity interleukin 2 receptors to a high affinity state following fusion of cell membranes. Proc Natl Acad Sci U S A 1986; 83:3992–6.
44. Robb RJ, Greene WC, Rusk CM. Low and high affinity cellular receptors for interleukin 2: implications for the level of Tac antigen. J Exp Med 1984; 160:1126–46.
45. Tsudo M, Kozak RW, Goldman CK, Waldmann TA. Demonstration of a non-Tac peptide that binds interleukin 2: a potential participant in a multichain interleukin 2 receptor complex. Proc Natl Acad Sci U S A 1986; 83:9694–8.
46. Teshigawara K, Wang H-M, Kato K, Smith KA. Interleukin 2 high-affinity receptor expression requires two distinct binding proteins. J Exp Med 1987; 165:223–8.
47. Weissman AM, Harford JB, Svetlik PB, et al. Only high-affinity receptors for interleukin 2 mediate internalization of ligand. Proc Natl Acad Sci U S A 1986; 83:1463–6.
48. Sharon M, Klausner RD, Cullen BR, Chizzonite R, Leonard WJ. Novel interleukin-2 receptor subunit detected by cross-linking under high-affinity conditions. Science 1986; 234:859–63.
49. Robb RJ, Rusk CM, Yodoi J, Greene WC. Interleukin 2 binding molecule distinct from the Tac protein: analysis of its role in formation of high-affinity receptors. Proc Natl Acad Sci U S A 1987; 84:2002–6.
50. Dukovich M, Wano Y, Thuy LTB, et al. A second human interleukin-2 binding protein that may be a component of high-affinity interleukin-2 receptors. Nature 1987; 327:518–22.
51. Tsudo M, Kozak RW, Goldman CK, Waldmann TA. Contribution of a p75 interleukin 2 binding peptide to a high-affinity interleukin 2 receptor complex. Proc Natl Acad Sci U S A 1987; 84:4215–8.
52. Sharon M, Siegel JP, Tosato G, Yodoi J, Gerrard TL, Leonard WJ. The human interleukin 2 receptor β chain: direct identification, partial purification, and patterns of expression on peripheral blood mononuclear cells. J Exp Med 1988; 167:1265–70.
53. Colamonici OR, Neckers LM, Rosolen A. Putative γ-subunit of the IL-2 receptor is detected in low, intermediate, and high affinity IL-2 receptor-bearing cells. J Immunol 1990; 145:155–60.
54. Sherr CJ. Colony-stimulating factor-1 receptor. Blood 1990; 75:1–12.
55. Ihle JN, Weinstein Y. Immunological regulation of hematopoietic/lymphoid stem cell differentiation by interleukin 3. Adv Immunol 1986; 39:1–50.
56. Suda T, Suda J, Ogawa M, Ihle JN. Permissive role of interleukin 3 (IL-3) in

proliferation and differentiation of multipotential hemopoietic progenitors in culture. J Cell Physiol 1985; 124:182–90.
57. Spivak JL, Smith RRL, Ihle JN. Interleukin 3 promotes the in vivo proliferation of murine pluripotent hematopoietic stem cells. J Clin Invest 1985; 76:1613–21.
58. May WS, Ihle JN. Affinity isolation of the interleukin-3 surface receptor. Biochem Biophys Res Commun 1986; 135:870–9.
59. Park LS, Friend D, Gillis S, Urdal DL. Characterization of the cell surface receptor for a multi-lineage colony-stimulating factor (CSF-2α). J Biol Chem 1986; 261:205–10.
60. Nicola NA, Peterson L. Identification of distinct receptors for two hemopoietic growth factors (granulocyte colony-stimulating factor and multipotential colony-stimulating factor) by chemical cross-linking. J Biol Chem 1986; 261:12384–9.
61. Sorenson P, Farber NM, Krystal G. Identification of the interleukin-3 receptor using an iodinatable, cleavable, photoreactive cross-linking agent. J Biol Chem 1986; 261:9094–7.
62. Sorenson P, Mui AL-F, Krystal G. Interleukin-3 stimulates the tyrosine phosphorylation of the 140 kD interleukin-3 receptor. J Biol Chem 1989; 264:19253–8.
63. Nicola NA, Metcalf D. Binding of the differentiation-inducer, granulocyte-colony-stimulating factor, to responsive but not unresponsive leukemia cell lines. Proc Natl Acad Sci U S A 1984; 81:3765–9.
64. Nicola NA, Metcalf D. Binding of ^{125}I-labeled granulocyte colony-stimulating factor to normal murine hemopoietic cells. J Cell Physiol 1985; 124:313–21.
65. Nicola NA, Begley CG, Metcalf D. Identification of the human analogue of a regulator that induces differentiation in murine leukemic cells. Nature 1985; 314:625–8.
66. Begley CG, Metcalf D, Nicola NA. Primary human myeloid leukemia cells: comparative responsiveness to proliferative stimulation by GM-CSF or G-CSF and membrane expression of CSF receptors. Leukemia 1987; 1:1–8.
67. Park LS, Waldron PE, Friend D, et al. Interleukin-3, GM-CSF, and G-CSF receptor expression on cell lines and primary leukemia cells: receptor heterogeneity and relationship to growth factor responsiveness. Blood 1989; 74:56–65.
68. Uzumaki H, Okabe T, Sakaki N, et al. Identification and characterization of receptors for granulocyte colony-stimulating factor on human placenta and trophoblastic cells. Proc Natl Acad Sci U S A 1989; 86:9323–6.
69. Gough NM, Nicola NA. Granulocyte-macrophage colony-stimulating factor. In: Dexter TM, Garland J, Testa N, eds. Colony-stimulating factors: molecular and cellular biology. New York: Marcel Dekker, 1989:111–53.
70. Nicola NA. Why do hemopoietic growth factor receptors interact with each other? Immunol Today 1987; 8:134–9.
71. DiPersio J, Billing P, Kaufman S, Eghtesady P, Williams RE, Gasson JC. Characterization of the human granulocyte-macrophage colony-stimulating factor receptor. J Biol Chem 1988; 263:1834–41.
72. Park LS, Friend D, Gillis S, Urdal DL. Characterization of the cell surface receptor for granulocyte-macrophage colony stimulating factor. J Biol Chem 1986; 261:4177–83.
73. Park LS, Friend D, Gillis S, Urdal DL. Characterization of the cell surface receptor for human granulocyte/macrophage colony-stimulating factor. J Exp Med 1986; 164:251–62.
74. Walker F, Burgess AW. Specific binding of radioiodinated granulocyte-macrophage colony-stimulating factor to hemopoietic cells. EMBO J 1985; 4:933–9.
75. Paul WE, Ohara J. B-cell stimulatory factor-1/interleukin 4. Annu Rev Immunol 1987; 5:429–60.

76. Park LS, Friend D, Grabstein K, Urdal DL. Characterization of the high-affinity cell surface receptor for murine B cell-stimulating factor 1. Proc Natl Acad Sci U S A 1987; 84:1669–73.
77. Ohara J, Paul WE. Receptors for B-cell stimulatory factor-1 expressed on cells of hematopoietic lineage. Nature 1987; 325:5337–40.
78. Park LS, Friend D, Sassenfeld HM, Urdal DL. Characterization of the human B cell stimulatory factor 1 receptor. J Exp Med 1987; 166:476–88.
79. Cabrillat H, Galizzi J-P, Djossou O, et al. High affinity binding of human interleukin 4 to cell lines. Biochem Biophys Res Commun 1987; 149:995–1001.
80. Lowenthal JW, Castle BE, Christiansen J, et al. Expression of high affinity receptors for murine interleukin 4 (BSF-1) on hemopoietic and nonhemopoietic cells. J Immunol 1988; 140:456–64.
81. Sanderson CJ, Campbell HD, Young IG. Molecular and cellular biology of eosinophil differentiation factor (interleukin 5), and its effects on human and mouse B cells. Immunol Rev 1988; 102:29–50.
82. Takatsu K, Tominaga A, Harada N, et al. T cell-replacing factor (TRF/IL-5): molecular and functional properties. Immunol Rev 1988; 102:107–35.
83. Rolink AC, Melchers F, Palacios R. Monoclonal antibodies reactive with the mouse interleukin 5 receptor. J Exp Med 1989; 169:1693–701.
84. Kishimoto T, Hirano T. Molecular regulation of B-lymphocyte response. Annu Rev Immunol 1988; 6:485–512.
85. Van Snick J. Interleukin-6: an overview. Annu Rev Immunol 1990; 8:253–78.
86. Taga T, Kawanishi K, Hardy RR, Hirano T, Kishimoto T. Receptors for B cell stimulatory factor 2: quantitation, specificity, distribution and regulation of their expression. J Exp Med 1987; 166:967–81.
87. Taga T, Hibi M, Hirata Y, et al. Interleukin-6 triggers the association of its receptor with a possible signal transducer, gp130. Cell 1989; 58:573–81.
88. Namen AE, Schmierer AE, March CJ, et al. B cell precursor growth-promoting activity: purification and characterization of a growth factor active on lymphocyte precursors. J Exp Med 1988; 167:988–1002.
89. Park LS, Friend DJ, Schmierer A, Dower SK, Namen AE. Murine interleukin 7 (IL-7) receptor: characterization of an IL-7-dependent cell line. J Exp Med 1990; 171:1073–89.
90. Yoshimura T, Matsushima K, Oppenheim JJ, Leonard EJ. Neutrophil chemotactic factor produced by lipopolysaccharide (LPS)-stimulated human blood mononuclear leukocytes: partial characterization and separation from interleukin 1 (IL 1). J Immunol 1987; 139:788–93.
91. Schroder J-M, Mrowietz U, Morita E, Christophers E. Purification and partial biochemical characterization of a human monocyte-derived, neutrophil-activation peptide that lacks interleukin 1 activity. J Immunol 1987; 139:3474–83.
92. Walz A, Peveri P, Aschauer H, Baggiolini M. Purification and amino acid sequencing of NAF, a novel neutrophil-activating factor produced by monocytes. Biochem Biophys Res Commun 1987; 149:755–61.
93. Grob PM, David E, Warren TC, DeLeon RP, Farina PR, Homon CA. Characterization of a receptor for human monocyte-derived neutrophil chemotactic factor/interleukin-8. J Biol Chem 1990; 265:8311–6.
94. Samanta A, Oppenheim JJ, Matsushima K. Interleukin 8 (monocyte-derived neutrophil chemotactic factor) dynamically regulates its own receptor expression on human neutrophils. J Biol Chem 1990; 265:183–9.
95. Samanta AK, Oppenheim JJ, Matsushima K. Identification of specific receptors for monocyte-derived neutrophil chemotactic factor (MDNCF) on human neutrophils. J Exp Med 1989; 169:1185–9.

96. Beutler B, Cerami A. Cachectin (tumor necrosis factor): a macrophage hormone governing cellular metabolism and inflammatory response. Endocr Rev 1988; 9:57–64.
97. Kull FC, Jacobs S, Cuatrecasas P. Cellular receptor for ^{125}I-labeled tumor necrosis factor: specific binding, affinity labeling, and relationship to sensitivity. Proc Natl Acad Sci U S A 1985; 82:5756–60.
98. Scheurich P, Ucer U, Kronke M, Pfizenmaier K. Quantification and characterization of high-affinity membrane receptors for tumor necrosis factor on human leukemic cell lines. Int J Cancer 1986; 38:127–33.
99. Smith RA, Kirstein M, Fiers W, Baglioni C. Species specificity of human and murine tumor necrosis factor. J Biol Chem 1986; 261:14871–874.
100. Yoshie O, Tada K, Ishida N. Binding and crosslinking of ^{125}I-labeled recombinant human tumor necrosis factor to cell surface receptors. J Biochem 1986; 100:531–41.
101. Tsujimoto M, Feinman R, Kohase M, Vilcek J. Characterization and affinity crosslinking of receptors for tumor necrosis factor on human cells. Arch Biochem Biophys 1986; 249:563–8.
102. Creasey AA, Yamamoto R, Vitt CR. A high molecular weight component of the human tumor necrosis factor receptor is associated with cytotoxicity. Proc Natl Acad Sci U S A 1987; 84:3293–7.
103. Shepherd VL, Abdolrasulnia R. Isolation of a receptor for tumor necrosis factor from human lung tissue. Cytokine 1989; 1:96.
104. Stauber GB, Aiyer RA, Aggarwal BB. Human tumor necrosis factor-α receptor. Purification by immunoaffinity chromatography and initial characterization. J Biol Chem 1988; 263:19098–104.
105. Kaur P, Saklatvala J. Interleukin 1 and tumour necrosis factor increase phosphorylation of fibroblast proteins. FEBS Lett 1988; 241:6–10.
106. Donato NJ, Gallick GE, Steck PA, Rosenblum MG. Tumor necrosis factor modulates epidermal growth factor receptor phosphorylation and kinase activity in human tumor cells. J Biol Chem 1989; 264:20474–81.
107. Engelmann H, Aderka D, Rubinstein M, Rotman D, Wallach D. A tumor necrosis factor-binding protein purified to homogeneity from human urine protects cells from tumor necrosis factor toxicity. J Biol Chem 1989; 264:11974–80.
108. Brockhaus M, Schoenfeld HJ, Schlaeger EJ, Honziker W, Lesslauer W, Loetscher H. Identification of two types of tumor necrosis factor receptors on human cell lines by monoclonal antibodies. Proc Natl Acad Sci U S A 1990; 87:3127–31.
109. Hohmann HP, Remy R, Brockhaus M, Van Loon APGM. Two different cell types have different major receptors for human tumor necrosis factor (TNF). J Biol Chem 1989; 264:14927–34.
110. Bazan JF. A novel family of growth factor receptors: a common binding domain in the growth hormone, prolactin, erythropoietin and IL-6 receptors, and the p75 IL-2 receptor β-chain. Biochem Biophys Res Commun 1989; 164:788–95.
111. Cosman D, Lyman SD, Idzerda RL, et al. A new cytokine receptor superfamily. Trends Biochem Sci 1990; 15:265–70.
112. Idzerda RL, March CJ, Mosley B, et al. Human interleukin 4 receptor confers biological responsiveness and defines a novel receptor superfamily. J Exp Med 1990; 171:861–73.
113. Stamenkovic I, Clark E, Seed B. A B-lymphocyte activation molecule related to the nerve growth factor, receptor and induced by cytokines in carcinomas. EMBO J 1989; 8:1403–10.
114. Kwon B, Weissman S. cDNA sequences of two inducible T-cell genes. Proc Natl Acad Sci U S A 1989; 86:1963–7.

115. Yarden Y, Ullrich A. Growth factor receptor tyrosine kinases. Annu Rev Biochem 1988; 57:443–82.
116. House C, Wettenhall TEH, Kemp BE. The influenc of basic residues on the substrate specificity of protein kinase C. J Biol Chem 1987; 262:772–9.
117. Gallis B, Pritchett KS, Jackson J, et al. IL-1 induces rapid phosphorylation of the IL-1 receptor. J Immunol 1989; 143:3235–40.
118. Matsushima K, Kobayashi Y, Copeland TD, Akahoshi T, Oppenheim JJ. Phosphorylation of a cytosolic 65-kDa protein induced by interleukin-1 in glucocorticoid pretreated normal human peripheral blood mononuclear leukocytes. J Immunol 1987; 139:3367–74.
119. Matsushima K, Shiroo M, Kung H, Copeland TD. Purification and characterization of a cytosolic 65-kilodalton phosphoprotein in human leukocytes whose phosphorylation is augmented by stimulation with interleukin-1. Biochemistry 1988; 27:3765–70.
120. Kaur P, Saklatvala J. Interleukin 1 and tumor necrosis factor increase phosphorylation of fibroblast proteins. FEBS Lett 1988; 241:6–14.
121. Evans SW, Farrar WL. Identity of common phosphoprotein substrates stimulated by interleukin 2 and diacylglycerol suggests a role of protein kinase C for IL 2 signal transduction. J Cell Biochem 1987; 34:47–59.
122. Ishii T, Kohno M, Nakamura M, Hinuma Y, Sugamura K. Characterization of interleukin 2-stimulated phosphorylation of 67 and 63 kDa proteins in human T cells. Biochem J 1987; 242:211–9.
123. Ferris DK, Willette-Brown J, Ortaldo JR, Farrar WL. IL-2 regulation of tyrosine kinase activity is mediated through the p70–75 β-subunit of the IL-2 receptor. J Immunol 1989; 143:870–6.
124. Asao H, Takeshita T, Nakamura M, Nagata K, Sugamura K. Interleukin 2 (IL-2)-induced tyrosine phosphorylation of IL-2 receptor p75. J Exp Med 1990; 171:637–44.
125. Sharon M, Gnarra JR, Leonard WJ. The β-chain of the IL-2 receptor (p70) is tyrosine phosphorylated on YT and HUT-102B2 cells. J Immunol 1989; 143:2530–3.
126. Koyasu S, Tojo A, Miyajima A, et al. Interleukin 3-specific tyrosine phosphorylation of a membrane glycoprotein of *Mr* 150,000 in multifactor-dependent myeloid cell lines. EMBO J 1987; 6:3979–84.
127. Sorenson PHB, Mui AL-F, Murthy SC, Krystal G. Interleukin-3, GM-CSF, and TPA induce distinct phosphorylation events in an interleukin 3-dependent multipotent cell line. Blood 1989; 73:406–18.
128. Isfort RJ, Stevens D, May WS, Ihle JN. Interleukin 3 binds to a 140-kDa phosphotyrosine-containing cell surface protein. Proc Natl Acad Sci U S A 1988; 85: 7982–6.
129. Lewis C, Mazzei G, Shaw A. Monoclonal antibodies reacting with the interleukin 1 receptor define a multi-molecular complex. Eur J Immunol 1990; 20:207–13.
130. Saragovi H, Malek TR. Evidence for additional subunits associated to the mouse interleukin 2 receptor p55/p75 complex. Proc Natl Acad Sci U S A 1990; 87: 11–5.
131. Mizel SB, Kilian PL, Lewis JC, Paganelli KA, Chizzonite RA. The interleukin 1 receptor. Dynamics of interleukin 1 binding and internalization in T cells and fibroblasts. J Immunol 1987; 138:2906–12.
132. Qwarnstrom EE, Page RC, Gillis S, Dower SK. Binding, internalization and intracellular localization of interleukin-1β in human diploid fibroblasts. J Biol Chem 1988; 263:8261–9.
133. Grenfell S, Smithers N, Miller K, Solar R. Receptor-mediated endocytosis and nuclear transport of human interleukin 1β. Biochem J 1989; 264:813–22.

134. Fujii M, Sugamura K, Sano K, Nakai M, Sugita K, Hinoma Y. High-affinity receptor-mediated internalization and degradation of interleukin 2 in human T cells. J Exp Med 1986; 163:550–62.
135. Galizzi J-P, Zuber CE, Cabrillet H, Djossou O, Banchereau J. Internalization of human interleukin 4 and transient down-regulation of its receptor in the CD23-inducible jijoye cells. J Biol Chem 1989; 264:6984–9.
136. Shepherd V. Receptor-mediated endocytosis. Life Chem Rep 1989; 6:317–65.
137. Miller DS. Stimulation of RNA and protein synthesis by intracellular insulin. Science 1988; 240:506–9.
138. Burwen SJ, Jones AL. The association of polypeptide hormones and growth factors with the nuclei of target cells. Trends Biochem Sci 1987; 12:159–62.
139. Rakowics-Szulczynska EM, Rodeck U, Herlyn M, Koprowski H. Chromatin binding of epidermal growth factor, nerve growth factor, and platelet-derived growth factor in cells bearing the appropriate surface receptors. Proc Natl Acad Sci U S A 1986; 83:3728–32.
140. Curtis BM, Widmer MB, deRoos P, Qwarnstrom EE. IL-1 and its receptor are translocated to the nucleus. J Immunol 1990; 144:1295–303.
141. Dingwall C, Laskey RA. Protein import into the cell nucleus. Annu Rev Cell Biol 1986; 2:367–90.
142. Lee H-K, Xia X, Choi YS. IL-4 blocks the up-regulation of IL-2 receptors induced by IL-2 in normal human B cells. J Immunol 1990; 144:3431–6.
143. Smith KA, Cantrell DA. Interleukin 2 regulates its own receptors. Proc. Natl Acad Sci U S A 1985; 82:864–8.
144. Saito Y, Sabe H, Suzuki N, et al. A larger number of chains (Tac) enhance the association rate of interleukin 2 to the high affinity site of the interleukin 2 receptor. J Exp Med 1988; 168:1563–72.
145. Smith KA. The interleukin 2 receptor. Annu Rev Cell Biol 1989; 5:397–425.
146. Yoshimoto T, Nabanishi K, Matsui K, et al. IL-5 up-regulates but IL-4 down-regulates IL-2R expression on a cloned B lymphoma line. J Immunol 1990; 144:183–90.
147. Martinez OM, Gibbons RS, Garovoy MR, Aronson FR. IL-4 inhibits IL-2 receptor expression and IL-2 dependent proliferation of human T cells. J Immunol 1990; 144:2211–5.
148. Scheurich P, Thoma B, Ucer U, Pfizenmaier K. Immunoregulatory activity of recombinant tumor necrosis factor (TNF)-α: induction of TNF receptors on human T cells and TNF-α-mediated enhancement of T cell responses. J Immunol 1987; 138:1786–90.
149. Le J, Fredrickson G, Reis LFL, et al. Interleukin 2-dependent and interleukin 2-independent pathways of regulation of thymocyte function by interleukin 6. Proc Natl Acad Sci U S A 1988; 85:8643–7.
150. Hancock WW, Muller WA, Cotran RS. Interleukin 2 receptors are expressed by alveolar macrophages during pulmonary sarcoidosis and are inducible by lymphokine treatment of normal human lung macrophages, blood monocytes, and monocyte cell lines. J Immunol 1987; 138:185–91.
151. Holter W, Goldman CK, Casabo L, Nelson DL, Greene WC, Waldmann TA. Expression of functional IL2 receptors by lipopolysaccharide and interferon-γ stimulated human monocytes. J Immunol 1987; 138:2917–22.
152. Espinoza-Delgado I, Ortaldo JR, Winkler-Pinkett R, Sugamura K, Varesio L, Longo DL. Expression and role of p75 interleukin 2 receptor on human monocytes. J Exp Med 1990; 171:1821–6.
153. Feldman GM, Finbloom DS. Induction and regulation of IL-4 receptor expres-

sion on murine macrophage cell lines and bone marrow-derived macrophages by IFN-γ. J Immunol 1990; 145:854–9.

154. Ohara J, Paul WE. Up-regulation of interleukin 4/B-cell stimulatory factor 1 receptor expression. Proc Natl Acad Sci U S A 1988; 85:8221–5.

155. Puri RK, Finbloom DS, Leland P, Mostowski H, Siegel JP. Expression of high affinity IL-4 receptors on murine tumor infiltrating lymphocytes and their upregulation by IL-2. Immunology 1990; 70:492–7

156. Snyers L, Dewit L, Content J. Glucocorticoid up-regulation of high-affinity interleukin 6 receptors on human epithelial cells. Proc Natl Acad Sci U S A 1990; 87:2838–42.

157. Bauer J, Lengyel G, Bauer TM, Acs G, Gerok N. Regulation of interleukin-6 receptor expression in human monocytes and hepatocytes. FEBS Lett 1989; 249:27–30.

158. Tsujimoto M, Feinman R, Vilcek J. Differential effects of type I IFN and IFNγ on the binding of tumor necrosis factor to receptors in two human cell lines. J Immunol 1986; 137:2272–6.

159. Aggarwal BB, Eessalu TE, Hass PE. Characterization of receptors for human tumor necrosis factor and their regulation by gamma-interferon. Nature 1985; 318:665–7.

160. Unglaub R, Maxeiner B, Thoma B, Pfizenmaier K, Scheurich P. Downregulation of tumor necrosis factor (TNF) sensitivity via modulation of TNF binding capacity by protein kinase C activators. J Exp Med 1987; 166:1788–97.

161. Johnson SE, Baglioni C. Tumor necrosis factor receptors and cytocidal activity are down-regulated by activators of protein kinase C. J Biol Chem 1988; 263:5686–92.

162. Aggarwal BB, Eessalu TE. Effect of phorbol esters on down-regulation and redistribution of cell surface receptors for tumor necrosis factor-α. J Biol Chem 1987; 262:16450–5.

163. Drapier J-C, Wietzerbin J. IFN-γ down-regulates expression of TNF receptors on murine macrophages. Cytokine 1989; 1:93.

164. Heyman SJ, Welborn MB, Shepherd VL. Characterization of TNF receptor binding in human endothelial cells and macrophages. Am Rev Respir Dis 1990; 141:A920.

165. Bielefeldt Ohmann H, Campos M, McDougall L, Lawman MJP, Babiuk LA. Expression of tumor necrosis factor-α receptors on bovine macrophages, lymphocytes and polymorphonuclear leukocytes, internalization of receptor-bound ligand, and some functional effects. Lymphokine Res 1990; 9:43–58.

166. Ding A, Sanchez E, Srimal S, Nathan CF. Macrophages rapidly internalize their tumor necrosis factor receptors in response to bacterial lipopolysaccharide. J Biol Chem 1989; 264:3924–9.

167. Owen-Schaub LB, Crump WL, Morin GI, Grimm EA. Regulation of lymphocyte tumor necrosis factor receptors by IL-2. J Immunol 1989; 143:2236–41.

168. Robb RJ, Kutny RM. Structure function relationships for the IL-2-receptor system. IV. Analysis of the sequence and ligand-binding properties of soluble Tac protein. J Immunol 1987; 139:855–62.

169. Maliszewski CR, Sato TA, Vanden Bos T, et al. Cytokine receptors and B cell functions. I. Recombinant soluble receptors specifically inhibit IL-1- and IL-4-induced B cell activities in vitro. J Immunol 1990; 144:3028–33.

170. Fernandez-Botran R, Vitetta ES. A soluble, high-affinity, interleukin-4-binding protein is present in the biological fluids of mice. Proc Natl Acad Sci U S A 1990; 87:4202–6.

171. Novick D, Engelmann H, Wallach D, Rubinstein M. Soluble cytokine receptors are present in normal human urine. J Exp Med 1989; 170:1409–14.

172. Seckinger P, Isaaz S, Dayer J-M. Purification and biologic characterization of a specific tumor necrosis factor inhibitor. J Biol Chem 1989; 264:11966–73.
173. Seckinger P, Zhang J-H, Hauptmann B, Dayer J-M. Characterization of a tumor necrosis factor α (TNF-α) inhibitor: evidence of immunological cross-reactivity with the TNF receptor. Proc Natl Acad Sci U S A 1990; 87:5188–93.

CHAPTER 28

CYTOKINES AND AIDS

Monique A. Berman and Christy I. Sandborg

California College of Medicine
University of California
Irvine, California

INTRODUCTION

The major disease manifestations of advanced human immunodeficiency virus (HIV) infection include opportunistic infections, central nervous system disorders, lymphadenopathy, cachexia, fever, and tumor development (reviewed in Refs. 1–4). In all the disease activities, cytokines can be implicated and may play essential roles in mediating these processes. This review examines the known effects of HIV infection on cytokine production in vivo and in vitro, the potential role of cytokines in the pathogenesis of acquired immunodeficiency syndrome (AIDS), and the effect of cytokines on HIV infection in vitro and in clinical trials.

The large number of immunological abnormalities that accompany HIV infection have mainly been attributed to the depletion and selective defect in the $CD4^+$ subset of lymphocytes (5). This subset of T lymphocytes, as well as monocytes-macrophages (Mϕ), are the predominant target cells for infection by HIV (6–17). Infection of the Mϕ system causing impaired Mϕ function and altered cytokine production has also been proposed as a mechanism to explain many of the immune defects and tissue injury associated with HIV infection (18). $CD4^+$ T lymphocytes and Mϕ interact directly in antigen-specific responses and are interdependent through Mϕ immunoregulatory factors, such as interferon-γ (IFN-γ), and T cell stimulatory factors, such as interleukins-1 and 6 (IL-1 and IL-6) and tumor necrosis factor α (TNFα). These and other cytokines have multiple effects on the immune system and many other cell types that also produce cytokines. Therefore, altered production of cytokines by monocyte-Mϕ (monokines) could result in the observed T cell defects and altered production of cytokines by T lymphocytes (lymphokines) could result in Mϕ dysfunction. Thus far it has not been possible to determine which cytokine defect(s) due to HIV infection initiate the abnormalities and which effects are secondary to these cytokine abnormalities.

HIV-1 infection generally exhibits three phases: (a) a phase of primary infection and viral replication and initiation of an immune response to HIV; (b) a long-lasting phase of virus containment with an immune response, including antibodies to HIV and $CD8^+$ cytotoxic lymphocytes against HIV structural and regulatory proteins; at this stage, low numbers of productively infected cells (1 in 10^5) are found in the circulation (19,20); and (c) a phase of advanced disease with high levels of virulent HIV production. In the circulation, T lymphocytes are the main population of cells infected and only a low percentage of monocytes carry HIV (20). In other tissues (brain, lung, and lymph nodes) the frequency of productively infected cells can be much greater (10,000-fold higher) than in the blood, and the infected cells in these sites are Mϕ (21–23).

In the early phases, the manifestations of HIV infection are hyperactivity and hyperplasia of certain immune cells, especially B cells, rather than deficiencies (24,25). Autoimmune manifestations may also be signs of hyperactivity (24–26). The majority of the increased Ig production is specific for HIV (27), suggesting that many of the observed activities and cytokine levels may represent part of a normal immune response to HIV, rather than an aberrant response. The strong and prolonged activation of the immune system may in turn trigger regulatory mediators that could result in suppression of the host's immune system. These multiple immunoregulatory signals are mediated in part by the cytokine network. Cytokines that stimulate B lymphocytes (e.g., interleukin-1, IL-6, and IL-4) could play a role in the B cell hyperactivity characteristic of AIDS-related complex (ARC), persistent generalized lymphadenopathy (PGL), and AIDS. T lymphocyte inhibitory cytokines [e.g., IL-1 inhibitors, IL-2 inhibitors, and transforming growth factor β (TGF-β)] may be involved in the defective antigen responsiveness of T cells in HIV infection. In addition to the immunoregulatory effects, cytokines have tissue growth and repair functions. Imbalance in the secretion of these factors could affect normal tissue function, the promotion of neoplasias, and repair after injury. Secretion of monokines, induced directly by HIV or HIV gene products, through secondary infections, or by lymphokines, may mediate the progressive cachexia and weight loss. To date, the study of cytokines in AIDS has been limited to some of the best known cytokines, mainly those produced by peripheral blood cells, therefore providing only an incomplete view of the role of cytokines in the pathogenic processes of HIV infection that affect many organ systems. Early studies included only cells from AIDS patients with advanced disease; more recent studies have examined cytokines in light of the different phases of HIV infection.

MONOKINE PRODUCTION IN HIV INFECTION

The presence of HIV in Mϕ and their specialized forms in the brain (11–13,28), lymph nodes (9,10,19), blood (6,7,20), skin (16), and lungs (14,15) of patients with AIDS has been clearly demonstrated. This wide distribution of infected Mϕ in different tissues may not only be important as a reservoir for virus, as has been suggested (8,18,29–31), but may directly affect Mϕ function and cytokine (monokine) production in many tissues (18).

Mϕ from HIV-infected individuals have been shown to be impaired in their accessory cell functions, which are essential for the initiation of immune responses (18,32–35). They also appear to be impaired in their maturation (36) and in effector functions (37–41). Since in the cytokine network Mϕ respond to signals from T cells [e.g., IFN, IL-2, IL-3, IL-4, and granulocyte-macrophage colony-stimulating factor (GM-CSF)], it is not clear if HIV-induced changes in T cells are responsible for altered Mϕ activities. Major changes in monokine secretion occur in vivo as evidenced by the studies on circulating cytokine levels. The in vitro studies using normal Mϕ infected with HIV in vitro show that HIV can under certain conditions directly alter monokine production, suggesting that this mechanism contributes to the cytokine abnormalities in vivo and disease manifestations.

Serum Levels of Cytokines in HIV Infection

Serum levels of cytokines in healthy individuals tend to be low or below the sensitivity of current assays. Therefore, only increases to detectable levels usually associated with disease states can be studied. Negative findings should be cautiously interpreted in view of the low sensitivity of immunoassays, interference by inhibitors in bioassays, and instability of protein factors upon storage in serum at room temperature.

Although the findings of impaired Mϕ activities could suggest decreased Mϕ activation, Mϕ appear to be strongly activated in HIV infection as manifested by the increased production of several Mϕ factors. Lysozyme, a product of activated monocytes, is increased in the serum of AIDS patients and correlates with disease progression (42). Neopterin, a pyrazinopyrimidine compound derived from GTP, is produced by human Mϕ upon stimulation with IFN-γ (43), and serum or urine neopterin levels can provide an assessment of Mϕ activation in disease states (44,45). In HIV-related disease, increased concentrations of neopterin are seen early in the course of the disease, usually before $CD4^+$ T cells begin to decrease (46). Levels of neopterin are further increased in patients with AIDS-related complex and are highest in patients with AIDS. In a study of 68 HIV-1-seropositive homosexuals over 6 years, the predictive value of urine neopterin levels for disease progression was found to be higher than that of $CD4^+$ T cell counts (47). Increased levels of serum neopterin in HIV-1-seropositive individuals also correlate with increased circulating IFN-γ (48) and deficient in vitro IL-2 production in response to soluble recall antigens (49). High levels of an unusual acid-labile IFN-α have been documented in patients with symptomatic HIV infection (50–53). No IFN was detectable in normal serum, but persistently elevated levels of IFN in patients with HIV infection are indicative of disease progression from ARC to AIDS (54). Thus the activated state of Mϕ appears to be associated with abnormal lymphokine production. Further evidence for Mϕ activation in HIV infection is the finding that monocytes from patients with AIDS express significant levels of IL-2 receptor and constitutively express steady-state levels of IL-2 receptor mRNA (55). The expression of IL-2 receptor on normal monocytes-Mϕ can be induced by LPS and IFN-γ (56–58). In HIV infection the mechanism for Mϕ activation has not been clearly defined but may at least in part result from increased stimulation by IFN-γ.

Serum levels of the monokines TNF-α, IL-1, IL-6, and IFN-α have also been investigated. In normal serum TNF-α is undetectable or present in very low concentrations, but high levels are associated with disease states in humans (59–61). Using a sensitive radioimmunoassay, Lahdevirta et al. (62) found that all AIDS patients studied had highly increased levels of serum TNF-α. An increase was also seen in about half of patients with ARC and in some patients with lymphadenopathy syndrome. Asymptomatic carriers of HIV exhibited low levels of TNF-α, whereas AIDS patients had the highest levels, suggesting a correlation with disease activity. Patients with anemia and lymphopenia were found to have higher serum levels of TNF-α than patients without these hematological disorders (63). In children with AIDS, elevated serum levels of TNF-α were found to be associated with progressive encephalopathy (64). However, TNF-α has not been detectable in cerebrospinal fluid from patients with AIDS dementia complex (65,66), although elevated levels of IL-1β, IL-6, and soluble IL-2 receptor were detectable in cerebrospinal fluid.

Serum levels of IL-1α and IL-1β in HIV-seronegative and HIV-seropositive IV drug abusers and homosexuals have been studied by Reddy and Grieco (67). In their study, high levels of IL-1α were found in normal control sera (359 ± 146 pg/ml, n = 26) but IL-1β concentrations were low in these sera (4.04 ± 1.4 pg/ml). IL-1α levels were decreased in seropositive individuals, but the mean IL-1β level showed a >10-fold increase in patients with AIDS (n = 89). Although the average serum IL-1β level for the entire group of AIDS patients was strongly increased, only 30% of these patients had IL-1β levels above the range of healthy seronegative controls. These data showing increased IL-1β in a portion of AIDS patients only suggest that other factors in addition to HIV infection alone influence serum IL-1 levels. The levels may reflect disease activity, different types of opportunistic infections, different viral strains, predominant tissue sites of HIV infection, or genetic differences in host cytokine responses.

Monokine Production by Peripheral Blood Mononuclear Cells (PBMC) from Individuals with HIV Infection

The evidence for defective T cell responses in AIDS prompted the initial studies of IL-1 production in AIDS. Since IL-1 produced by Mϕ induces IL-2 production and proliferation of T lymphocytes (68–71), it was proposed that a decrease in IL-1 production might contribute to the T cell defect in AIDS. The early reports on spontaneous IL-1 production by fresh PBMC in short-term cultures showed no change, decreased, or slightly increased release of IL-1 activity by PBMC from AIDS patients compared to PBMC cultures from healthy controls (72–75). In these studies IL-1 activity in Mϕ culture supernatants was measured using the murine thymocyte proliferation assay. However, thymocyte proliferation, even in the presence of IL-1, can be inhibited by factors including prostaglandins and inhibitory cytokines present in supernatants from activated PBMC (76–78). These inhibitors can mask IL-1 activity in culture superatants (76). It is therefore necessary either to use immunoassays, which are generally less sensitive, or to separate IL-1 from inhibitors for the assessment of IL-1 levels in the bioassays for IL-1.

The use of chromatographic separation of supernatant from unstimulated Mϕ allowed the detection of greatly increased IL-1 activity released by PBMC from AIDS patients and the identification of inhibitors of thymocyte proliferation (79,80). An inhibitor of 7 kD (6–9 kD) was found to be greatly increased in unstimulated PBMC or Mϕ cultures from AIDS patients (79,80). This factor strongly inhibits thymocyte proliferation and antigen-induced T cell proliferation and has no effect on phytohemagglutinin (PHA)-induced PBMC proliferation (76,81). The high levels of this factor in AIDS may play a role in the impaired T cell maturation and in the selective impairment of antigen-specific responsiveness of T cells in AIDS. More recent studies using radioimmune assays also demonstrated strongly increased IL-1 release by monocytes in AIDS (82,83). Weiss et al. (83) investigated the production of cell-associated IL-1 in fresh, uncultured unstimulated adherent monocytes from HIV-infected patients. This approach reflects ongoing generation of IL-1 by the cells in vivo. High levels of cell-associated IL-1 activity and IL-1α and IL-1β antigen were found in monocytes from HIV-infected patients compared with normal monocytes. In serum-free cultures (24 h), only monocytes from HIV-infected individuals released high levels of IL-1, whereas no release occurred from normal cells. Stimulation with LPS in this study resulted in the release only of IL-1β by normal cells, but IL-1α and IL-1β were released by monocytes from HIV-infected individuals.

In some studies of PBMC and alveolar Mϕ, no increased IL-1 was detectable in HIV-infected individuals (84–86). The absence of increased IL-1 in these studies may be due to the use of reagents that are specific for IL-1β only (84); IL-1α may be preferentially activated. Further, the use of lipopolysaccharide (LPS) as a stimulant in vitro (85,86) may obscure the high spontaneous cytokine release by Mϕ from AIDS patients.

PBMC and adherent PBMC (Mϕ) from HIV-infected donors have also been shown to produce high levels of IL-6 in 24 h cultures (87,88). Further, freshly isolated unstimulated PBMC from HIV-seropositive donors and patients with ARC and AIDS were shown to express high levels of IL-6 mRNA but no IL-6 mRNA was detectable in PBMC from healthy donors (87).

TNF-α (cachectin) has also been found strongly increased in monocytes-Mϕ from peripheral blood of AIDS patients (82,86,89,90). As discussed for IL-1 production, only *spontaneous* TNF-α release appears to be strongly increased. Investigators who used LPS or PHA and phorbol myristate acetate (PMA) to stimulate PBMC found strongly decreased TNF-α levels in PBMC cultures from patients with symptomatic HIV infection compared with stimulated normal PBMC (86,91). Monocytes, which are activated in vivo, may be unable to respond to a subsequent stimulant. In vitro this may be manifested by lower levels of transcription and production of cytokines in response to stimuli, such as PHA, PMA, or endotoxin added as a stimulus or present in fetal calf serum. In vivo this refractory state may compromise the host defense mechanisms, particularly against the secondary opportunistic diseases associated with AIDS.

Several studies have examined the association of spontaneous monokine release with other disease markers and with the stage of HIV infection. Increased spontaneous release of IL-1, TNF-α, and IL-6 was found to correlate with the stage of HIV infection (80,82,86,87,89,92). Sandborg et al. showed that patients with AIDS produced the highest levels of IL-1 and of a 7 kD T cell inhibitory monokine

(TCIM). These levels were independent of concurrent active opportunistic infection or antibiotic therapy. Patients with persistent generalized lymphadenopathy (PGL) also produced increased levels of IL-1 and 7 kD TCIM, whereas ARC patients showed a wide range of responses. Asymptomatic seropositive patients produced less IL-1 and 7 kD TCIM than controls. The mechanism for the decreased release of these factors in asymptomatic infection is not known. Perhaps T lymphocytes, which stimulate the production of monokines, are activated during this early stage of HIV infection and produce lymphokines, such as IL-4 that inhibit IL-1 secretion (93–97).

Similar to the studies on IL-1, TNF-α was found to correlate with symptomatic HIV infection (82,86,89). Further, patients who displayed augmented in vitro secretion of TNF-α had elevated levels of TNF-α in sera (81). Levels of IL-6 mRNA in freshly isolated, unstimulated PBMC also correlate well with plasma IL-6 levels and were found elevated in HIV-infected individuals and undetectable in controls (87). In contrast to IL-1 and TNF-α, however, IL-6 plasma levels, IL-6 mRNA, and IL-6 bioactivity released in 24 h PBMC or Mϕ cultures were highly increased early in the course of HIV infection, at the asymptomatic, non-ARC/AIDS stage (87). Further, plasma IL-6 levels in HIV-infected donors with coinfections, such as tuberculosis, candidiasis, syphilis, and *Pneumocystis* pneumonia, were found in the same range as seen in HIV-infected donors who had no documented coinfections (87). These findings suggest that HIV infection alone may be essential in inducing IL-6 production in vivo.

Effect of In Vitro HIV Infection on Monokine Secretion

Since in vivo activation of Mϕ and subsequent spontaneous release of cytokines by monocytes-Mϕ ex vivo does not correlate with the presence of detectable opportunistic infection or other coinfections, different activating mechanisms must be considered. Currently it remains to be clarified if HIV infection of monocytes-Mϕ is directly responsible for the enhanced production of monokines or whether abnormal activation is a consequence of immune dysregulation.

The hypothesis proposing direct activation of Mϕ by HIV has been tested by studying cytokine production after infection of normal Mϕ with HIV-1 in vitro. It has been shown that normal human peripheral blood-derived macrophages can be infected with various isolates of HIV-1 (15,17,98–100). Certain isolates are strongly monocytes-Mϕ tropic and replicate effectively in these cells (e.g., HTLV-III Ba-L); other HIV-1 isolates, such as HTLV-IIIB, have been adapted for in vitro culture in T cells and replicate less efficiently in fresh human Mϕ. The use of different isolates and different experimental protocols for the study of in vitro induction of cytokines by HIV have produced conflicting results.

Roy et al. (101) infected human peripheral blood-derived Mϕ with HIV (HTLV IIIB) and measured IL-1 activity in supernatants after 1 or 2 days of culture in the presence of LPS or latex beads using the thymocyte proliferation assay. The results showed strongly decreased IL-1 activity in cultures exposed to infectious HIV compared with cultures stimulated with LPS or latex in the absence of HIV. In this system, HIV infection may have resulted in the production of relatively more IL-1 inhibitor(s) that masked IL-1 activity, as has been observed by Berman et al. (79) using PBMC from AIDS patients. A similar IL-1 inhibitor is also produced by in vitro HIV-infected Mϕ cultures and can mask IL-1 activity in bioassays (102). Using partially purified HIV derived from T cell cultures to infect normal Mϕ, Merrill et al. (103) reported increased TNF-α and IL-1 release in infected Mϕ cultures. Competition with soluble CD4, the receptor for HIV (104) inhibited this effect. Monoclonal antibody to CD4 (OKT4A) alone also induced these cytokines, suggesting that HIV envelope gp120-CD4 interaction is required to induce these monokines. Wahl et al. (105) examined the direct effect of purified viral envelope protein gp120 on IL-1 and prostaglandin E_2 (PGE_2) release by Mϕ. Both these mediators were strongly increased in 24 h cultures. This study shows that the interaction of viral envelope gp120 and CD4 is sufficient to trigger the activation of monocytes-Mϕ. The effect of gp120 was shown to be inhibited by specific antiserum to gp120. Similar levels of IL-1 and PGE_2 could be induced by monoclonal antibodies to CD4 (either OKT4 or OKT4A), further supporting the finding that IL-1 production and PGE_2 release can be mediated through CD4 on monocytes. Purified HIV has also been shown to increase IL-6 messenger RNA and IL-6 secretion in Mϕ cultures (106).

In contrast to the reports showing induction of monokines by HIV or HIV envelope glycoprotein, recent reports have not confirmed these findings. Molina et al. (107) studied fresh PBMC, 9 day adherent PBMC cultures, and the monocytic leukemia line THP-1 infected in vitro with monocytotropic HIV-1 (HIV-1-Ba-L and HIV-1-SF162) (108), T cell-derived HIV-1 (HTLVIIIB/H9), or recombinant gp120 (109). No increased release of TNF-α, IL-1β, or IL-6 was observed in the HIV-infected or gp120-stimulated Mϕ cultures. Another study, using fibronectin-adherent precultured adherent normal Mϕ infected in vitro with monocytes-Mϕ tropic HIV-1, also failed to detect altered production of TNF-α or TNF-α mRNA using a highly sensitive polymerase chain reaction (PCR) technique. Despite the highly productive HIV infection and giant cell formation by infected Mϕ observed in these studies, no induction of TNF-α, IL-1, IL-6, or tissue factor genes was detectable (110,111).

At present the explanation for these different results in cytokine production following in vitro infection of Mϕ with HIV-1 is uncertain. Some investigators have attributed the increased cytokine release to the presence of contaminating endotoxin in culture media or viral preparations (109,110). Other explanations may lie in the different experimental systems used. Studies with positive results, showing induction of cytokines, have used partially purified virus preparations of HIV-1 propagated in T cells (103,105,106). Thus it may be important to separate virus particles from certain cellular factors (e.g., IFN) that could interfere with induction. Alternatively, viral isolates that have been adapted for in vitro propagation in Mϕ may have lost their ability to induce monokines. Further studies are needed to demonstrate the exact requirements for in vitro monokine induction by HIV. Certain viral characteristics, cofactors, such as lymphokines, or host cell characteristics may be required for altered monokine release.

ROLE OF CYTOKINES IN THE IMPAIRED GROWTH AND RESPONSIVENESS OF T CELLS IN HIV INFECTION

T Cell Growth

The loss of $CD4^+$ T (helper) lymphocytes from the blood and tissues is a prominent consequence of advanced HIV infection that is still not clearly understood.

Low CD4$^+$ T cell counts (less than 200 mm^{-3}) are often an indication of the development of AIDS with opportunistic infections (112). In advanced AIDS with opportunistic infections, the depletion often includes CD8$^+$ T (cytotoxic-suppressor) T cells and all lymphoid populations (112). Infection of CD4$^+$ T lymphocytes with HIV can be directly cytopathic by lysis (113) or syncytia formation (114), yet in light of the low number of productively infected cells, except in the stage of advanced AIDS, the direct cytopathic effects alone cannot explain the massive loss of CD4$^+$ T cells. [It has been calculated that a decrease from the normal 1000 CD4$^+$ T cells mm^{-3} of blood to 500 represents a loss of 2.5×10^9 cells, which must operate continuously, since about 5×10^8 CD4$^+$ lymphocytes are normally produced daily (115).] In addition to direct cytopathic effects by HIV, mechanisms to prevent the production of CD4$^+$ T cells from stem cells or to continuously destroy or inhibit the expansion of CD4$^+$ cells are likely to contribute (116–118).

Defective growth (119) and abnormalities in maturation of different hematopoietic lineages have been observed in AIDS (120–126). Even before the stage of AIDS and in the absence of cytotoxic therapy, a significant loss of hematopoietic progenitors, including granulocyte-macrophage colony-forming units (CFU), megakaryocyte CFU, and erythroid progenitors, can be detected in peripheral blood (127). Decreased in vitro colony formation by PHA-stimulated T lymphocytes is also an early abnormality after HIV infection (128). Progenitors of T cells in the bone marrow have been found to be susceptible to HIV infection (129,130) and may be directly affected by HIV. However, the defective production of other lineages is more likely to involve inadequate stimulation by hematopoietic cytokines (e.g., colony-stimulating factors and interleukins). More cytokine studies are needed to establish their role in the mechanism of impaired hematopoiesis. In addition to impaired stimulation or responsiveness, inhibitory cytokines spontaneously produced by adherent Mϕ from AIDS patients may play a role in the decreased proliferation of T colony-forming cells (T-CFC). Lunardi-Iskandar et al. (131) showed that the removal of adherent cells from peripheral blood mononuclear cells can enhance the in vitro proliferation of T-CFC from AIDS patients. Adherent cells from AIDS patients or conditioned media from these cells were found to inhibit T-CFC from HIV-negative individuals. In these studies, both IL-2 receptor expression and IL-2 production of normal mitogen-stimulated T cells were also inhibited by the adherent cell-conditioned media. Not only CD4$^+$ T cells but also CD8$^+$DR$^+$ T cells from AIDS patients are defective in their capacity to form colonies in vitro (132). This impaired proliferation of CD8$^+$DR$^+$ T cells cannot be corrected by stimulation with exogenous IL-2 or anti-CD3 monoclonal antibody and IL-4 (132). The CD8$^+$DR$^+$ IL-2R subset of T lymphocytes, which may be important in the control of viral infection, may be preactivated in vivo and refractory to further activation signals in vitro. Alternatively, this subset may be regulated by inhibitory cytokines, such as TGF-β (133), which can be selectively induced in this subset. In contrast to these studies, which used bulk mononuclear cells as feeder cell for T clones, Langhoff et al. (134) used dendritic cell-enriched fractions from normal PBMC as feeders for T cells from AIDS patients and controls. Dendritic cells are efficient antigen-presenting accessory cells derived from bone marrow precursors. In the presence of normal dendritic cells, CD4$^+$ T cells from HIV-seropositive individuals, even those with

AIDS and reduced CD4$^+$ T cell numbers compared to controls, exhibited a normal cloning efficiency and proliferative capacity. Further, when high doses of HIV-1 were added to T cell clones from control subjects, no cytopathic effects were observed in the presence of dendritic cells, but CD4$^+$ T cells were markedly reduced in bulk mononuclear cell cultures. These experiments suggest that growth inhibitory effects associated with HIV infection may be mediated through cytokines produced by certain mononuclear cells, including adherent monocyte-macrophages (Mϕ), and other accessory cells, the nonadherent dendritic cells, can provide growth-promoting cytokines.

T Cell Responses in HIV Infection

The process of specific T cell activation and expansion requires the production of IL-2 by T cells and expression of high-affinity T cell receptors (135). Abnormalities of IL-2 receptor expression (136) and defects in the ability of T lymphocytes from AIDS patients to generate the cytokines IL-2 and IFN-γ upon stimulation (73,136–141) have been proposed to play an important role in the pathogenesis of AIDS (1). However, the assessment of T cell function in AIDS is complicated by the loss of CD4$^+$ T cells, and studies carried out on heterogeneous cell populations with abnormal CD4/CD8 T cell ratios and monocyte populations are difficult to interpret because they do not provide information on the proportion of cells expressing a given function. In some studies using equivalent numbers of T cells from AIDS patients and controls stimulated with mitogen in vitro, similar levels of IL-2 production were found in the two groups (141). Tumor cell lines infected with HIV in vitro were also shown to produce similar levels of IL-2 mRNA compared to uninfected cells (142). Using cloned T cells from peripheral blood of AIDS patients, Maggi et al. (120) found that the majority of the cloned cells produced lower amounts of IFN-γ and IL-2 but showed normal or enhanced production of lymphokines promoting B cell proliferation.

Defective IL-2 production and responsiveness of T cells in HIV infection appear to be limited to certain stimuli. Studies have shown that the in vitro proliferative response to pokeweed mitogen (PWM) and antigen presented in the context of self MHC (major histocompatibility complex) can be lost early in HIV infection, even in the absence of a numerical loss of CD4$^+$ T cells (141,143). Similarly, T cells from certain AIDS patients showed defective IL-2 production and proliferation in the autologous mixed lymphocyte response (144,145). The response to allogeneic cells and PHA decreases at later stages of HIV infection, as clinical symptoms occur (143,146,147). An early selective defect in the T cell antigen receptor (TCR)-mediated activation of T cells was also observed using immobilized anti-CD3 monoclonal antibody-induced T cell proliferation and differentiation to cytotoxic effector cells (148). The decreased response to antigen or anti-CD3 is associated with decreased IL-2 production (148–150) and can, at least in vitro, be largely restored by addition of recombinant IL-2 (143,148). T cell responsiveness to soluble antigen and cytotoxic T cell production can also be restored by costimulation with alloantigens (143,151) or monoclonal antibody to CD45 (152). This suggests that antigen-specific T cells are present (at least at earlier stages of HIV infection) but cannot be fully activated by addition of antigens alone. As in impaired hematopoiesis, the mechanism for the selective defect in T cell responsiveness needs further investigation. Some findings suggest that suppressive cells or cytokines may be involved in the selective impairment of antigen-specific T cell responses but not in the loss of mitogen (PHA) responsiveness seen in advanced disease (153). A number of factors that inhibit T cell responses associated with HIV infection have been found in serum (154–156) and PBMC cultures from AIDS patients (79,80,157–161). In later stages of infection, when not only memory cells but also naive T cells are depleted (162–164), T cells deteriorate further and appear to exhibit intrinsic activation defects (1,148). Signal transduction may be affected by HIV or viral products (e.g., envelope gp120). In vitro studies suggest that gp120 can cause activation of T cells, B cells, and Mϕ. These chronically activated cells may become unresponsive to other stimuli (reviewed in Ref. 165).

ROLE OF CYTOKINES IN AIDS-RELATED KAPOSI'S SARCOMA

An important aspect of AIDS is its association with malignant disease, primarily Kaposi's sarcoma (KS) and malignant lymphoma. Several lines of evidence suggest that cytokines may play an essential role in the development of KS. When grown in vitro, cells derived from KS lesions of AIDS patients release several cytokines, including IL-1, basic fibroblast growth factor (bFGF) (166), and IL-6 (167). IL-6 can also be detected in sections from tumor-involved areas (167). AIDS KS cells express IL-6 receptors, and their growth can be stimulated by IL-6 (167). Further, the HIV-1 *tat* gene introduced into the germline of mice induced skin lesions resembling KS (168). The *tat* gene product (Tat) can also directly stimulate proliferation of AIDS KS cells in vitro (168). Although these in vitro experiments cannot definitively prove a mechanism for tumorigenesis in vivo, they suggest a role for HIV-Tat and cytokines (IL-6, IL-1, and bFGF) in the induction and/or progression of KS in HIV-1-infected individuals. An analogous mechanism involving the release of Tat and cytokines from HIV-1-infected Mϕ or T cells may also contribute to the development of AIDS-associated B cell lymphomas.

EFFECT OF CYTOKINES ON HIV REPLICATION

The reactivation of a latent or low-level chronic infection to a highly productive infection appears to be a central feature in the pathogenesis of AIDS. Several lines of evidence demonstrate that viral replication is enhanced by cellular activation signals, including mitogen stimulation (113,169,170), phorbol esters (171), and antigen stimulation (172). An understanding of how cellular activation signals interact with HIV gene activation is essential to developing strategies to control HIV replication. The role of cytokines in cellular activation has prompted investigation into whether various cytokines can directly or indirectly enhance or inhibit HIV gene transcription and viral replication.

Of the cytokines studied, TNF-α and the colony-stimulating factors appear to have the most consistent effect on upregulation of HIV replication, but these effects differ depending on the type of HIV-infected cell studied. Several studies have shown that TNF-α is the major cytokine that enhances HIV replication in

T cells. In chronic infection of the T cell lines, MOLT-4, Jurkat, H9, and CCRF-CEM, enhancement of viral replication was induced with TNF-α, and this effect was correlated with increased sensitivity to TNF-induced cytotoxicity (173). TNF-α also upregulated viral replication in acutely infected MOLT-4 cells (174) and completely blocked the antiviral activity of azidothymidine (AZT) in infected MOLT-4 cells (175). Supernatants from LPS- and viral antigen-stimulated monocyte cultures upregulated HIV reverse transcriptase (RT) expression in chronically infected promonocytic (U1) and T cell (ACH-2) lines (176,177). Reversal of TNF-α activity by a neutralizing antiserum to TNF-α inhibited the upregulation of HIV replication induced by crude supernatants of LPS-stimulated macrophages in ACH-2 cells, indicating that TNF-α was the major cytokine in these supernatants responsible for this upregulation (176). Direct addition of recombinant TNF-α and TNF-β were found to stimulate viral replication in ACH-2, whereas PDGF, IFN-γ, IL-4, IL-3, IL-2, or IL-1 had no effect (178). IL-1 has been shown to have a weak enhancing effect on HIV transcription and to synergize with TNF-α in a chronically infected T cell line MOLT-4 (179).

Although TNF appears to be the major cytokine capable of significantly enhancing viral replication in T cell models of chronic HIV infection, other cytokines in addition to TNF appear to upregulate viral expression in acute and chronically infected monocytes and monocytoid cell lines. TNF-α and GM-CSF increased HIV RT activity in the chronically infected promonocytic cell line U1 (180,181). The colony-stimulating factors, M-CSF, GM-CSF, and IL-3, enhanced HIV p24 production in normal blood monocytes acutely infected with a monocytotropic HIV strain (182). Perno et al. (100) extended this observation, showing that although GM-CSF potentiated viral antigen expression in infection in vitro of peripheral blood monocyte cultures with both monocytotropic and lymphocytotropic strains of HIV, GM-CSF enhanced the antiviral effect of AZT. These studies suggest that GM-CSF alters the metabolism of AZT and endogenous deoxynucleotide triphosphates, which results in enhanced antiviral activity. CSF-1 treatment of peripheral blood monocyte cultures was found to enhance the susceptibility of these cultures to HIV infection by peripheral blood mononuclear cells from HIV-infected patients (98). IL-6 has been shown to upregulate HIV replication reflected by RT activity in an acutely infected promonocytic cell line THP-1 (183) and synergize with TNF-α and GM-CSF in viral expression in U1 cells by a posttranscriptional mechanism (184).

Although most studies support the observation that TNF and colony-stimulating factors can enhance viral replication, some studies report conflicting results. In one study, high concentrations of TNF-α caused inhibition of HIV replication in an acutely infected T cell line (HUT 78 and T cells cloned from healthy seronegative individuals) (180), and Hammer et al. (185) reported that GM-CSF downregulated HIV RT activity and viral antigen expression in a model of an acutely infected promonocytic cell line U937. It is not yet known whether these differences arise from the differences in model systems being studied or represent the complex interaction of multiple factors.

The enhancer region of the long terminal repeat (LTR) region of the HIV genome contains multiple elements that are binding sites for cellular nuclear binding factors. Cellular activation can lead to activation and induction of nuclear proteins, and this may be one mechanism by which cellular activation can enhance viral transcription. The phorbol ester PMA has been shown to upregulate viral replication and to activate a DNA binding protein indistinguishable from the nuclear factor κB (NF-κB) (171,186). This cellular factor binds to an 11 base pair sequence present in the immunoglobulin light-chain enhancer and related sequences in other cellular and viral enhancers. NF-κB can activate viral transcription by binding to NF-κB-like sites in the HIV enhancer of the long terminal repeat region of HIV (186). The cytokines TNF-α and IL-1β have been shown to be physiological activators of NF-κB and can activate the HIV LTR in cells transfected with HIV constructs (187,188). Gel mobility shift assays have demonstrated that TNF-α enhancement of HIV replication in ACH-2 cells is associated with the induction of nuclear factors binding to NF-κB sites of the HIV LTR (189).

Although the cytokines GM-CSF, TNF-α, and IL-6 appear to upregulate HIV genome expression, others, most notably members of the interferon family, appear to downregulate HIV replication under certain conditions. Pretreatment of cells with IFN inhibited infection, reflected by viral antigen expression, release of infectious virus, or viral mRNA in acutely infected T cell lines (H9, HUT 78, and $CD4^+$ T cell clones from an HIV-seronegative individual) (180,190). Pretreatment with IFN-γ and α suppressed viral expression in acutely infected PBMC, T cell lines, and U937 cell lines (191). However, IFN-γ had a minimal effect against viral infection in acutely infected peripheral blood mononuclear cells. IFN-α, β, and γ inhibited acute HIV infection in normal monocytes purified from peripheral blood from a seronegative individual when added as late as 3 days after infection (192). Koyanagi et al. (182) similarly demonstrated IFN-γ suppression of p24 antigen release when IFN-γ was continuously added following infection. IFN-γ also inhibited viral RT release by a chronically infected promonocytic cell line (U937) (185). Pretreatment and continued exposure with both these cytokines completely inhibited viral replication. When the cytokine exposure was discontinued, however, viral replication ultimately reached the same level as untreated cultures, suggesting that viral binding and entrance into the cell was not affected (185). Similarly, viral antigen expression in an acutely infected T cell line MT-4 was transiently suppressed by IFN-γ but returned to untreated levels after day 5 following infection (193). Poli et al. (194) showed that IFN-γ suppressed the release of viral antigens and virions in the chronically infected cell lines U1 and ACH-2, but increased cell-associated viral proteins were found, implying that IFN-γ inhibits a late stage of HIV replication. These in vitro studies clearly demonstrate that cessation of addition of IFN to culture medium permits viral replication to proceed, prompting different approaches to maintain or amplify the inhibitory effect of IFN-γ. Bednarik et al. (195) developed a model linking IFN-α_2 production to HIV replication in a T cell line and demonstrated complete inhibition of viral replication over a 14 day period. Johnson et al. (196) reported long-term (>28 day) suppression of viral replication in the H9 T cell line when a combination of IFN-α, AZT, and recombinant soluble CD4 was added at the time of viral infection.

Recent work has suggested that TGF-β can selectively inhibit GM-CSF- and IL-6-induced viral replication in U1 cells but appears to upregulate viral expression in acutely infected cells (197). TGF-β was found to have no effect on

TNF-α-induced viral expression, suggesting that the site of action of TGF-β is likely to be posttranscriptional.

CYTOKINE THERAPY IN AIDS

The development of effective therapies to correct immune defects and suppress HIV replication is a major goal in the treatment of patients with HIV-associated disease. Cytokines that stimulate defective immune mechanisms and hematopoiesis as well as cytokines that inhibit viral replication could be of great benefit.

Interleukin-2

The potential of IL-2 administration in restoring the diminished $CD4^+$ T cell population and defective T cell responses has been examined in several clinical trials (198–200). These studies determined the maximum tolerated dose for rIL-2 but did not establish a beneficial effect of recombinant IL-2 (rIL-2) therapy. In a study with 87 patients with AIDS receiving intravenous rIL-2 three times a week for 8 weeks, no changes in T cell numbers and responsiveness were observed and there was no clinical benefit (201). In a similar study it was noted that serum INF-γ activity was increased significantly following IL-2 infusion, but T cell numbers and subsets did not change (202). Murphy et al. (203) found that serious nonopportunistic bacterial infection was an unexpectedly frequent complication during intravenous IL-2 therapy. This finding cannot be explained by any known IL-2 effects. Further studies are needed to explain the in vivo effects of IL-2. However, with these results strongly suggesting deleterious effects of IL-2, studies must examine other cytokines or cytokine combinations involving IL-2 for restorative effects in HIV infection.

Interferons

Based on their antiviral, antiproliferative, and immunomodulatory properties in many in vivo and in vitro systems, interferons have received major attention as potential therapeutic agents in AIDS. Ho et al. (191) demonstrated that recombinant interferon-αA (rIFN-αA) inhibited HIV replication in peripheral blood mononuclear cells in vitro, and the combination of interferon-α and antiviral drugs can result in synergistic inhibition (196,204,205).

Studies of animal retroviruses have shown that interferons are active antiviral agents that appear to act at the level of assembly and release of virus particles (206). With in vivo treatment in an experimental murine model 4 h after retrovirus exposure, combined interferon-α and AZT therapy was protective against disease and rechallenge in mice infected with the Rauscher leukemia virus (207). Such encouraging results suggest that early combination therapy may also have the potential to prevent disease activities in HIV infection.

Interferon-α preparations were studied for the treatment of AIDS-associated Kaposi's sarcoma as early as 1981. Krown et al. (208) reported that rIFNA-α induced various degrees of tumor regression, including complete remission in several patients with Kaposi's sarcoma. Since this study, several reports have shown the efficacy of IFN-α treatment in some patients with Kaposi's sarcoma, showing tumor regression in 24–42% of patients (208–212). Studies combining IFN-α with AZT are also in progress (213).

Fibroblast IFN-β has many of the same effects as IFN-α but appears to be better tolerated at high doses than IFN-α (214). Initial trials in patients with Kaposi's sarcoma showed some antiretroviral activity but only minimal antitumor activity (214).

IFN-γ produced by T lymphocytes has been shown in animal models to stimulate macrophage tumoricidal and microbicidal activity (215,216), natural killer (NK) cell activity, and T and B lymphocyte responses (217–219). With cells from AIDS patients, significant enhancing effects of IFN-γ on monocyte microbicidal and tumoricidal activity, surface HLA-DR expression of monocytes-macrophages, and T lymphocyte responsiveness in vitro were observed (reviewed in Ref. 220). Other in vitro studies demonstrated that IFN-γ inhibits virus production in infected peripheral blood monocytes-Mφ and in latently infected U1 promonocytic cells (derived from the U937 tumor cell line).

These in vitro findings showing both immunostimulatory and antiretroviral effects support the study of IFN-γ in HIV-infected individuals. A phase I trial in patients with Kaposi's sarcoma and AIDS showed considerable dose-dependent toxicity and depression of granulocyte and lymphocyte counts (221). Some evidence of enhancing activity on monocyte-mediated cytotoxicity was found, but no clinically apparent tumor regression was noted.

In a phase I/II study of IFN-γ in 21 patients with AIDS, antiviral toxicity was observed (220). A clinical response was found in 3 of 17 patients with Kaposi's sarcoma. Although these studies failed to show consistent clinical responses, further studies are needed to include longer courses of therapy and the effect of IFN-γ in patients at less advanced stages of HIV infection.

Colony-Stimulating Factors (CSF)

CSFs are cytokines required for in vitro proliferation and differentiation of hematopoietic precursor cells (222,223). Since hematopoiesis is frequently impaired in HIV infection and may be further exacerbated by AZT, CSFs could be beneficial by stimulating hematopoiesis and correcting the cytopenias associated with AIDS. Trials involving granulocyte-macrophage CSF have resulted in dose-dependent increases in circulating leukocytes with increases in mature and immature neutrophils, eosinophils, and monocytes (224,225). Prolonged therapy in leukopenic HIV-infected patients increased leukocyte counts and showed no adverse effects of long-term (6 month) administration (226). There was no consistent modulation of HIV p24 antigen levels in this study. This point is of major concern for therapy in view of the in vitro activities of GM-CSF on HIV expression. As discussed previously, GM-CSF can suppress virus expression in the promonocytoid U937 tumor cell line (185) but has also been found to enhance virus production in primary monocytes and cell lines (100,181,182).

Current and future therapeutic approaches include the combination of cytokines (e.g., G-CSF and erythropoietin) and cytokines known to influence primitive hematopoietic cells, including IL-3 and IL-1 (227), IL-4 (228–230), and IL-6 (231,232). Combination therapy with cytokines and pharmacological agents that affect different steps in the HIV infective and replicative cycle also hold promise in the treatment of this disease (196).

SUMMARY

Studies on the immune dysfunction in HIV infection have shown early defects in antigen-specific responses by $CD4^+$ helper T cells. The mechanism for this selective impairment has not yet been clearly established. Cytokine studies show defective IL-2 induction and production and at least partial restoration with IL-2 and stimulation of impaired T cell growth by dendritic cells. Cytokines released by activated Mϕ from AIDS patients can selectively inhibit antigen-specific responses and may contribute to the immunodeficiency.

The studies of Mϕ in HIV infection have provided evidence for Mϕ activation and increased monokine release in vivo and in vitro. The well-characterized monokines that have been found to be elevated (to date mainly, IL-1, IL-6, and TNF-α) are known to stimulate B lymphocytes and to mediate fever and cachexia. These factors are likely to act as mediators in B cell hyperactivity, fever, and tissue destruction, which are prominent symptoms of AIDS.

The effects of cytokines on the enhancement of HIV replication appear to act at different regulatory sites in the HIV infectious cycle. TNF-α appears to upregulate HIV genome expression by activating cellular transcriptional factors that bind to the HIV enhancer region, and some studies have suggested that GM-CSF and IL-6 act posttranscriptionally. The cytokines IFN and TGF-β, which downregulate HIV replication, appear to act posttranscriptionally, and IFN appears to prevent the release of virus from the cell but does not prevent infectious virus from being assembled intracellularly (21).

HIV replication and cytokine production and activity appear to be interconnected, supporting the concept that HIV infection subverts the cellular activation machinery to help direct viral gene expression. Predicting the net effects of different cytokines on in vivo HIV infection based on in vitro studies may be misleading because of the complexity of the cytokine network and the pleiotropic activities of most cytokines. Many cytokines work in a paracrine or autocrine fashion and can lead to the concurrent presence of multiple factors with sometimes opposing effects on cell activation and HIV replication. In the future, however, understanding the interdependence of HIV infection and cytokines and the immune system may lead to the development of therapeutic strategies aimed at treatment of HIV-related disease.

REFERENCES

1. Margolick JB, Lane HC, Fauci AS. Immunopathogenesis of HTLV-III/LAV infection. In: Gallo RC, Haseltine W, eds. Viruses and human cancer. New York: Alan R. Liss, 1987:59–79.
2. Ho DD, Pomerantz RJ, Kaplan JC. Pathogenesis of infection with human immunodeficiency virus. N Engl J Med 987; 317:278–86.
3. Seligmann M, Pinching AJ, Rosen FS, et al. Immunology of human immunodefi-

ciency virus infection and the acquired immunodeficiency syndrome. An update. Ann Int Med 987; 107:234–42.

4. Levy JA. The human immunodeficiency viruses: detection and pathogenesis. In: Levy JA, ed. AIDS: pathogenesis and treatment. New York: Marcel Dekker. 1989:159–229.
5. Fauci AS. The human immunodeficiency virus: infectivity and mechanism of pathogenesis. Science 1988; 239:617–22.
6. Klatzmann D, Barre-Sinoussi F, Nugeyere MT, et al. Selective tropism of lymphadenopathy associated virus (LAV) for helper-inducer T lymphocytes. Science 1984; 255:59–63.
7. Gallo RC, Salahuddin SZ, Popovic M, et al. Frequent detection and isolation of cytopathic retroviruses (HTLV-III) from patients with AIDS or at risk for AIDS. Science 1984; 224:500–3.
8. Ho DD, Rota TR, Hirsch MS. Infection of monocyte/macrophages by human lymphotropic virus type III. J Clin Invest 1986; 77:1712–5.
9. Armstrong JA, Horne R. Follicular dendritic cells and virus-like particles in AIDS-related lymphadenopathy. Lancet 1984; 2:370–2.
10. Tenner-Racz K, Racz P, Schmidt H, et al. Immunohistochemical, electron microscopic and in situ hybridization evidence for the involvement of lymphatics in the spread of HIV-1. AIDS 1988; 2:299–309.
11. Koenig S, Gendelman HE, Orenstein JM, et al. Detection of AIDS virus in macrophages in brain tissue from AIDS patients with encephalopathy. Science 1986; 233:1089–93.
12. Wiley CA, Schrier RD, Nelson JA, Lambert PW, Oldstone MBA. Cellular localization of human immunodeficiency virus infection within the brains of acquired immune deficiency virus patient. Proc Natl Acad Sci U S A 1986; 83:7089–93.
13. Meyenhofer MF, Epstein LG, Cho E-S, Sharer LR. Ultrastructural morphology and intracellular production of human immunodeficiency virus (HIV) in brain. J Neuropathol Exp Neurol 1987; 46:474–84.
14. Chayt KJ, Harper ME, Marselle LM, et al. Detection of HTLV-III RNA in lungs of patients with AIDS and pulmonary involvement. JAMA 1986; 256:2356–9.
15. Salahuddin SZ, Rose RM, Groopman JE, Markham PD, Gallo RC. Human T lymphotropic virus type III. Infection of human alveolar macrophages. Blood 1986; 68:281–4.
16. Tschachler E, Groh V, Popovic M, et al. Epidermal Langerhans cells. A target for HTLV-III/LAV infection. J Invest Dermatol 1987; 88:233–7.
17. Gartner S, Markovits P, Markovits M, Kaplan H, Gallo RC, Popovic M. The role of mononuclear phagocytes in HTLVIII/LAV infection. Science 1986; 223:215–9.
18. Pauza CD. HIV persistence in monocytes leads to pathogenesis and AIDS. Cell Immunol 1988; 112:414–24.
19. Harper M, Marselle L, Gallo R, Wong-Staal F. Detection of lymphocytes expressing human T-lymphotropic virus type III in lymph nodes and peripheral blood from infected individuals by in situ hybridization. Proc Natl Acad Sci U S A 1986; 83:772–6.
20. Schnittman SM, Psallidopoulos MC, Lane HC, et al. The reservoir for HIV-1 in human peripheral blood is a T cell that maintains expression of CD4. Science 1989; 245:305–8.
21. Koenig S, Gendelman HE, Orenstein JM, et al. Detection of AIDS virus in macrophages in brain tissue from AIDS patients with encephalopathy. Science 1986; 233:1089–93.
22. Cameron PU, Dawkins RL, Armstrong JA, Bonifacio E. Western blot profiles, lymph

node ultrastructure and viral expression in HIV infected patients; a correlative study. Clin Exp Immunol 1987; 68:465–78.
23. Plata F, Autran B, Martins L, et al. AIDS virus-specific cytotoxic T lymphocytes in lung disorders. Nature 1987; 328:348–51.
24. Bowen DL, Lane HC, Fauci AS. Immunologic features of AIDS. In: DeVita JVT, Hillman S, Rosenberg SA, eds. AIDS: etiology, diagnosis, treatment and prevention. Philadelphia: J. B. Lippincott, 1985: 89–109.
25. Mizuma H, Litwin S, Zolla-Pazner S. B cell activation in HIV infection: relationship of spontaneous immunoglobulin secretion to various immunologic parameters. Clin Exp Immonol 1988; 71:410–6.
26. Edelman AS, Zolla-Pazner S. AIDS: a syndrome of immune dysregulation, dysfunction, and deficiency. FASEB J 1989; 3:22–30.
27. Amadori A, Zamarchi R, Ciminale V, et al. HIV-1-specific B-cell activation: a major constituent of spontaneous B cell activation during HIV-1 infection. J Immunol 1989; 143:2146–52.
28. Gabauzda D, Ho D, de la Monte S, Hirsch M, Rota T, Sobel R. Immunohistochemical identification of HTLV-III antigens in brains of patients with AIDS. Ann Neurol 1986; 20:289–95.
29. Klatzmann D, Gluckman JC. HIV infection: facts and hypotheses. Immunol Today 1986; 7:291–6.
30. Sei Y, Petrella RJ, Tsang P, Bekesi JG, Yokohama MM. Monocytes in AIDS. N Engl J Med 1986; 315:1611–2.
31. Davidson BL, Kline PL, Rowland J, Quinn TC. Surface markers of monocyte function and activation in AIDS. J Infect Dis 1988; 158:483–6.
32. Eales L-J, Farrant J, Helbert M, Pinching AJ. Peripheral blood dendritic cells in persons with AIDS and AIDS related complex: loss of high intensity class II antigen expression and function. Clin Exp Immunol 1988; 71:423–7.
33. Rich EA, Toossi Z, Fujiwara H, Hanigosky R, Lederman MM, Ellner JJ. Defective accessory function of monocytes in human immunodeficiency virus-related disease syndromes. J Lab Clin Med 1988; 112:174–81.
34. Prince HE, Moody DJ, Shubin BI, Fahey JL. Defective monocyte function in acquired immune deficiency syndrome (AIDS): evidence from a monocye-dependent T-cell proliferative system. J Clin Immunol 1985; 5:21–5.
35. Mann DL, Gartner S, LeSane F, Blattner WA, Popovic M. Cell surface antigens and function of monocytes and a monocyte-like cell line before and after infection with HIV. Clin Immunol Immunopathol 1990; 54:174–83.
36. Offenberger J, Lieu T, Frick O, Ammann AJ. Impaired monocyte-to-macrophage maturation in patients with lymphadenopathy syndrome. J Clin Immunol 1986; 6:467–71.
37. Smith P, Ohura K, Masur H, Lane HC, Fauci AS, Wahl SM. Monocyte function in acquired immunodeficiency syndrome: defective chemotaxis. J Clin Infect 1984; 74:2121–8.
38. Washburn RG, Tuazon CU, Bennett JE. Phagocytic and fungicidal activity of monocytes from patients with acquired imunodeficiency syndrome. J Infect Dis 1985; 151:565–6.
39. Poli G, Bottazzi B, Acero R, et al. Monocyte function in intravenous drug abusers with lymphadenopathy syndrome and in patients with acquired immunodeficiency syndrome: selective impairment of chemotaxis. Clin Exp Immunol 1985; 62:136–43.
40. Bender BS, Davidson BL, Kline R, Brown C, Quinn TC. Role of the mononuclear phagocyte system in the immunopathogenesis of human immunodeficiency virus

infection and the acquired immunodeficiency syndrome. Rev Infect Dis 1988; 10:1142–54.

41. Estevez ME, Ballart IJ, Diez RA, Planes N, Scaglione C, Sen L. Early defect of phagocytic cell function in subjects at risk for acquired immunodeficiency syndrome. Scand J Immunol 1986; 24:215–21.
42. Grieco MH, Reddy MH, Kothari HG, Lange M, Buimovici-Klein E, William D. Elevated β_2-microglobulin and lysozyme levels in patients with acquired immune deficiency syndrome. Clin Immunol Immunopathol 1984; 32:174–84.
43. Huber C, Batchelor JR, Fuchs D, et al. Immune response-associated production of neopterin. Release from macrophages primarily under control of interferon-gamma. J Exp Med 1984; 160:310–6.
44. Fuchs D, Hansen A, Reibnegger G, Werner ER, Dierich MP, Wachter H. Neopterin as a marker for activated cell-mediated immunity: application in HIV infection (review). Immunol Today 1988; 9:150–5.
45. Wachter H, Fuchs D, Hansen A, Reibuegger G, Werner ER. Neopterin as marker for activation of cellular immunity: immunological basis and clinical application (review). Adv Clin Chem 1989; 27:81–141.
46. Bogner JR, Matuschke A, Heinrich B, Eberle E, Goebel FD. Serum neopterin levels as predictor of AIDS. Klin Wochenschr 1988; 66:1015–8.
47. Fuchs D, Spira TJ, Hansen A, et al. Neopterin as a predictive marker for disease progression in human immunodeficiency virus type 1 infection. Clin Chem 1989; 35:1746–9.
48. Fuchs D, Hansen A, Reibnegger G, et al. Interferon-gamma concentrations are increased in sera from individuals infected with human immunodeficiency virus type 1. J AIDS 1989; 2:158–62.
49. Fuchs D, Shearer GM, Boswell RN, Clerici M, Reibnegger G, Werner R. Increased serum neopterin in patients with HIV-1 infection is correlated with reduced in vitro interleukin-2 production. Clin Exp Immunol 1990; 80:44–8.
50. DeStefano E, Friedman RM, Friedman-Kien AE, et al. Acid labile human leukocyte interferon in homosexual men with Kaposi's sarcoma and lymphadenopathy. J Infect Dis 1982; 146:451–5.
51. Eyster ME, Goedert JJ, Poon MC, Preble OT. Acid-labile alpha interferon: a possible marker for the acquired immune deficiency syndrome in hemophiliac patients. N Engl J Med 1983; 309:583–6.
52. Capobianchi MR, DeMarco F, DiMarco P, Dianzani F. Acid-labile human interferon alpha production by peripheral blood mononuclear cells stimulated by HIV-infected cells. Arch Virol 1988; 99:9–19.
53. Lau AS, Livesey JF. Endotoxin induction of tumor necrosis factor is enhanced by acid-labile interferon-α in acquired immunodeficiency syndrome. J Clin Invest 1989; 84:738–43.
54. Read SE, Williams BRG, Coates RA, et al. Elevated levels of interferon-induced 2-5A synthetase in generalized persistent lymphadenopathy and AIDS. J Infect Dis 1985; 152:466–72.
55. Allen JB, McCartney-Francis N, Smith PD, et al. Expression of interleukin 2 receptors by monocytes from patients with acquired immunodeficiency syndrome and induction of monocyte interleukin 2 receptors by human immumodeficiency virus in vitro. J Clin Invest 1990; 85:192–9.
56. Hermann F, Cannistra SA, Levine H, Griffin JD. Expression of interleukin-2 receptors and binding of interleukin-2 by gamma interferon-induced human leukemic and normal monocytic cells. J Exp Med 1985; 162:1111–6.
57. Wahl SM, McCartney-Francis N, Hunt DA, Smith PD, Wahl LM, Katona IM. Mon-

ocyte interleukin-2 receptor gene expression and interleukin-2 augmentation of microbicidal activity. J Immunol 1987; 139:1342–7.
58. Holter W, Goldman CK, Casabo L, Nelson DL, Green WC, Waldman TA. Expression of functional IL-2 receptors by lipopolysaccharide and interferon-stimulated human monocytes. J Immunol 1987; 138:2971–2.
59. Waage A, Halstensen A, Espevik T. Association between tumor necrosis factor in serum and fatal outcome in patients with meningococcal disease. Lancet 1987; 1:355–7.
60. Balkwill F, Burke F, Talbot D, et al. Evidence for tumour necrosis factor/cachectin production in cancer. Lancet 1987; 2:1229–32.
61. Scuderi P, Lam KS, Ryan KJ, et al. Raised serum levels of tumour necrosis factor in parasitic infections, Lancet 1986; 1:1364–5.
62. Lahdevirta J, Maury CPJ, Teppo A-M, Repo H. Elevated levels of circulating cachetin/tumor necrosis factor in patients with acquired immunodeficiency syndrome. Am J Med 1988; 85:289–91.
63. Maury CPJ, Lahdevirta J. Correlation of serum cytokine levels with haematological abnormalities in human immunodeficiency virus infection. J Intern Med 1990; 227:253–7.
64. Mintz M, Rapaport R, Oleske JM, et al. Elevated serum levels of tumor necrosis factor are associated with progressive encephalopathy in children with acquired immunodeficiency syndrome. Am J Dis Child 1989; 143:771–4.
65. Gallo P, Piccinno MG, Krzalic L, Tavolato B. Tumor necrosis factor alpha (TNFα) and neurological diseases. Failure in detecting TNFα in the cerebrospinal fluid from patients with multiple sclerosis, AIDS dementia complex, and brain tumors. J Neuroimmunol 1989; 23:41–4.
66. Gallo P, Frei K, Rordorf C, Lazdins J, Tavolato B, Fontana A. Human immunodeficiency virus type 1 (HIV-1) infection of the central nervous system: an evaluation of cytokines in cerebrospinal fluid. J Neuroimmunol 1989; 23:109–16.
67. Reddy MM, Grieco MH. Neopterin and alpha and beta interleukin 1 levels in sera of patients with human immunodeficiency virus infection. J Clin Microbiol 1989; 27:1919–23.
68. Gery I, Lepe-Zuniga JL. Interleukin 1: uniqueness of its production and spectrum of activities. Lymphokines 1984; 9:109–25.
69. Dinarello CA. Interleukin-1. Rev Infect Dis 1984; 6:51–95.
70. Oppenheim JJ, Kovacs EJ, Matsushima K, Durum SK. There is more than one interleukin 1. Immunol Today 1986; 7:45–56.
71. Mizel SB. Interleukin-1, and T cell activation. Immunol Rev 1982; 63:51–72.
72. Enk C, Gerstoft J, Moller S, Reinvig L. Interleukin 1 activity in the acquired immunodeficiency syndrome. Scand J Immunol 1986; 23:491–7.
73. Alcocer-Varela J, Alarcon-Segovia D, Abud-Mendoza C. Immunoregulatory circuits in the acquired immune deficiency syndrome and related complex. Production of and response to interleukins 1 and 2, NK function and its enhancement by interleukin-2 and kinetics of mixed lymphocyte reaction. Clin Exp Immunol 1985; 60:31–8.
74. Gupta S, Vayuvegula B, Ruhlig M, Thornton M. Interleukin 1 and interleukin 2 production in the acquired immune deficiency syndrome (AIDS) and AIDS-related complex. J Clin Lab Immunol 1987; 22:113–6.
75. Lepe-Zuniga JL, Mansell PWA, Hersh EM. Idiopathic production of interleukin-1 in acquired immune deficiency syndrome. J Clin Microbiol 1987; 25:1695–700.
76. Berman MA, Sandborg CI, Calabia BS, Andrews BS, Friou GJ. Studies of an interleukin 1 inhibitor: characterization and clinical significance. Clin Exp Immunol 1986; 64:136–45.

77. Arend WP, Joslin FG, Thompson RC, Hannum CH. An IL-1 inhibitor from human monocytes. Production and characterization of biologic properties. J Immunol 1989; 143:1851–8.
78. Larrick JW. Native IL-1 inhibitors. Immunol Today 1989; 10:61–2.
79. Berman MA, Sandborg CI, Calabia BS, Andrews BS, Friou GJ. Interleukin 1 inhibitor masks high interleukin 1 production in acquired immunodeficiency syndrome (AIDS). Clin Immunol Immunopathol 1987; 42:133–40.
80. Sandborg CI, Berman MA, Imfeld KL, Cesario TC, Zaldivar F Jr. Interleukin-1 and a 7-kDA T-cell inhibitory monokine reflect disease activity in infection with HIV-1. J AIDS 1990; 3:1148–54.
81. Berman MA, Sandborg CI, Imfeld KL, Zaldivar F Jr. 8 K MW interleukin 1 (IL-1) inhibitor stimulates polyclonal antibody production and inhibits antigen-specific responses. FASEB J 1988; 2:A902.
82. Roux-Lombard P, Modoux C, Cruchaud A, Dayer J-M. Purified blood monocytes from HIV-1-infected patients produce high levels of TNFα and IL-1. Clin Immunol Immunopathol 1989; 50:374–84.
83. Weiss L, Haeffner-Cavaillon N, Laude M, Gilguin J, Kazatchkine MD. HIV infection is associated with the spontaneous production of interleukin-1 (IL-1) in vivo and with an abnormal release of IL-1 alpha in vitro. AIDS 1989; 3:695–9.
84. Lathey JL, Agosti JM, Nelson JA, et al. A selective defect in tissue factor mRNA expression in monocytes from AIDS patients. Clin Immunol Immunopathol 1990; 54:1–13.
85. Cox RA, Anders GT, Cappelli PJ, et al. Production of tumour necrosis factor-alpha and interleukin-1 by alveolar macrophages from HIV-1-infected persons. AIDS Res Hum Retroviruses 1990; 6:431–41.
86. Hober D, Hague A, Wattre P, Beaucaire G, Mouton Y, Capron A. Production of tumour necrosis factor-alpha (TNF-α) and interleukin-1 (IL-1) in patients with AIDS. Enhanced level of TNF-α is related to higher cytotoxic activity. Clin Exp Immunol 1989; 78:329–33.
87. Breen EC, Rezai AR, Nakajima, et al. Infection with HIV is associated with elevated IL-6 levels and production. J Immunol 1990; 144:480–4.
88. Volkman DJ, Schultz J. IgG production in vitro by B cells from HIV infected donors is directed against HIV envelope proteins and correlated to high levels of IL-6 production. FASEB J 1990; 4:3278A.
89. Wright SC, Jewett A, Mitsuyasu R, Bonavida B. Spontaneous cytotoxicity and tumor necrosis factor production by peripheral blood monocytes from AIDS patients. J Immunol 1988; 141:99–104.
90. Agostini C, Zambello R, Trentin L, et al. Alveolar macrophages from patients with AIDS and AIDS-related complex constitutively synthesize and release tumor necrosis factor alpha. Am Rev Resp Dis 1991; 144:195–201.
91. Ammann AJ, Palladino MA, Volberding P, Abrams D, Martin NL, Conant M. Tumor necrosis factor alpha and beta in acquired immunodeficiency syndrome (AIDS) and AIDS-related complex. J Clin Immunol 1987; 7:481–5.
92. Voth R, Rossol S, Klein K, et al. Differential gene expression of IFN-α and tumor necrosis factor-α in peripheral blood mononuclear cells from patients with AIDS related complex and AIDS. Immunology 1990; 144:970–5.
93. Donnelly RP, Fenton MJ, Finbloom DS, Gerrard TL. Differential regulation of IL-1 production in human monocytes by IFN-gamma and IL-4. J Immunol 1990; 145:569–75.
94. te Velde AA, Huijbens RJ, Heije K, de Vries JE, Figdor CG. Interleukin-4 (IL-4) inhibits secretion of IL-1 beta, tumor necrosis factor alpha, and IL-6 by human monocytes. Blood 1990; 76:1392–7.

95. Zlotnik A, Fischer M, Rochin N, Zipori D. Evidence for effects of interleukin 4 on macrophages: enhancement of antigen-presenting ability of bone marrow-derived macrophages. J Immunol 1987; 138:4275–9.
96. Hart PH, Vitti, GJ, Burgess DR, Whitty GA, Piccoli DS, Hamilton JA. Potential antiinflammatory effects of interleukin 4: supression of human monocyte tumor necrosis factor A, interleukin 1, and prostaglandin E_2. Proc Natl Acad Sci U S A 1989; 86:3803–7.
97. Essner R, Rhoades K, McBride WH, Morton DL, Economon JS. IL-4 down-regulates IL-1 and TNF gene expression in human monocytes. J Immunol 1989; 142:3857–61.
98. Gendelman HE, Orenstein JM, Martin MA, et al. Efficient isolation and propagation of human immunodeficiency virus on recobminant colony-stimulating factor 1-treated monocytes. J Exp Med 1988; 167:1428–41.
99. Nicholson JKA, Cross GD, Callaway CS, McDougal JS. In vitro infection of human monocytes with human T lymphocytotropic virus type III/lymphadenopathy-associated virus (HTLVIII/LAV). J Immunol 1986; 137:323–9.
100. Perno C-F, Yarchoan R, Cooney DA, et al. Replication of human immunodeficiency virus in monocytes. Granulocyte/macrophage colony-stimulating factor (GM-CSF) potentiates viral production yet enhances the antiviral effect mediated by 3′-azido-2′3′-dideoxythymidine (AZT) and other dideoxynucleoside congeners of thymidine. J Exp Med 1989; 169:933–51.
101. Roy S, Fitz-Gibbon L, Poulin L, Wainberg MA. Infection of human monocytes/macrophages by HIV-1: effect on secretion of IL-1 activity. Immunology 1988; 64:233–9.
102. Locksley RM, Crowe S, Sadick MD, et al. Release of interleukin 1 inhibitory activity (contra-IL-1) by human monocyte-derived macrophages infected with human immunodeficiency virus in vitro and in vivo. J Clin Invest 1988; 82:2097–105.
103. Merrill JE, Koyanagi Y, Chen ISY. Interleukin-1 and tumor necrosis factor α can be induced from mononuclear phagocytes by human immunodeficiency virus type 1 binding to the CD4 receptor. J Virol 1989; 63:4404–8.
104. Klatzman D, Champagne E, Chamaret S, et al. T-lymphocyte T4 molecule behaves as the receptor for human retrovirus LAV. Nature 1984; 312:763–7.
105. Wahl LM, Corcoran ML, Pyle SW, Arthur LO, Harel-Bellan A, Farrar WL. Human immunodeficiency virus glycoprotein (gp 120) induction of monocyte arachidonic acid metabolites and interleukin 1. Proc Natl Acad Sci U S A 1989; 86:621–5.
106. Nakajima K, Martinez-Maza O, Hirano T, et al. Induction of IL-6 (B cell stimulatory factor/IFN-β_2) production by HIV. J Immunol 1989; 142:531–6.
107. Molina J-M, Scadden DT, Byrn R, Dinarello CA, Groopman JE. Production of tumor necrosis factor α and interleukin 1β by monocytic cells infected with human immunodeficiency virus. J Clin Invest 1989; 84:733–7.
108. Molina J-M, Schindler R, Ferrini R, et al. Production of cytokines by peripheral blood monocytes-macrophages infected with human immunodeficiency virus type 1 (HIV-1). J Infect Dis 1990; 161:888–93.
109. Molina J-M, Scadden DT, Amirault C, et al. Human immunodeficiency virus does not induce interleukin-1, interleukin-6, or tumor necrosis factor in mononuclear cells. J Virol 1990; 64:2901–5.
110. Munis JR, Richman DD, Kornbluth RS. Human immunodeficiency virus-1 infection of macrophages in vitro neither induces tumor necrosis factor (TNF)/cachectin expression nor alters TNF/cachectin induction by lipopolysaccharide. J Clin Invest 1990; 85:591–6.
111. Kornbluth RS, Munis JR, Oh PS, Meyland PR, Richman DD. Characterization of a macrophage-tropic HIV strain that does not alter macrophage cytokine production

yet protects macrophages from superinfection by vesicular stomatitis virus. AIDS Res Hum Retroviruses 1990; 6:1023–6.
112. Lane HC, Masur H, Gelman EP. Correlation between immunologic function and clinical subpopulations of patients with the acquired immune deficiency syndrome. Am J Med 1985; 78:417–22.
113. Zagury D, Bernard J, Leonard R, et al. Long-term cultures of HTLV-III-infected T cells: a model of cytopathology of T-cell depletion in AIDS. Science 1986; 231:850–3.
114. Lifson JD, Reyes GR, McGrath MS, Stein BS, Engleman EG. AIDS retrovirus induced cytopathology: giant cell formation and involvement of CD4 antigen. Science 1986; 232:1123–6.
115. Montagnier L. Virological and immunological factors of AIDS pathogenesis. In: Girard M, Valette L, eds. 4e Colloque des cent gardes. Retroviruses of human AIDS and related animal diseases. Lyon, France: Fondation Merieux, 1989:11–7.
116. Haase AT. Pathogenesis of lentivirus infections. Nature 1986; 322:130–6.
117. Klatzman ND, Montagnier L. Approaches to AIDS therapy. Nature 1986; 319:10–1.
118. Zinkernagel RM. Virus-triggered AIDS: a T cell-mediated immunopathology? Immunol Today 1988; 9:370–2.
119. Pantaleo G, Koenig S, Baseler M, Lane HC, Fauci AS. Defective clonogenic potential of $CD8^+$ T lymphocytes in patients with AIDS. Expansion in vivo of a nonclonogenic $CD3^+CD8^+DR^+CD25^-$ T cell population. J Immunol 1990; 144:1696–704.
120. Maggi E, Macchia D, Parronchi P, et al. Reduced production of interleukin 2 and interferon-gamma and enhanced helper activity for IgG synthesis by cloned $CD4^+$ T cells from patients with AIDS. Eur J Immunol 1987; 17:1685–90.
121. Spivak JL, Selonick SE, Quinn TC. Acquired immune deficiency syndrome and pancytopenia. JAMA 1983; 250:3084–7.
122. Spivak JL, Bender BS, Quinn TC. Hematologic abnormalities in the acquired immune deficiency syndrome. Am J Med 1984; 77:224–8.
123. Schneider DR, Picker LJ. Myelodysplasia in the acquired immune deficiency syndrome. Am J Clin Pathol 1985; 84:144–52.
124. Osborne BM, Guarda LA, Butler JJ. Bone marrow biopsies in patients with the acquired immunodeficiency syndrome. Hum Pathol 1984; 15:1048–53.
125. Geller SA, Muller R, Greenberg ML, Siegal FP. Acquired immunodeficiency syndrome. Distinctive features of bone marrow biopsies. Arch Pathol Lab Med 1985; 109:138–41.
126. Leiderman IZ, Greenberg ML, Adelsberg BR, Siegal FP. Defective myelopoiesis in acquired immune deficiency syndrome (AIDS). IN: Gottlieb MS, Groopman JE, ed. Acquired immune deficiency syndrome, UCLA symposium on molecular and cellular biology. New York: Alan R Liss, 1984:281–9.
127. Bagnara GP, Zauli G, Giovannini M, Re CM, Furlini G, LaPlaca M. Early loss of circulating hemopoietic progenitors in HIV-1 infected subjects. Exp Hematol 1990; 18:426–30.
128. Windelstein A, Klein RS, Evans TL, Dixon BW, Holder WL, Weaver LD. Defective in vitro T cell colony formation in the acquired immunodeficiency syndrome. J Immunol 1985; 134:151–6.
129. Folks TM, Kessler SW, Orenstein JM, Justement JS, Jaffe ES, Fauci AS. Infection and replication of HIV-1 in purified progenitor cells of normal human bone marrow. Science 1988; 242:919–22.
130. Lunardi-Iskandar Y, Nugeyerc MT, Georgoulias V, Barre-Sinonssi F, Jasmin C, Chermann JC. Replication of the human immunodeficiency virus 1 and impaired differentiation of T cells after in vitro infection of bone marrow immature T cells. J Clin Invest 1989; 83:610–5.

131. Lunardi-Iskandar Y, Georgoulias V, Vittecoq D, et al. Peripheral blood adherent cells from AIDS patients inhibit normal T-colony growth through decreased expression of interleukin 2-receptors and production of interleukin 2. Leuk Res 1987; 11:753–60.
132. Pantaleo G, Koenig S, Baseler M, Lane HC, Fauci AS. Defective clonogenic potential of $CD8^+$ T lymphocytes in patients with AIDS. Expansion in vivo of a nonclonogenic $CD3^+CD8^+DR^+CD25^-$ T cell population. J Immunol 1990; 144:1696–704.
133. Kehrl JH, Wakefield LM, Roberts AB, Jakowlew S, Alzarez-Mon M. Production of transforming growth factor β by human T lymphocytes and its potential role in the regulation of T cell growth. J Exp Med 1986; 163:1037–50.
134. Langhoff E, McElrath JH, Bos J, et al. Most $CD4^+$ T cells from human immunodeficiency virus-1 infected patients can undergo prolonged clonal expansion. J Clin Invest 1989; 84:1637–43.
135. Greene WC, Depper JM, Kronke M, Leonard WJ. The human interleukin-2 receptor: analysis of structure and function. Immunol Rev 1986; 92:29–48.
136. Prince HE, Kermani-Arab V, Fahey JL. Depressed interleukin 2 receptor expression in acquired immune deficiency and lymphadenopathy syndromes. J Immunol 1984; 133:1313–7.
137. Tsuchiya S, Imaizumi M, Minegishi M, et al. Lack of interleukin-2 production in a patient with $OKT4^+$ T cell deficiency. N Engl J Med 1983; 308:1294.
138. Hauser GJ, Bino T, Rosenberg H, et al. Interleukin-2 production and response to exogenous interleukin-2 in a patient with the acquired immune deficiency syndrome (AIDS). Clin Exp Immunol 1984; 56:14–7.
139. Ebert EC, Stoll DB, Cassens BJ, et al. Diminished interleukin production and receptor generation characterize the acquired immunodeficiency syndrome. Clin Immunol Immunopathol 1985; 37:283–97.
140. Murray HW, Welte K, Jacobs JL, et al. Production of and in vitro response to interleukin 2 in the acquired immunodeficiency syndrome. J Clin Invest 1985; 76:1959–64.
141. Lane HC, Depper JM, Greene WS, Whalen G, Waldmann TA, Fauci AS. Qualitative analysis of immune function in patients with the acquired immunodeficiency syndrome. Evidence for a selective defect in soluble antigen recognition. N Engl J Med 1985; 313:79–84.
142. Arya SK, Gallo RC. Human T-cell growth factor (interleukin 2) and gamma interferon genes: expression in human T-lymphotropic virus type III- and type I-infected cells. Proc Natl Acad Sci U S A 1985; 82:8691–5.
143. Shearer GM, Bernstein DC, Tung KSK, et al. A model for the selective loss of major histocompatibility complex self-restricted T cell immune responses during the development of acquired immune deficiency syndrome (AIDS). J Immunol 1986; 137:2514–21.
144. Smolen JS, Bettelheim, Koller U. Deficiency of the autologous mixed lymphocyte reaction in patients with classic hemophilia treated with commercial factor VIII concentrate. J Clin Invest 1985; 75:1828–37.
145. Garbrecht FC, Siskind GW, Wexler ME. Lymphocyte transformation induced by autologous cells. XVIII. Impaired autologous mixed lymphocyte reaction in subjects with AIDS-related complex. Clin Exp Immunol 1987; 67:245–51.
146. Hofmann B, Lindhardt BO, Gerstoft J, et al. Lymphocyte transformation response to pokeweed mitogen as a predictive marker for development of AIDS and AIDS related symptoms in homosexual men with HIV antibodies. Br Med J 1987; 295: 293–6.
147. Clerici M, Stocks N, Zajac RA, et al. Detection of three distinct patterns of T helper cell dysfunction in asymptomatic, human immunodeficiency virus-seropositive pa-

tients. Independence of CD4$^+$ cell numbers and clinical staging. J Clin Invest 1989; 84:1892–9.

148. Gruters RA, Terpstra FG, DeJong R, Van Noesel CJM, VanLier RAW, Miedema F. Selective loss of T cell function in different stages of HIV infection. Eur J Immunol 1990; 20:1039–44.

149. Luria S, Chambers I, Berg P. Expression of the type 1 immunodeficiency virus Nef protein in T cells prevents antigen receptor-mediated induction of interleukin 2 mRNA. Proc Natl Acad Sci U S A 1991; 88:5326–30.

150. Schellekens PTA, Roos MTL, De Wolf F, Lange JMA, Miedema F. Low T-cell responsiveness to activation via CD3/TCR is a prognostic marker for acquired immunodeficiency syndrome (AIDS) in human immunodeficiency virus-1 (HIV-1)-infected men. J Clin Immunol 1990; 10:121–7.

151. Clerici M, Stocks NI, Zajac RA, Boswell RN, Shearer GM. Accessory cell function in a symptomatic human immunodeficiency virus-infected patients. Clin Immunol Immunopathol 1990; 54:168–73.

152. Harris PE, Strba-Cechva, Rubinstein P, Mann D, King DW, Suciu-Foca N. Amplification of T cell blastogenic responses in healthy individuals and patients with acquired immunodeficiency syndrome. J Clin Invest 1990; 85:746–56.

153. Hofmann B, Odum N, Jakobsen BK, et al. Immunological studies in the acquired immunodeficiency syndrome. II. Active suppression or intrinsic defect-investigated by mixing AIDS cells with HLA-DR. Scand J Immunol 1986; 23:669–78.

154. Cunningham-Rundles S, Michelis M, Masur H. Serum suppression of lymphocyte activation in vitro in acquired immunodeficiency disease. J Clin Immunol 1983; 3:156–65.

155. Miller LE, Hennig AK, John PA, Loster BE, Tomar RH. Serologic factors in the pathogenesis of AIDS. In: Wormser GP, Stahl RE, Bottone GJ, eds. AIDS and other manifestations of HIV infection. Park Ridge, IL: Noyes, 1987:380–96.

156. Farmer JL, Gottlieb AA, Nishira T. Inhibition of interleukin 2 production and expression of the interleukin 2 receptor by plasma from acquired immune deficiency syndrome patients. Clin Immunol Immunopathol 1986; 38:235–43.

157. Laurence J, Mayer L. Immunoregulatory lymphokines of T hybridomas from AIDS patients: constitutive and inducible suppressor factors. Science 1984; 225:66–9.

158. Stella CC, Ganser A, Hoelzer D. Defective in vitro growth of the hemopoietic progenitor cells in the acquired immunodeficiency syndrome. J Clin Invest 1987; 80:286–93.

159. Leiderman IZ, Greenberg ML, Adelsberg BR, Siegal FP. A glycoprotein inhibitor of in vitro granulopoiesis associated with AIDS. Blood 1987; 70:1267–72.

160. Ratner L, Polmar SH, Paul N, Ruddle N. Cytotoxic factors secreted by cells infected by human immunodeficiency virus type 1. AIDS Res Hum Retroviruses 1987; 3:147–55.

161. Ammar A, Cibert C, Bertoli A-M, Tsilivakos V, Jasmin C, Georgoulias V. Biological and biochemical characterization of a factor produced spontaneously by adherent cells of human immunodeficiency virus-infected patients inhibiting interleukin-2 receptor chain (Tac) expression on normal T cells. J Clin Invest 1991; 87:2048–55.

162. De Paoli P, Battistin S, Crovatto M, et al. Immunologic abnormalities related to antigenaemia during HIV-1 infection. Clin Exp Immunol 1988; 74:317–20.

163. de Martini RM, Turner RR, Formenti SC, et al. Peripherial blood mononuclear cell abnormalities and their relationship to clinical course in homosexual men with HIV infection. Clin Immunol Immunopathol 1988; 46:258–71.

164. Van Noesel CJM, Gruters RA, Terpstra FG, Schellekens PTA, van Lier RAW, Miedema F. Functional and phenotypic evidence for a selective loss of memory T

cells in asymptomatic human immunodeficiency virus-infected men. J Clin Invest 1990; 86:293–9.

165. Pinching AJ, Nye KE. Defective signal transduction a common pathway for cellular dysfunction in HIV infection. Immunol Today 1990; 11:256–9.
166. Ensoli B, Nakamura S, Salahuddin SZ, et al. AIDS-Kaposi's sarcoma-derived cells express cytokines with autocrine and paracrine growth effects. Science 1989; 243:223–6.
167. Miles SA, Rezai AR, Salazar-Gonzales JF, et al. AIDS Kaposi sarcoma-derived cells produce and respond to interleukin 6. Proc Natl Acad Sci U S A 1990; 87:4068–72.
168. Ensoli B, Barillari G, Salahuddin SZ, Gallo RC, Wong-Staal F. Tat protein of HIV-1 stimulates growth of cells derived from Kaposi's sarcoma lesions of AIDS patients. Nature 1990; 345:84–6.
169. McDougal JS, Mawle A, Cort SP, et al. Cellular tropism of the human retrovirus HTLV-III/LAV. I. Role of T cell activation and expression of the T4 antigen. J Immunol 1985;135:3151–62.
170. Folks TM, Kelly J, Benn S, et al. Susceptibility of normal human lymphocytes to infection with HTLV-III/LAV. J Immunol 1986; 136:4049–53.
171. Harada S, Koyanayi Y, Nakashima H, Kobayashi N, Yamamoto N. Tumor promoter, TPA, enhances replication of HTLV-III/LAV. Virology 1986;154:249–58.
172. Margolick J, Volkman DJ, Folks TM, Fauci AS. Amplification of HTLV-III/LAV infection by antigen-induced activation of T cells and direct suppression by virus of lymphocyte blastogenic responses. J Immunol 1987; 138:1719–23.
173. Matsuyama T, Hamamoto Y, Soma G-I, Mizuno D, Yamamoto N, Kobayashi N. Cytocidal effect of tumor necrosis factor on cells chronically infected with human immunodeficiency virus (HIV): enhancement of HIV replication. J Virol 1989; 63:2504–9.
174. Ito M, Baba M, Sato A, et al. Tumor necrosis factor enhances replication of human immunodeficiency virus (HIV) in vitro. Biochem Biophys Res Commun 1989; 158:307–12.
175. Ito M, Baba M, Mori S, et al. Tumor necrosis factor antagonizes inhibitory effect of azidothymidine on human immunodeficiency virus (HIV) replication in vitro. Biochem Biophys Res Commun 1990; 166:1095–101.
176. Clouse KA, Powell D, Washington I, et al. Monokine regulation of human immunodeficiency virus-1 expression in a chronically infected human T cell clone. J Immunol 1989; 142:431–8.
177. Clouse KA, Robbins PB, Fernie B, Ostrove JM, Fauci AS. Viral antigen stimulation of the production of human monokines capable of regulating HIV-1 expression. J Immunol 1989; 143:470–5.
178. Folks TM, Clouse KA, Justement J, et al. Tumor necrosis factor α induces expression of human immunodeficiency virus in a chronically infected T-cell clone. Proc Natl Acad Sci U S A 1989; 86:2365–8.
179. Kobayashi N, Hamamoto Y, Koyanagi Y, Chen ISY, Yamamoto N. Effect of interleukin-1 on the augmentation of human immunodeficiency virus gene expression. Biochem Biophys Res Commun 1989; 165:715–21.
180. Wong GHW, Krowka JF, Stites DP, Goeddel DV. In vitro anti-human immunodeficiency virus activities of tumor necrosis factor-α and interferon-gamma. J Immunol 1988; 140:120–4.
181. Folks TM, Justement J, Kinter A, Dinarello CA, Fauci AS. Cytokine-induced expression of HIV-1 in a chronically infected promonocyte cell line. Science 1987; 238:800–2.
182. Koyanagi Y, O'Brien WA, Zhao JQ, Golde DW, Gasson JC, Chen ISY. Cytokines

alter production of HIV-1 from primary mononuclear phagocytes. Science 1988; 241:1673–5.
183. Tsunetsugu-Yokota Y, Honda M. Effect of cytokines on HIV release and IL-2 receptor α expression in monocytic cell lines. J AIDS 1990; 3:511–6.
184. Poli G, Kinto A, Bressler P, Justement JS, Timmer WC, Fauci AS. Interleukin 6 (IL-6) induces HIV expression and synergizes with other cytokines at transcriptional and post-transcriptional levels. Sixth International Conference on AIDS, San Francisco, CA 1990:Vol. 3:161, abstract S.A.318.
185. Hammer SM, Gillis JM, Groopman JE, Rose RM. In vitro modification of human immunodeficiency virus infection by granulocyte-macrophage colony stimulating factor and gamma interferon. Proc Natl Acad Sci U S A 1986; 83:8734–8.
186. Nabel G, Baltimore D. An inducible transcription factor activates expression of human immunodeficiency virus in T cells. Nature 1987; 326:711–3.
187. Osburn L, Kunkel S, Nabel GJ. Tumor necrosis factor α and interleukin 1 stimulate the human immunodeficiency virus enhancer by activation of the nuclear factor kappa B. Proc Natl Acad Sci U S A 1989; 86:2336–40.
188. Israel N, Hazan U, Alcami J, et al. Tumor necrosis factor stimulates transcription of HIV-1 in human T lymphocytes, independently and synergistically with mitogens. J Immunol 1989; 143:3956–60.
189. Duh EJ, Maury WJ, Folks TM, Fauci AS, Rabson AB. Tumor necrosis factor α activates human immunodeficiency virus type 1 through induction of nuclear factor binding to the NF-kappa B sites in the long terminal repeat. Proc Natl Acad Sci U S A 1989; 86:5974–8.
190. Hartshorn KL, Neumeyer D, Vogt MW, Schooley RT, Hirsch MS. Activity of interferons alpha, beta and gamma against human immunodeficiency virus replication in vivo. AIDS Res Hum Retroviruses 1987; 3:125–33.
191. Ho DD, Rota TR, Kaplan JC, et al. Recombinant human interferon alpha-A suppresses HTLV-III replication in vitro. Lancet 1985; 1:602–4.
192. Kornbluth RS, Oh PS, Munis JR, Cleveland PH, Richman DD. Interferons and bacterial lipopolysaccharide protect macrophages from productive infection by human immunodeficiency virus in vitro. J Exp Med 1989; 169:1137–51.
193. Nakashima H, Yoshida T, Harada S, Yamamoto N. Recombinant human interferon gamma suppresses HTLV-III replication in vitro. Int J Cancer 1986; 38:433–6.
194. Poli G, Orenstein JM, Kinter A, Folks TM, Fauci AS. Interferon gamma but not AZT suppresses HIV expression in chronically infected cell lines. Science 1989; 244:575–7.
195. Bednarik DP, Mosca JD, Raj NBK, Pitha PM. Inhibition of human immunodeficiency virus (HIV) replication by HIV-trans-activated α_2-interferon. Proc Natl Acad Sci U S A 1989; 86:4958–62.
196. Johnson VA, Barow MA, Merrill DP, Chou T-C, Hirsch MS. Three-drug synergistic inhibition of HIV-1 replication in vitro by zidovudine, recombinant soluble CD4, and recombinant interferon-alpha A. J Infect Dis 1990; 161:1059–67.
197. Kinter A, Poli G, Justement JS, Kehrl JH, Fauci AS. Opposite effects of transforming growth factor-β (TGFβ) on HIV infection in chronically versus acutely infected monocytic cells. In Sixth international conference on AIDS 1990; abstract SA319.
198. Lane HC, Siegel JP, Rook AH. Use of interleukin 2 in patients with the acquired imunodeficiency syndrome. J Biol Response Mod 1984; 3:512–6.
199. Rook AH, Masur H, Lane HC. Interleukin 2 enhances the depressed natural killer and cytomegalovirus-specific cytotoxic activities of lymphocytes from patients with the acquired immune deficiency syndrome. J Clin Invest 1983; 72:398–403.
200. Ernst M, Kern P, Ilad HD, Ulmer AJ. Effects of systemic in vivo interleukin-2 reconstitution in patients with acquired immunodeficiency syndrome (AIDS) and

AIDS-related complex (ARC) on phenotypes and functions of peripheral blood mononuclear cells (PBMC). J Clin Immunol 1986; 6:170–81.

201. Volberding P, Moody DJ, Beardlee D, Bradley EC, Wofsy CB. Therapy of acquired immune deficiency syndrome with recombinant interleukin 2. AIDS Res Hum Retroviruses 1987; 3:115–24.

202. Murray HW, DePamphilis J, Schooley RT, Hirsch MS. Circulating interferon-gamma in AIDS patients treated with interleukin-2 (letter). N Engl J Med 1988; 318:1538–9.

203. Murphy PM, Lane HC, Gallin JI, Fauci AS. Marked disparity in incidence of bacterial infections in patients with the acquired immunodeficiency syndrome receiving interleukin-2 or interferon-gamma. Ann Intern Med 1988; 108:36–41.

204. Hartshorn KL, Vogt MW, Chou TC, et al. Synergistic inhibition of human immunodeficiency virus in vitro by azidothymidine and recombinant alpha A interferon. Antimicrob Agents Chemother 1987; 31:168–72.

205. Vogt MW, Durno AG, Chou TC, et al. Synergistic interaction of 2′,3′-dideoxycytidine and recombinant interferon-alpha-A on replication of human immunodeficiency virus type 1. J Infect Dis 1988; 158:378–85.

206. Pitha P, Bilello JA, Riggin CH. Effect of interferon on retrovirus replication. Tex Rep Biol Med 1981–2; 41:603.

207. Ruprecht RM, Chou T-C, Chipty F, et al. Interferon-α and 3′-azido-3′-deoxythymidine are highly synergistic in mice and prevent viremia after acute retrovirus exposure. J AIDS 1990; 3:591–600.

208. Krown SE, Real FX, Cunningham-Rundles S, et al. Preliminary observations on the effect of recombinant leukocyte A interferon in homosexual men with Kaposi's sarcoma. N Eng J Med 1983; 308:1071–6.

209. Gelmann EP, Preble OT, Steis R, et al. Human lymphoblastoid interferon treatment of Kaposi's sarcoma in the acquired immune deficiency syndrome. Am J Med 1985; 78:737–41.

210. Groopman JE, Scadden DT. Interferon therapy for Kaposi sarcoma associated with the acquired immunodeficiency syndrome (AIDS). Ann Intern Med 1989; 110:335–7.

211. Lane CH, Feinberg J, Davey V, et al. Antiretroviral effects of interferon-α in AIDS-associated Kaposi's sarcoma. Lancet 1988; 2:1218–2.

212. De Wit R, Boucher CAB, Veenhof KHN, Schattenkerk JKME, Bakker PJM, Danner SA. Clinical and virological effects of high-dose recombinant interferon-α in disseminated AIDS-related Kaposi's sarcoma. Lancet 1988; 2:1214–7.

213. Kovacs JA, Deyton L, Davey R, et al. Combined ziduvodine and interferon-α therapy in patients with Kaposi sarcoma and the acquired immunodeficiency syndrome (AIDS). Ann Intern Med 1989; 111:280–7.

214. Miles SA, Wang H, Cortes E, Carden J, Marcus S, Mitsuyasu RT. Beta-interferon therapy in patients with poor-prognosis Kaposi sarcoma related to the acquired immunodeficiency syndrome (AIDS). Ann Intern Med 1990; 112:582–9.

215. Pace JL, Russel SW, Torres BA, Johnson HM, Gray PW. Recombinant mouse gamma interferon induces the priming step in macrophage activation for tumor cell killing. J Immunol 1983; 130:2011–3.

216. Schreiber RD. Identification of gamma-interferon as a murine macrophage-activating factor for tumor cytotoxicity. Contemp Top Immunobiol 1987; 17: 1183.

217. Welsh R. Natural cell-mediated immunity during viral infections. Curr Topics Microbiol Immunol 1981; 92:83–106.

218. Frasca D, Adorini L, Landolfo S, Doria G. Enhancing effect of IFN-gamma on helper T cell activity and IL-2 production. J Immunol 1985; 134:3907–11.

219. Nakamura M, Manser T, Pearson GDN, Daley MJ, Gefter ML. Effect of IFN-gamma on the immune response in vivo and on gene expression in vitro. Nature 1984; 307:381–2.
220. Heagy W, Groopman J, Schindler J, Finberg R. Use of IFN-gamma in patients with AIDS. J AIDS 1990; 3:5840–90.
221. Lane HC, Davey RT, Sherwin SA, et al. A phase I trial of recombinant human interferon-gamma in patients with Kaposi's sarcoma and the acquired immunodeficiency syndrome (AIDS). J Clin Immunol 1989; 9:351–61.
222. Metcalf D. The granulocyte-macrophage colony-stimulating factors. Science 1985; 229:16.
223. Clark SC, Kamen R. The human hematopoietic colony-stimulating factors. Science 1987; 236:1229–37.
224. Groopman JE, Molina JM, Scadden DT. Hematopoietic growth factors. Biology and clinical applications. N Engl J Med 1989; 321:1449–59.
225. Baldwin GC, Gasson JC, Quan SG, et al. Granulocyte-macrophage colony-stimulating factor enhances neutrophil function in acquired immunodeficiency syndrome patients. Proc Natl Acad Sci U S A 1988; 85:2763–6.
226. Miles SA, Mitsuyasu RT, Lee K, et al. Recombinant human granulocyte colony-stimulating factor increases circulating burst forming unit-erythron and red blood cell production in patients with severe human immunodeficiency virus infection. Blood 1990; 75:2137–42.
227. Iscove NN, Yan X-Q. Precursors (pre-CFC multi) of multilineage hemopoietic colony-forming cells quantitated in vitro. J Immunol 1990; 145:190–5.
228. Rennick D, Yang G, Muller-Sieburg C, et al. Interleukin 4 (B-cell stimulatory factor 1) can enhance or antagonize the factor-dependent growth of hemopoietic progenitor cells. Proc Natl Acad Sci U S A 1987; 84:6889–93.
229. Peschel C, Paul WE, Ohara J, Green I. Effects of B cell stimulatory factor-1/interleukin 4 on hematopoietic progenitor cells. Blood 1987; 70:254–63.
230. Kishi K, Ihle JN, Urdal DL, Ogawa M. Murine B-cell stimulatory factor-1 (BSF-1)/interleukin-4 (IL-4) is a multilineage colony-stimulating factor that acts directly on primitive hemopoietic progenitors. J Cell Physiol 1989; 139:463–8.
231. Wong GG, Clark SC. Multiple actions of interleukin 6 within a cytokine network. Immunol Today 1988; 9:137–9.
232. Ikebuchi K, Ihle JN, Hirai Y, Wong GG, Clark SC, Ogawa M. Synergistic factors for stem cell proliferation: further studies of the target stem cells and the mechanism of stimulation by interleukin-1, interleukin-6, and granulocyte colony-stimulating factor. Blood 1988; 72:2007–14.

INDEX

About the Editors

STEVEN L. KUNKEL is a Professor of Pathology in the Department of Pathology at The University of Michigan Medical School, Ann Arbor. The author of numerous papers in professional journals, he is a member of the American Association of Immunologists, the American Association of Pathology, the American Society for Microbiology, the American Heart Association, and the American Thoracic Society. In addition, he is an associate editor of four scientific journals. Dr. Kunkel received the B.S. (1973) and M.S. (1974) degrees in microbiology–immunology from North Dakota State University, Fargo, and the Ph.D. degree (1978) in microbiology from the University of Kansas, Lawrence.

DANIEL G. REMICK is an Assistant Professor of Pathology and the Director of Autopsy Service in the Department of Pathology at The University of Michigan Medical School, Ann Arbor. He is the author of a number of professional papers and a member of the American Association of Pathologists, the International Academy of Pathology, the Shock Society, and the American Association of Immunologists. Dr. Remick received the B.S. degree (1978) in chemistry from the University of Minnesota at Duluth, and the M.D. degree (1982) from the Mayo Medical School, Rochester, Minnesota.